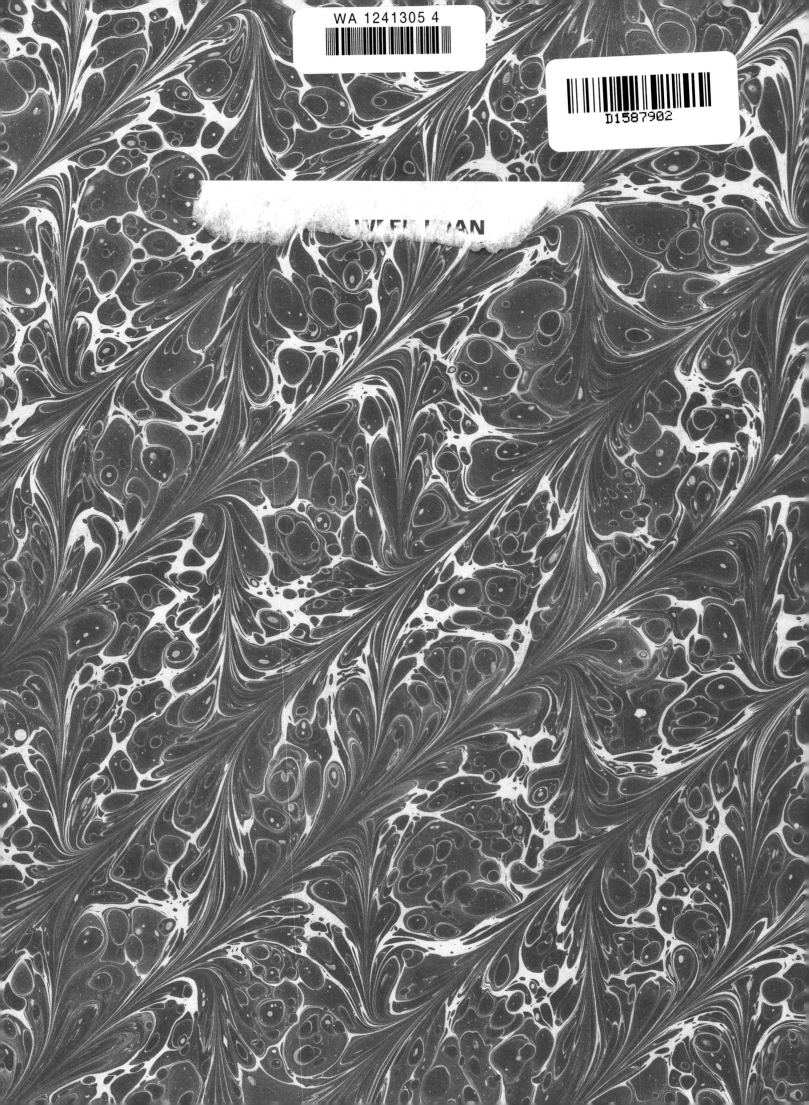

CHIROPRACTIC

An Illustrated History

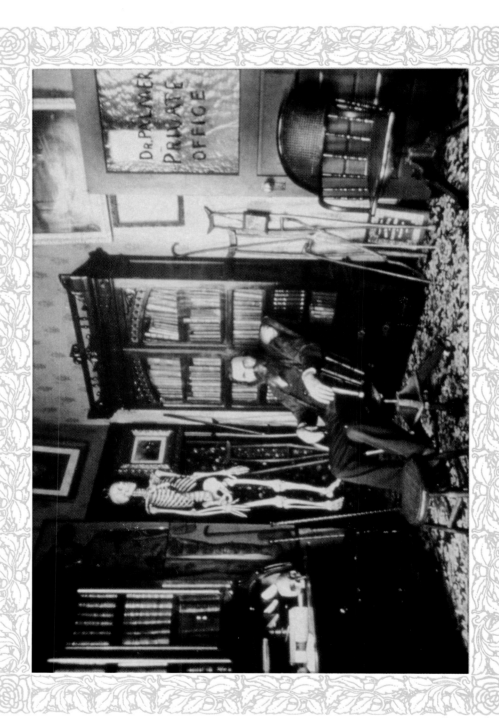

CHIROPRACTIC

An Illustrated History

Dennis Peterson, M.A.
Director
David D. Palmer Health Sciences Library
Palmer College of Chiropractic
Davenport, Iowa

Glenda Wiese, M.A.
Archivist and Special Collections Librarian
David D. Palmer Health Sciences Library
Palmer College of Chiropractic
Davenport, Iowa

This project has been developed and written with
the cooperation and endorsement of
the Association for the History of Chiropractic and
the Chiropractic Centennial Foundation.

with 939 *illustrations*

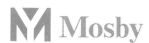

St. Louis Baltimore Berlin Boston Carlsbad Chicago London Madrid
Naples New York Philadelphia Sydney Tokyo Toronto

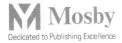

Executive Editor: Martha Sasser
Associate Developmental Editor: Kellie F. White
Project Manager: Carol Sullivan Weis
Senior Production Editor: Linda McKinley
Designer: Betty Schulz

Copyright © 1995 by Mosby–Year Book, Inc.

Printed in the United States of America
Composition by The Clarinda Company
Color separation by Accu-Color, Inc.
Printing/binding by Walsworth Publishing Company

Mosby–Year Book, Inc.
11830 Westline Industrial Drive
St. Louis, Missouri 63146

Library of Congress Cataloging in Publication Data

Peterson, Dennis.
   Chiropractic: an illustrated history / Dennis Peterson, Glenda Wiese.
      p.   cm.
  Includes bibliographical references and index.
  ISBN 0-8016-7735-1
  1. Chiropractic--History. I. Wiese, Glenda. II. Title.
RZ221.P48 1995
615.5'34'09--dc20
                                   94-22834
                                     CIP

94 95 96 97 98 / 9 8 7 6 5 4 3 2 1

CONTRIBUTORS

Stanley P. Bolton, D.C.
Philosopher of Chiropractic
Fellow, Palmer Academy of Chiropractic
Private Practice
Sydney, Australia

Alana Callender, M.S.L.S.
Associate Professor and Director
Department of Admissions
Palmer College of Chiropractic
Davenport, Iowa

Robin Canterbury, D.C.
Professor and Chairman
Department of Radiology
Palmer College of Chiropractic
Davenport, Iowa

Mary-Anne Chance, D.C.
Editor, *Chiropractic Journal of Australia*
Secretary/Treasurer, Association for the History of
    Chiropractic—Australia
Wagga Wagga, Australia

Carl Cleveland III
President
Cleveland College of Chiropractic—Kansas City
Cleveland College of Chiropractic—Los Angeles
Kansas City, Missouri

Meridel Gatterman, D.C.
Director
Chiropractic Sciences Division
Canadian Memorial College of Chiropractic
Toronto, Ontario, Canada

Pierre Louis Gaucher-Peslherbe, D.C., Ph.D.
Maitre es Lettres (Anglais), Directeur de Recherche
Institut Pour L'Etude de la Statique et de la Dynamique
    du Corps Humain
Lyons, France

Russell Gibbons
Editor, *Chiropractic History*
Pittsburgh, Pennsylvania

Joseph C. Keating Jr., Ph.D.
Portland, Oregon

John S. Kyneur, D.C.
Private Practice
New Lambton, New South Wales, Australia

Herb Lee, D.C., F.I.C.C.
Professor Emeritus
Clinical Education Department
Canadian Memorial Chiropractic College
Toronto, Ontario, Canada

George McAndrews, J.D.
McAndrews, Held & Melloy
Chicago, Illinois

Jerome F. McAndrews, D.C.
Vice President for Professional Affairs
American Chiropractic Association
Arlington, Virginia

Rolf Peters, B.Sc., D.C.
Editor, *Chiropractic Journal of Australia*
President, Association for the History of
    Chiropractic—Australia
Wagga Wagga, Australia

Dennis Peterson, M.A.
Associate Professor and Director
David D. Palmer Health Sciences Library
Palmer College of Chiropractic
Davenport, Iowa

William S. Rehm, D.C.
Private Practice, Chiropractic Historian
Baltimore, Maryland

William G. Rothstein
Professor of Sociology
Department of Sociology
University of Maryland—Baltimore County
Baltimore, Maryland

Herbert J. Vear, D.C., F.C.C.S., L.L.D.
President Emeritus
Western States Chiropractic College;
Dean Emeritus
Canadian Memorial Chiropractic College;
Past President, Association of Chiropractic History
Pickering, Ontario, Canada

Walter I. Wardwell, Ph.D.
Professor Emeritus of Sociology
University of Connecticut
Storrs, Connecticut

Glenda Wiese, M.A.
Archivist and Special Collections Librarian
David D. Palmer Health Sciences Library
Palmer College of Chiropractic
Davenport, Iowa

For
Paula, Ryan, and Kyle
and
Carl, Elizabeth, and Audrey

PREFACE

On the eve of its second century of service, the Chiropractic profession has treated and helped relieve the suffering of hundreds of millions of people worldwide. The story of chiropractors' dedication to serving their patients and helping "sick people get well" is a genuine, heartfelt, and inspiring story, a story that especially touches those of us directly involved with educating today's students of Chiropractic.

To the editors and contributors, it would seem the world should already know the story about this natural healing art and its struggle to win a place in a very competitive health care marketplace. However, even among those who use chiropractic care, there is little awareness of the profession's colorful 100 years of history.

The chiropractic profession had its beginnings in America at the end of the nineteenth century when an industrious, intelligent, home-schooled Canadian immigrant who was living in the middle of rural America on the banks of the bustling upper Mississippi River Valley town of Davenport, Iowa, made a historic leap of reason. At the time, the milieu of the world's political, social, and economic events were profoundly changing America and the world. These events would propel humanity down an inevitable number of new and global pathways, the consequences of which no previous era in history could match. There was the discovery and development of Edison's electricity, Bell's telephone, Benz's automobile, Wright's airplane, Still's osteopathy, Roentgen's radiology, and Palmer's chiropractic, all of which have had a tremendous hand in shaping today's reality.

We have invited some of the most knowledgeable writers and scholars involved with Chiropractic to help tell chiropractic's story. The reader must recognize that one short text cannot tell the *whole* of the chiropractic story. The story is continually unfolding as archival and historical collections are made available to scholars. We have been in a privileged position to edit this history given the rich chiropractic environment of Palmer College and Davenport, Iowa, and given the ample historical resources available in the David D. Palmer Health Sciences Library. Using these resources and the expertise of our contributors, we have attempted to capture a snapshot of Chiropractic's legacy.

This book is organized by relating chronological highlights of chiropractic's first 100 years, including a short biography of the Founder, Daniel David Palmer. Then follow chapters on equipment, technique, and radiology—the major components of the profession and aspects that are uniquely chiropractic and set the profession apart from traditional medicine and surgery. Next we focus on a number of individuals who have had a hand in shaping chiropractic's early story, with chapters on chiropractic education, past chiropractic leaders, women in chiropractic, and those involved with the political side of the profession through national associations. Last, we end the story of Chiropractic with an epilogue on what the twenty-first century may hold for the future of the profession by a sociologist who has been writing about Chiropractic for over 40 years. We hope you enjoy this pictoral history of the chiropractic profession. ∾

ACKNOWLEDGMENT

This project has been a joy to develop. The joy is in dealing with the people of the profession, who helped to lovingly and passionately craft this work. There are many people who have gone beyond their personal obligations to help ensure the creation of this work. And there has been the joy of working with the rich historical chiropractic resources available at the David D. Palmer Health Sciences Library. The manuscripts, correspondence, books, pamphlets, journals, photographs, and clippings gathered and kept by both D.D. and B.J. Palmer and other chiropractors throughout their lifetimes has left a profound and inestimable record of this profession's young heritage.

We would like to acknowledge and thank our contributing authors for their work, without whom the text could not have encompassed so much history. A number of authors and scholars have been of tremendous help and encouragement to us, especially Walter Wardwell of Storrs, Connecticut; Joseph C. Keating Jr. of Los Angeles, California; and Pierre Louis Gaucher-Peslherbe of Lyons, France.

We also wish to acknowledge and thank Palmer College of Chiropractic for allowing us to draw on the vast historical chiropractic resources of the Special Collection Department of the David D. Palmer Health Sciences Library. We appreciate the cooperation and support from the President, Dr. Donald Kern; the office of the Vice President for Academic Affairs; R. Douglas Baker; D.C.; and Donald Betz, Ph.D. for allowing us to craft this book over the past 2 years.

We also must acknowledge several David D. Palmer Health Sciences Library staff members for their contributions. Special appreciation goes to Jetta Nash, Sofya Spector, and Cindi Williams of the Library's Special Collections and Archives department, whose help has been invaluable in the location of illustrations. We want to acknowledge Jim Bandes and his staff from the Library's Instructional Media Services office, Dr. Larry Sigulinsky of the Health Science Illustration Office, and Wanda Simmons of Palmer University's Marketing and Communications Department for their work and assistance in the preparation of the book's illustrations. We also wish to acknowledge the assistance of individuals, organizations, and the chiropractic colleges in locating and reproducing historical photographs, especially the resources provided to us by Vi Nickson, archivist at Logan Chiropractic College; Carl Cleveland, III, President of the Cleveland Chiropractic Colleges; Ron Beideman, archivist at National College of Chiropractic; Bill Rehm of Baltimore, Maryland; and Russell Gibbons of Pittsburgh, Pennsylvania. Thank you for digging into your archives of historical illustrations and sharing them with us. We also want to acknowledge the support and guidance given by our editors at Mosby–Year Book, Martha Sasser and Kellie White, who have been so supportive and understanding about deadlines and the coordination of gathering our resources from all over the world.

Finally, the editors want to give a special acknowledgment about the support and encouragement we received from our families over the past 3 years when we first began writing this book. Thank you to Paula, Ryan, and Kyle and Carl, Elizabeth, and Audrey. Without your love, understanding, and encouragement, this project would not have been nearly so rewarding. ∾

Dennis Peterson
Glenda Wiese

CONTENTS

1   **ANTECEDENTS TO CHIROPRACTIC**   1
A Cultural Approach from Ancient Myths to Modern Mythologies
Pierre Louis Gaucher-Peslherbe

2   **AMERICAN MEDICINE IN THE NINETEENTH CENTURY**   30
Experimentation and Consolidation
William G. Rothstein

3   **DANIEL DAVID PALMER**   56
"Old Dad Chiro," the Founder of Chiropractic
Glenda Wiese, Dennis Peterson

4   **THE AGE OF WONDERMENT—CHIROPRACTIC IN THE EARLY TWENTIETH CENTURY**   90
Health Care in the Midwest at the Turn of the Century
Joseph C. Keating Jr.

5   **PATHWAY TO IDENTITY FOR A NEW HEALING ART**   124
Chiropractic's Maturation: 1910-1929
Russell W. Gibbons

6   **CHIROPRACTIC'S CRUCIBLE**   152
Surviving the Great Depression and World War II: 1930-1945
Russell W. Gibbons

7   **THE POSTWAR YEARS**   180
1945-1973
Carl S. Cleveland III, Joseph C. Keating Jr.

8   **CHIROPRACTIC'S RENAISSANCE**   214
From 1963 to 1993
Jerome F. McAndrews, George P. McAndrews

9   **CHIROPRACTIC ADJUSTING TECHNIQUES**   240
The Rock That Anchors Chiropractic
Herb Lee, Meridel Gatterman

10 **CHIROPRACTIC EQUIPMENT** 262
"Clothes Maketh the Man"
John S. Kyneur, Stanley P. Bolton

11 **RADIOGRAPHY AND CHIROPRACTIC SPINOGRAPHY** 288
Robin Canterbury

12 **CHIROPRACTIC SCHOOLS AND COLLEGES** 338
"To Teach and to Practice Chiropractic"
Glenda Wiese, Dennis Peterson

13 **CHIROPRACTIC'S PATHFINDERS** 388
Images and Legacies
William S. Rehm

14 **CHIROPRACTIC PROFESSIONAL ASSOCIATIONS** 420
The Names and Politics That Have Forged Present Pathways
Joseph C. Keating Jr.

15 **WOMEN IN CHIROPRACTIC** 444
Alana Callender

16 **CHIROPRACTIC AROUND THE WORLD** 462
Herbert J. Vear, Pierre Louis Gaucher-Peslherbe, Rolf Peters, Mary-Ann Chance, Glenda Wiese

17 **EPILOGUE** 488
Walter I. Wardwell

BIBLIOGRAPHY 497

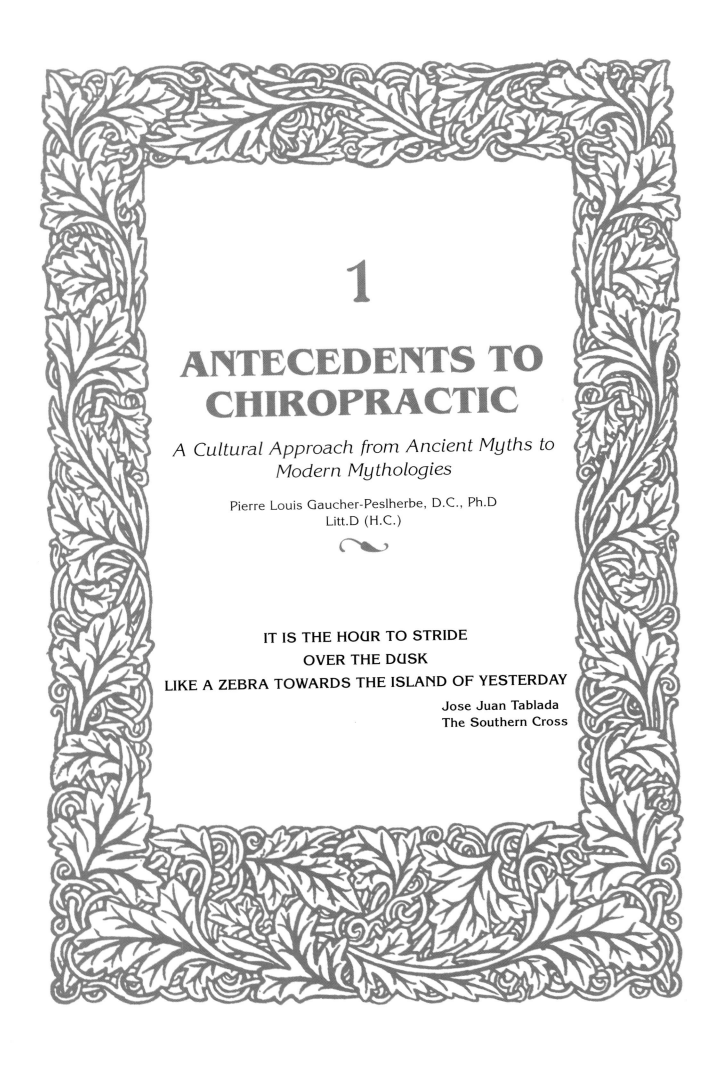

1

ANTECEDENTS TO CHIROPRACTIC

A Cultural Approach from Ancient Myths to Modern Mythologies

Pierre Louis Gaucher-Peslherbe, D.C., Ph.D
Litt.D (H.C.)

IT IS THE HOUR TO STRIDE

OVER THE DUSK

LIKE A ZEBRA TOWARDS THE ISLAND OF YESTERDAY

Jose Juan Tablada
The Southern Cross

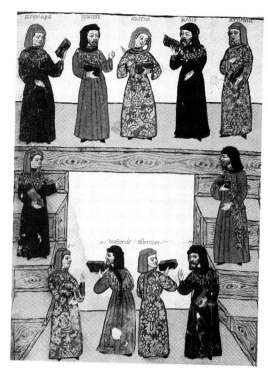

Western medicine has achieved astounding supremacy over most healing practices, mostly because of an exclusion of other approaches based on prejudice.[1] Medicine has a history of celebrating great classical figures such as Hippocrates, Galen, Ibn Sinna, Ambroise Pare, Sydenham, Jenner, Magendie, Claude Bernard, and Pasteur. However, claims to preeminence by medical doctors have often preceded the deeds that justify such esteem.[2] Many medical doctors attempted to curtail the development of other healing arts, the services of which the public requested. To write a history of any aspect of Western medicine therefore frequently requires describing the various deceptions used by regular practitioners to keep others subservient, unworthy of the regular practitioners' lofty considerations and privileges.

In antiquity and the Middle Ages, progress in medicine meant adding new commentaries to former great writers whose books were a compulsory and frequently only basis in teaching the art. Pictured here (from left to right and from top to bottom) are Asclepios, Hippocrates, Avicenna, Rhazes, Aristotle, Ibn Sarabyun, Galen, Mesuah, Dioscorides, Albertus Magnus, and Macer (G. Cademosto).
Courtesy Bibliothèque Nationale, Paris.

Along with the great doctors of a more classical age, there were a host of practitioners who were often called "quacks" because they used their hands to heal. Physicians were taught in great universities where they received an education emphasizing logic and doctrine, whereas the other classes were apprenticed to learn a craft through practice. A difference was further made between those who worked *cum defecto* (amputation of a part) and those who practiced *ad integrum* (merely setting the parts right).[3] Bonesetters who treated while preserving the integrity of the body were considered to have a lowlier status than those who did not.

The survival of conservative health care has to be assessed against this cultural background. The consequence for the patient is best seen in the surprising reluctance of doctors to treat pain when, for example, the wide use in antiquity of nepenthe and the Memphis stone can be cited to demonstrate that the means were available. However, "medicine in medieval and classical times reduced the ancient use of natural analgesics, anesthetics and narcotic substances (mandrake, henbane, poppy, ivy, hemlock)."[4] From 1810 to 1846 and even later, "the long episode of the militant refusal of anesthesia in surgical operations by the highest medical authorities of both worlds, when the appropriate chemical substances (nitrogen protoxide, ether, morphine, chloroform) were known, is a striking case in itself."[4]

Although the heart of most acknowledged medical modes of practice is in Greece, their roots go back to early myths.[5] The people who made the cave paintings had to hunt and fight for themselves and for their clans.[6] They showed a daring ability to perform complex neurosurgical operations such as with trephining (i.e., opening parts of the skull for medical or religious reasons). By sheer necessity, they could also perform much simpler and more obvious interventions. They also had to face the world in an erect posture; the skeletons of even the very young showed signs of severe osteoarthrosis of the spine, dislocations, luxations, and

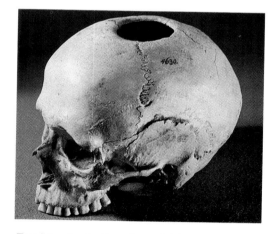

Trephined skulls of neolithic period may show healed wound edges indicating recovery from operation whose purpose, whether medical or magical, remains unknown.
Courtesy Nationalmuseet, Copenhagen.

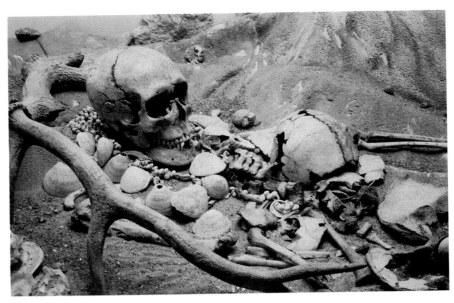

This Hoedic burial site in Britanny, reconstituted by A.E. Riskine, dates from 4600 BC. Important mesolithic (nomadic) personalities were buried with antlers, collars made with precious stones, or various shells. Longevity was not much more than 25 to 30 years, and the infantile mortality rate was extremely high. The woman was about 25 years old and her child 3 years old.

Courtesy A.E. Riskine, Musée de Préhistoire, Carnac, France.

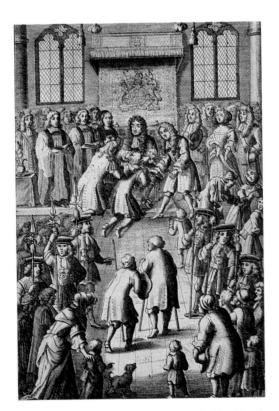

In France and England, the "royal gift of healing" was considered an undisputed medication against scrofula (ganglionic tuberculosis). It was often described as morbus regium (R. White).

Courtesy British Library, London.

fractures. In some cases, there are signs of successful manipulation,[7] which might explain why throughout history and in every culture, a symbolic significance has been attributed to bones and joints, either the whole skeleton or parts of it.[8]

Egyptians and Aztecs believed that the soul rested in the bones and that they were to be revived from the grave. Ezechiel is known to have prophetized over scattered bones and, at the Lord's bidding, to have revived them, flesh and all. In Iran, bones were carefully laid aside lest the devil break them and let the soul wander in the wild. In some Christian mystical experiences, one of the surest ways to spiritual life was to visualize oneself as a skeleton. To the Eskimo, the same effort signaled a mystical rebirth within the original matrix of animal life.[9]

Mythical notions of how the human body acquired joints began in pre-recorded history. In Mexico the Purapechas believed that when the gods first created humans, joints were lacking; the entire world had to be destroyed three times before normal joints were included.[10] It was believed in Tibet that Devas had first created humans with a diaphanous body, which Asuras then tried to petrify into a solid skeleton. To undo the spell, Devas had to break the bones and hence the joints.[11] Curiously, the last tale very nearly parallels Lavoisier's intuition that humans were created out of solidified gases.

This description of bones and joints shows that it was only gods or demigods who had permission to tamper with the way the skeleton worked. This is one reason the results of the bonesetters were marvelled at rather than studied in primitive societies. Many centuries later in France and England, the bonesetter's way of touching people was even compared with the King's touch against scrofula.[12] Bonesetting then clearly appeared to be a sacred art. However, it had already been established in

Greece that an art could never become a science.[13] Even hippocratic medicine was never socially allowed to achieve that status.

The most important question to consider is whether Western medicine as a discipline has properly described the nature of things or whether chiropractic described some human feature altogether or partly missed by medicine; that is, whether chiropractic has been properly considered despite it upsetting the established professional order. Both chiropractic and medicine promote values that are universal. Their approaches to these values vary; some are totally contrary. Therefore it is necessary to return to original sources and to attempt to untangle the progress of both disciplines. "It is as if there was an analogy between the psychological structure of remnants from antiquity and the structure of constituting material in modern man."[14] ༄

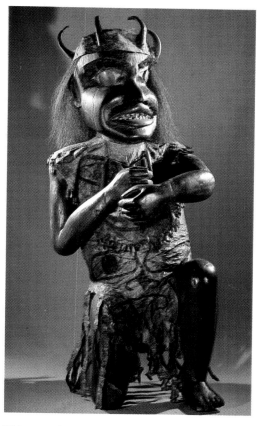

This wood and leather statue of a shaman is from British Columbia in Canada. Healing priests would ward off sickness or evil sprits through various forms of protective magic. This awe-inspiring figure also indicates that practices could be aggressive.
Courtesy Musée de l'Homme, Paris.

PRIMITIVE MEDICINES

Shamanism

One of the beliefs of shamanism is that the body of a shaman is not an instrument used by the spirit to ride. After rigorous training and a proper ceremony, the shaman's body lies motionless so that the soul may soar to some other sphere of spiritual life and influence the course of disease. Because of this initiation, the healer has a recognized ability to speak the language of animals and is free to fly from heaven to hell and back to earth again. Shamans dream that their bodies are dismembered and their flesh eaten by ancillary spirits. They have to name each bone before the bones are reunited and made fast again with iron links; they have to become strong enough to face any future ordeal. To prove they have experienced this ritual, shamans might wear special garments with displays of bones sewn on them. According to primitive calendar symbols, shamans could also become a bird, lion, or snake, (i.e., a master of all the times).[15]

In older societies, medicine men occupied an important place on a par with war leaders. *Medicine* meant "force" and "power" in the context. Still, there are great differences between shamans from Northern America and those from the Southern part of the continent, both socially and religiously, and also between an Andean shaman and a Siberian one.[16] The Siberian shaman is closer to the Amazonian counterpart because religious responsibilities exceed real medical functions for both. In all cases, a shaman strives to retrieve lost harmony on behalf of the tribe, often by fighting to reintegrate the tribe's primitive condition in a lost paradise. It amounts to the myth of the eternal return.

On his way to China in 1273 in a province situated south of Tibet, Marco Polo wrote that when someone there is ill, relatives call in enchanters: "Their instruments blare forth and they sing and dance and swing all around the place for a long time until one of them falls on his back foaming at the mouth and looking as if he were dead. Dancing is brought to a standstill and they pretend that the evil spirit had moved into him who fell."[17] This is a clear case of medical shamanism.

Neither of the priests P. Le Jeune in 1634 nor J.F. Lafitau more than a half century later were fully convinced of the therapeutic value of the approaches they observed in native societies around Caughnawaga in Canada[18]:

One would think that a sick person would request rest more than anything else . . . the din would be sufficient to cause death. But the din itself is not much. The poor wretched souls are at the discretion of empiricists who blow on them, press them with frenetic violence in the parts which are ailing most. . . . They exhaust them to such an extent that they are more diseased to have been shaken than because of their sickness.

Le Jeune and Lafitau also noted that the natives had "endless secrets for curing illnesses that up to now we had practically no way of curing." Moreover, "the savages are equally successful with ruptures and prolapses, dislocations, luxations, and fractures. Cases are known of broken bones that have been set and are fully restored to use in a week."[19]

These surprising cures introduce yet another difference between medicine and bonesetting. The practitioner of the former discusses the patient's pulse, excreta, and humours and refers to fluids that circulate around the body, whereas the practitioner of the latter applies procedures on localized and solid parts. The second is an antimedical approach. The antimedical label could also be applied to surgeons even though they work with knife and fire.[20] It is not surprising that these differing disciplines with such antagonistic foundations should progress at different rates and that their respective languages, descriptions, and achievements should not meet, let alone be properly understood by each other. Such antagonism leads to blind prejudice when learning is used as a weapon of social power.[21]

Traditional Pharmacopoeia

It has been observed that chimpanzees will fight intestinal parasitism by sucking some twigs that they have first stripped of their bark; otherwise the plant is deadly poisonous. The young are trained to do it properly, but captive animals will eat the whole specimen and die. *Homo erectus* is almost 2 million years old, whereas *Homo sapiens* has survived the Ice Age for more than 200,000 years. Mastery of fire allowed *Homo erectus* to cook plants; experiment with various forms of macerations, infusions, and decoctions; and observe their properties.

An orally transmitted tradition arose that has been described as the "traditional pharmacopoeia."[22] Great civilizations codified it in various compendiums from 6000 to 3000 BC. One of the oldest documents is the Sumer tablet at the University Museum in Philadelphia, which deals with straight pharmacological remedies.[23] The cultures of Sumer and Egypt knew how to use "lion oil" (poppy), Egyptians and Indians knew about different types of colchicum (alkaloids) as well as scilla (glucosides) among other types of liliaceae, the Chinese promoted the use of artemisia (wormwood), and the people of the Incan empire reserved the use of quinquina (antifever) and huanarpo (aphrodisiac) almost exclusively for their rulers.[24]

In northern Argentina, *Ruda chalepensis* is noted for its specific effects on heart disease.[25] With a high dose, it also becomes a powerful abortive. It complements any other infusion by increasing the efficiency of the infusion. The plant is also believed to cast out evil spirits and to calm unexpected visitors. Each effect is approached as part of the plant's natural properties. Infusions are believed to cleanse all veins and arteries in the body and to drive out disease. To achieve these effects, the plant's efficiency must be increased through certain rituals. It is advisable to select three buds oriented to the east and other similar specifications. To

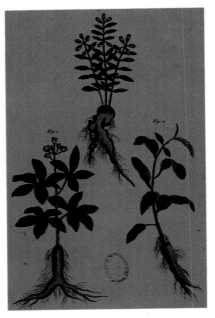

The gingseng root (man-shaped root) was considered in China to have quite miraculous properties to treat a wide range of diseases from sexual asthenia to tuberculosis and diabetes. Only jewels were as expensive as this root (P.J. Buc'hoz).

Courtesy Bibliothèque Interuniversitaire de Médecine, Paris.

do that will not invest the plant with qualities it would otherwise lack, but it will help increase its specific virtues in perfect harmony with the underlying cause of disease. Classical medicine might use the same plant to treat the poor, but the symbolic aspects were usually suppressed, whereas primitive medicine would rely heavily on them. Rather than just diagnose disease, the primitive medicine man would try to discover how a diseased person relates to the surrounding magical forces. The ailment is exactingly localized, together with the reason for its being present.

Only remnants of American Indian medical traditions were preserved after the genocide of the native tribes after Columbus. Hence in most of Latin America the approach to health is founded on hippocratic traditions brought by European settlers. Importing African slaves did not affect medical approaches because Africans could only participate in very primitive forms of hygiene and disease prevention. What has survived today has been modified by four centuries of adaptation.[26]

In traditional Andean societies, disease is feared but also has a social function. A mentally and physically healthy individual is considered socially alien and dangerous; a diseased condition is preferred because it shows that the individual is under the influence of the powers that rule the universe.[27] Incan traditions and influence also extended east to the Amazon tribes, as evidenced by the use of imported chicha rituals (corn beer), potteries, and masks.[28]

Incan populations continue to practice coca leaves divination (katipa). The Incans believe that the human body is made up of several material and immaterial envelopes organized around a hollow tube.[29] Energy came from the dead, who were responsible for fertility in both people and the earth. The whole of nature is considered to be animated with spirits that could be appeased through ritual drunkenness.[30]

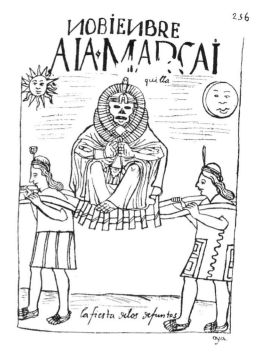

Celebrating the dead in Peru implied that embalmed corpses were carried from house to house and were offered gifts or prayers. The celebration took place in November each year, long before the Catholic calendar reached the area (F.G. Poma de Ayala).
Courtesy Institut d'Ethnologie, Paris.

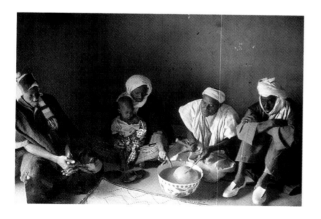
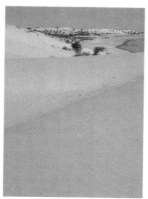
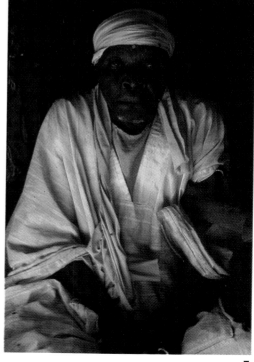

The River Niger is said to be alive with genii or **Ghimbala.** *In Western Mali, the spirits can be summoned through water drums. If the drummer is not very careful about the rhythm and types of beats used, the drummer may become possessed. A cure can last up to several months, after which the patient becomes the healing priest's obligee or* male bania *forever.*
Courtesy Catherine and Bernard Desjeux, Paris.

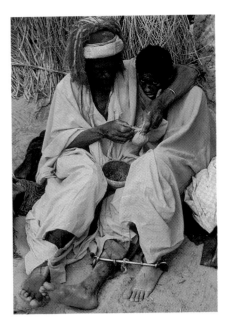
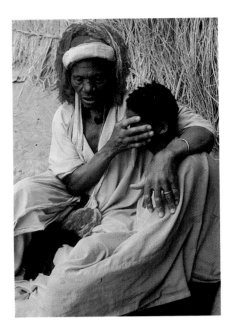

Fumigating to diagnose the case and then gently coaxing an insane patient are only parts of a very complex ceremony that can become very violent.
Courtesy Catherine and Bernard Desjeux, Paris.

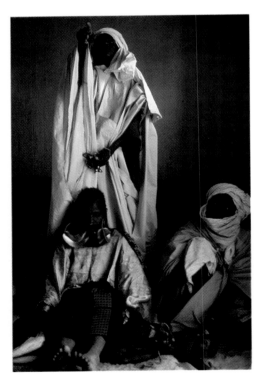

In the yare ritual, a goat is an introductory gift and one of the means to achieve a cure. The healing priest or gaw summons the spirits from all corners of the world, and the offending one is then ordered into the goat, which is eaten in common afterward.
Courtesy Catherine and Bernard Desjeux, Paris.

African Medicine

Some of the oldest organized societies occurred in Africa, where medical customs have always been traditional. For the natives, nature is full of powers that must be recognized. People are considered to be structured around three elements: the breath of life, the physical body, and the ethereal replica of the body. To kill someone, a wizard eats the ethereal replica because only the insane can live without it. Diagnosing what has possessed the diseased person is the main approach.[31]

Normally, bonesetters in Africa are trained by older practitioners. They set the bones and immobilize the broken limbs with splints. However, none of these actions are considered effective and practitioners are in danger of being bewitched if their hands have not been ointed with the collected sap of a specific liana while praying that the force in it was channeled to the sick. This rite is performed before healers are allowed to function. Another example of a very complex occult initiation performed before healing is from the Musey country of Tchad[32]:

> The bonesetter's hands had to be smeared several times with a mixture made of karite nut oil (gluey and sticking well), lalamara roots (which do not break easily), sewena roots (aerial creepers which have to reach the ground), mason-bee earth (very hard when it dries). All this means that the bones he shall set will stick and become solid again. . . . To inherit the ability to heal and to practice properly, a youth must be initiated through the whole process.

Bonesetting therefore clearly amounts to a well-defined and limited specialty. Its technical expertise is very coherent even by modern standards; it is logically and physiologically organized with perfectly mastered steps.[33]

Just as logically organized is the complex practice that deals with ge-

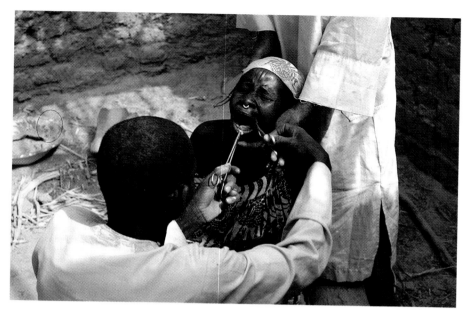

Divination by cauris or dinlogun. *Cauris are first shaken and directed toward each cardinal point; they are then brought three times to the forehead before they are thrown onto the floor. What their position is and whether they are closed or opened indicate what is to be decided. They may have to be thrown several times depending on the ritual.*

Courtesy Catherine and Bernard Desjeux, Paris.

nii. It sometimes requires a large assembly, such as in the Songhays cult in Mali. Each patient is possessed by a spirit, and the cure takes place through a crisis that leads to an initiation. If the crisis does not occur, the possessed person would become insane and might even die. It is a complex way to deal with the cure or at least prevention of mental disease. However, possession cults are not as widely practiced today. This is partly due to the low incomes of most people, who can no longer afford the costs, and partly due to a growing Muslim intolerance toward the cults. Traditional therapies give a name to a disease, whereas Muslim therapies strive to cleanse what has been polluted, which has meaning only in a religious sense.[34] Attempts to name a common psychiatric link between traditional practitioners and clinical medicine have mostly emphasized the political aspects of such a collaboration rather than its medical value.[35]

The obvious events that surround the onset of a disease are not believed to fully identify all its underlying causes, even more so when the disease has mysterious peculiarities or lasts longer than expected. In the Yoruba religion in Nigeria, the "master of the mysteries" is in charge of explaining the disease. An *Ifa* tray is used to score marks from a pattern made by several throws of kola nuts. This type of divination is similar to the Chinese *I Ching.* The resulting pattern refers to a specific verse in *Odu,* their book of sayings, which is then explained by the priest.[36]

For example, if a person breaks a leg after falling from a tree, the bonesetter is first called to reduce the break. *Ifa* is then consulted to find out why Eshu, the trickster god, created havoc out of a quiet pursuit. The real cause has to be expressed in terms of spiritual influence, which may emanate from the dead, the Orisha (gods), or some malevolent living person. This influence is believed to have created the sickness.[37]

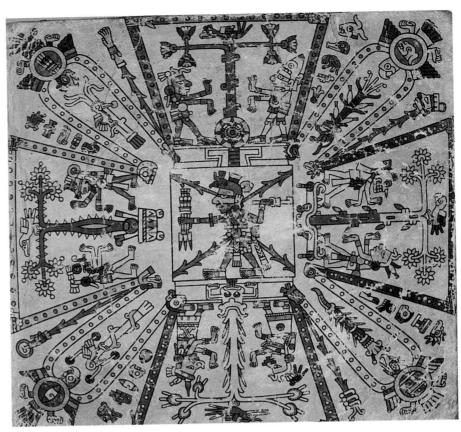

Mixtec map of the five world regions. It identifies the four past worlds at cardinal points and the present one in the center. Each one is represented by a god who directs the history and gives its specific pattern to the universe.

Courtesy Merseyside County Museums, Liverpool, England.

Nahuatl (Aztec) Medicine

Aztecs achieved great feats in astronomy, architecture, and many other areas, including medicine. The North American continent was populated by a medley of isolated cultures; more than 2000 different languages were spoken, each in a very limited area. The conquest by the Spanish decimated all the different cultures.[38]

Nonetheless, Nahuatl medicine had many interesting and original features. Both men and women could practice. Disease was considered the consequence of a violation of religious rules (e.g., rheumatism) or a choice by some god (e.g., dropsy). Even fractures were deemed to result from some spirit who had tripped the wounded person. Medicine, religion, and black magic were closely related. The Aztecs knew the use of mushrooms (e.g., peyote, ololiuhqui) to procure visions and hallucinations. The notions of heat and cold were deeply ingrained in their medical approach to disease and drugs. Other than a real competence in anatomy, surgery, and dissections (partly because of ritual cannibalism), Aztecs also used an extensive pharmacopoeia, as shown in the celebrated *Libellus de medicinalibus Indorum herbis,* written in 1552.[39]

One of the most interesting aspects of their medical beliefs was the notion of *tonalli,* which can be compared with the Musey ethereal body in Africa. More mysterious still, the person who practiced medicine could be a good and learned practitioner *(nanahualtin)* or someone who could make anyone the victim of illness *(tecocoliani)*. Many different sorts of diviners were consulted to diagnose a case, but in very serious cases, only the *paini* (a shaman who could fly to the other world) could deal with the disease.[40]

According to Brother Sahagun, it seems probable that the physicians *(titici)* were on the brink of realizing some sort of hippocratic revolution of their own when the Spanish arrived. Aztec physicians should then be defined as *tlaiximatini* (one who knows the nature of things through experience).[41] C.W. Weiant notes an amusing mistake in which the bonesetter was called *medico verdadero* (true doctor) by the Spanish invaders because the bonesetter knew how "to concert the bones" (i.e., to make the joints work properly). In the minds of the Spanish, the priest was too cruel to deserve the title.[42] The evolution of Nahuatl medicine ended with the Spanish invasion.

Kanaka Medicine

Kanaka medicine represents one of the most poetical approaches ever devised.[43] The people of the Melanesian Islands do not consider the body to exist as a self-governing entity or to have any kind of reality. Its existence is intertwined with the trees and vegetation that surround and almost choke it because of their luxuriance. The word *kara* refers to both the bark of a tree and the skin of a person, another word refers to both the pulp of a fruit and human flesh, and another word to both heart-wood and bones. Glandular organs are given a fruit name, and lungs are named after the Kanaka totem tree *(kuni)*. Intestines are named after the lianas that twine around everything in the forest. It amounts to a complete identity of substance that creates a deep solidarity between people and the environment. M. Leenhardt wrote that a child, like a young shoot, is said to grow from an aqueous state in which the child is full of sap to a hard and ligneous condition.[44] Another tradition is to bury an umbilical cord and plant a tree above it.

To those who use Kanaka medicine, death is not a passage to annihilation. When alive, people are reflections of their effects on others; when dead, people may come back under various forms as *bao*. Medicine in this context relates to plants, possession rites, and also bonesetting. Contrary to most other cultures, bonesetting in the Melanesian Islands is practiced by women, who act as a group.

EASTERN MEDICINE

Tibetan Medicine

At least one form of learned medical tradition was fully influenced by all medical traditions that prevailed at the time. It happened in Tibet as the outcome of a consciously devised policy.[45] During the seventh century the ruler of the kingdom decided to import technology and the method to compute the five elements from China, the Buddhist religion from India, many worldly treasures from Nepal, and law treatises from Byzantium. The king then invited three physicians to travel and confer with him—one from India, one from China, and one from Persia (a Nestorian Christian). Many foreign physicians continued to be invited in later

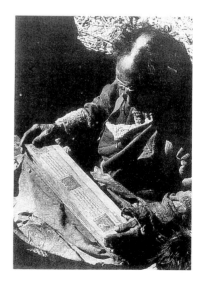

Tibetan practitioner or am-chi *reading the* Four Treatises (Rgynd-bzhi), *a medical compendium in verse that has been claimed to be of sanskrit origin.*

Courtesy Centre National de la Recherche Scientifique (CNRS), Paris.

9

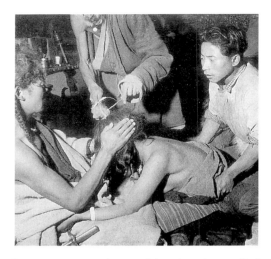

Ignipuncture with a red hot iron is applied here to the top of the skull. The specific point to be treated has first been recognized because pressing on it with the fingertip gave relief to the patient.

Courtesy Centre National de la Recherche Scientifique (CNRS), Paris.

The Master of the Signs, *Chinese calligraphy from a painting by Chen Dehong (1984).*

Courtesy Editions Syros, Paris.

centuries, and many Tibetans were sent to India or China. A great number of translations of medical books were completed as a result (e.g., Vagbhata's translation).

The *Rgynd-brhi* (four treatises) is a fundamental medical compendium in verse that supposedly has a sanskrit origin and was introduced in the eighth century. During the eleventh century, one of the foremost ayurvedic works was also translated. Because of these influences, medical practice in Tibet can be referred to as a form of Tibetan ayurveda (i.e., knowledge of longevity).[46] This, together with Chinese sources that introduced pulse examination, ignipuncture, and a knowledge of visceral organization, finalized the Tibetan tradition as it is known today in the monasteries.

As in Buddhism, ignorance is considered the general cause of disease. Particular causes are the three poisons that affect the seven tissues and excreta. These poisons circulate through channels in the body, particularly in the three main channels along the vertebral column. Additional causes of disease are the ways people eat and live. After a proper urine examination has been performed, disease processes are considered to result from some excess. Hence therapeutic regimens mostly remove, cleanse, and eliminate. All procedures are rationally devised: "Techniques are innumerable but they would amount to a shot in the dark if a principle was lacking."

Tibetan medicine has a very rich tradition involving antagonistic treatments, modifications in lifestyle and diet, medicines, and external interventions. Surgery was used only when all else had failed. No medical profession ever existed in Tibet, only a variety of practitioners *(am-chi)* who ranged from the very learned monk with Buddhist grounding to simple village healers who relied mostly on taoism. There were no taboos about bodies. F. Meyer[47] observed that the way death is represented in the Tibetan tradition has been the only thing preventing a transformation of the immediate tradition through a proper understanding of anatomical knowledge the way it happened in Western medicine before the Renaissance. Nonetheless, Tibetan medicine created a remarkable symbiosis between religion and traditional medicine.

Chinese Medicine

Herbal remedies have always been the most prevalent mode of treatment in Chinese medicine. The Chinese character for the word *medicine* is made up of a *yi,* which expresses the shaman's cry, above a *you,* which refers to fermented drugs.[48] Medicine originally consisted of shakings, wailings, massages, punctures with stone bradawls, ignipuncture, and sacrificial beverages. In China, physicians did not rank above ordinary craftspeople and were despised by the literate class of Mandarins. For all practical purposes, orthodox Chinese medicine was established between the third century BC and the seventh century AD. The Han dynasty ordered *The Classical Treatises* to be compiled. This collection dealt with acupuncture, pulse taking, pharmacology, anesthesiology, preventive medicine and gymnastics, and therapeutic manipulations.

Ayurvedic principles reached China during the Sui dynasty, at which time Buddhist monks from India were welcomed guests. However, Buddhist principles never overruled original Chinese concepts. On the contrary, they were forcefully restated in major works on acupuncture, pulse recording, and pharmacology. According to these Chinese concepts, the body receiving treatment is assimilated to the universe as well as the kingdom or state. To treat and to rule is the same. Confucian principles of the sacredness of the body prevented the development of a promising tradition in surgery. Orthodox Chinese medicine finally only resorted to concoctions to treat internal organs and acupuncture to deal with external diseases. Ancient sages would rather instruct those who were not ill in how to remain healthy or order things before the disease appeared.

In Chinese medicine, joints are the civil servants of the human body, and blood is its minister. In this system, anatomical structures are not referred to as organic except for the way they may energetically interrelate. In other words, the body is approached as the place in which the various breaths are balanced. For example, bone is related to the kidney, but as a skeletal structure, it is governed by the bladder point in the upper thoracic area. The axis *shaoyin* deals with inner vitality and joint motion, whereas the axis *shaoyang* prevents the joints from becoming lax and the bones from loosening so that the body totters.[49] Muscles relate to the spleen and tendons to the liver. Joints are assimilated to a barrier in which energy is believed to concentrate.

All these points are governed by the stomach point, which is situated on the shinbone. Furthermore, the original breath *(yuen-tchi)* is also related to the kidney and is described as the "root" of a person.[50] Joint manipulations were and are widely used. They were extensively developed during the Mongol dynasty and were particularly recorded by We Yilin in the *Shiyi dexiao fang*. In one section, he wrote on various wounds, luxations, and reduction of fractures; he gave advice on manipulation and established an analgesic formula based on the roots aconite and mandarave.[51] Manipulations were also approached as the choice therapeutic modality in central China.

Fundamental concepts in Chinese medicine are directly related to taoism and stem from a unique principle, "the essence of which is the

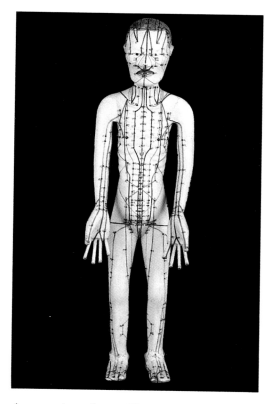

Acupuncture figure. This important Chinese therapeutic modality has been continually used for thousands of years to treat various organs, often quite distant from the punctured point.

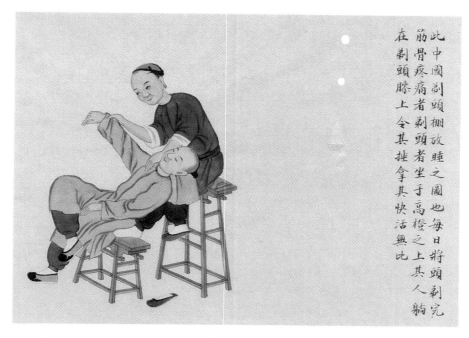

A patient receiving manipulation of the shoulder. Joint manipulation has always been an important feature of Chinese medical treatment.

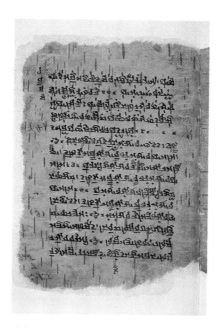

Breathing exercises have been mostly developed by one of the two main tao schools. They are still widely practised as qigong *today.*

center of the circle corresponding to the endless changes."[52] These changes are ordained by the *I Ching*: its hexagrams characterize the dynamic properties of the whole world. The entire universe is made up of a vast collection of breaths that, when pure, help to shape the skies and, when adulterated, belong to the earth. People are caught between the two, and striving for a very long life is the only valid accomplishment.[53] There were two main Tao schools in China, one that developed many breathing exercises still widely practiced today as *qigong* and the other dedicated to develop a form of medicine working with talismans.

Orthodox Chinese medicine is one of the most sophisticated systems ever devised. Modern applications are countless and effective provided Chinese practices are properly applied and not merely introduced as an additional medical procedure. D.D. Palmer[54] cites the case of a Chinese houseboy sick with cholera: "a native physician was prodding him under the tongue with a long needle." He also refers to a "queer" physiological chart covered with black spots, "made up from millions of experiments during the past 2000 or 3000 years from patients who had died or recovered." Once in Shanghai, a chiropractor witnessed a very clever chiropractic adjustment. He asked how long the Chinese had been practicing these moves. The reply was, "At least 5000 years."

Indian Medicine

In India, religion is a prevalent factor in all aspects of life. From prehistoric times onward, Vedas (compiled sacred hymns) were integral parts of many rituals. Social organization in India imposes caste distinctions because of *Jati* (pure birth). Castes alone may allow a person to properly cultivate knowledge. The Brahmins who perform the Vedas would never do the work of a *shudra* (who cannot be born twice). However, the potter's hand is equated to the sacred words of the Vedas, and the potter is also frequently a bonesetter. In *Shatapatha Brahmana* the potter's method in moulding the vessel holding the sacrificial fire is strictly defined and is symbolically equivalent to the creation of the world. In bonesetting, "Things can be repaired by acting on their clay representation; that is why the reduction of a fracture is considered to be on par with pottery making."[55]

In contrast, the usual mode of practice when joints were manipulated was taken care of by bath attendants.[56] A.H. Anquetil-Duperron, a French orientalist and the translator of *Zend Avesta* in the eighteenth century, relates how in Bombay he was given no peace until his attendant had made his spine crack. "He kneels on the small of your back, grasps your shoulders and makes your spine crack by moving all the vertebrae."[57] Manipulation was no longer a medically advised prescription but a mere habit of hygiene.

In Vedic times, the making of herbal elixirs led to the concoction of fermented sacrificial liquors and magical drugs. However, brahmanical medicine prevailed as the real science of life (i.e., ayurveda). It classified vital breaths as they circulated along channels that were under the control of specific centers known as *wheels* or *lotus*. Other than exogenous diseases, all conditions were thought to stem from a disturbed element in the seven organic compounds that constituted the body. Three of these compounds known as *tri-dosha* (three troubles) were involved when disease occurred, and three compounds *(tridhatu)* were involved when a person was healthy. The various disease-producing combinations have been recorded in major treatises or *samhita,* which were written from tra-

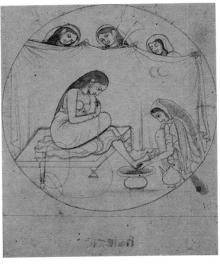

This seventeenth century Mughal miniature illustrates the necessity of bodily cleanliness as a preventive means to protect health in Indian medical thought.

Courtesy British Museum, London.

dition by Charaka and Sushruta, presumably in Galen's time (about the second century). There was also a surgical treatise attributed to Nagar-juna.[58] Indian medicine taught the Arabs to differentiate between the physician and the surgeon. They transmitted this distinction to medieval European medicine, where it happened to agree with Roman Church prohibitions to clergy and monks. Arabic medicine also left a medical tradition of repute in Northern India, where it is still commonly practiced. It is now known as *Unani* or Greco-Arab medicine.[59]

Two factors should be emphasized in Indian medicine. One is the importance given to hygiene, diet, proper living, and preventive means to protect health. The other is that Indian medicine never purported that the influence of spirits or evils produces disease. A belief in such influence was considered by ayurvedic practitioners in much the same way that scientific medical practitioners treat alternatives to medicine today. Indian biological concepts had a vitalistic grounding, whereas concepts in the west remained mechanistic. The consequence was very different scientific approaches and different values and intuitions. P. Masson-Oursel[60] pleads for more critical criteria to properly understand this approach, which is several millennia old and founded on observations.

ARABIC MEDICINE

The case has been made that Arabic medicine never existed—that it was a misnomer. On the other hand, science would never have developed in Europe the way it did if not for the Arabic approach to medicine. Arabic medicine refers only to those medical treatises that were written in the Arabic language or that have survived because they were translated into Arabic. This is the case regardless of the author's language or creed, that is, whether Syriac, Pahlavi, Aramaic, or Hebrew was spoken in everyday life and whether the religion was Muslim, Christianity, or Judaism. Islam is the religion of the Koran, and during the medieval period, it was also the culture of the science of alchemy; all practical sciences were organized around Islam. It implied a different perception of the world and a language of its own. Spiritual and physical objects were described as beams of light. Life was considered to progress toward an increased process of densification that, if continued, led to matter in crystal form. Alchemists contended that the process could be reversed.

Alchemy fostered the promotion of a number of sciences. The relationship between archetypes and plants led to the development of botany and pharmacology; the relationship that was supposed to exist between angelical and animal worlds encouraged the profound study of the medical sciences.[61] These specific fields of knowledge were considered to be the points where "forces" and "bodies" could meet and artificial channels could be made to exist through art. Alchemy was at the heart of all transmutations by which solid bodies could be penetrated by subtle forces. All these movements also had to be mathematically established because they were in the celestial sphere. As a result, astronomy was the other omnipresent science of the time.

Because of alchemy, medicine was never allowed to develop along the lines proposed by al-Biruni in the tenth century. He refused all metaphysical speculations and endorsed only scientific conclusions drawn from observation alone. He was ignored in a world in which even scientific activity was to be entirely submissive to God.[62] As a sufin, Ibn Khal-

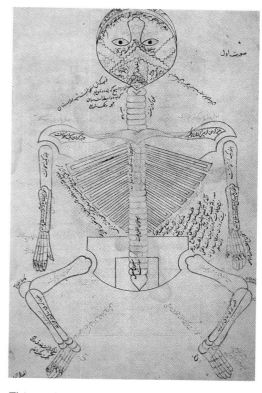

This arabic, almost birdlike representation of the human frame emphasizes the fact that exactness in anatomy was not an issue during the Middle Ages. Only the study of macrocosm was thought to enlighten the physiology and pathology (microcosm) of humans (M. Shirazi).

Courtesy Bibliothèque Nationale, Paris.

dun, the father of sociology in the fourteenth century, could not envisage science other than as a mystical experience.[63] The consequence was that aristotelian logic ruled the organization of all knowledge, including medicine. Medical matters were fully revolutionized because they had to be assessed by a thorough mathematical analysis. The methodologic results were amazing, but very little knowledge of these results came to the Western world. Only 40 Arabic medical treatises (out of more than a thousand known today) were translated into Latin. Hence very few changes would ensue in Western medicine despite the breakthroughs in Arabic medicine.[64]

The only real exception was az-Zahrawi, better known as Albucasis. He had died in 1009 and was a surgeon, not a physician. Spinal manipulative techniques were considered part of surgery and were more prevalent, along the lines of Greek, Byzantine, and Hindu medicines. Oribasius, Paul of Aegina, Apollonius of Kitium, and Sushruta were the main sources cited. Observations made by Albucasis were frequently quoted by Chauliac, Vidius, and Paré, but there was no real improvement in either technique or concepts. Learning in this area seemed set—a usually fatal blow in science. Travelers to Turkey and Egypt in the nineteenth century only knew of spinal manipulations because they were exposed to them by bath attendants.

The Arabs left yet another legacy to the world of science. Beyond their description of harmony in natural phenomena, they also emphasized tension as a characteristic of all phenomena pertaining to life. This notion of tension opened the way to mysticism, its pathos, and its revolts in the Western world before it also influenced the biological sciences, including chiropractic, much later. Palmer declared that "life is based on tone," and the concept of axial tension, when operative in the central nervous system, is still very prevalent in many research works.[65]

MANIPULATING THE SPINE IN THE WESTERN WORLD

From Greece to the Renaissance Age

Well into the seventeenth century and regardless of whether they were Greek, Roman, Byzantine, Cretan, Arabic, Spanish, Turkish, Italian, French, or German, all published authors resorted to the same method. The patient was bandaged and lay on a board; traction was applied toward the head and feet while pressure was exerted onto a selected spinal area. From available illustrations, the lumbo-dorsal area was most frequently involved in these attempts. Then the thrust was directed toward either the head or hips. Pressure was made by using the hands or feet or by sitting on the spine to move it and correct a disturbed lumbar lordosis. A piece of wood could also be used as a lever to apply sustained pressure to the diseased part of the back while the patient was lying prone.

K.A. Ligeros[66] claims that Greek physicians actually manipulated the spine as chiropractors do today. The method just described was used in cases in which there was a dislocation, luxation, or fracture of the spine, that is, a major displacement with possible spinal cord damage and paralysis or death as a likely outcome. Treatment could amount to a harsh form of punishment. For example, in some cases the patient was tied onto a ladder, which then fell to the floor. Nonetheless, there are a few indications supporting Ligeros's view that minor spinal displacements (i.e., the

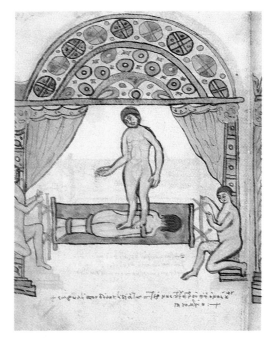

The hippocratic method to manipulate the spine relied on combined traction applied with a thrust or sustained pressure. Traction was by means of a windlass or from a folded cloth pulled by helpers. The thrust could come from a person sitting or standing on the back of a patient or by means of a board acting as a lever (Apollonius of Cyprus).

Courtesy Piccarda Quilici, Lucia Parmiggiani, and Jean-Paul Jolivet, Biblioteca Universitaria, Archiginnasio de Bologna, Bologna, Italy.

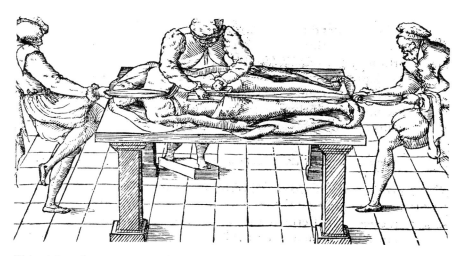

This sixteenth century woodcut describing a method still being used and advised by Ambroise Paré (1517-1590) to "restore a thoracic vertebra in its proper place."
Courtesy François Deguilly, Bibliothèque Municipale, Orléans, France.

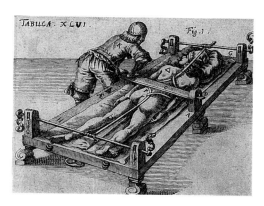

A notable evolution results from the introduction of a spring-loaded apparatus that is fixed onto a bed and that allows for traction and thrust to be controlled by a single person (J. Scultetus).
Courtesy Bibliothèque Interuniversitaire de Médecine, Paris.

hippocratic *pararthremata*) were also recognized and treated by ancient practitioners. That could be the case on the votive tablet from the Aesculapium of Piraeus (600 BC). However, the case treated by Galen was irrefutable. The patient complained of numbness and tingling in the fingers of the left hand after a fall. Treatment consisted of a single manipulation to the patient's neck, yet simple as it was, it still required Galen's expertise to be successful. Medicine in Europe then entered a very dark age.

In 587, Bishop Gregory of Tours[67] became indignant at a bonesetter because he pretended to call on the assistance of saints to achieve his cures. He would publicly treat people using helpers to pull his patient's arms and legs for him. They would stretch the body with so much force that it was feared the nerves would be torn. Gregory concluded, "The poor

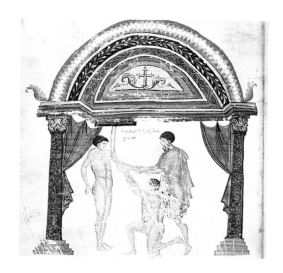

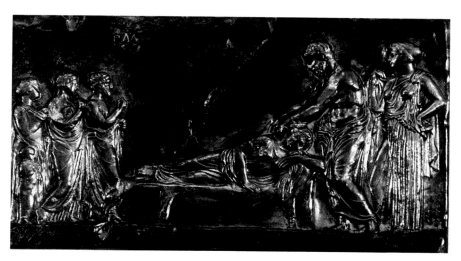

Minor spinal displacements may be the modern counterparts of Aesculapian manipulations. Proper adjustments may also be illustrated on a number of votive tablets recovered from Asclepieion in Piraeus (600 BC).
Courtesy Logan College of Chiropractic, Chesterfield, Missouri.

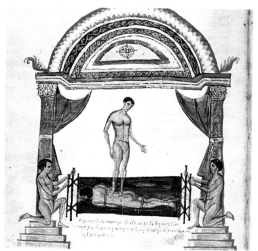

Examples of Roman manipulation.
Courtesy Ministerio per Beni Culturi e Ambinetali, Bologna, Italy.

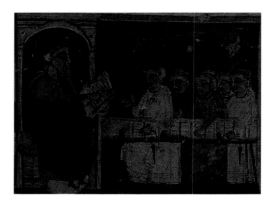

From the eleventh century, medicine was taught in universities. There were numerous masters in Salerno, and their teachings were influenced by Constantinus Africanus, then Rolando of Parma. The same applied to Guglielmo Scalicetti in Bologna, Guido Lanfranchi in Paris, and Johannes Yperman in the Netherlands. It was the tradition to present renowned teachers in illuminationsas frontispieces in their main published works.

Courtesy Bibliothèque Interuniversitaire de Médecine, Paris.

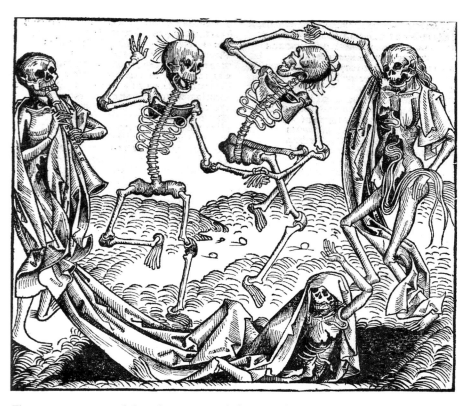

The reappearance of the plague in mid–fourteenth century Europe resulted in a full social, economical, and cultural collapse. The danse macabre became a subject of artistic presentation. The knee and elbow joints are pictured as coupling shafts, whereas the pelvic girdle is a T-shaped double hinge-joint (H. Schedel).
Courtesy Bibliothèque Interuniversitaire de Médecine, Paris.

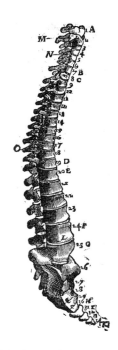

By the mid–sixteenth century, Ambroise Paré (1561) among others had pictured a proper anatomical likeness of the human spine. Charles Estienne (1539-1545) and Andréas Vesalius (1543) published their epoch-making works that signaled an important cultural shift and investigations relying fully on firsthand observations.

Courtesy François Deguilly, Bibliotèque Municipale, Orléans, France.

soul was left lying unconscious on the ground, if he were not cured." The fact that a number of patients were healed was an even greater offense, since Didier the bonesetter was a lay healer. At the time, medicine had been declared the exclusive domain of Church secular activities. A number of methods in use to treat the sick were completely irrational; when this was recognized, the irrationality was forcefully condemned but only when the practice was a lay practice. On a par with Jewish or heathen physicians, lay healers were declared to practice in a state of "canonical inability" to heal.

Eleventh century translations from the Arabic by Constantinus Africanus did not improve the situation. The aim of the translations was not to understand the Arabs' contribution to medicine but to retrieve Galen's teachings as they had been known in Alexandria.[68] Another purpose was to promote the physician's social status to that of a counselor in all facets of life (e.g., in his translation of Ibn Gazzar's *De coitu*). However, most Arabic treatises had been written or inspired by the works of dissenting Christians who had fled after the Council of Chalcedon (451 AD). Whether they settled in Persia, India, or China, they were still heretics, and the Arabs were dreaded infidels. Many misconceptions and misquotes dotted these translations.

Nevertheless, there were other important and more justly famous physicians in Salerno and the new universities.[69] *Chirurgia* (1210) by Rolando da Parma proposed several methods to treat spinal dislocations that were not surpassed until the early twentieth century. Among them was one procedure a number of chiropractors would ascribe to Bohemian bonesetters because it required the use of a folded cloth to manipulate

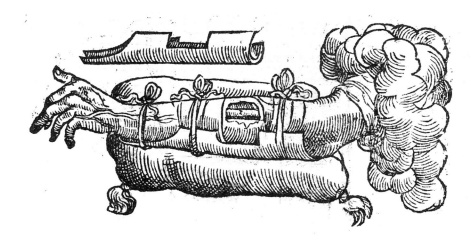

Paré's teachings in the vernacular were easily understood by most country and army surgeons. He used ligatures instead of a cauterizing iron to stop hemorrhage. He was credited with having discovered this method even though it had been advised before by Oribasius and Scalicetti among others. The method was then abandoned until the nineteenth century.

Courtesy François Deguilly, Bibliothèque Municipale, Orléans, France.

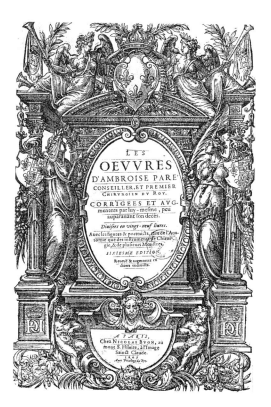

Sixteenth century clinical surgery was entirely reformed almost single-handedly by a former barber apprentice with no academic training who had become a military surgeon. Ambroise Paré (1517-1590) then became first surgeon to the King of France. His works were not written in Latin, as were all works for physicians then, but in the vernacular French.

From Pare A: *Collected works*, ed 6, 1607.

the spine. This is the way Frank Dvorski was reported to practice, and it was once claimed that D.D. Palmer did get his inspiration from Dvorski.[70] It amounted to giving a rough pull to the spine or a dislocated jaw with the cloth rather than delivering a proper adjustment.

The creation of great medieval universities also led to the exclusion of women doctors. All minor operative crafts were also excluded but were later assembled under the heading "practical medicine." Clergy and monks were requested to deal only with spiritual matters, but clerical medicine survived to some extent.[71]

The new hierarchy in medieval medicine was established at a great cost, and bonesetters suffered greatly from the process.[72] However, bonesetters were also partly to blame. For example, a family of bonesetters from the Pays de Caux in Normandy knew how to treat disjunctions of bones or fractures resulting from a violent fall or severe blow.[73] They also could remedy bruised nerves and limbs, bring the bone into its joint again, and restore the body to its original vigor.[74] They were summoned to the French Court to treat all types of sprains and fractures, and they also occupied the highest offices: chaplain to the King, gentleman of the Privy Chamber, High Court President, and Finance Superintendent.

So it happened in their case, bonesetters were also socially superior to any medical doctor. That period lasted from Henry II to Louis XIII—from 1547 to 1643. During this time, these bonesetters had every opportunity to introduce a proper academic background and to make the craft into a full profession but failed to do so. Instead, they were content with being celebrated among the "Illustrious of Gaul."[75] These socially respected bonesetters abandoned the practice and now rank among the many "hereditary physicians" whose families flourished in France until the seventeenth century and who touched for dog bites and other mishaps.[76]

The Age of Enlightenment

When the Enlightened Age arose in medicine in the seventeenth and eighteenth centuries, bonesetters were thrown off hospital wards in which

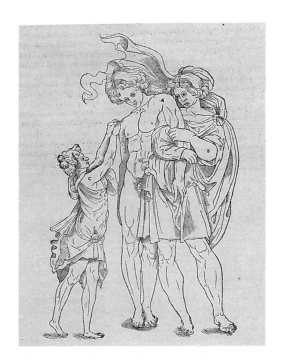

Fifteenth and sixteenth century Renaissance artists became increasingly involved in the serious pursuit of anatomical knowledge. As a medical man, Guido Guidi (1508-1569) used these artists' works when he translated Nicetas's Surgical Collection *from Greek into Latin (F. Salviati).*

Courtesy Bibliothèque Interuniversitaire de Médecine, Paris.

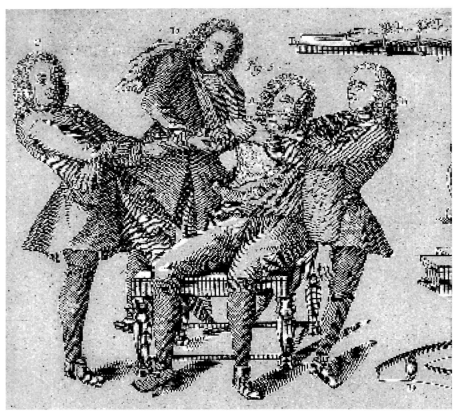

In the seventeenth century, iatromechanists applied mechanical principles to medicine. It led to a search for new methods to improve on former knowledge and practices and a reliance on reasoning from facts rather than assuming the validity of ancient teachers out of respect for them (J. Scultetus).

Courtesy Bibliothèque Interuniversitaire de Médecine, Paris.

access had previously been granted. This action was done in the name of science, although it was no more than medical prejudice at work. Bonesetters were never again seen in the wards, and hospital privileges for chiropractors in the United States are only very recent acquisitions. At about the same time, a major change in medical concepts led physicians and surgeons to approach the body as a set of levers worked by muscles; they considered muscle function to brace the spine. Muscles were seen as the new centers of reference, and spinal dislocations were abandoned as explanations for diseases. Massages and frictions were the new recommended treatments, whereas joint reductions were condemned.[77]

Three main concepts against bonesetting precluded a proper appraisal of the art. One was the belief that there always was a fracture of the vertebrae whenever a lesion occurred as the result of enforced movement. Luxations were seen only as an indication for major surgery. There was no question of the possibility of a graded response, in which the degree of luxation would be taken into account to determine appropriate treatment. Manipulating the spine was branded a rash and dangerous maneuver that could result in instant death. What doctors were really condemning were the earlier hippocratic modes of practice. By a convenient extrapolation, any other technique was also condemned, and that included the practice of bonesetters.[78]

The second concept arose because of the prevalence of tuberculous

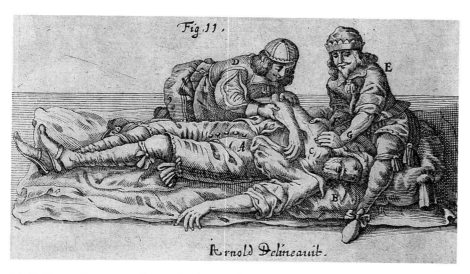

Until the rediscovery of anesthesia in 1842, the setting of a dislocated limb by surgical means required great exertion from both surgeon and helpers. Bonesetters who knew better had been refused access to hospitals and were forcefully denounced as incompetent charlatans.

Courtesy Bibliothèque Interuniversitaire de Médecine, Paris.

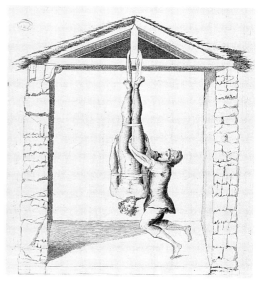

From Appollonius of Cyprus (circa 60 AD) to Nicetas (tenth century AD) and from Guido Guidi (sixteenth century) to E.F.M. Bosquillon (eighteenth century), the same methods of Hippocrates and Byzantium were used to manipulate the human frame. Here a hip luxation is set according to Guidi as reprinted in Bosquillon's compilation (F. Salviati).

Courtesy Bibliothèque Interuniversitaire de Médecine, Paris.

lesions of the spine. It was thought that any sore spot might indicate purulent vertebral decay and that manipulation might induce a full collapse of the suspected caries. Only red hot iron and major surgery were advised, and resorting to mechanical means to attempt a reduction was forbidden.[79]

The last concept was that a hump was suspected to indicate sexual deviation, especially in the youth; this idea also resulted in the introduction of totally misguided procedures.[80]

Curiously, at the same time that missionaries to America and elsewhere were sternly condemning shaking a patient by shamans, Wrinkler wrote that by violently shaking a man suffering from an ear fluxion, he relieved him of his ailment. He considered that these violent moves had shaken the nerves and activated their juices. Treatment could be harsher still: J.F. Paullini resorted to the whip and rod to cure scores of intractable illnesses, deafness among them. The innocent ruse of an old doctor, told by J.C. Tissot, is another example. The doctor did not believe that taking the waters was of any value, but he advised his patient to do so. No sooner had the patient arrived at a spa than the doctor sent him off to another one "for in his opinion the cure depended more on the jolting of the carriage than on taking the waters."[81]

At the time, there were many illnesses that doctors could do little about, but a treatment was available for disorders of the back that would ensure success almost every time it was used. Medical practitioners would violently shake and whip the animal spirits in the various parts of their patients' bodies only because they refused to accept let alone comprehend something that pertained to another field of knowledge. They thought it was real progress over the wickedness of those who pretended to reduce luxated joints. R.T. Anderson aptly stated the following[82]:

> [from then on] bonesetting became identified with the humble oral tradition of uneducated peasants and working people. That identification became a stigma ... and status alone blinded professional borrowers who might be tempted to bring it back to respectability.

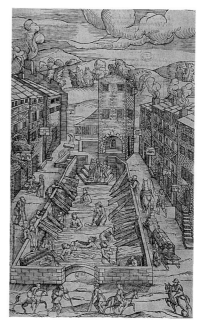

Hydrotherapy and public baths were a very common feature of Roman life. Some thermal springs continued into late antiquity in Campania, Italy. They were rediscovered during the Middle Ages, but most new resorts had very rudimentary constructions.

Courtesy Bibliothèque Interuniversitaire de Médecine, Paris.

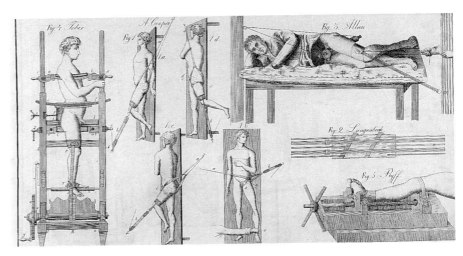

During the nineteenth century, many mechanical devices were invented to treat joint dislocations. All these machines worked on the basis of a forcible operation (A.L. Richter).

Courtesy Bibliothèque Interuniversitaire de Médecine, Paris.

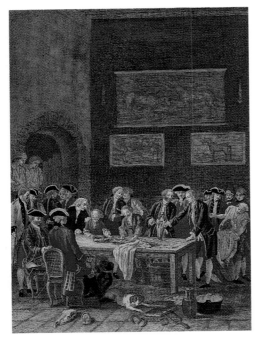

The art of veterinary surgery was first defined as a profession in Lyon in 1761 and then in Paris in 1766. It was first taught along the lines of a project by Georges Louis Buffon. Animal and even human dissections were carried to a subtly refined art. On this frontispiece, teaching appears to have been somewhat careless, with book strewn over the floor alongside horseshoes and bones for dogs (C. de Lafosse).

Courtesy Bibliothèque Interuniversitaire de Médecine, Paris.

Medical doctors were not the only ones to denigrate bonesetting to assert their own progress toward professionalization and to further disqualify the art. Midwives retained the use of medieval techniques to manipulate the spines of newborns; it was a cultural and social demand to give the child a human form. The reasons midwives had for performing the proceduce further concealed the therapeutic benefits of bonesetting; it made the practice medically meaningless. On the other end of the professional spectrum, surgeons claimed the sole right to treat fractures and sprains. The outcome was frequently an aggravation of the lesion the patient suffered from because the surgeons were not very successful; the contractures and spasms induced by the machinery they used to make a reduction often had an adverse effect on proper mending of bone fragments. Still, surgeons would unabashedly denounce bonesetters as uncouth outcasts to promote their own professionalization process. Meanwhile they would compel bonesetters to pay a fee to their association.[83]

The aspects leading to the creation of the new profession of veterinary surgeon are another example. French authorities decided to create the new profession of veterinary surgeon. Country folks had always managed by themselves or with specialized help from gelders or farriers. To impose the new practitioners on farmers, the authorities decided that veterinary services would cost nothing because veterinary surgeons were to be made functionaries of the Crown. Veterinary training would also include specific subjects such as learning how to deliver a baby, resuscitating a drowned person, and *setting bones*. The French authorities believed that thrift in the peasant world would induce the farmers to call one free practitioner instead of the two or three who would claim fees. No one knows how the veterinary surgeons were taught, but it proved even bonesetting could be taught in a university.[84]

The French revolution that shortly followed may have helped to further modify the situation, since academic medical qualifications were suspended by the revolution and later suppressed for all health professions. However, the opposite happened.[85] The new clinical concepts sweeping the medical scene implied that at long last physicians were interpreting their science in the light of surgical knowledge, which proved to be very fruitful.[86] School teachers began condemning bonesetting in the name of progress.[87] The condemnation was associated with a blind faith in the promises made "in the name of science."

BONESETTING

Regardless of the prevailing thought of the time, some patients and even medical doctors were open to alternative methods of healing. Most practitioners denied the possibility of different approaches, an opinion disregarding the fact that any approach might prove as effective as current methods provided it was given an appropriate setting. However, those who disagreed, notably the better educated class in Western societies, led the return to mechanical measures.

Captain Cook's experience of *rumi* after he had reached Tahiti in 1777 has been frequently told. Being "much out of order," he was taken care of by women who made a perfect mummy of his flesh until his bones cracked. The procedure gave him immediate relief. The same kind of "pumelling and squeezing" was also observed by R.T. Anderson[88] in Hawaii, where it is known as *lomilomi*. The procedure is used to soothe pain and limber up any stiffened muscle; it involves hard deep kneading of the flesh and tissues performed with a remarkable skill. The main feature is walking on the patient's back aided by two canes, and it is said to be related to *momi-ryoji* in Japan.

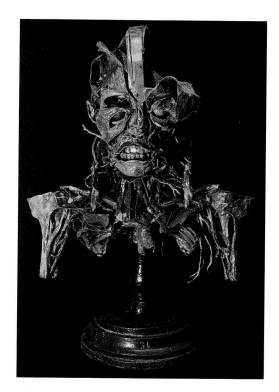

The cousin of the painter, Honoré Fragonard (1732-1799) was a confirmed anatomist and taught at the Alfort veterinary school specializing in morphological studies. A true artist, he managed to "concert" his dissections into real works of art that sought to show life, even beyond death.

Courtesy Editions Jupilles, LeMans, France.

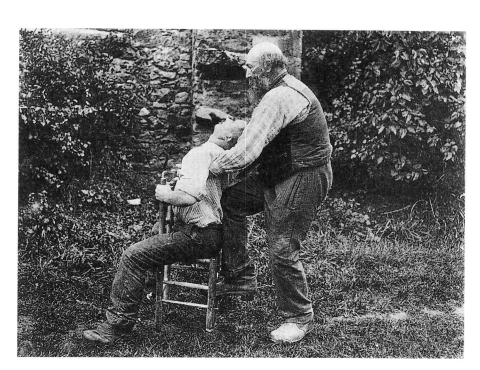

This French postcard shows a bonesetter treating a lumbago or acute low back pain. It was shot in Britanny, France, near Vannes circa 1880.

Courtesy Musée des Arts et Traditions Populaires, Paris.

21

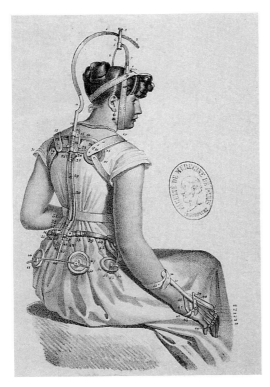

American surgeon Robert W. Lovett once described the nineteenth century as "a most confusing period. The theorist and the apparatus-inventor went mad and every form of device appeared. Braces and corsets infinitely complicated, worse than useless, appeared by the dozen" (P.N. Gerdy).

Courtesy Bibliothèque Interuniversitaire de Médecine, Paris.

Treading on the backbone of a prone patient has been documented the world over. The only difference from former hippocratic methods was that traction was not applied. For the process to be successful, different cultures required that the trampler be a virgin or the mother of twins or to be born foot-first. Ritual formulae were often exchanged between the patient and the healer during the performance to make it more effective. It might also be advised that the performer be of the opposite sex or, as in many rural areas, to be very young. It has been pointed out that such manipulations were also used for prevention or for their general stimulating effects. E. Schiotz[89] describes a witchcraft trial in Norway in 1662 during which the accused explained her method for relieving back pain: since the age of 3 years she had trodden on the backs of sufferers from rheumatism, but now she could do it better with her hand.

W.M. Thackeray reported that manipulation was used in Turkey, and E. Harrison and N. Andry de Boisregard commented on what was known as "Paris massage." However, these modalities were sometimes considered too brutal because they were frequently practiced by "hefty and ignorant helpers."[90] Another major influence swept the medical scene—the new concept of "spinal irritation." However, it is to be emphasized that neither osteopathy nor chiropractic were really influenced by the concept toward the end of the nineteenth century.[21] At the time, the spinal cord was visualized by some to be the locus of a "spinal soul" *(Ruckenmarksseele)*[21]; only for most physiologists, *soul* was a convenient word that meant "sensory function."[91]

J.E. Riadore, an English physician, noted that from Rufus the Ephesian to Charles Bell, no attempt had been made to explain nervous diseases on the basis of anatomical observations. "Many," he said, "ridicule the idea of examining the spine. . . . If overlooked, the patient's affliction will continue to baffle all remedies."[92] To support his argument, he referred to E. Harrison, who had described what he called an incomplete luxation or subluxation of the vertebrae. P. Pott believed that for the most part the source of spinal trouble was in connecting ligaments losing their power to hold the bones together. The spine thus lost its natural firmness, and the distortion became permanently established.[93] J.E. Riadore concluded the following[94]:

> The cause is never suspected to be in the spine, and the latter is never examined; the subluxated vertebra is never replaced in its original linear direction . . . to a degree sufficient to prevent the spinal cord or a nerve to be unduly pressed at its exit, to cause constitutional or local irritation in some organ to which the irritated nerves are distributed.

Treatment consisted essentially of an orthopedical mixture of procedures, despite the fact that it was prescribed along the lines of a neurological analysis. These ideas sound in many ways like D.D. Palmer's theories, but there is no mention of the neuroskeleton, axial tension bearing on the structures, or the spine being a regulator of tension.[95]

Another neurological area that has not received its share of attention refers to pain and the way it reaches consciousness. J. Hilton, an English surgeon, observed that after a fall, a person may feel a peculiar sensation in the hands and feet; the next morning, that person is unable to arise. He wrote that the little filaments in the sensory and motor nerves had been put in a state of extreme tension as they passed through the intervertebral foramina and that the immediate parts were necessarily stretched. He considered these symptoms to be the result of some structural disturbance, although he could not ascertain what the injury was. He never considered the joints, despite his advice that the nerves should be traced to

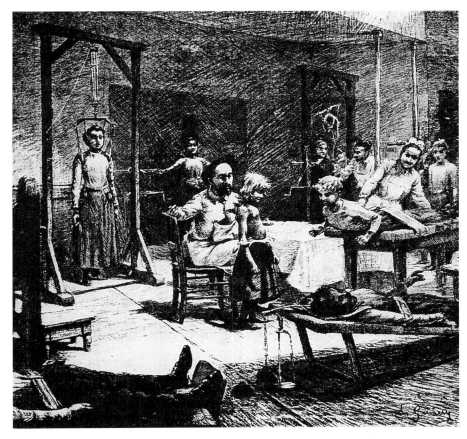

The orthopaedic ward of rue Denfert-Rochereau in nineteenth century Paris shows that the patients were left bruised by the conflicting theories of the times.
Courtesy Bibliothèque Interuniversitaire de Médecine, Paris.

arrive at the part of diseased spine causing the pain.[96] Galen did the same when diagnosing the cause of the cervicobrachial neuralgia, which had baffled his fellow physicians. Only he knew how to manipulate the offending vertebra.

Bonesetters could have experienced the same medical development from their concepts as the surgeons had after the French revolution except for medical prejudice. This was fully documented by R.T. Anderson[97] in the case of Herbert Barker, the most famous English bonesetter at the turn of this century. W.I. Wardwell[98] quotes a 1925 editorial of the *Lancet:* "The medical profession of the future will have to record that our profession has greatly neglected this important subject. . . . That by our faulty methods we are largely responsible for its very existence."

THE AGE OF MEDICAL DISSENT

A key is needed to organize the cultural traits that may explain the emergence of chiropractic as a unique science.[99] In the Indo-European tradition as recorded by G. Dumezil,[100] disease is focused around three poles:(1) god-induced disease (treatment through charms), (2) traumatisms (treatment by violence in return), and (3) wasting diseases (treat-

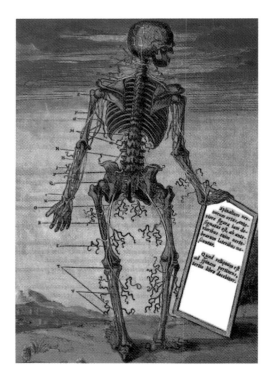

Sixteenth century anatomist Charles Estienne (1504-1564) wished that "truth be shown to the eye through dissection." He was the first to propose a clear description of the sympathetic and parasympathetic nervous systems. He was also the first to introduce Renaissance anatomical discoveries in Renaissance landscapes. He beautifully illustrated the neuro-skeleton that was to become the basis of D.D. Palmer's many teachings.

Courtesy P.L. Gaucher-Peslherbe, LeMans, France.

ment by medicinal plants). A similar organization has been proposed for popular traditions in healing: (1) to break a spell, (2) to set bones, and (3) to medicate with herbs.[101] It might be more appropriate to consider traditional practices through the classifications applied to popular religion, since traditional medical habits are also a method by which a culture can be expressed.[102]

Chiropractic was never an unscientific cult, only a different science.[103] When Palmer proposed chiropractic to the world, he had been a professional mesmerist (magnetic healer) for 9 years. Mesmerism can be considered the most pervasive form of medical dissent in modern times.

The scientists and academians who assembled to judge Mesmer's new mode of healing refused to acknowledge facts that did not fit the established classification of laws, that is, those laws they had themselves established. Mesmerists requested a proper science be constituted to study those irregularities and abnormalities that could not be explained by established laws.[104]

Mesmer's quest was not unreasonable, but it disturbed too many reasonable people who felt threatened by it. Jussieu was the only naturalist in the commission, and he was the only one to comment on a medicine that would touch for health *(médecine d'attouchements)*. He observed the following[105]:

> It has been practiced in all times and in every nation. It has always languished in obscurity because it was abandoned into improper hands to direct it, administered without method, and relegated to popular and limited techniques. . . . It is now high time that we endeavored to establish a medicine that touches for health on a firmer basis and that we perfected it since it is already so useful and since it will be even more the case when it is better known.

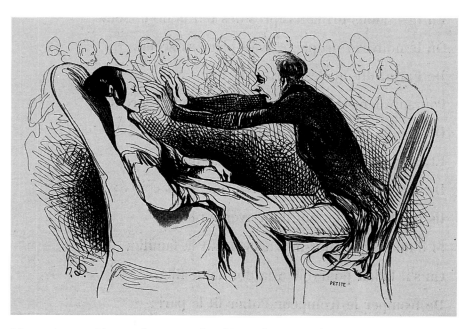

Mesmerism and hypnotism were the object of satire and a number of caricatures during the nineteenth century. François Fabre was the editor of the Lancette Française, *and he wrote in a sarcastic and pseudodemocratic vein to promote the interests of the medical profession. He was born in Marseille as was his friend Honoé Daumier, who illustrated his* Némésis médicale.

Courtesy Bibliothèque Interuniversitaire de Médecine, Paris.

When this was written in 1784, the field of mesmerism was open and the opportunities it offered were unlimited, both in the scientific and occult domains.

One fundamental feature of health practice cannot be overemphasized—the belief that illness, wherever it appears and whatever form it takes, is first and foremost a loss in vitality, so remedies are only considered effective if they help nature. As described by W.G. Rothstein,[106] the end result is a search for a therapeutic method that treats the cause rather than symptoms arising from the cause. This attitude can easily lead to endless efforts to identify the cause. It is also most desirable to locate it anatomically so that a specific method of treatment can be defined.

Such an attitude existed at the end of the nineteenth century. The reason D.D. Palmer was motivated to propose chiropractic is best understood by a reference written in 1891 to the prevalent craze in medical circles dealing with "traumatic hysteria": "The true nature of some paralysis after a traumatism (is to be compared) to the paralysis occurring with mesmerism."[107] Chiropractic should be approached as an answer to the deficiencies in medical concepts that existed.

This chapter is dedicated to the memory of Katell Legall, a Doctor of Chiropractic in the loftiest aspects the calling implies. My deepest appreciation is expressed to Professor Walter I. Wardwell, Dr. Sylvie Leturmy, and Professor David Le Breton for their help and comments. Neither they nor the other authors of this book should bear any responsibility for the contents of this chapter.

ANNOTATED REFERENCES

1. Clavreul J: *L'ordre médical*, Paris, 1978, Editions du Seuil; Leonard J: *La médecine entre les savoirs et les pouvoirs; histoire intellectuelle et politique de la médecine francaise au XIX siecle*, Paris, 1981, Aubier-Montaigne.

2. Rothstein WG: *American physicians in the 19th century: from sects to science*, Baltimore, 1972, Johns Hopkins Press; McLahan G, McKeown T, editors: *Medical history and medical care*, Oxford, 1971, Oxford University Press; Carr-Saunders AM, Wilson PA: *The professions*, London, 1933, Oxford University Press, p 304.

3. Cosmacini G: *Soigner et réformer; médecine et santé en Italie de la grande peste à la premierè guerre mondiale*, Paris, 1992, Editions Payot, p 60; Pouchelle MC: *Corps et chirurgie à l'apogée du Moyen Age*, Paris, 1983, Editions Flammarion.

4. Peter JP: Western medicine in its history, a winding path between knowledge and misunderstanding. In Gaucher-Peslherbe PL, editor: *Health and marginality: a source of misunderstanding,* Annals of the Walter Wardwell Conference, Orleans, 1992, Editions Grandvaux, pp 17-27.

5. Mohen JP, editor: *Le temps de la préhistoire*, Paris, 1989, Société Prehistorique Française et Archeologia; Leroi-Gourhan A: *Les religions de la préhistoire*, Paris, 1964, Presses Universitaires de France; Riskine AE: *Carnac, l'armée de pierres*, Paris, 1992, Imprimerie Nationale.

6. Leroi-Gourhan A: *Le geste et la parole: techniques et langage*, Paris, 1964-1965, Editions Albin Michel; Gaucher G: *Methodes de recherche en prehistoire*, Paris, 1990, Les Presses du Centre National de la Recherche Scientifique.

7. Brothwell D, Sandison AT: *Diseases in antiquity: a survey of the diseases, injuries and surgery of early populations*, Springfield, Ill, 1967, Charles C. Thomas; Lançon B: Tactus salubritate, manipulative medicine in late antiquity Gaul, personal communication, 1986. With the proviso that they were soothing techniques rather than cure, mere mending is more frequently encountered.

8. Eliade M: *Traité d'histoire des religions*, Paris, 1986, Editions Payot; Jarcho S: *Human paleopathology*, New Haven, Conn, 1966, Yale University Press; Binford PL: *Bones, ancient men and modern myths*, New York, 1981.

9. Eliade M: *Le chamanisme et les techniques archaïques de l'extase*, Paris, 1978, Editions Payot.

10. Ramirez F: Relación sobre la Residencia de Michoacan. In *Monumenta mexicana*, Rome 1959. (Quoted by Le Clezio JMG: *Le rêve mexicain ou la pensée interrompue*, Paris, 1988, Editions Gallimard, p 234.)

11. Burckhardt T: Cosmologie et science moderne. In *Les etudes traditionnelles*. (Quoted by Canteins J: *Sauver le mythe. I. Le potier démiurge*, Paris, 1986, Editions Maisonneuve et Larose.)

12. Bloch M: *Les rois thaumaturges: étude sur le caractere surnaturel attribué à la puissance royale particulièrement en France et en Angleterre*, Paris, 1983, Editions Gallimard, pp 382-383.

13. Finley MI: *Les anciens Grecs: une introduction à leur vie et à leur pensée*, Paris, 1981, F Maspéro, p 113; Vernant JP: *Figures, idoles et masques*, Paris, 1990, Editions Julliard; Graves R: *The Greek myths*, Harmondsworth, 1978, Penguin Books.

14. Ricoeur P: Introduction. In *Les cultures et le temps*, Paris, 1975, Editions Payot/Les Presses de l'Unesco, pp 19-41; Valabrega JP: *Phantasmes, mythes, corps et sens: une théorie psychanalytique de la connaissance*, Paris, 1992, Editions Payot.

15. Eliade M: *Le chamanisme*, op cit, pp 128-153; Graves R: *The Greek Myths*, op cit, vol 1, 108(27.4), 124(37.7), 254(72.2); vol 2, 106(123.1). They were calendar emblems of the tripartite year, which were later partly reused by the four evangelists.

16. Hargous S: *Les appeleurs d'âmes: l'univers chamanique des Indiens des Andes*, Paris, 1985, Editions Albin Michel, pp 88, 248.

17. Etiemble: *L'Europe chinoise. I. De l'Empire Romain à Leibniz*, Paris, 1988, Editions Gallimard, p 127.

18. Lafitau JF: *Moeurs des sauvages Américains comparés aux moeurs des premiers temps*, Paris, 1983, F Maspéro, pp 127-128; Le Jeune P: *Relation de ce qui s'est passé en la Nouvelle France en l'année 1634*, vol 2, p 126; Fenton WN, Moore EL, editors: *Customs of primitive times by Father Joseph-Francois Lafitau*, 2 vols, Toronto, 1974, Champlain Society.

19. Lafitau JF: op cit, p 119; Thwaites RG, editor: *The Jesuits' relations and allied documents, 1610-1791,* New York, 1959, Pageant Book.

20. Cosmacini G: *Soigner et réformer*, op cit, pp 59, 106-108.

21. Gaucher-Peslherbe PL: *Chiropractic early concepts in their historical setting*, Lombard, 1993, National College of Chiropractic.

22. Pelt JM: L'ethnopharmacologie à l'aube du troisième milléaire. In Fleurantin J, editor: *Ethnopharmacologie: Sources, méthodes, objectifs,* Paris, 1991, Orstom/Societe Francaise d'Ethnopharmacoloqie, pp 20-25.

23. Kramer SH: *L'histoire commence à Sumer*, Paris, 1986, Editions Arthaud, pp 80-83.

24. Gaignault JC, Diers J: L'homme, la plante et le médicament. In *Ethnobotanique, pharmacopée et thérapeutes traditionnels*, ISERM/CHU, Necker, 1992.

25. Sturzenegger O: Les plantes dans la pharmacopée traditionnelle: de l'empirique au symbolique, *La Revue du Praticien* 93:65-67, 1993.

26. Peeters A in Retel-Laurentin A editor: *Une anthropologie médicale en France?* Paris, 1983, Editions du Centre National de la Recherche Scientifique, p 16.

27. Hargous S: *Les appeleurs d'âmes*, op cit, p 43; Reichel-Dolmatoff GA: Nivel de salud y medicina popular en una aldea mestiza de Columbia, *Rev Colomb Antrop* 7, 1958.

28. Erikson P: Qu'importe donc l'ivresse tant qu'on a le breuvage: fermentation, tempérance et rituel chez les Matis d'Amazonie brésilienne, *Cahiers de Sociologie Economique et Culturelle: Ethnopsychologie* 18:89-97, 1992.

29. Alt FNC: Body and soul in Quechua thought, *Journal of Latin American Lore* 179-196, 1982; Bernard C: *Les Incas: peuple du soleil*, Paris, 1990, Editions Gallimard.

30. Saignes T: Boire dans les Andes, *Cahiers de Sociologie Economique et Culturelle: Ethnopsychologie* 18:53-62, 1992. The author rightly points out that a discourse on alcohol is also a discourse on society and that it justifies ensuing modes of exclusion.

31. Diawara I: Les cultes de possession avec transes au Niger, *Cahiers de Sociologie Economique et Culturelle: Ethnopsychologie,* 9:67-80, 1988; Bhely-Quenum O: *L'initié*, Paris, 1979, Présence Africaine.

32. Louatron J: *Wakonga femme prestigieuse de Holom: une annee dans la vie d'une "possédée" Musey (au Tchad), Avril 1969-Avril 1970*, Paris, 1983, Ecole des Hautes Etudes en Sciences Sociales, pp 55-57.

33. Gaucher-Peslherbe PL: Réflexions sur l'emploi des thérapies manipulatives chez les Bananas du Tchad (rencontres audiovisuelles ethnographiques), *Troisième Congrès International des Médecines Traditionnelles*, 1991.

34. Zempleni A in Retel-Laurentin A, editor: *Une anthropologie medicale en France?* Paris, 1983, Editions du Centre National de la Recherche Scientifique, p 37; Castelain JP: L'ethnomédecine, ethnoscience et anthropologie de la maladie, *Cahiers de Sociologie Economique et Culturelle: Ethnopsychologie* 8:15-20, 1987.

35. Tall EK: L'anthropologue et le psychiâtre face aux médecines traditionnelles: récit d'une expérience, *Cahier des Sciences Humaines* 28(1):67-81, 1992; Sow I: *Les structures anthropologigues de la folie en Afrique Noire*, Paris, 1978, Editions Payot.

36. Rouch J. *La religion et la magie Songhay,* Paris, 1960, Presses Universitaires de France; Gibbal JM: *Guérisseurs et magiciens du Sahel,* Paris, 1984, Editions AM Montaillé.
37. Verger P: *Notes sur le culte des Orisha et Vodun,* Dakar, 1957, Institut Francais d'Afrique Noire. pp 51, 246-253. Maclean U: Magic and medicine: In Regush NM, editor: *Frontiers of healing: new dimensions in parapsychology,* New York, 1977, Avon, pp 89-100; Sindzingre N, Zempleni A: Anthropologie de la maladie, *Bulletin d'Ethnomédecine* 15:8, 1982; Verger P: *Orisha: les dieux Yorouba en Afrique et au Nouveau Monde,* Paris, 1982, Editions AM Montaillé.
38. Sioui GE: *Pour une autohistoire amérindienne: essai sur les fondements d'une morale sociale,* Quebec, 1989, Les Presses de l'Université Laval; Todorov T: *La conquête de l'Amérique: la question de l'autre,* Paris, 1982, Editions du Seuil.
39. Baudot G: Maladies et medecine en Amérique précolombienne. In Sendrail M: *Histoire culturelle de la maladie,* Toulouse, 1980, Editions Privat, pp 251-274; La Cruz M: *Libellus de medicinalibus Indorum herbis,* Mexico, 1964, Instituto Mexicano del Seguro Social.
40. Cline HF: *Guide to ethnohistorical studies.* In *Handbook of the Middle American Indians,* vols 12 to 15, Austin, Tex, 1972-1975, University of Texas Press; Coury C: *La médecine de l'Amérique précolombienne,* Paris, 1963, Editions Roger Dacosta.
41. Sahagun Fray B: *Histoire Générale des choses de la Nouvelle Espagne,* Paris, 1981, F Maspéro; Leon-Portilla M: *Aztec thought and culture: a study of the ancient Nahuatl mind,* Norman, Okla, 1963, University of Oklahoma Press.
42. Weiant CW: *Medicine and chiropractic,* Lombard, 1975, The National College of Chiropractic, p 69.
43. Le Breton D: *Anthropologie du corps et modernité,* Paris, 1990, Presses Universitaires de France, pp 16-18.
44. Leenhardt M: *Do kamo,* Paris, 1947, Editions Gallimard, pp 54-70.
45. Meyer F: *Gso-ba-rig-pa: le système médical tibétain,* Paris, 1988, Presses du Centre National de la Recherche Scientifique, pp 79-80.
46. Tibetan humoral theory entirely arises from ayurvedic medicine. *Sushruta Su,* 21, 35, 46; *Ni,* 1, 4; *Charaka Su,* 20; *Vi,* 8 as quoted by F. Meyer. Food is listed in the Tibetan treatises with the variety it has in India instead of the monotony it has in Tibet. However, "vulnerable spots" are not identical, a fact that emphasizes the originality of Tibetan tradition in anatomy.
47. *Sushruta Su,* 29; *Charaka In,* 1-2 as quoted, pp 151-152. An excellent English summary is provided on pp 211-213.
48. Despeux C: Histoire de la médecine chinoise. In *Encyclopédie des médecines naturelles: acupuncture et médecine traditionnelle Chinoise,* Paris, 1989, Editions Techniques; Granet M: *La pensée Chinoise,* Paris, 1968, Editions Albin Michel; Huard P, Bossy J: Souffrance et maladie dans le monde Chinois. In Sendrail M: *Histoire culturelle de la maladie,* op cit, 291-310; Veith I: *The yellow emperor's classic of internal medicine,* Berkeley, Calif, 1972, University of California Press, pp 117-118.
49. Guillaume G: Rhumatologie et médecine traditionnelle Chinoise. In *Encyclopédie des médecines naturelles: acupuncture et médecine traditionnelle Chinoise,* Paris, 1989, Editions Techniques; Faubert AM: *Traité didactique d'acupuncture traditionnelle Chinoise,* Paris, 1977, Editions Christian Trédaniel.
50. Guillaume G, Mach Chieu: *Rhumatologie et médecine traditionnelle Chinoise: acupuncture,* 2 vols, Paris, 1990, Editions de la Tisserande; Kespi JM: *L'acupuncture,* Moulin les Retz, 1982, Editions Maisonneuve.
51. Despeux C: Personal communication, Jan 19, 1992; Ng SY: A brief review of manipulation in Chinese history, *Bulletin of the European Chiropractors' Union* 28(2):24-29, 1980.
52. Maspero H: *Le taoisme et les religions chinoises,* Paris 1971, Editions Gallimard; Despeux C: *Zao-bichen: traité d'alchimie et de physiologie taoiste,* Paris, 1979, Editions Les Deux Océans; Schipper K: *Le corps taoiste,* Paris, 1982, Editions Fayard.
53. Etiemble: *L'Europe Chinoise,* op cit, 396-406; Moraze C: *Les origines sacrées des sciences modernes,* Paris, 1986, Editions Fayard; Mussat M: *Energétique des systèmes vivants,* Paris, 1982, Editions Medsi.
54. Palmer DD: Queer notions of the Chinese. In *Textbook of the science, art, and philosophy of chiropractic for students and practitioners: founded on tone (the chiropractor's adjustor),* Portland, Ore, 1910, Portland Printing House, p 858.
55. Hocart as quoted by Canteins J: *Le potier démiurge,* op cit; 100; Masson-Oursel P: *L'Inde antique et la civilisation indienne,* Paris, 1951, Editions Albin Michel, pp 44-47; Coomaraswamy AK: *Aspects de l'hindouisme,* Milano, Italy, 1988, Editions Arche.
56. Gaucher-Peslherbe PL: *Chiropractic: early concepts,* op cit, 76-82; Zimmer H: *Hindu medicine,* Baltimore, 1948, Johns Hopkins Press; Huard P, Bossy J, Mazars G: *Les médecines de l'Asie,* Paris, 1978, Editions du Seuil.
57. Anquetil-Duperron AH as quoted by Estradere J: *Du massage: son historique, ses manipulations, ses effets physiologiques et thérapeutiques,* Paris, 1863, Editions A Delahaye; Ming Wong, Huard P: *Soins et techniques du corps en Chine, au Japon et en Inde,* Paris, 1971, Editions Berg International.
58. Bhishagratna KKL: *The sushruta samhita,* Calcutta, 1907-1916; Bose JN, Kaviratna AC: *The charaka samhita,* Calcutta, 1896-1913; Charkravarti, Kaviratna as quoted by Lyons AS, Petrucelli RJ: *Medicine: an illustrated history,* New York, 1978, Harry N Abrams; Agarwal RS: *Secrets of Indian medicine,* Pondicherry, 1971, Sri Aurobindo Ashram.
59. Pugh J: The semantics of pain in Indian culture and medicine, *Culture, Medicine and Psychiatry* 15:4, 1991; Mazars G: Souffrance et maladie dans le monde Indien. In Sendrail M: *Histoire culturelle de la maladie,* op cit, 275-290.
60. Masson-Oursel P: *L'Inde antique,* op cit, 246; Reeves H et al: *La synchronicité, l'âme et la science,* La Varenne Saint Hilaire, 1990, Editions Seveyrat; Eliade M: *Briser le toît de la maison: la créativité et ses symboles,* Paris, 1986, Editions Gallimard.
61. Corbin H: *Alchimie comme art hiératique,* Paris, 1986, Editions de l'Herne; Lory P: *Alchimie et mystique en terre d'Islam,* Lagrasse, 1989, Editions Verdier; Halleux R: *Les textes alchimiques,* Turnhout, 1979, Brepols; Eliade M: *Forgerons et alchimistes,* Paris, 1977, Editions Flammarion.
62. Arnaldez R: La science arabe à travers l'oeuvre de Biruni. In *Lumières arabes sur l'Occident médiéval,* Paris, 1978 as quoted by Jacquart D, Micheau F: cf infra; Gardet L: Vues musulamanes sur le temps et l'histoire (essai de typologie culturelle). In Ricoeur P et al: *Les cultures et le temps,* Paris, 1975, Payot/Les Presses de l'Unesco, pp 223-255.
63. Lacoste Y: *Ibn Khaldoun: naissance de l'histoire, passé du Tiers-Monde,* Paris, 1966, F Maspéro; Ajerar H: Politique et prophétie: Islam et Occident, *Cahiers de Sociologie Economique et Culturelle: Ethnopsychologie* 17:79-91, 1992.
64. Jacquart D, Micheau F: *La médecine arabe et l'Occident médiéval,* Paris, 1990, Editions Maisonneuve et Larose.
65. Gaucher-Peslherbe PL: *A phenomemological approach to the pathogenesis of chiropractic lesions as aetiologically involved in vertebrogenous pain syndromes,* Bournemouth, England, 1972, Anglo-European College of Chiropractic; Bongioanni F, Illi C: Chiropractic rehabilitation after spinal surgery. In Gaucher-Peslherbe PL, editor: *Health and marginality,* op cit, 51-58.
66. Ligeros KA: *How ancient healing governs modern therapeutics: the contribution of hellenic science to modern medicine and scientific progress,* New York, 1937, GP Putnam, pp 420, 464-465. Niketas of Byzantium's *Surgical Collections* (ninth century AD) have been published by E.F.M. Bosquillion in the eighteenth century and by H. Schöne in 1896. The drawings are by Apollonius of Kitium (second century BC).

67. Gregory of Tours: *Liber historiarum*, IX, 6; Lançon B: *Maladies, malades et thérapeutes en Gaule à la fin de l'Antiquité*, Paris, 1991, Sorbonne; Gaucher-Peslherbe PL: La médecine a l'épreuve du reboutage: physiologie du rhabillage, *Cahiers de Sociologie Economique et Culturelle: Ethnopsychologie* 15:105-119, 1991; Rousselle A: *Croire et guérir: la foi en Gaule dans l'Antiquité tardive*, Paris, 1990, Editions Fayard.

68. Jacquart D, Micheau F: *La médecine arabe*, op cit, 96-107.

69. Cosmacini G: *Soigner et réformer*, op cit, 40-45; Jacquard D, Micheau F: op cit, 167-203.

70. Bennet G: History. In Howorth MB, Petrie JG, Bennet G: *Injuries of the spine*, Baltimore, 1964, Williams & Wilkins, pp 1-59. The use of a folded cloth never originated as a Dvorski's method or feature.

71. Delaunay P: *La médecine et l'église: contribution a l'histoire de l'exercice médical par les clercs*, Paris, 1948, Editions Hippocrate.

72. Vigarello G: *Le corps redressé: histoire d'un pouvoir pédagogique*, Paris, 1978, Editions Jean-Pierre Delarge; Maffesoli M: *Logique de la domination*, Paris, 1976, Presses Universitaires de France.

73. Bloch M: *Les rois thaumaturges: etude sur le caractère surnaturel attribué à la puissance royale particulièrement en France et en Angleterre*, Paris, 1983, Editions Gallimard, pp 382-383.

74. Sweet Waterman: *An essay on the science of bonesetting*, Providence, RI, 1833, Marshall & Hammond; Palmer DD: The natural bonesetters. In *Textbook of the Science, Art*, op cit, pp 543-549.

75. Sammarthanus S: *Gallorum doctrina illustrium*, 1598 (Translated by Colletet as Scevole [ou Gaucher] de Sainte Marthe: *Eloge des hommes illustres*, Paris, 1644, 55ff as quoted by Bloch M: op cit, 382).

76. Dupront A: *Du sacré: croisades et pélerinages, images et langages*, Paris, 1987, Editions Gallimard, pp 419-466; Loux F: *Pratiques et savoirs populaires: le corps dans la société traditionnelle*, Paris, 1979, Editions Berger-Levrault, pp 146-154.

77. Georgii A: *Kinetic jottings: miscellaneous extracts from medical literature, ancient and modern, illustrating the effects of mechanical agencies in the treatment of diseases*, London, 1880, H Renshaw; Estradere J: *Du massage: son historique, ses manipulations, ses effets physiologiques et thérapeutiques*, Paris, 1863, A Delahaye; Vigarello G: *Le corps redressé*, op cit, 63-69.

78. Bonnet A: *Traité des maladies et articulations*, 2 vols, Lyon, 1845, Ch Savy Jeune; Cooper AP: *A treatise on dislocations and on fractures of the joints*, London, 1823, The Author; Malgaigne JF: *Traité des fractures et des luxations*, 2 vols, Paris, 1847 and 1855, JB Baillière.

79. Pott P: *Remarks on that kind of palsy of the lower limb which is frequently found to accompany a curvature of the spine and is supposed to be caused by it: together with its method of cure, to which are added observations on the necessity and propriety of amputation in certain cases and under certain circumstances*, London, 1779, J Johnson.

80. Veith I: *Histoire de l'hystérie*, Paris, 1973, Editions Seghers; Deslandes L: *De l'onanisme et autres abus vénériens*, Paris, 1835; Zambaco D: *Onanisme avec troubles nerveux chez deux petites filles*, Paris, 1882; Bonnet A: *Traité des maladies*, op cit, 522.

81. Tissot JC: *Gymnastique médicinale et chirurgicale: ou essai sur l'utilité du mouvement, ou des différents exercices du corps, et du repos dans la cure des maladies*, Paris, 1780, Chez Bastien, pp 318-319.

82. Anderson RT: On doctors and bonesetters in the 16th and 17th centuries, *Chiropractic History* 3:13-14, 1983.

83. Case brought by the municipal magistrates of the City of Blois against master-surgeons who were suing a bonesetter, Pierre Regnard, who would call himself a "restorer of the bones in the human body" (18 July 1619), *Archives du Département de Loir et Cher*, France.

84. Bedel C, Huard P: *Médecine et pharmacie au XVIII siècle*, Paris, 1986, Editions Hermann.

85. Ackerknecht EH: *La médecine hospitalière à Paris (1794-1848)*, Paris, 1986, Editions Payot.

86. Foucault M: *La naissance de la clinique: une archéologie du regard médical*, Paris, 1975, Presses Universitaires de France; Peter JP: L'histoire par les oreilles: notes sur l'assertion et le fait dans la médecine des Lumières, *Le Temps de la Réflexion* 1:273-314, 1980; Leonard J: *La médecine entre les savoirs*, op cit.

87. Chapiseau F: *Le folklore de la Beauce et du Perche*, 2 vols, Vendôme, 1983, Editions du Cherche-Lune, pp 160-162; Lewis B: *Physiologie du Bourbonnais*, Moulins, 1842, PA Desrosiers, p 151.

88. Anderson RT: Hawaiian therapeutic massage, *Worldwide Report* (1982) 24, 5:4A, 1982; Schiötz E: The history of manipulation. In *Manipulation, past and present*, London, 1975, William Heinemann, pp 5-27.

89. Schiötz E: op cit, 17.

90. Lomax E: Manipulative therapy: a historical perspective. In Buerger A, Tobis JS, editors: *Approaches to the validation of manipulative therapy*, Springfield, Ill, 1977, Charles C Thomas, pp 205-216; Harrison E: *Pathological and practical observations on spinal diseases, illustrated with cases and engravings: also an enquiry into the origin and cure of distorted limbs*, London, 1827, T & G Underwood.

91. Riadore JE: *Treatise on irritation of spinal nerves as the source of nervousness, indigestion, functional and organical derangements of the principle organs of the body, and on the modifying influence of temperament and habits of man over disease, and their importance as regards conducting successfully the treatment of the latter and on the therapeutic use of water*, London, 1842, J Churchill; Canguilhem G: *La formation du concept de réflexe au XVII et XVIII siècles*, Paris, 1977, Librairie Philosophique J Vrin; Temkin O: The classical roots of Glisson's doctrine of irritation, *Bull Hist Med* 4:38, 1964; Schiller F: Spinal irritation and osteopathy, *Bull Hist Med.* 45:250, 1971; Pflüger E: *Die Sensorischen Functionen des Ruckenmarks der Wierbeltiere nebst einer neuen Lehre über die Leitungsgesetze der reflexionen*, Berlin, 1853, as quoted by Canguilhem G: *Etudes d'histoire et de philosophie des sciences*, Paris, 1975, Librarie Philosophique J Vrin, p 301.

92. Riadore JE: op cit, 84-85.

93. Pott P: *Some few general remarks on fractures and dislocations*, London, 1769, L Hawes; Dods A: *Patholocial observations on the rotated or contorted spine, commonly called lateral curvature: deduced from practice*, London, 1824, T Caddel; Shaw J: *On the nature and treatment of the distortions to which the spine and the bones of the chest are subject: with an enquiry into the merits of several modes of practice which have hitherto been followed in the treatment of distortion*, London, 1823-1824, Longman; Serny JB: *Spinal curvature, its consequence and its cure: illustrated by the history of thirty-three cases successfully treated*, London, 1840, Sherwood.

94. Gaucher-Peslherbe PL: Chiropractic, an illegitimate child of science? I. De nervorum descriptio. II. De opprobria medicorum, *Europ J Chiropractic* 34(1):40-45; 34(2):98-106, 1986.

95. Palmer DD: *The chiropractor's adjustor*, op cit; Palmer DD: *The chiropractor*, Los Angeles, 1914, Beacon Light Printing; Gaucher-Peslherbe PL: Defining the debate: exploration of the factors that influenced chiropractic's founder, *Chiropractic History* 8(1): 14-18, 1988.

96. Hilton J: *On rest and pain: a course of lectures on the influence of mechanical and physiologial rest in the treatment of accidents and surgical diseases, and the diagnostic value of pain*, New York, 1879, William Wood; Breig A: *Adverse mechanical tension in the C.N.S.*, New York, 1970, Wiley; Clarke E, Jacyna LS: *Nineteenth century origins of neuroscientific concepts*, Berkeley, Calif, 1987, University of California Press; Gauchet M: *L'inconscient cérébral*, Paris, 1992, Editions du Seuil.

97. Anderson RT: Bonesetting: a medical bone of contention, *ACAJ* 18(10):91-100, 1981.

98. Wardwell WI: *Chiropractic: history and evolution of a new profession*, St Louis, 1992, Mosby, p 24.

99. Illi FW: *La vérité sur la chiropractique,* Bern, 1938, Association des Chiropraticiens Suisses; Weiant CW et al: *The case for chiropractic in the literature of medicine,* New York, 1945, The New York State Chiropractic Society; Verner JR: *The science and logic of chiropractic,* Englewood, 1950, The Author; Schwartz HS, editor: *Mental health and chiropractic: a multidisciplinary approach,* New York, 1973, Sessions Publishers; Wilks CA: *Chiropractic speaks out: a reply to medical propaganda, bigotry and ignorance,* Park Ridge, 1973, Wilks Publishing; Dintenfass J: *Chiropractic: a modern way to health,* New York, 1975, Pyramid Books; Janse J: *Principles and practice of chiropractic: an anthology,* Lombard, 1976, National College of Chiropractic; Gibbons RW: The evolution of chiropractic: medical and social protest in America: notes on the survival years and after. In Haldeman S, editor: *Modern developments in the principles and practice of chiropractic,* New York, 1980, Appleton Century Crofts, pp 3-24; Wardwell WI: *Chiropractic: history and evolution of a new profession,* St Louis, 1992, Mosby.

100. Dumezil G: La médecine et les trois fonctions, *Magazine Littéaire* p 229, 1986.

101. Vivier M: Le jardin, garde-manger et pharmacie, *Cahiers de Sociologie Economique et Culturelle: Ethnopsychologie* 8:57-82, 1987

102. Dupront A: *Du sacré,* op cit, 420-422; Bouteiller M: *Médecine populaire d'hier et d'aujourd'hui,* Paris, 1966, Maisonneuve et Larose.

103. Caplan RL: Chiropractic. In Salmon JW, editor: *Alternative medicines: popular and policy perspectives,* New York, 1984, Tavistock, pp 80-113.

104. Azouvi F: Introduction. In de Villers C: *Le magnétiseur amoureux,* Paris, 1978, Librairie Philosophique J Vrin; Miller G: Le secret de Mesmer, *Ornicar* 5:46-59, 1977; Amadou R, editor: *F.-A. Mesmer: le magnétisme animal,* Paris, 1971, Editions Payot; Darnton R: *La fin des lumieres: le mesmérisme et la révolution,* Paris, 1984, Librairie Academique Perrin; Peter JP: Un intermédiaire mal perçu: Franz Anton Mesmer (1734-1815)—médecin trop guérisseur, guérisseur trop médecin, *Actes du Colloque du Centre Mérigional d'Histoire Sociale, des Mentalités et des Cultures* pp 141-153, 1978.

105. Jussieu AL: *Rapport de l'un des Commissaires chargés par le Roi de l'examen du magnétisme animal,* Paris, 1784, Veuve Hérissan; Chertok L, Stenger I: Ecouter Jussieu? In *Le coeur et la raison: l'hypnose en question, de Lavoisier à Lacan,* Paris, 1989, Editions Payot, pp 31-37.

106. Rothstein WG: *American physicians in the 19th century: from sects to science,* Baltimore, 1972, Johns Hopkins University Press.

107. Duplay S, Reclus P: *Traité de chirurgie,* vol 3, Paris, 1891, Editions G Masson, pp 695-698; Powles J: On the limitations of modern medicine, *Sci Med Man* 1(1):1-30, 1973.

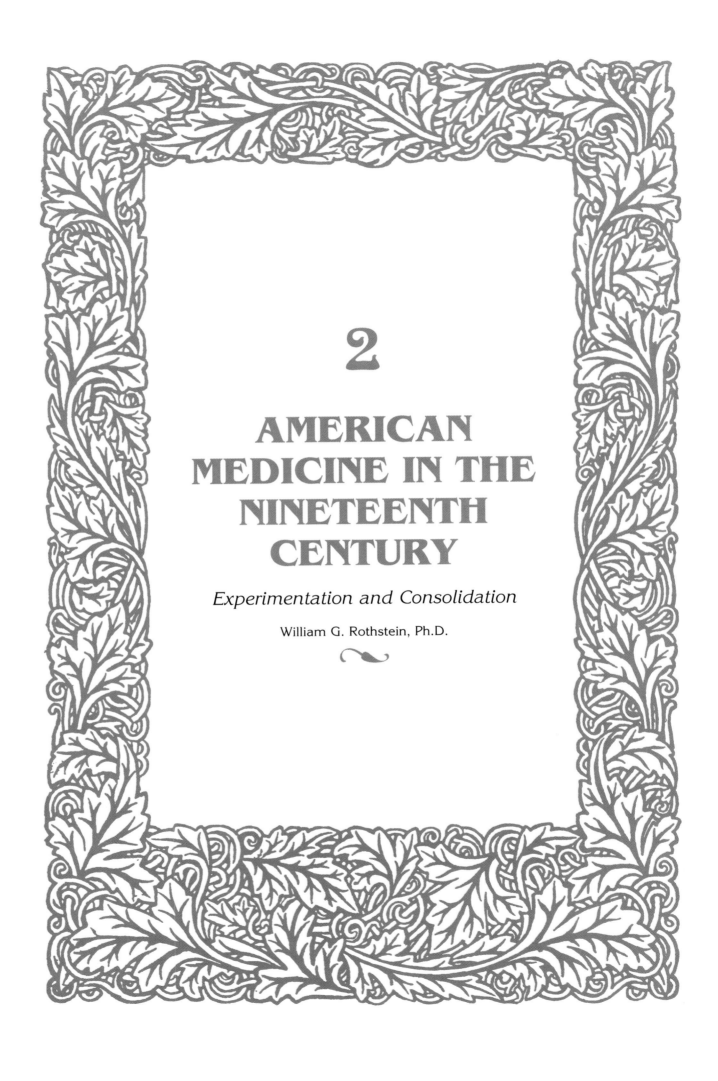

2

AMERICAN MEDICINE IN THE NINETEENTH CENTURY

Experimentation and Consolidation

William G. Rothstein, Ph.D.

Throughout most of the nineteenth century, medicine could do little to prevent illness or restore the health of the sick. At the beginning of the century, many different kinds of treatments existed, with no one system assuming a dominant role. As towns and cities grew, the number of physicians increased and more medical care was provided. Physicians adopted a set of distinctive treatments known as "heroic therapy" that aroused public opposition and persuaded many patients to turn to botanical medicine, homeopathy, and other alternatives. After the midcentury, medical care became institutionalized with the growth of hospitals and dispensaries and the professionalization of the major groups of physicians. In the last two decades of the century, bacteriology provided a scientific basis for the diagnosis, etiology, and prevention of infectious diseases and, together with anesthesia, permitted the expansion of surgery. These developments led the major groups of physicians to unite around an approach to medical care based on the biological sciences. This new approach was not successful in treating all types of illnesses, and some patients turned to other forms of treatment, including chiropractic.

THE STATE OF MEDICAL CARE IN 1800

By 1800, North America had been settled continuously for almost two centuries. During that time, three major traditions of medical care had come into widespread use—European folk medicine, native American Indian medicine, and European professional medicine. Each was associated with specific types of healers and methods of self-treatment.

European folk medicine was the dominant form of medical care used in the colonies, especially in the self-medication that has characterized the first line of treatment of the sick in all ages. The colonists brought with them many botanicals used to make folk medicines in England, including such well-known plants as dandelion, mustard, horseradish, sarsaparilla, and mints. The plants were grown in family gardens, harvested, and prepared in a variety of ways, such as by brewing the leaves to make teas; boiling roots or leaves in water, wine, or brandy to make a syrup; and cooking roots or leaves with fats or oils to make ointments. Recipes were handed down and printed in books and almanacs.

Folk medicine was practiced by several types of healers. Many lay healers, often called "root and herb" or "botanical" doctors, limited their treatments to botanical medicines. Most lay healers were untrained, but some had studied with other healers. Nursing of the sick was performed

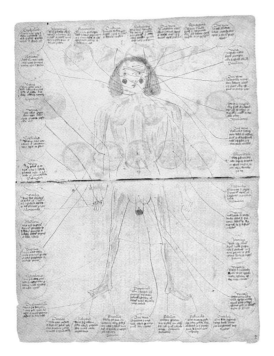

A fifteenth century anatomically realistic chart showing points for bloodletting, a common practice in the colonies.
Courtesy Biblioteca Apostolica Vaticana, Rome.

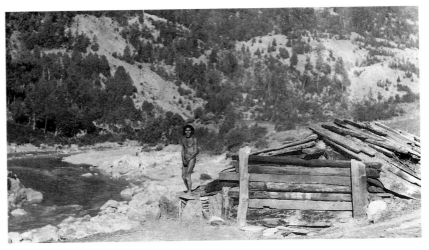

A member of the Karok tribe in Oregon or California leaving a sweat lodge, where men from the tribe gathered for heat treatment thought to maintain health and cure illness.
Courtesy National Anthropological Archives, Smithsonian Institution, Washington, DC.

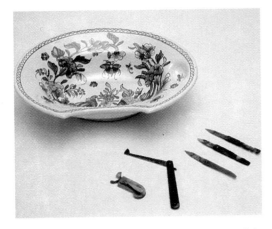

Bowls and lancets like these were used in bloodletting.
Courtesy Pearson Museum, School of Medicine, Southern Illinois University, Springfield, Illinois.

by women who relied on folk practices. Babies were delivered by midwives who used folk practices.

The second tradition was native American Indian medicine. The Indians had developed their own system of medical care, which included a variety of botanical drugs and other treatments, such as steam baths in specially designed huts where water was poured over heated rocks, a custom that also existed in northern Europe. Many colonists believed that the Indians had developed treatments that were especially useful for the illnesses of North America and accepted Indian medicine as a valid form of medical care. Although few Indians practiced medicine among the colonists, some lay healers claimed that they had learned their methods of healing from the Indians and called themselves "Indian doctors."

The third tradition was English professional medicine based on the classic medical theories as they evolved from Hippocrates and Galen to Sydenham, Boerhaave, and others. This tradition had little direct impact on the colonists. Few English physicians emigrated to the colonies, and only a small number of Americans went to England or other European countries to study medicine. These physicians not only played a minor role as providers of medical care, but they trained few American physicians through the apprenticeship system. Colonial physicians were rarely able to earn a livelihood by practicing medicine, and many of them engaged in other occupations, such as farming or business. Clergymen often had some knowledge of European medicine and practiced medicine in addition to their clerical responsibilities.

Physicians spent their days visiting the homes of the sick, seeing a few patients in their own homes, and preparing drugs for patients. Drug preparation was especially important because few pharmacies existed in colonial America. Patients purchased drugs from physicians in the same way that people patronize pharmacies today.

The influence of the classic European medical tradition extended beyond the activities of physicians. Some lay healers acquired a limited knowledge of European medicine and incorporated it in their practices. For example, bloodletting was practiced by "bleeders" and others in the colonies. European folk medicine also absorbed many elements of the classic medical tradition.

Classic European medicine had its greatest impact in books written by English physicians to advise lay persons on medical care and self-treatment, including methods of preparing botanical medicines. Some of these books were reprinted in America, frequently with supplements by American physicians describing American diseases and American botanical drugs.

The usefulness of each of these traditions can be understood only in the context of the illnesses and treatments of the time. The major causes of sickness and death throughout the colonial period and until the end of the nineteenth century were infectious diseases such as pneumonia, influenza, tuberculosis, smallpox, and yellow fever. Many infants died from "cholera infantum," a general name for gastrointestinal diseases such as diarrhea and dysentery caused by ingesting spoiled milk and other foods contaminated with excessive bacteria.

Physicians of the time had no knowledge of the role of bacteria in causing disease and therefore knew nothing about the significance of personal contact, insect vectors, or other means by which infectious diseases spread. Many diseases that are known to be contagious today, such as tuberculosis, were not thought to be so by physicians of the time. Personal habits to prevent the spread of disease that are taken for granted, such as not sharing a drinking cup or a spoon with others, were unknown.

Physicians had no treatments that cured diseases. The prevailing approach to treatment in both folk and professional medicine was based on the belief that diseases consisted of the sum of their symptoms. Because physicians did not have modern diagnostic instruments, symptoms were defined very crudely. For example, thermometers were not used to measure body temperature, so that fevers were defined subjectively, such as a feeling of feverishness by the patient. Conditions with similar symptoms were considered to be the same disease, so all fevers were considered subclasses of a disease called "fever."

Using the logic that removing the symptoms cured the disease, physicians designed treatments to have a direct impact on the symptoms. Unfortunately, few of them had a beneficial effect on the patient. The most common drugs were harsh purgatives and emetics that were designed to clean out the patient's system. If the patient had a fever, the physician might employ bloodletting, which reduced fever, although with harmful side effects. Patients recovering from illnesses would be given tonics, an ill-defined class of drugs designed to improve the appetite or strength. The major tonics in the colonial period were teas from local herbs and berries and alcoholic beverages. Other medications included salves and astringents for wounds, drugs to promote perspiration, and mints and rhubarb for indigestion. Few of these drugs are currently used, and most did more harm than good.

The major drugs of the period considered to be of value today were cinchona (or Peruvian) bark and opium, from which quinine and morphine were isolated in the early nineteenth century, respectively. Cinchona, an effective treatment for the symptoms of malaria, and opium, an analgesic, were (like all botanicals) administered in their crude state. Cinchona was prepared by grinding the bark of the cinchona tree and mixing it with water or wine, which the patient then drank. The bark contained only a small amount of the active ingredient, and its bitter taste often induced vomiting, which negated its value. As a result, even these drugs were of limited benefit before their active ingredients were isolated.

The other major medical procedures were obstetric deliveries, which were usually performed by midwives, and surgical procedures. Because no anesthetics had been discovered to alleviate pain during operations

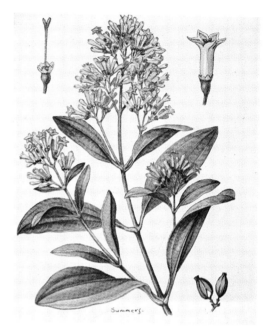

The cinchona plant—the source of the bark powder that for centuries was known as a miracle cure for malaria.

From Krug E: *An introduction to materia medica and pharmacology.*

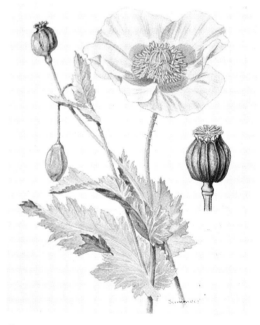

Opium poppy. Opium, from which morphine is derived today, was one of the major drugs used during the Colonial period.

From Krug E: *An introduction to materia medica and pharmacology.*

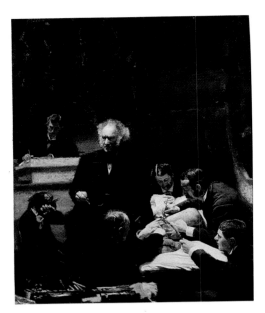

The Gross Clinic *by American painter Thomas Eakins. In this oil portrait the noted American surgeon Samuel Gross is demonstrating a surgical procedure. Notice his assistants are not wearing gowns, nor is the family member who is sitting nearby.*
Courtesy Jefferson Medical College of Thomas Jefferson University, Philadelphia.

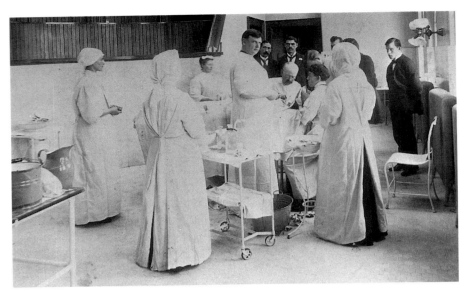

Dr. John Fulton and Dr. Charles Wheaton in the St. Joseph's Hospital operating room of St. Paul, Minnesota, circa 1890. Note the use of gowns, caps, and gloves.
Courtesy Minnesota Historical Society, St. Paul, Minnesota.

and because the causes and methods of preventing postoperative infections were unknown, operative surgery was undertaken only as a last resort. The most common surgical procedures were lancing boils, setting fractures, reducing dislocations, extracting teeth, sewing up wounds, and amputating limbs. Any operation on the cranium, thorax, or abdomen was invariably fatal, so few were performed. Major amputations and other dangerous surgical procedures were shunned by most physicians and were performed in the eighteenth and early nineteenth centuries by a small number of master surgeons who traveled regularly throughout a region of the country amputating limbs, removing some kinds of tumors, and operating for cataract. Some master surgeons performed thousands of operations during their careers.

The greatest medical development of the period was vaccination with cowpox to prevent smallpox, a procedure that was first tested scientifically in the late 1790s by Edward Jenner, an English physician. Because smallpox was a widespread and deadly disease, vaccination rapidly became widely used and was the first great contribution of medicine to public health. Vaccination was performed by both physicians and lay persons.

CHANGES IN MEDICAL CARE IN THE EARLY NINETEENTH CENTURY

The growth of cities and towns in the eighteenth century weakened the rural traditions that sustained folk medicine and provided opportunities for full-time careers for physicians.

As people moved from rural areas to towns and cities, they adopted new customs and gave up traditional ones like folk medicines. Urban residents had less opportunity than those in rural areas to grow, gather, and prepare their own botanical medicines. Their higher incomes enabled

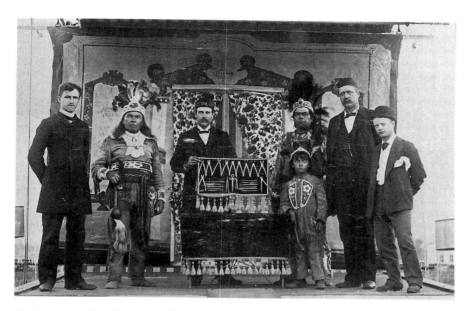

Kickapoo Indian Medicine Show, an 1890 photograph taken in Marine, Minnesota. The public was often taken in by the claims and cures promised by the traveling medicine shows and preferred the taste of their tonics to the often bitter tasting botanical remedies.
Courtesy Minnesota Historical Society, St. Paul, Minnesota.

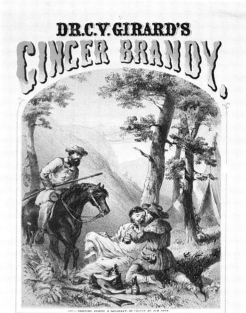

A colorful nineteenth century advertisement for a patent medicine from a period without government regulation of ingredients or verification of claims.
Courtesy Library of Congress, Washington, DC.

them to purchase manufactured drugs, which led to the rise of the patent medicine industry. Each patent medicine claimed to have a distinctive set of ingredients, which were seldom revealed or printed on the label. The manufacturers advertised widely, especially in the newly popular newspapers, and often claimed that the undisclosed ingredients in their products had unique powers to cure or relieve illnesses. Some patent medicines were as good as drugs prepared by physicians and most were more palatable because they contained sweeteners or used a sugar coat-

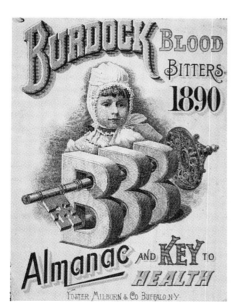

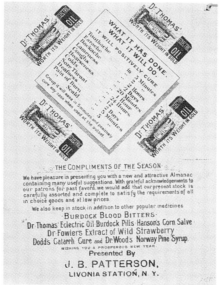

Burdock's Almanac. *An example of a proprietary medicine-maker's advertising almanac. Note the promises to cure almost every disease within a matter of days.*
Courtesy Palmer College of Chiropractic Archives, Davenport, Iowa.

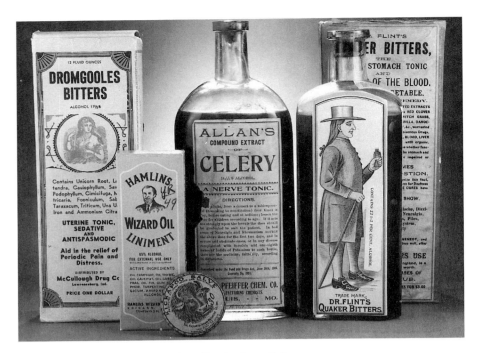

A sampler of patent medicines.
Courtesy Smithsonian Institute, Washington, DC.

ing on the pills. Many contained dangerous drugs that were not revealed on the label, like morphine, or made fraudulent claims, such as the ability to cure cancer or tuberculosis.

Patent medicines became popular in cities and towns, often at the expense of folk healers, whose drugs were bitter and often nauseating. Patent medicines also made the public more receptive to the idea of medical care as a commercial or professional activity.

Urbanization also strengthened the medical profession, which had a high status in the colonial era. Local governments employed physicians to care for the sick poor and asked their advice on public health matters. Some colonial physicians were political leaders, and a few became nationally prominent. As the urban population and urban wealth increased at the turn of the nineteenth century, more physicians were able to earn their livelihood practicing medicine. This encouraged many young men to train for medicine as a career.

Medical Education in North America

Until the end of the eighteenth century, formal medical education in America consisted of 3 years of apprenticeship training with a physician, who was called a *preceptor*. Any physician could serve as a preceptor, and any student who could find a preceptor could undertake an apprenticeship. The student read the preceptor's few books, ground and prepared drugs, served as a nurse and aide, and traveled with the preceptor on visits to patients. After completing the apprenticeship, the student received a certificate from the preceptor and opened a practice or became a junior partner of some physician.

The apprenticeship system was formalized by the local medical societies. As the number of physicians in a community increased, they organized medical societies with two major functions. One was to establish

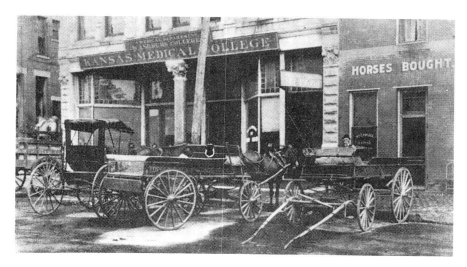

Kansas Medical College of Topeka, one of many unregulated proprietary schools that sprang up all over the United States.
Courtesy Kansas State Historical Society, Topeka, Kansas.

"boards of censors" to examine and award certificates or licenses to students who completed apprenticeships. In this respect they acted as formal licensing agencies in those states where the boards were given licensing authority by the state governments and as informal agencies elsewhere. (There were no significant penalties for practicing without a license.) Their other major function was to admit to membership only those physicians whom the members considered qualified practitioners. In an era without meaningful licensing laws, membership in a medical society was evidence to the public of a physician's competence and distinguished those physicians from other practitioners in the community.

The major drawback of apprenticeship training was the limited theoretical knowledge of most preceptors. The average preceptor knew little about anatomy or theories of disease and was ignorant of the latest medi-

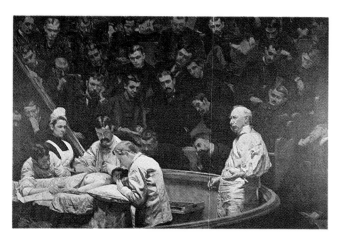

The Agnew Clinic, an 1889 painting by Thomas Eakins. Note how the surgeon and assistants are gowned. It illustrates the progress antiseptic surgery had made in the 14 years since Eakins depicted the Gross Clinic.
Courtesy University of Pennsylvania, School of Medicine, Philadelphia.

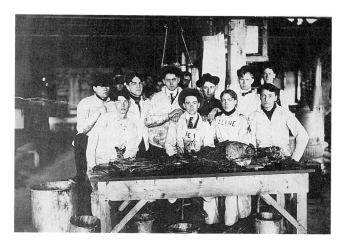

Photograph circa 1900 of a dissection class at the University of Iowa, School of Medicine.
Courtesy University of Iowa Archives, Iowa City, Iowa.

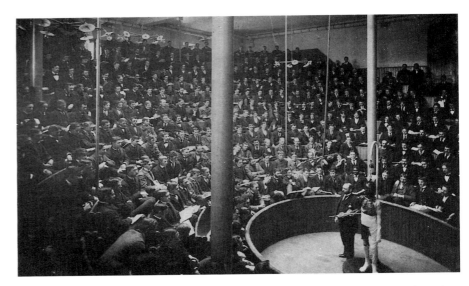

Before operations on live patients became a standard part of medical education, cadavers were used. Here, a professor of anatomy gives a demonstration in the "bull pit."
Courtesy Edward G. Miner Library, University of Rochester, Rochester, New York.

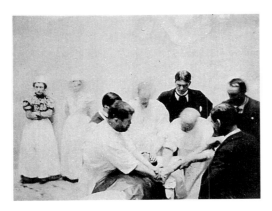

Photograph circa 1900 of a surgery at the Univerity of Iowa School of Medicine. Note that the assistants are neither gowned nor gloved for their procedures.
Courtesy University of Iowa Archives, Iowa City, Iowa.

cal knowledge. One reason for the slow diffusion of medical knowledge among physicians was the small number of medical journals.

To deal with the poor scientific and theoretical training of most preceptors, leading physicians established medical schools in the largest cities beginning late in the eighteenth century. The medical schools, which were owned by the physicians who taught in them, had two major requirements for the M.D. degree. One was attendance at two terms of medical school lectures to learn the theoretical side of medicine. The other was a 3-year apprenticeship with a physician of the student's choice to learn the practical side.

Medical schools revolutionized medical education. For the first time, many students had the opportunity to study with the nation's leading physicians. A degree from a medical school was highly prestigious, enabling the new graduates to gain the confidence of their patients. Medical schools were inexpensive to operate. The classes consisted entirely of lectures (with the exception of a course in dissection) and required only a lecture hall. The physicians who taught in the medical schools used their faculty appointments to enhance their professional reputations and were not overly concerned with the profits of the medical school. For all these reasons, the 4 medical schools in operation in 1800 increased to 42 in 1850, and the number of graduates rose from 343 in the years from 1800 to 1809 to over 17,000 between 1850 and 1859. Perhaps as many students attended a year of medical school lectures but did not graduate.

One consequence of the increased number of physicians was that professional medical care became available for the poor as well as those who could afford to pay. Hospitals, which had been built in a few cities as charities for the poor, appointed physicians to treat their patients. Dispensaries employed physicians, usually recent graduates of medical schools who wanted practical experience, to provide medical care and drugs to the needy who came to the dispensary office. Dispensary physicians also visited patients in their homes to deliver babies and care for the bedridden sick. Because dispensaries were much cheaper to operate and more popular with patients, many of them were opened by governments or private charities. Few hospitals were built before the Civil War.

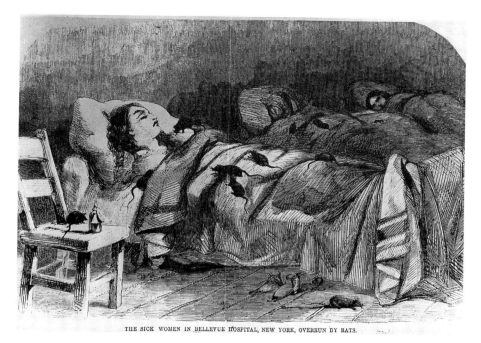

THE SICK WOMEN IN BELLEVUE HOSPITAL, NEW YORK, OVERRUN BY RATS.

Bellevue Hospital: Sick Women in Ward, Overrun by Rats. *An 1860 engraving from* Harper's Weekly *portraying the substandard conditions patients confronted.*
Courtesy Museum of the City of New York, New York.

Heroic Therapy

Medical schools, textbooks, societies, and journals had another significant impact on the profession: they standardized medical practice in the first decades of the nineteenth century. Before that time, apprentices learned the idiosyncratic practices of their preceptors and had little subsequent contact with other physicians to influence them to change their approaches. Now, thousands of medical students studied the same textbooks and listened to lectures from the same physicians. They read the same medical journals and discussed their cases with other physicians in medical society meetings. The effect was to standardize medical care among physicians.

This new standardized system of therapeutics was called "heroic therapy." Heroic therapy was characterized by the unremitting use of bloodletting, purgatives, emetics, blistering (the pus emitted when the blister was broken was considered beneficial), and other drastic treatments. Almost all patients were given harsh purgatives and emetics by the spoonful, patients with fevers and other conditions were frequently bled until they fainted, and few patients were allowed to escape the clutches of the physician unharmed. The drug that became the hallmark of heroic therapy was calomel, a salt of mercury that acted as a strong purgative. The continued use of calomel produced mercurial poisoning, which was characterized by excessive salivation, swelling of the gums, ulceration of the mouth, loss of teeth, and even worse consequences. Several other poisons, including antimony (used as an emetic) and arsenic (used as a tonic), were also part of the materia medica of the time.

The rationale behind heroic therapy was that infectious diseases, with a few exceptions such as tuberculosis, have a rapid onset and reach their critical stage within a matter of hours or days. The outbreaks were even more terrifying in the epidemics of yellow fever, cholera, and other diseases that killed many thousands of Americans during the first half of the nineteenth century. Physicians reasoned that it was essential to use medicines with a rapid effect on the patient if death were to be avoided. Most physicians of the time had little faith in the healing powers of nature and believed that drugging and bleeding were essential to save lives. Indeed, therapeutic activism was the hallmark of heroic therapy.

THE REBELLION AGAINST HEROIC THERAPY

Patients soon realized that heroic therapy effected no cures, produced an excessive number of deaths, and tormented them with the long-term effects of poisons on their gastrointestinal systems and other organs. The result was a populist rebellion against the medical profession that brought forth a new generation of practitioners who denounced regular physicians and presented themselves as providers of safer forms of treatment.

The major alternative to regular medicine was botanical medicine, which continued to be popular among patients, particularly in rural areas, who could not afford to employ physicians. Many botanical practitioners advertised their medicines as containing "no calomel" to attract patients who refused heroic therapy.

Thomsonism

The most successful botanical practitioner opposing heroic therapy was Samuel Thomson (1769-1843), an itinerant healer who developed a botanical system of treatment. His major treatments were lobelia, an herb that acted as a powerful emetic, steam baths, cayenne pepper dissolved in hot water to warm the patient, teas using botanical drugs, and tonics combining botanicals with wine or brandy. Thomson's medicines were administered in a specific order or "course" of treatments designed to clean out, warm, and finally strengthen the patient. Thomson wrote a book, *New Guide to Health,* that described his treatments, provided detailed methods of obtaining and preparing good quality drugs, and contained advice on healthy living. He also established a system of Friendly Societies, groups of lay Thomsonians who met regularly and assisted each other in times of illness. Thomson employed a number of salesmen throughout the country to sell his books and drugs.

"Thomsonism," as the system was called, became a huge success throughout rural and frontier America in the 1830s. The drugs were inexpensive and, if used in moderation, gentler than heroic therapy. Thomsonism soon extended beyond a system of medical care to become a social movement that held national conventions in the 1830s and undertook a program of political activism to reduce the power of the regular profession. The popularity of Thomsonism also produced a number of professional Thomsonian healers who assumed leadership of the movement. Thomson, who advocated self-help, strongly opposed efforts to professionalize his movement.

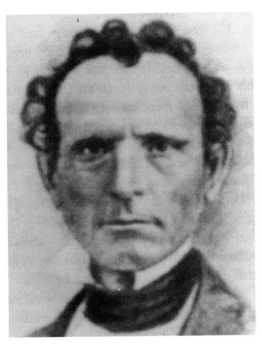

Sylvester Graham (1794-1851), originator of the Graham cracker, was a proponent of natural healing.

Courtesy National Library of Medicine, Bethesda, Maryland.

The Homeopathic Movement

Albeit the most popular, Thomsonism was only one of a number of health movements that arose in reaction to heroic therapy. Most of the others appealed to the urban working and middle classes and purported that nature was beneficent and that disease was caused by disregarding natural laws. They stressed pure foods, personal hygiene, and abstinence from stimulants such as alcohol, tea, coffee, tobacco, and sometimes meat. The most important health movements were Grahamism, founded by Sylvester Graham (after whom the Graham cracker is named) and William Andrus Alcott, and hydropathy, which originated in Europe and advocated water cures using baths, wet sheets, and douches. Hydropathy was sufficiently popular that over 200 water cure establishments were opened during the nineteenth century. Even patent medicines appealed to the critics of heroic therapy by placing "no calomel" on their labels, although the drugs used instead were often equally harmful.

Eventually the desire for reform reached the medical profession itself and led some regular physicians to turn to homeopathy, a system of medicine devised by Samuel Hahnemann (1755-1843). As a young physician in Germany, Hahnemann became a critic of regular medicine and its use of cathartics, bloodletting, and polypharmacy (combining different drugs in the same prescription). To test the effects of individual medicines, Hahnemann took cinchona bark for several days to ascertain its effect on a healthy person. He found that it made him feverish and flushed and gave him other symptoms such as those of patients with malaria. He concluded that cinchona bark, which all physicians believed was a cure for malaria (it actually only relieves the symptoms), had given him, a healthy person, the symptoms of malaria and therefore malaria.

Hahnemann's experience led him to formulate the basic law of homeopathy: drugs that produce certain symptoms in healthy people will cure those same symptoms in the sick. He then discovered that minuscule doses of homeopathic drugs were more effective than large doses. This led to his second principle: homeopathic drugs should be administered in infinitesimal doses. Hahnemann also advocated fresh air, bed rest, proper diet, sunshine, and public hygiene at a time when many physicians denied their value. Homeopathy was remarkably successful in treating patients. Regular physicians claimed that homeopathic doses had no

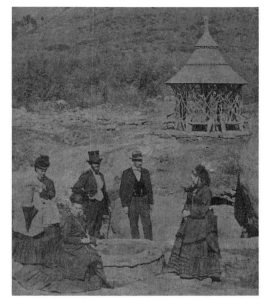

Visitors "taking the waters" during the late 1900s at Navajo Soda Springs, Manitou Springs, Colorado.

Courtesy Denver Public Library, Western History Department, Denver.

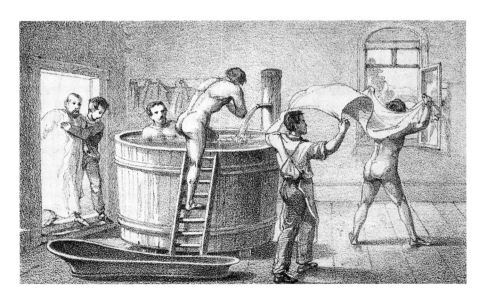

Curative baths, one form of hydrotherapy, was a popular form of natural healing in the late nineteenth century.

Courtesy Wellcome Institute Library, London.

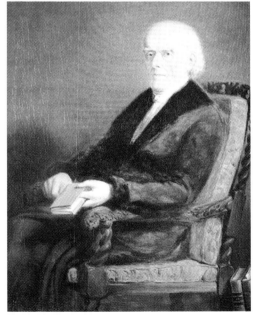

Dr. Samuel Hahnemann (1755-1843) founded homeopathy on the premise that drugs producing certain symptoms in healthy people will cure those same symptoms in the sick.

From Richardson S: *Homeopathy, the illustrated guide.*

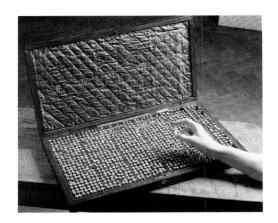

Samuel Hahnemann's remedy box. Many homeopaths kept their remedies in a similar box, but few had one that was so splendid.
From Richardson S: *Homeopathy, the illustrated guide.*

conceivable physiological effect on the patient and that homeopathy's success was actually due to the healing powers of nature. The more perspicacious observers realized Hahnemann demonstrated that the healing powers of nature were far superior to the regular treatments of the time, especially heroic therapy.

Homeopathy became popular among the European aristocracy in the 1830s and was soon brought to the United States. Unlike Thomsonism, homeopathy had the intellectual and social credentials to appeal to educated physicians and laymen, for whom it was a welcome change from the excesses of heroic therapy. Homeopathy rapidly gained a substantial following among some regular physicians and middle- and upper-income urban patients.

Regular physicians who practiced homeopathy came under attack from their colleagues and were ostracized because of homeopathy's rejection of heroic therapy. Homeopathic members of regular medical societies were expelled, and those seeking admission were rejected. Apprentices of homeopathic physicians were denied admission to regular medical schools. The movement to rid the medical profession of homeopaths was a major factor in the organization of the American Medical Association in 1847, which established a code of ethics banning professional ties between regular physicians and homeopaths.

Expulsion from the regular medical profession forced the homeopaths to establish homeopathic medical societies, medical schools, and later hospitals and dispensaries. Eventually, homeopathic physicians had a full range of medical institutions that paralleled those of the regular medical profession. Because homeopathic physicians had many middle income and wealthy patients, their institutions had the financial resources to maintain parity with those of regular physicians.

The Eclectic Movement

Meanwhile, the professional botanical practitioners were proceeding along the same lines. They also recognized that medical schools and medical societies were essential to their survival. Most groups of botanical physicians were short lived, but one, the eclectics, became a legitimate alternative to the regulars and homeopaths. Their use of the term *eclectic* was intended to mean that they accepted all valid treatments in any form of medicine. In practice, they remained true to their botanical origins, and most eclectic physicians limited themselves to botanical medicine. Eclectics tended to practice in small towns and villages and among lower-income patients, so eclectic medicine lacked the resources of homeopathic and regular medicine.

Thus by midcentury the spectrum of health care providers was quite broad. There were three major groups of physicians: the regulars, who were the largest and most influential; the homeopaths, who were numerous in urban areas in the Northeast and Midwest; and the eclectics, who usually practiced in the rural Midwest and parts of the South. Each had its own therapeutic philosophy, its own medical schools and medical societies, and its supporters among the public. Another group of practitioners, midwives, delivered many babies in rural areas and urban immigrant communities. On the fringes of the medical care system were other botanical practitioners, hydropaths, faith healers, and health reformers, all of whom were highly individualistic and unwilling to unite. They played a lesser and steadily declining role as providers of health care.

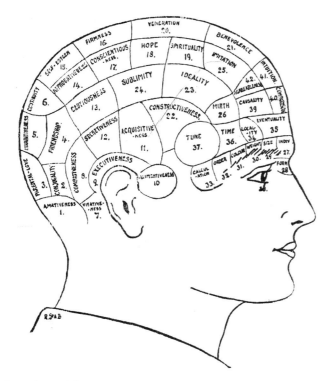

Location of the organs of phrenology. In the late nineteenth century, the theory of phrenology proposed that the conformation of the skull was indicative of mental ability and character.

From Severn JM: *The life story and experiences of a phrenologist,* 1929.

MEDICAL CARE AFTER THE CIVIL WAR

The decades after the Civil War were a period of formalization of medical care that strengthened professional physicians and weakened the individual healers, social movements, and health fads so influential in the first half of the century.

The three major sects continued to compete for public favor. The regulars, who composed 85% of the approximately 120,000 physicians in 1900, sought to control the medical care system, whereas the homeopaths, with about 10% of all physicians, and the eclectics, with less than 5%, argued for freedom of choice for the patient. The homeopaths and eclectics were strong enough to defend themselves against the regulars. Both had national, state, and in some cases, local medical societies that paralleled the regular medical societies. Their patients supported them enthusiastically in battles with the regulars and usually thwarted any proposed legislation designed to weaken them.

Because each sect depended on its ability to recruit students for its survival, the most important institution in each sect was its medical schools. Medicine, like other professions, grew in popularity after the Civil War, and medical schools proliferated to take advantage of the growing demand. Each sect was able to have numerous medical schools because they were proprietary institutions that survived on tuition income alone. This was feasible because medical education continued to consist primarily of lectures delivered to large classes, which kept costs low. Although the largest medical schools were quite profitable to their physician owners, the major financial benefits to most teachers came from consultations with former students and fees from patients attracted to physicians who had faculty appointments.

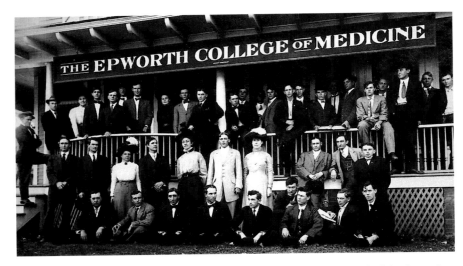

Epworth College of Medicine, a typical proprietary medical school of the late nine-teenth century. Few students were rejected from admission, and nearly all enter-ing students graduated after two sessions of medical school and 3 years' appren-ticeship with a physician.

The medical schools of each sect differed in the quality of education they provided. Beginning about 1880 a few elite medical schools offered a longer and more thorough education to those students who could afford it. The majority of the schools provided a decent education to the great mass of students, whereas some marginal schools and diploma mills admitted many students but graduated very few. Both the regulars and homeopaths had medical schools at all three quality levels, but the eclectics had only one medical school that was above average.

As medical knowledge increased, the three sects grew more similar in their practices. They all accepted surgery, which was revolutionized in the 1850s by the discovery of ether, nitrous oxide, and chloroform. These

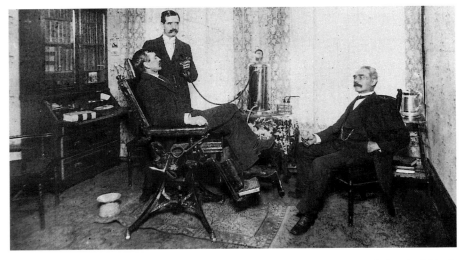

Dr. Joseph Hunter, a graduate of the University of Pennsylvania School of Medi-cine, administering nitrous oxide in 1873.

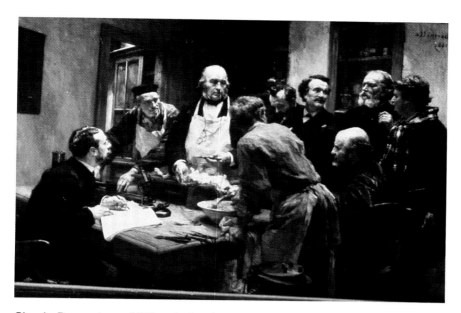

Claude Bernard, *an 1889 painting by Louis Lhremite, showing the physiologist Claude Bernard, who explained many functions of the internal organs, at work on an experimental vivisection.*
Courtesy Palais de la Decouverte, Paris.

anesthetics enabled patients to undergo operations without pain for the first time, which permitted surgeons to work more slowly and carefully and led to new kinds of operations. Anesthetics had no effect on postoperative infection, which continued to be the major cause of death in surgery and retarded its development.

The three sects also accepted the new specialties that originated in Europe and were brought to the United States by American physicians who studied in European hospitals to learn the newest methods of medical care. The first specialty was ophthalmology; others that followed were concerned with different parts of the body, with techniques such as surgery and obstetrics, with particular diseases, and with specific kinds of

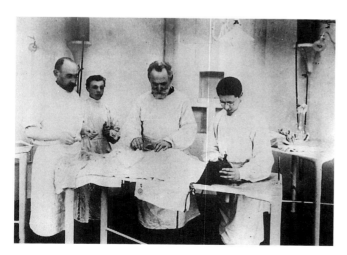

Ivan Pavlov, seen here with his co-workers, carrying out a demonstration of his theory of the conditioned reflex. Pavlov further contributed to psychiatry by showing that neuroses could be artificially produced in dogs.
Courtesy World Health Organization, Geneva, Switzerland.

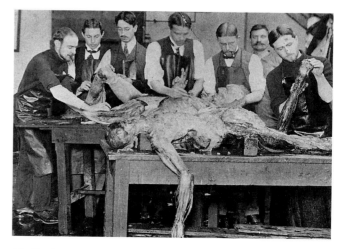

Medical students at work on a cadever circa 1890 as anatomical dissection was becoming an essential part of medical education.
Courtesy Minnesota Historical Society, St. Paul, Minnesota.

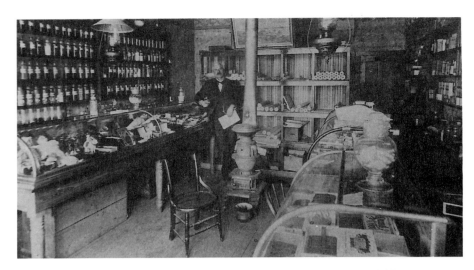

Dr. James Raizon of Trinidad, Colorado, in his drug store circa 1880.
Courtesy Colorado Historical Society of Colorado, Denver.

patients such as children. Even though the overwhelming majority of physicians in the nineteenth century continued to be general practitioners, specialists moved to the forefront of the profession in terms of influence, appointments to hospital staffs and medical school faculties, and leadership in medical societies.

Last, all sects shared the same views toward the medical sciences, which were being revolutionized at this time. Anatomy, the primary medical science in the eighteenth century, was joined in the nineteenth century by physiology, pathology, bacteriology, and at the end of the century, pharmacology and biochemistry. The medical schools of all three sects taught these subjects similarly, often using the same textbooks. All three sects also had identical views on public health.

The sects remained divided over drug therapy. The regulars, capitulating to public opposition to heroic therapy, abandoned it in the 1850s and 1860s. New developments in pharmacology brought many new synthetic drugs to market, but their effects on the patient remained symptomatic and their side effects could be as harsh as those of earlier drugs.

The urban working classes and the poor continued to receive most of their medical care in dispensaries. By now, every major city had numerous dispensaries, some of which provided care in a particular specialty. The specialty dispensaries, or clinics, were established by physicians interested in becoming specialists. By studying many patients with the same medical problems, the physicians could learn more about them. Hospital physicians also placed patients with the same condition together in wards to study them. By the end of the century, dispensaries and hospitals were the primary locations for training specialists and increasing clinical knowledge, a position they continue to hold today.

The Growth of Hospitals

The institution that grew most rapidly in the last quarter of the nineteenth century was the hospital. Public hospitals evolved out of the almshouses established by towns and cities in the eighteenth and nineteenth centuries to care for the sick poor, the elderly, orphans, the home-

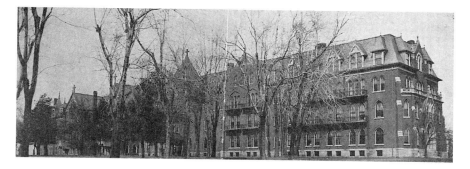

An exterior view of Mercy Hospital, Davenport, Iowa, circa 1890, typical of hospitals in smaller midwestern communities.

Courtesy Special Collections Room, Davenport Public Library, Davenport, Iowa.

less, the insane, and others. As the almshouse population increased in a city, separate institutions were established to care for each group. One of these was the public hospital to care for the sick poor.

About this same time, private voluntary hospitals were built in a few cities. The first ones were sponsored by philanthropic groups, often with government support, but after the Civil War, religious groups became the major force in the voluntary hospital movement. By the 1880s, many large cities had public and voluntary hospitals, both of which often received public funds. At the turn of the century the hospital movement spread to the smaller towns.

During most of the nineteenth century the major function of the hospital was to provide food, shelter, and bed rest to the needy. Hospitals were not popular with those who could afford to be cared for at home because hospital care was no better than home care and hospital patients had a greater risk of contracting infections from other patients in an era when their mode of transmission was unknown. Consequently, most hospital patients were the poor or those who lost their jobs when ill and were forced to accept charity.

Other factors also fostered the growth of hospitals. Large-scale immigration to cities from overseas and rural areas increased the number

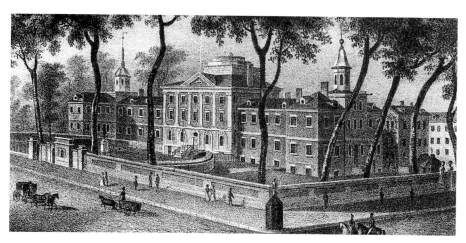

The Pennsylvania hospital, circa 1800, America's first hospital.

Courtesy The Pennsylvania Hospital, Philadelphia, Pennsylvania.

47

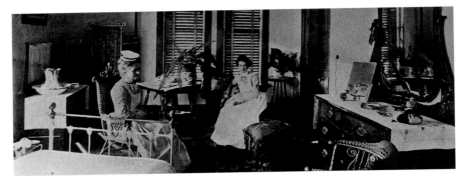

A view of the interior of Mercy Hospital, Davenport, Iowa, circa 1890.
Courtesy Special Collections Department, Davenport Public Library, Davenport, Iowa.

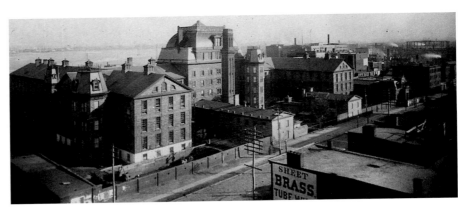

A view of Bellevue Hospital, New York City, circa 1885. Bellevue Hospital traces its beginnings back to 1685 when the British West Indies Company established a small hospital. It had several different locations in the city, and eventually the City of New York helped with the cost of running the hospital. It served as an almshouse, a "pesthouse" for yellow fever victums, and a penitentiary and had wards for the sick and insane.
Courtesy Collection of The New-York Historical Society, New York.

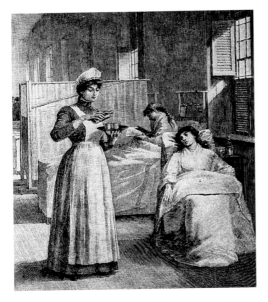

Nurse Administering Medicine to an Ailing Girl, *a woodcut circa late nineteenth century.*
Courtesy the Bettman Archive, New York.

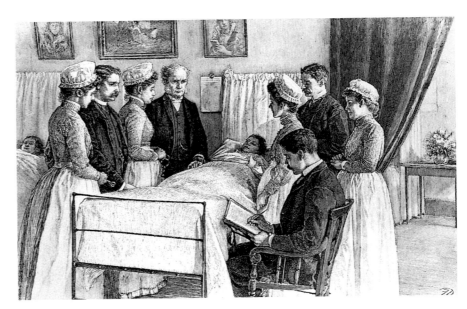

A Critical Case—A Bedside Consultation for the Benefit of Students and Nurses at Bellevue Hospital, *an engraving from 1890.*
Courtesy the Bettman Archive, New York.

of people who needed to be cared for when they became ill. The expansion of factories and railroads multiplied the number of industrial accidents. Crowded city streets led to streetcar and other accidents and more people who became ill while away from home. All of them needed a place to go for care.

The hospital movement had a major impact on the dispensary. Toward the end of the century, many hospitals opened outpatient departments to care for patients who did not need hospitalization. Because outpatient departments used the facilities of the hospital, they provided better care than the independent dispensaries and soon replaced them. By the beginning of the twentieth century, most independent dispensaries had either gone out of business or merged with hospitals.

The expansion of hospitals led to the need for trained nurses to care for hospital patients. Previously, hospital nursing was performed by unskilled workers or recuperating patients, a situation that became less satisfactory as the number of hospital patients increased. Meanwhile, after the Civil War, more women entered the labor force, and many of them sought new and interesting skilled occupations. These two factors coalesced to create a new profession—nursing. Following the model established by Florence Nightingale in England, American hospitals set up training schools for nurses beginning in the 1870s. The students spent 2 and later 3 years in the hospital gaining practical experience in nursing and hearing occasional lectures by the physicians on the hospital staff. Hospitals were more interested in obtaining cheap labor than in providing the students with a satisfactory education, a situation that plagued nursing education for many decades.

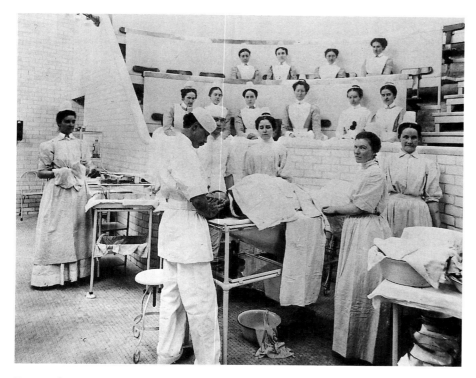

Doctor Operating with Women Nursing Students Observing, *a photograph by R.F. Turnbull taken in St. Luke's Hospital of New York City in 1899.*
Courtesy Museum of the City of New York, New York.

Because of their nursing schools, hospitals employed graduate nurses only as supervisors and teachers. This forced most nursing school graduates to work as private duty nurses in homes. Some became "visiting" (now public health) nurses employed by governments or charities to care for the sick poor. Hospital nursing did not become a major vocation for graduate nurses until the 1930s.

The last decades of the century saw a greater concern with the mentally ill. The standard treatment developed during the nineteenth century for the mentally ill was institutional care. Early in the century a few private mental hospitals for the wealthy were constructed, and some decades later public hospitals were built in most states to care for the great majority of the mentally ill. This was a great advance over earlier treatment, which often consisted of physical restraint. The superintendents of these hospitals were physicians, who were the first specialists in mental disorders. Late in the century, the concept of mental illness expanded to include patients with neuroses as well as psychoses, which led to an interest in noninstitutional treatment. The first psychiatrists, in the modern sense of the term, provided this kind of care.

Bacteriology and Medicine

Medicine and public health in the late nineteenth century were transformed by the discovery of the bacterial nature of many infectious diseases, which was the greatest achievement of the medical sciences up to that time. The acceptance of scientific medicine led to physician licensing laws, the closing of the weaker medical schools, the widespread adoption of scientific medicine by social institutions, and the merging of the major sects. It also led to the emergence of new types of health care providers to care for patients who were not satisfied with this new approach to medicine.

After 1850, improved microscope lenses and better methods of refracting light in the microscope enabled scientists to observe microorganisms with greater precision than ever before. The researches of Louis Pasteur, Robert Koch, and other European scientists from the 1860s to the end of the century showed that specific bacteria were present in the blood-

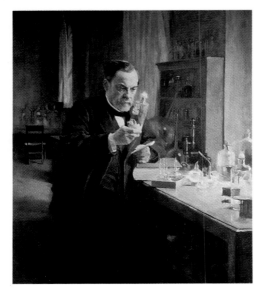

Louis Pasteur in His Laboratory, *an oil portrait by Albert-Gustaf Edelfelt. Pasteur was responsible for laying the groundwork of modern immunity theory and immunization.* Courtesy Musee Pasteur, Institut Pasteur, Paris.

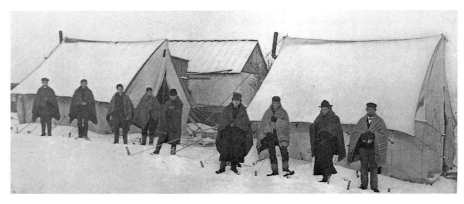

Tent life at 28 degrees below zero. The White Haven Tuberculosis Sanitorium, circa 1904.

From *The Annual Report of the Free Hospital for Poor Consumptives,* Feb 1904. Courtesy College of Physicians of Philadelphia Historical Collections.

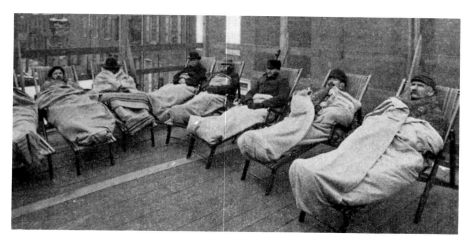

Patients suffering from tuberculosis (or consumption), the most common cause of death in the United States throughout the nineteenth century. After the discovery of the tubercle bacillus, physicians realized the condition was infectious and began treating consumption in sanitoriums using a regimen of fresh air, nutritious food, and supervised rest and exercise.

From *The Annual Report of the Philadelphia Protestant Episcopal City Mission,* 1906. Courtesy College of Physicians of Philadelphia Historical Collections.

streams and bodies of animals and humans with certain diseases. When scientists removed blood containing the bacteria from animals with one of these diseases, cultured the bacteria to purify them, and then injected the bacteria into the bodies of experimental animals without the disease, the experimental animals contracted the disease. These experiments demonstrated that bacteria played a key role in many infectious diseases.

As a result of this revolutionary finding, physicians for the first time understood a key factor in the etiology of the most common diseases of the time. The greatest and most immediate impact was on public health. The discovery that disease-causing bacteria were present in water supplies, milk, and foods; that some bacteria were conveyed from person to person through the air and others were transmitted by means of insects and other vectors; and that proper disposal of human waste and other kinds of sewage could prevent the spread of bacteria made it possible to design public health programs to prevent the spread of disease.

Another fundamental bacteriological breakthrough occurred in surgery when the English physician Joseph Lister discovered in the late 1860s that the serious and often fatal postoperative infections experienced by many patients were caused by bacteria that entered the wound during the operation. In the next several decades, these bacteria were found to be present on the hands and clothing of the surgeon, the body of the patient, and the surgical instruments and dressings. This led to a new kind of aseptic surgery in which everything that came into contact with the patient during the operation was sterilized or disinfected to minimize the risk of postoperative infection.

Aseptic surgery made it possible to operate on the cranium, thorax, and abdomen for the first time. Although many of these new operations were life saving, others were less beneficial. In some cases, it appeared that heroic therapy had been replaced by heroic surgery.

The effect of bacteriology on other kinds of treatment was much more limited. No one knew how to kill the disease-causing bacteria in the patient's body without harming the patient. The first bacteriological treatments that actually cured diseases were tetanus antitoxin, introduced in

1890, and diphtheria antitoxin, introduced in 1894. Diphtheria antitoxin, which cured a terrifying and fatal children's disease, demonstrated the great possibilities of bacteriology, even to its critics. Broad-based antibiotics, however, were not developed until the sulfa drugs of the 1930s and penicillin in the 1940s.

Bacteriology revolutionized diagnosis. Before bacteriology, it did not matter whether diphtheria, for example, was diagnosed accurately or not. Once bacteriologists showed that diphtheria was an infectious disease that could be spread from child to child, the need to isolate the patient was recognized, and this necessitated an accurate diagnosis of diphtheria. After diphtheria antitoxin became available, accurate diagnosis was essential to ensure that the drug would be used properly. Furthermore, antitoxin was effective only if administered early in the course of diphtheria, which made a prompt diagnosis as important as an accurate one. Physicians also had to know how to prepare cultures from the throats of diphtheria patients to send to laboratories so that an accurate diagnosis could be made.

Clearly, bacteriology and the other medical sciences required physicians to have a level of medical and scientific knowledge formerly considered superfluous for a general practitioner. This realization led to the enactment of licensing laws to evaluate the graduates of all medical schools. Previously, each sect insisted that only its physicians could evaluate the competence of its medical school graduates, which made it impossible to enact uniform licensing laws. Now graduates of all medical schools could be examined on their knowledge of the medical sciences and the specialties without reference to drug treatment. This enabled states to enact laws requiring all physicians to obtain licenses before practicing medicine.

In this and other ways the new scientific medicine reformed medical education. Medical students now sought out medical schools with the laboratories and other equipment necessary to learn about the new and

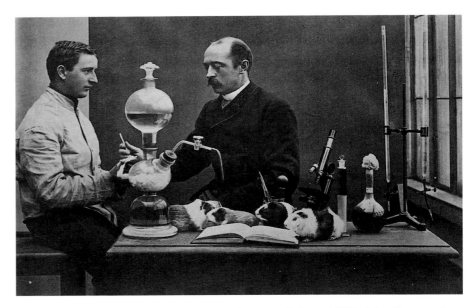

Emil von Behring in His Laboratory, *a photograph from 1890 of the German bacteriologist Emil von Behring in the laboratory.*
Courtesy Stock Montage, Chicago.

exciting areas of medicine, partly to become good physicians and partly to pass the licensing examinations. Many medical schools of all sects could not afford to make these changes and closed. The remaining medical schools affiliated with private or public universities to obtain the necessary financial resources.

Bacteriology also had a dramatic impact on sectarian therapeutics. Physicians discovered that most of the drugs used by the regulars, homeopaths, and eclectics were ineffective or provided only symptomatic relief. They also realized that treatments based solely on symptoms had no scientific validity. Reducing a patient's fever need not affect the disease that caused the fever. The sects grudgingly admitted that the principles of drug action over which they fought so bitterly for almost a century all lacked scientific validity.

Although regular physicians initially resisted accepting homeopaths and eclectics as colleagues, they gradually realized that the public would not give them a monopoly over such key issues as licensing physicians, accrediting medical schools, and public health. Regular physicians then agreed to serve on licensing and public health boards with homeopaths and eclectics and ultimately opened their medical societies to them. Gradually the three sects merged and adopted the same approach to medicine.

The new scientific medicine soon affected most medical institutions. Physicians were playing a greater role as providers of health care in hospitals, the armed forces, and industry and as examiners of applicants for life insurance policies. Nurses used scientific medicine in their roles as hospital, private duty, and public health nurses. The growing field of public health, which affected the lives of all Americans, was based almost exclusively on applied bacteriology.

As scientific medicine expanded its role in patient care, it became evident that it did not meet all the needs of patients. The new diagnostic techniques failed to discover the causes of many patient complaints. Furthermore, as public health and the rising standard of living reduced death rates from infectious diseases, people lived longer and contracted chronic and degenerative diseases. The medical model that worked so well with infectious diseases was less successful for these diseases. For this and other reasons, some patients turned elsewhere for either some or all of their medical care.

ALTERNATIVE HEALERS

Several new types of healers came forth to care for these patients. Unlike the sects of the early nineteenth century, which were based on conflicting theories of drug action, these new healers espoused drugless therapy. The most successful groups, besides chiropractic, were Christian Science and osteopathy.

Christian Science

Christian Science was founded by Mary Baker Eddy in the 1870s as part of the long tradition of faith healing in America. Eddy believed that health problems have no existence in physical reality but result from im-

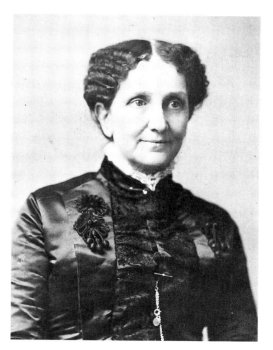

Mary Baker Eddy, founder of Christian Science.
Courtesy Library of Congress, Washington, DC.

proper mental influences. They can be cured by recognizing and dealing spiritually with these mental influences. Christian Science was popularized at the turn of the century through the activities of many Christian Science practitioners who undertook to heal the sick professionally. It was stimulated even more when it became a formal religion and opened churches. Christian Science thus became both a method of healing and a religion, a position that has created strains for its members because many Christian Scientists emphasize one dimension more than the other.

Osteopathy

Osteopathy was "flung to the breeze" by Andrew Taylor Still in 1874. Still was familiar with the long tradition of drugless healing in America and with the bonesetters who reduced dislocations and set fractures. He discovered that the manipulations of bonesetters had a beneficial impact that extended beyond the problems they were intended to solve. Building on this, he developed a system of medicine called *osteopathy*. During the twentieth century the education of osteopaths expanded to include the new scientific medicine. In most respects today, osteopathic medicine is part of conventional medicine.

The Physical Culture Movement

Besides these groups, faith healers, health reformers, and advocates of natural treatments attracted substantial followings at the end of the century. These groups refashioned many themes that had been popular in the early nineteenth century. Sylvester Graham had insisted that wheat containing the bran be used in baking as a wholesome alternative to meat; decades later, J. H. Kellogg created the first cold breakfast cereals with precisely the same rationale. The early nineteenth century emphasis on personal hygiene evolved into a concern with physical fitness, exemplified by the popularity of the bicycle and the physical culture movement.

Over the course of the twentieth century, the domain of scientific medicine has expanded beyond infectious diseases to include many other ailments, such as cardiovascular diseases and cancer. However, scientific medicine has not been able to cure most of these disorders; its goal has been to stabilize the condition of patients so that their lives can be as close to normal as possible indefinitely. The dearth of curative treatments has created opportunities for groups outside the medical profession to offer different modes of treatment, among them chiropractic. Unlike the nineteenth century when different methods of treatment existed within and outside the medical profession, the divergent groups in the twentieth century have all been outside the medical profession. For this reason the rapprochement that occurred among the sects in the nineteenth century has not recurred in the twentieth.

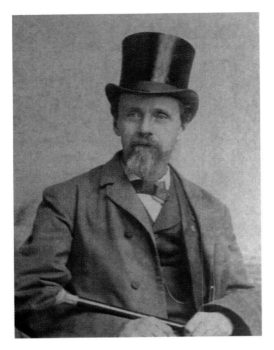

A portrait of A.T. Still, the founder of osteopathy, circa 1900.
Courtesy Kirksville College of Osteopathy, A.T. Still Memorial Library, Arichives Department, Kirksville, Missouri.

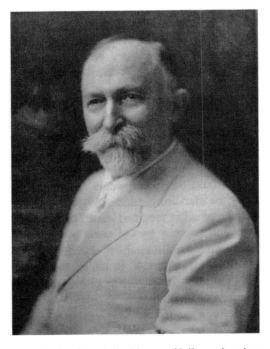

A portrait of Dr. John Harvey Kellogg, brother to the Kellogg of breakfast cereal fame and a physical culture movement proponent.
Courtesy Historical Society of Battle Creek, Battle Creek, Michigan.

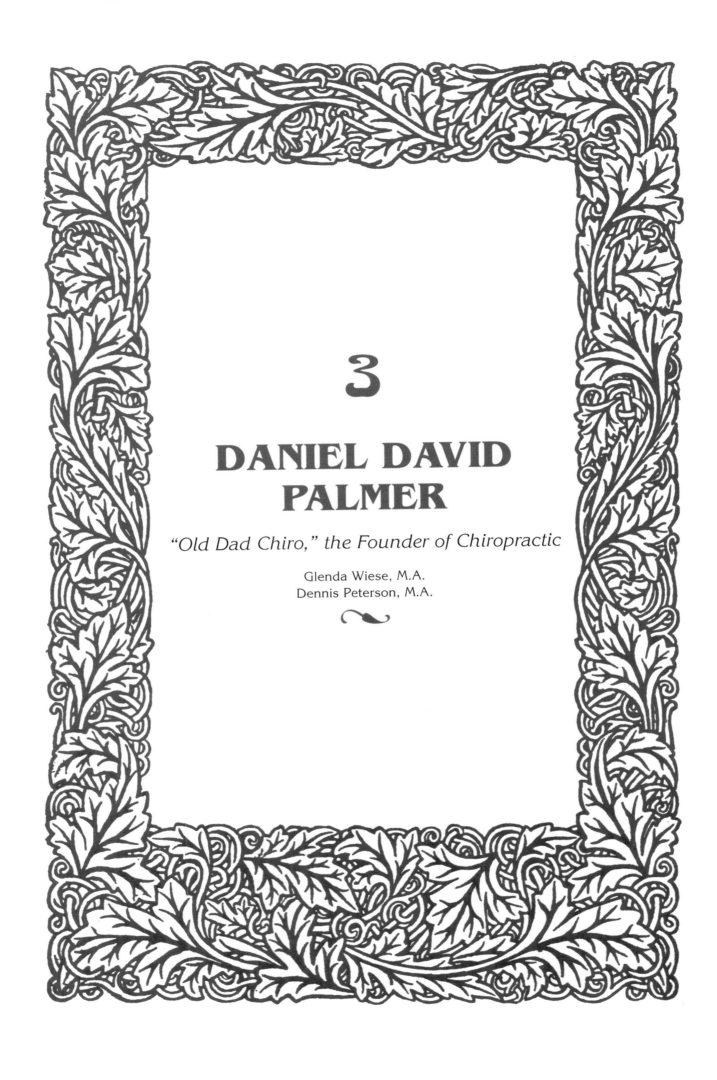

3

DANIEL DAVID PALMER

"Old Dad Chiro," the Founder of Chiropractic

Glenda Wiese, M.A.
Dennis Peterson, M.A.

The full family history of Daniel David Palmer can be traced from the British Isles in the seventeenth century to early New England settlements in the colonies of Massachusetts, Pennsylvania, and New York. D.D.'s grandfather, Stephen Palmer, then emigrated from New England to "Canada West," much of it later to be the province of Ontario. Just why Stephen Palmer emigrated is not known.

D.D. Palmer's father, Thomas, was born in 1823 in Prince Edward province. Little is known of his early years; it is assumed he lived most of his younger years in English Canada, moving at some point to Ontario. Thomas settled in an area now known as Port Perry, Ontario, just outside the newly declared province capital of York, which is now Toronto. Port Perry was laid out by an industrious Peter Perry and formally incorporated in 1845. The local economy was primarily agricultural, with a strong timber and sawmill industry. Thomas became a shoemaker and later a grocer and for a time was also a Port Perry school director and the postmaster.

Thomas and his wife, Catherine McVay, had three sons and three daughters. Daniel David was born March 7, 1845. He was followed by his brothers Thomas J. and Bartlett. His three sisters were named Lucinda Mariah, Hanna Jane, and Catherine. Commenting on the circumstances of his birth, D.D wrote the following:

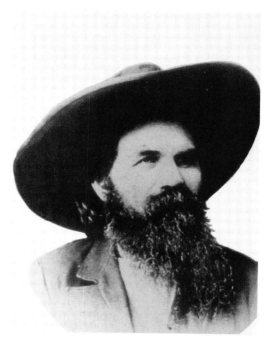

D.D. Palmer circa 1870.
Courtesy Palmer College of Chiropractic Archives, Davenport Iowa.

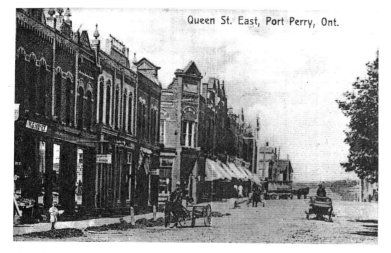

Port Perry, Ontario, Canada, circa 1865, about the time D.D. left for the United States.
Courtesy Scugog Shores Museum, Port Perry, Ontario.

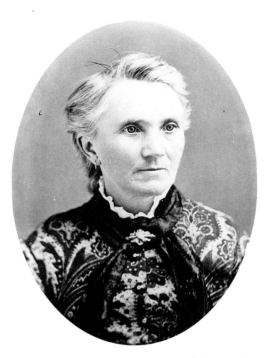

D.D.'s mother, Catherine McVay Palmer, circa 1890.
Courtesy Palmer College of Chiropractic Archives, Davenport, Iowa.

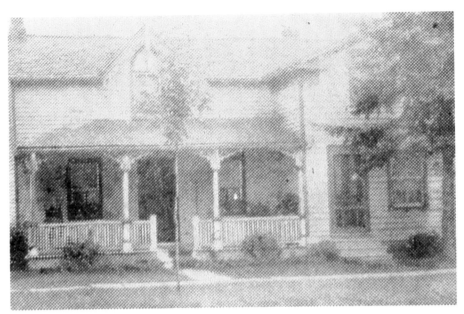

The house in which D.D. was born, circa 1945.
Courtesy Port Perry Star, Port Perry, Ontario.

My ancestors were Scotch and Irish on my maternal and English and German on my paternal side. When my grandparents settled near the now beautiful city of Toronto, there was but one log house, the beginnings of that great city [Toronto]. . . .

I came within one of never having a mama. My mother was one of a pair of twins, one of which died. The one which lived only weighed one and a half pounds. When I was a baby I was cradled in a piece of hemlock bark. My mother was as full of superstition as an egg is full of meat, my father was disposed to reasons on the subjects pertaining to life.

In Thomas J. Palmer's autobiography, Thomas describes how both he and D.D. had acquired the equivalent of an eighth grade education by the time they were 9 and 11, respectively, and were well on the way into

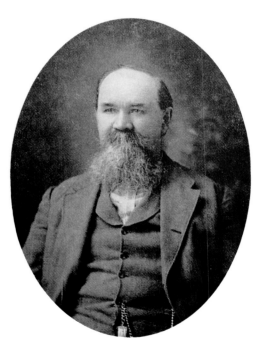

Thomas J. Palmer, D.D.'s younger brother, was the editor of several midwestern newspapers.
From *The Chronicles of Oklahoma*, Winter, 1950-1951.

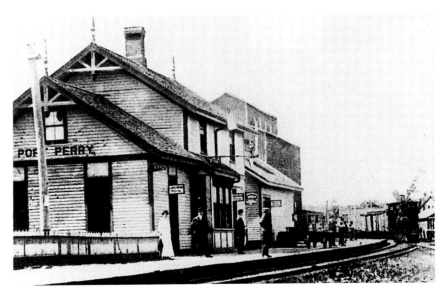

Port Perry, Ontario, Circa 1880.
Courtesy Russell Gibbons, Pittsburgh.

high school subjects, including natural sciences and classical languages, when their education was cut short. Their father's business failed in 1856, and the family moved to the United States, leaving 11-year-old D.D. and 9-year-old Thomas behind in Port Perry. Their schooling was intermittent; they had to work in a stave and match factory to support themselves.

With the downturn of the Port Perry economy, the two young men (now aged 20 and 18) left Port Perry in 1865 and walked to Whitby, Ontario, and bought a boat passage across Lake Ontario to the United States landing at Buffalo, New York. From Buffalo the young men traveled to Detroit and then to Chicago. From Chicago they were able to ride a returning Civil War troop train west to Iowa. Almost 3 months after they had begun their journey and after several years separation, they rejoined Thomas and Catherine and their siblings in south central Iowa in the heartland of rural America.

THE SCHOOLMASTER

Approximately 8 months after he arrived in the United States, 21-year-old D.D. became the schoolmaster of a one-room schoolhouse on the prairies of Muscatine County, Iowa. He taught 50 pupils ranging in age from 5 to 20 years during February and March of 1866. After this first teaching position, D.D. taught in nearby Concord Township, Louisa County, Iowa. The 7-month term with 80 pupils began January 1867. The next year, D.D. taught 47 students of District Two, Jefferson Township, Louisa County, with the term ending on March 17, 1868. By 1871, D.D. had become an experienced and veteran schoolmaster with 5 years of service. His next position was with 53 youths of the Intermediate Department in New Boston, Illinois, a bustling Mercer County Mississippi River port.

The move to Mercer County, Illinois, set the stage for yet another interesting facet in the life of the man who would eventually discover chiropractic. D.D. was teaching school in January and February of 1871 when he married his first wife, Abba Lord.

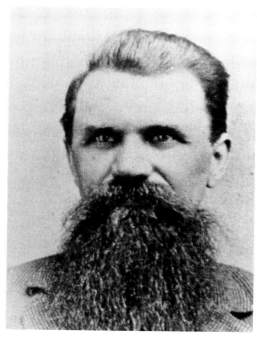

D.D. Palmer about the time he would have been serving as a schoolmaster in Louisa County, Iowa.

Courtesy Palmer College of Chiropractic Archives, Davenport, Iowa.

HORTICULTURALIST FARMER AND BUSINESSMAN

After 6 years of teaching school, D.D. thought it was time to seek a more profitable occupation. School teachers were not paid well, earning about the same as a skilled farmhand. At this time, unimproved land sold for $10 an acre, and improved farm land was being sold on both sides of the Mississippi River as fast as it could be cleared. Louisa County, Iowa, just across the river from Mercer County, was nine-tenths cleared and predominantly fenced.

In November 1871, D.D. and his wife Abba purchased 10 acres of land located in Eliza Township, Mercer County, Illinois, several miles north of New Boston. The small piece of land embraced a steep hill that sloped to the edge of the wet sloughs along the Mississippi River. On their farm, D.D. planted and cultivated over 30 varieties of fruit trees, including Bartlett's, Sheldon, Clapp's Favorite, Heath Free, and Heath Cling. D.D.

also planted a wide variety of evergreens not indigenous to the area. These included balsam fir, savin spruce, black spruce, blue spruce, white spruce, hemlock, red cedar, white pine, and scotch pine. He was also very interested in cultivating bees.

During this first 1½ years of farming, D.D.'s first marriage to Abba Lord ended in divorce. After 6 months, D.D. married Louvenia Landers in New Boston. Louvenia was reputed to be a downriver Southerner who had an infant son Frank by a previous marriage. She was described as short, round, dark eyed, and dark haired and was considered a woman of both culture and tenderness. D.D.'s only three children were born to he and Louvenia. There were two daughters born in New Boston—May in 1876 and Jessie in 1880. D.D.'s only son was born in What Cheer, Iowa, in 1882. His given name was Joshua Bartlett, but he preferred to be known as Bartlett Joshua, or just B.J.

Farming was tremendously risky, and D.D. had both successes and failures. In his journal, D.D. kept accurate records about his beekeeping business, which at times was very successful:

> Fall and Winter of 1871 left my bees out on stands—lost some with disease. . . . Winter of 1872 lost all (about) 50 on stands with disease. . . . Spring of 1873 went to Kentucky, got about 90 hives, 40 of them for me, increased to 100—wintered in cellar came out with 35 in Spring of '74. Increased to 100, put in cellar and came out with 55, disease again. . . . Year of 1875 increased to 100, etc.

In one of the last beekeeping entries for 1877, D.D. notes "took car load of honey—18,600 lb—to New York City—car cost $232—done fair." But a few years later, the 1880 and 1881 journal entries were not encouraging: "May 1 [1880], 12 hives dead out of 209. . . . June 17, water coming up in (river) bottom. Water came up the highest ever known by whites. . . . Aug. 25, no surplus yet. . . . Jan. 10 [1881], 26 below 0, was 30 below once. . . . Apr. 14, 20 degrees. Bees all dead."

Even with the eventual misfortunes of his beekeeping venture, D.D. was successful with his nursery ventures. Tedious hours of painstaking

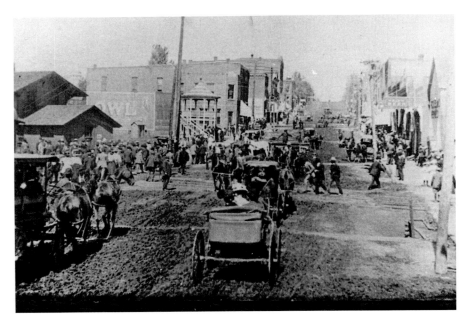

What Cheer, Iowa, about the time D.D. and his family lived there, circa 1880.
Courtesy Larry and Phyllis Nicholson, What Cheer, Iowa.

effort created a nursery operation of sufficient magnitude that the resolute D.D. was able to sell raspberry and other fruit bushes and trees to individuals and nursery operators all over the United States. D.D. noted the following in his journal:

> In the spring of 1874 I got (as was supposed) a plant of Lumm's [sic] Everbearer. Spring of 1875 I got 22 plants and it proved to be a seedling. Spring of 1876 I got 50 plants. In 1877 I got 28 plants from the original bush and 585 in all. In 1875 I had about 2500 plants, pollinated 2000 and on balance in 1879. . . .

D.D. evidently was skilled in the careful art of propagating the raspberries. Although hardy in maturity, raspberry shoots must be properly watered and carefully tended after being transplanted. Besides being a stalwart worker, one of D.D.'s advantages was the rich soil of his land, an area presumably untouched by the plow until his working of the land.

D.D. cultivated a mutation from his original raspberry plants, which developed extraordinary well-bearing large black raspberries that became known as "Sweet Home." He was very proud of his Sweet Home Raspberry, which was to be very successful. The Sweet Home received the top billing of all his marketing and sales efforts for his shoots. In addition to Sweet Home, D.D. grew and sold six other varieties of raspberries, concord grapes, Snyder blackberries, and strawberries and apple, crab apple, pear, plum, and cherry tree shoots.

Despite the successes, on December 31, 1881, D.D. sold Sweet Home for $1000 to John Glancy. From there he moved his family back to the prosperous and booming coal mining town of What Cheer, Iowa, where his parents and two brothers were still living. In its glory days of the 1880s, What Cheer boasted a population of nearly 8000, with nearly 100 coal mines in the area. The city and county was populated by people of mostly English, Scottish, Welsh, and Irish decent and boasted some 50 manufacturing plants producing everything from bicycles to wagons and clay

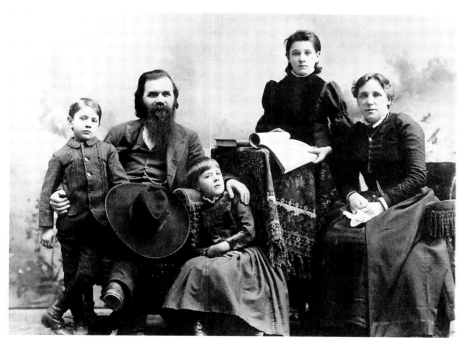

D.D. and his family in 1890. From left to right: B.J., D.D., Jessie, May, and Villa.
Courtesy Palmer College of Chiropractic Archives, Davenport, Iowa.

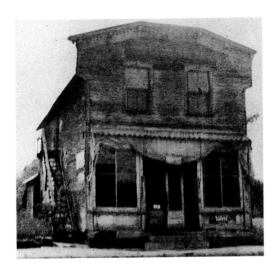

The building in which D.D. had his grocery store, taken many years after D.D.'s occupancy of it.

From Drain J: *Man tomorrow.*

products to wood stoves. There were 20 saloons, two gambling houses, a brewery, a soft drink manufacturer, an opera house, three major railroad lines, and an annual visit by the Ringling Brothers' wagon show, the forerunner to the Ringling Brothers' Circus.

D.D.'s brother Thomas was the editor of What Cheer's newspaper, the *What Cheer Patriot,* and his brother Bartlett worked as a liveryman in a local stable. D.D. opened a grocery in What Cheer, with his family living in the back of the store that was situated next to the post office and just south of the Rock Island Railroad depot. D.D. also taught school at the nearby community of Letts. The grocery sold all the necessities and bought and sold the local farmers' produce. D.D. also sold goldfish for which he maintained exacting records of births, deaths, and diseases, just as he had done for his beekeeping and nursery operations on his New Boston farm. In 1882, his only son B.J. was born on September 14 in What Cheer.

Amid this prosperity, tragedy struck 2 years later in 1884 when Louvenia died. With three children to care for, a business to maintain, and his teaching duties to uphold, 40-year-old D.D. married his third wife, 26-year-old Martha Henning, 6 months later in 1885.

SPIRITUALISM AND MAGNETIC HEALING

During the time D.D. lived in New Boston, he became interested in spiritualism. As uncharacteristic for a small Illinois river town as it may sound, spiritualism had a stronghold on several staunch New Bostonians, including some of its most prominent and wealthy citizens. Spiritualism as a religious concept was a form of Christianity, which held that although the body dies and does not survive, the spirit of the individual lives on. Communication with these spirits was possible through mediums who could contact this other world through sittings. The mediums at a sitting would either place themselves in a trance to contact the other world or hold a seance in which the medium becomes the vehicle through which the spirit makes contact with the corporeal world.

Spiritualism's writings and rise to acceptance is traced primarily to the Swedish scientist and mystic, Emmanuel Swedenborg. The German physician-scientist Franz Mesmer is also connected to its basic beliefs and structure. A later development of Spiritualism is directly tied to "spirit healing," in which mediums are believed to have special healing powers because of their abilities to contact the spirit world. Mesmer believed he had special powers when in an hypnotic state that allowed him to help in the diagnosis and treatment of disease.

The discussions of Spiritualism's rationale and its mystery appealed to an already deeply religious and perpetually curious D.D. He had always been an avid reader, especially of his Bible, in which he had underlined lines and verses to such an extent the entire book was black with markings. Regular Spiritualism meetings were held to debate the religion, which was at its height of popularity in the second half of the nineteenth century, and D.D. frequently entered into the discussions. He may have even walked the 6 or 7 miles from his farm into New Boston to attend these meetings. Recollections of D.D. Palmer were passed down through the generations by New Bostonians who tell of his short height and broad stature. He was always neatly dressed in clean, conservative clothes that were not necessarily fashionable. He was generally thought of as gracious and kind and was well-regarded by his neighbors. However, on occasion when deep in thought as he walked the lonely rural road, he would not lift his head to nod to fellow travelers. This gave rise to comments and opinions about D.D. being standoffish and arrogant.

These discussions of and experiences with Spiritualism undoubtedly led D.D. to his interest in magnetic healing. Because of his lifelong reading and study habits, word of an extraordinary magnetic healer in nearby Ottumwa, Iowa, was viewed with exceptional interest by the grocer and teacher. D.D. Palmer's keen interest in science and humanity was again challenged.

Paracelsus, a fifteenth century Austrian philosopher and alchemist, believed all matter—organic and inorganic—to be endowed with its own spirits. He also concluded that people possess magnetic powers capable of attracting either good or evil. He taught his followers that a "magnetic field" exuded from people; it could be guided by their wills, influencing the minds and bodies of others.

Two centuries later, Franz Anton Mesmer passed his medical examinations after first earning degrees in both philosophy and law and became interested in what he termed "animal magnetism." He chose this term for two reasons: First, there was a similiarity between the human organism and the iron magnet—both adhered to natural law. Second, "magnetism of the living" was "animal" from the Latin *anima* meaing "soul." Animal magnetism translated as Mesmer did indicated his interest was in "soul magnetism." He believed that magnetic properties could be used to treat various parts of the body if the magnets were shaped to conform to the size of the organ or external anatomy. Later he dropped the concept of magnets. Mesmer's ideas and concepts have been recognised in the development of the theory of modern hynopsis.

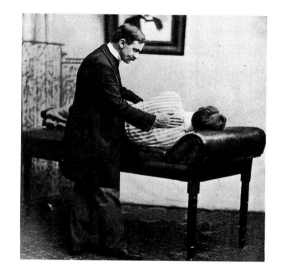

Magnetic healing was introduced in the United States in the late 1830s by Charles Poysen. One of his students, Phineas P. Quimby, treated Mary Baker Eddy, who was later to found the Christian Scientist faith. Magnetic healing used the healing anima power through a medium's hands. Magnetic healers would pass their hands over their patients' bodies, a continuation of the "laying on of the hands" healing that had been used since well before Hippocrates. Magnetic healing quickly spread around the nation.

During the time D.D. returned to What Cheer and was teaching in nearby Letts, a man by the name of Paul Caster in nearby Ottumwa, Iowa, died. Dr. Caster had made his mark as an "outstanding healer" and had built an extremely large practice as a magnetic healer. Blessed with a keen sense of public relations and the support of the local press, Caster was also widely known as a respected lecturer and constructed a large, four-story brick building that was later to become Ottumwa's first public hospital.

Caster's effectiveness as a healer was documented in an 1874 newspaper:

> Patients who have been bedridden for years and others who had for so long been hobbling about on crutches as to have lost all hope of health or soundness, have gone from him like the lame man at the beautiful gate of the temple, "walking and leading and praising God. . . ."

With his voracious appetite for reading and learning, D.D. Palmer came into contact with this most successful healer and found his work interesting. He was very impressed with Paul Caster's procedures, magnitude of practice, and the public reception Caster received. The philosophical concepts of magnetic healing were also attractive to D.D. In

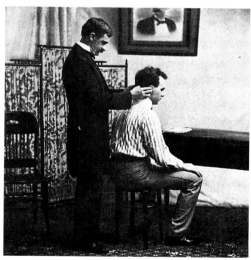

S.A. Weltmer demonstrating two magnetic healing positions.

From *Professor S.A. Weltmer's revised and illustrated mail course of instruction in magnetic healing,* 1901.

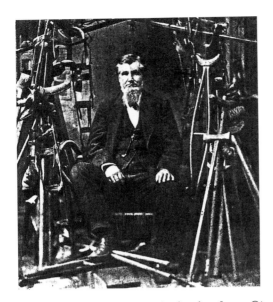

Paul Caster, the magnetic healer from Ottumwa, Iowa, who first interested D.D. in magnetic healing, taken with a few of the canes and crutches his patients discarded after his successful magnetic healing treatments.

Courtesy Palmer College of Chiropractic Archives, Davenport, Iowa.

many ways, this form of health treatment paralleled D.D.'s religiousity. An avid reader of the Bible and books on spiritualism, he also pursued more esoteric work. In his book collection was a text acquired in 1873 entitled *The Moral Aphorisms and Terseological Teachings of Confucius, The Sapient Chinese Philosopher.*

Palmer's quest for knowledge also led him to read scientific volumes of the period. D.D. was living at a time of experimentation in all areas of health care, from the philosophy of vitalism to the pragmatics of science. There was latitude for investigation in many directions, with little interference of any kind. Phrenology, naturopathy, allopathy, eclectic medicine, homeopathy, physical therapeutics, and osteopathy were present or on the horizon. D.D.'s natural intellectual affinity attracted him to the concepts of magnetic healing. He studied it and began its practice in Burlington, Iowa, along the banks of the Mississippi River.

When D.D. moved to Burlington in 1886, it was a bustling river town with a population of slightly over 25,000. He opened his offices in the business section of Burlington as "D.D. Palmer, Vital Healer." At the time, Burlington had magnetic healers, including J.S. Caster (the son of Paul Caster); eclectics; homeopaths; allopaths; and botanic and occultist practitioners. Details about D.D.'s time in Burlington are sketchy, probably because he was there only a few months before deciding to move upriver to Davenport, Iowa, sometime in 1887.

THE MOVE TO DAVENPORT

The 1887 Davenport City Directory contains an advertisement for the 42-year-old D.D. Palmer that read the following:

> D.D. Palmer
> Cures without Medicine
> Ryan Block Building
> Publisher of the *Educator*

Davenport, Iowa, and Moline and Rock Island, Illinois, were the "Tri-Cities." They were growing communities, with a good mixture of farm implement and railroad manufacturing, a strong surrounding agricultural base, and supporting businesses. The federal Rock Island Arsenal was growing from the small Fort Armstrong into a major military complex. D.D. probably felt his future would be more secure in Davenport with the larger Tri-Cities population, even though his start was a bit faltering. D.D. found himself with financial problems almost immediately and was sued to collect an unpaid promissory note.

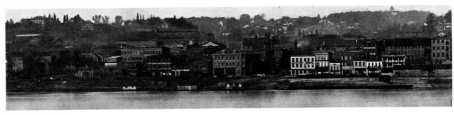

A view of Davenport, Iowa, from Rock Island, Illinois, looking across the Mississippi, circa 1880, about the time D.D. moved to the Tri-Cities.

Courtesy Special Collections, Davenport Public Library, Davenport, Iowa.

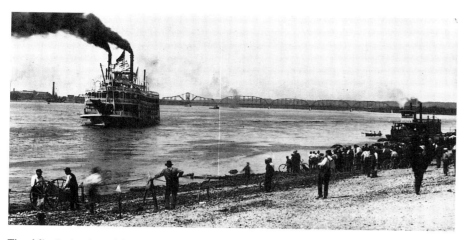

The Mississippi and its riverboats from the Davenport levy.
Courtesy Special Collections, Davenport Public Library, Davenport, Iowa.

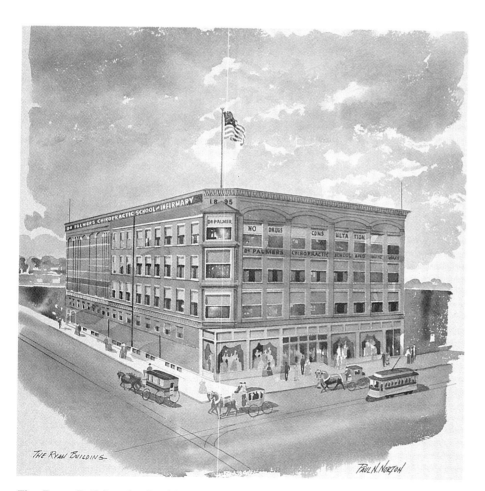

The Ryan Building by Paul Norton, where D.D. practiced magnetic healing and developed his theory of chiropractic.
Courtesy Palmer College of Chiropractic Archives, Davenport, Iowa.

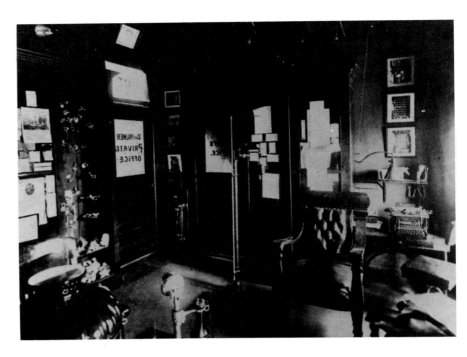

D.D.'s private office in the block of rooms he leased on the fourth floor of the Ryan Building.

Courtesy Palmer College of Chiropractic Archives, Davenport, Iowa.

D.D. Palmer's practice in the Ryan Building grew quickly. His finances began to improve, and the advertising program he created was substantial and far reaching. An advertisement dated June 30, 1888, was complete with case histories:

> Bertie Norling, 8 years old, of Davenport, Iowa, was in bed 3 days with fever. After one treatment he got up, ate his dinner and went to school.
> A.E. Stiles, of Muscatine, Iowa, was cured of indigestion, in two magnetic treatments.
> Mrs. Coval, of Burlington, had been unable to turn over in bed for 4 years; cured in one treatment.
> Mrs. E. M. Hoxie, 75 years old, of Burlington, was to use her words, "raised from death unto life," in six treatments.
> Where can you get cured quicker or for less money and without making a drug store of yourself? It may not be popular to be cured without medicine, but who cares so long as the sick will get well? Fashionable style has never cured any of suffering humanity, but it has killed thousands. . . .

After the reports, D.D. wrote the following:

> My office is centrally located, being two blocks from the ferry, where you can cross the river for 5 cents; two lines of street cars pass outdoors and a third, one block away; the depots are three and four blocks off. If patients at a distance will write to me, I will secure board and rooms for them. Board can be got at $2.50 per week and up.
> Consultations and treatment for the deserving poor are free. Price of treatments, $1 each at my room; $2 to $5 at patient's residence. Come and see me or write to me, giving me your case briefly as you see it and not what doctors have said, for they are often mistaken. I may not be able to cure you, and if not I don't want your case, and I may have on hand all I can treat; if so, I may require you to wait until I get room for you, looking for some other better way to get cured than by taking medicine, which often does harm and no good.

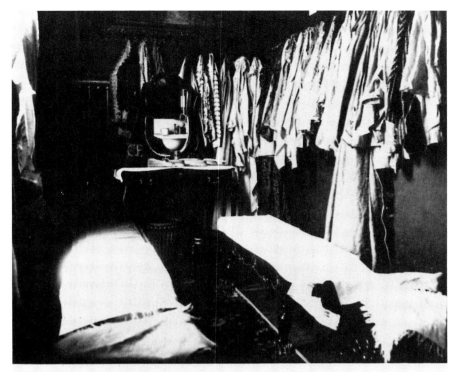

IT WAS ON THESE VERY TABLES THAT 11,389 ADJUSTMENT.
(so called treatments) WERE GIVEN IN 1902.

The interior of one of D.D.'s adjusting rooms in the Ryan Building. Note the cap-
tion below the photograph, written in D.D.'s own hand.
Courtesy Palmer College of Chiropractic Archives, Davenport, Iowa.

At this time, D.D. had Rooms 7, 11, 12, and 13 in the Ryan Building at the corner of Second and Brady Streets. In this suite of rooms, he also prepared another publication, the *Educator*, which he advertised and distributed successfully. Copy about his business appeared in the *Educator*:

> Dr. D.D. Palmer is not only doing a great work in Davenport, Iowa, with his magnetic healing, but somehow he finds time to issue a good looking little monthly folio, called the *Educator*. His *Educator* is designed especially to educate the world on the science of magnetic healing—an education the world needs. There are hundreds of healers who know nothing of the laws underlying their work; they accidentally heal many cases, but they are accidents; and if they understood the law underlying these accidents, and knew how to apply it, they might do much more good than they do.
>
> The *Educator*, besides educating the world on that subject, is a fighter. It fights the vaccination wickedness. While vaccination may, and to our minds does, in many instances, take the edge off of that terrible scourge, small-pox, it imparts in thousands of instances worse and more lasting ills. These things the *Educator* shows up. As the *Educator* is only 25 cents a year, the reader is advised to send and test it for himself or herself.

In 1888, D.D. Palmer had promotional expenses of $150, but his investment was paying dividends. Patients were flocking into his office from not only the Tri-Cities but also many communities that were a day's trip away by horse and buggy.

D.D.'S MAGNETIC HEALING PRACTICE

At age 43, D.D Palmer entered into what could be described as his "golden decade." With his growing magnetic healing practice, additional rooms were leased in 1888. D.D. married his fourth wife, Villa Amanda Thomas of Rock Island, Illinois, who was to be a helpmate to her husband. She assisted him in his practice, taking over the role of manager and tending to patients requiring overnight care and accommodations.

To a large extent, advertising techniques were important to the success of any healing arts practitioner, regardless of the type. Medical doctors often advertised their specialties along with offers of free consultations and examinations. Competition was intense with patent medicines that proclaimed the total efficacy of the products to cure all forms of ailments, real or imaginary. Among these miracle cures were Taylor's Cherokee Remedy and Ayers Sarsaparilla. Many of these nostrums were made of bitter herbs and roots suspended in an alcohol solution of extremely high proof.

In a brochure entitled *The Sick Get Well by Magnetism,* D.D. stated the following:

> There is one great difference in the application of magnetism and medicine. Magnetism is applied directly to the part diseased; but with drugs, the poor stomach has to take the dose, whether guilty or not.
>
> Some of our objectors, when convinced of our cures, say they are not lasting. A careful investigation of the following [testimonials] will convince anyone that they are not only lasting, but that we don't make one disease to cure another.

The best description of D.D.'s personal method of working with his patients comes from his grandson, Dr. David Palmer. In his book, *The Palmers,* Dr. Dave wrote the following:

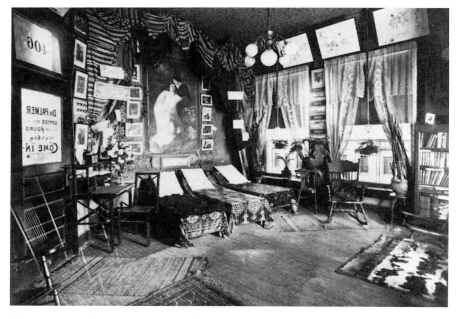

The rather opulent waiting room D.D. provided for his patients in the Ryan Building.

Courtesy Palmer College of Chiropractic Archives, Davenport, Iowa.

D.D. described his method of practicing magnetic healing. He would develop a sense of being positive within his own body; sickness being negative. He would draw his hands over the area of the pain and with a sweeping motion stand aside, shaking his hand and fingers vigorously, taking away the pain as it were drops of water.

About 4 years after he first arrived in Davenport, D.D. again expanded his facilities. An article in a What Cheer newspaper related D.D.'s father's reaction to his visit to Davenport:

> Mr. T. Palmer returned home last Saturday from a 7 weeks stay at Dr. Palmer's Magnetic Cure and Infirmary. . . .
>
> He says . . . He [Dr. Palmer] has 14 rooms which are crowded. He has now rented all the fourth floor, 66 × 76 feet, which will make 24 rooms. . . . His cures are made by the use of his hands only. He treats the cause of disease and not the effects. In finding the cause of disease, or as a physician would say in diagnosing, he often tells patients of their disease or ailments instead of the sick telling him. By this gift of knowing and being able to tell the sick how and where they are diseased better than they can themselves, he often finds causes which other doctors have failed to discover. . . . He wants cases which other doctors cannot cure, and judging by the ones I saw there, he certainly gets them. . . . His patients are mostly from the three cities, but many are from a distance, who board and sleep at the Infirmary. . . . His patients are of all classes, rich and poor, doctors, druggists, preachers and all classes, who cannot be cured by their family physicians. He does not cure all kinds of diseases, not all persons, but most of his patients are cured.

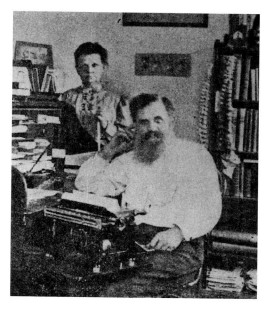

D.D. and his fifth wife, Mary "Molly" Hudler.
Courtesy Palmer College of Chiropractic Archives, Davenport, Iowa.

The sun was shining on D.D. Palmer's life. According to a listing of his accounts, he averaged between $3000 and $4000 per year income at a time when a suit cost $6, a 3-lb tin of baked beans was $0.10, and a hotel room was $2 a day.

There were problems of course. Barbs were often thrust toward D.D. personally and professionally. Inevitably, his response would be quick and vehement. He continued his reading of books, newspapers, and periodicals. D.D. kept careful watch on all forms of health practice so that he could publicly say he was conversant with all healing approaches. Palmer had to study the scientific and the metaphysical to satisfy his two intel-

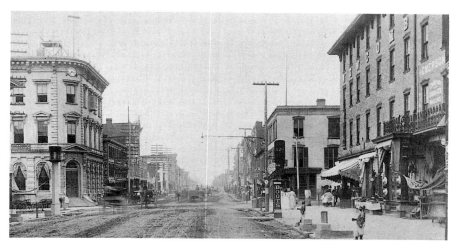

Second Street in Davenport, about the same view that D.D. would have seen when he stepped out of the Ryan Building and looked west.
Courtesy Special Collections, Davenport Public Library, Davenport, Iowa.

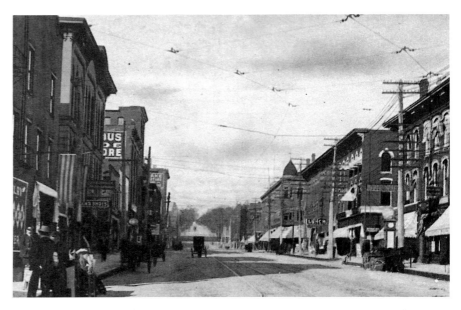

A view of Brady Street in Davenport, about the same view that D.D. would have had when he left the Ryan Building and headed north.

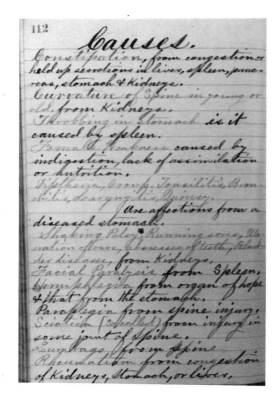

D.D.'s journal, where he recorded his bee-keeping and raspberry-growing data and later kept records of his patients.

lectual sides. Eventually the pragmatic and abstract were to meld in the creation of a dramatic healing art—chiropractic.

During this period of magnetic healing, D.D. Palmer kept news clippings that add insight into his personality and interests. Several clippings appear against vivisection. He also kept and pasted in his journal an editorial referring to him as an ex-coal digger, a quack, and a crank. Another article describes his collection of 80 animal heads in detail. Three articles tell of the 18-year-old May Palmer running away from home and being married to Niles Brownell, a businessman from Pomeroy, Iowa. Another accuses D.D. of treating a patient who later died. D.D.'s small collection of newspaper articles reveals him as a strong personality with conviction. He was willing to speak out on issues important to him and, like many heads of households, was at times unable to cope graciously with his offspring.

THE EVOLUTION OF CHIROPRACTIC

Even though he said it about himself, it may be somewhat improper to herald D.D. Palmer as the *discoverer* of chiropractic. There is an implied connotation of a subtle intellectual enlightenment or revelation. D.D.'s concept was the culmination of years of study in many fields. This may have included knowledge of crude physical manipulations that had been attempted in the past.

The word *invent* also does not totally apply. Palmer's healing art unfolded slowly, spawned from a variety of thought-provoking avenues. His creation was the sum of many parts.

History repeatedly indicates that a broad range of physical manipulations were used to help the ailing throughout the world. Hippocrates, the American Indian, Chinese, and Africans used a form of manipulation.

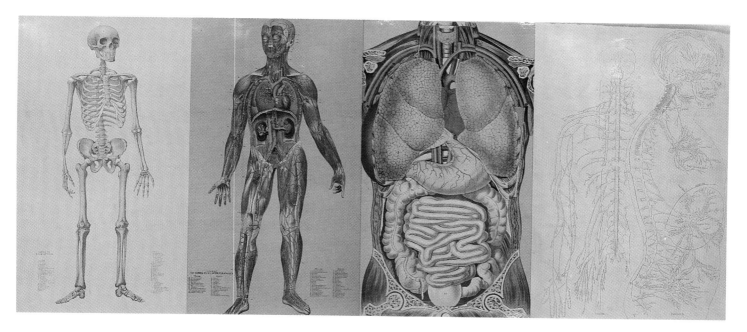

Examples of illustrations from Yaggy's Anatomical Study *by L.W. Yaggy & James J. West, 1885. D.D. probably would have used a chart similar to this one in his office.*

Courtesy Palmer College of Chiropractic Archives, Davenport, Iowa.

At the time of the American Revolution, Dr. Benjamin Rush, noted physician and politician, briefly delved into the field with a fellow scientist in Scotland. In the early nineteenth century, evidence suggests medical practitioners experimented with manipulation.

The first chiropractic adjustment was important. However, D.D. Palmer's major contribution to the health field was the codification of the philosophy, science, and art of chiropractic. His contemplative nature was a strength as he devised the philosophy of the new health art. The scientific rationale was wrested from a background of systematic study in anatomy and physiology. The art of chiropractic began with the very first spinal adjustment and developed from it.

D.D. performed the initial chiropractic adjustment in September 1895. In *The Chiropractor's Adjustor,* he wrote the following:

> Harvey Lillard, a janitor in the Ryan Block, where I had my office, had been so deaf for 17 years that he could not hear the racket of a wagon on the street or the ticking of a watch. I made inquiry as to the cause of his deafness and was informed that when he was exerting himself in a cramped, stooping position, he felt something give in his back and immediately became deaf. An examination showed a vertebra racked from its normal position. I reasoned that if that vertebra was replaced, the man's hearing should be restored. With this object in view, a half-hour' talk persuaded Mr. Lillard to allow me to replace it. I racked it into position by using the spinous process as a lever and soon the man could hear as before. There was nothing "accidental" about this, as it was accomplished with an object in view, and the result expected was obtained. There was nothing "crude" about this adjustment; it was specific, so much so that no Chiropractor has equaled it.

This classic chiropractic statement reveals an assured and self-confident D.D. Palmer. It is a carefully pruned presentation with the mark of D.D.'s skillful way with words. From other accounts, it is a truthful rendition of events as they occurred, perhaps omitting any uncertainty that D.D. may have had at the time of this first experiment.

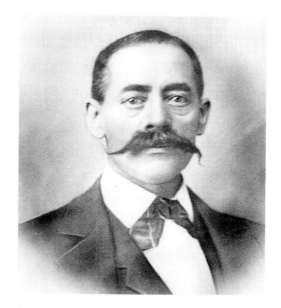

Harvey Lillard, an African-American who operated a janitorial service in the Ryan building, was D.D.'s first chiropractic patient. Ironically, it would be over 50 years before the Palmer School would admit African-Americans.

Courtesy Palmer College of Chiropractic Archives, Davenport, Iowa.

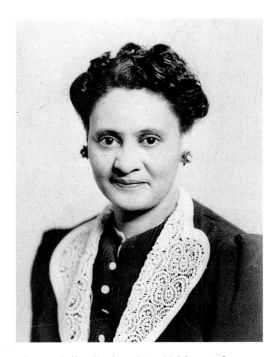

Harvey Lillard's daughter, Valdeenia Simons.
Courtesy Palmer College of Chiropractic Archives, Davenport, Iowa.

Harvey Lillard had been under care at D.D.'s Infirmary and Cure. Palmer was perplexed with Lillard's case. He had treated the janitor by a series of magnetic healing passes over the spine. In doing so, he had noticed a "peculiar bump" on the man's back. When he rubbed this area, he determined there was something "out of place." He then carefully palpated the spine to confirm his thoughts.

D.D. tried to reduce the "bump" over a period. As his various approaches failed, he became more positive and direct in his attempts, and ultimately the vertebra slipped in place. Within a couple of minutes, Lillard could hear a watch ticking a foot and a half from his ear with the other ear blocked.

Harvey Lillard's daughter, Mrs. Valdeenia Simons, recalled what had been told to her by her father many years before. According to Mrs. Simons, her father and a friend were telling humorous stories outside the open doorway leading to D.D. Palmer's office. D.D. was reading a book in his favorite chair. Overhearing the loud conversation, Palmer decided to join the two men and walked into the hall where they were standing.

Obviously enjoying the story's climax, D.D., laughing heartily, struck Harvey on the back with the book he had carried with him. Several days later, Lillard commented to Palmer that he thought he could hear a bit better following the merriment of the storytelling and the back-slapping incident.

D.D. commented, "We'll try to do something about that." Shortly, he began working with Lillard to restore his hearing. Valdeenia's explanation of the circumstances leading to the first adjustment is supportive of Palmer's comment that the first adjustment was "accomplished with an object in view."

Harvey Lillard later left Davenport, spending much of his life in Seattle where he continued to work as a janitor. He died on September 7, 1925.

As D.D. explored further, his attitude became more emphatic on his next adjustment. Of it he wrote the following:

> Shortly after this relief from deafness, I had a case of heart trouble which was not improving. I examined the spine and found a displaced vertebrae pressing against the nerves which innervate the heart. I adjusted the vertebra and gave immediate relief—nothing "accidental" or "crude" about this. Then I began to reason if two diseases, so dissimilar as deafness and heart trouble, came from impingement, a pressure on

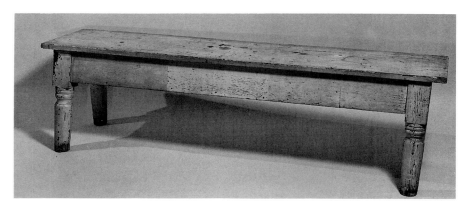

The table upon which D.D. delivered the first adjustment.
Courtesy Palmer College of Chiropractic Archives, Davenport, Iowa.

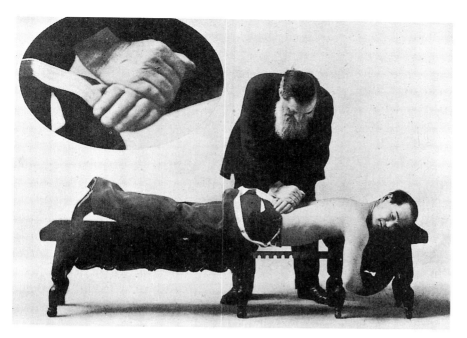

One of the few photographs of D.D. Palmer giving an adjustment.
From Palmer DD, Palmer BJ: *The science of chiropractic; it's principles and adjustments,* 1906.

nerves, were not other diseases due to a similar cause? Thus the science (knowledge) and art (adjusting) of chiropractic were formed at that time. I then began a systematic investigation for the cause of all diseases and have been amply rewarded.

With the conviction he had indeed made a profound inroad on the mysteries of health, D.D. now became quite secretive. His experimentation was done in private and in almost complete obscurity. The rooms in which he worked were darkened. Heavy drapes were drawn over the windows. Observations of his palpations and adjustments were impossible to discern by others who might be in the room.

His grandson, David D. Palmer, noted the following about D.D.:

Patients were adjusted lying face downward on the floor. (The adjusting table had not been thought of as yet.) Many of the patients left my grandfather's office with sore noses and jaws. Not a few left the office with a telltale red handkerchief held to their noses.

My grandfather was a practical practitioner and having had a lot of experience with people over his 50 years felt this new "discovery" to be so simple he was afraid someone would see how it was done and become a competitor in Davenport. He wanted to keep the discovery for himself.

This all seems pretty humorous to us now, but in those days, "bone setters" were apt to try to keep their ability from others by claiming that their success was due to an inherent sense of "feel" or as in grandfather's case, a magnetic ability not teachable or transferable to others.

To illustrate this point, Dad once told me this story. In D.D.'s treatment room there used to hang a long mirror which was used to see the patient's facial expressions during the adjusting thrust. The patient's face was always carefully kept turned the other way so he could not see the adjustment. And, I think, if it was necessary for the patient to face the mirror, D.D. stood between the patient and mirror.

This became a bother after a time. One day D.D. forgot his customary precaution. He noticed the patient carefully studying him. D.D. took the mirror from the wall and broke it into a thousand pieces. After that no mirror was allowed in the treatment room.

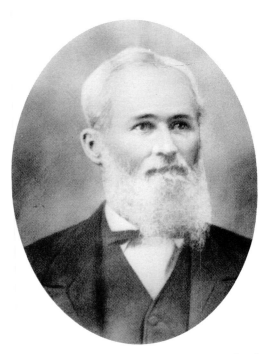

Samuel Weed, a Presbyterian minister, Greek scholar, and patient of D.D.'s who helped name chiropractic.

Courtesy Palmer College of Chiropractic Archives, Davenport, Iowa.

Previous writings such as in *The Magnetic* indicate D.D. was looking toward the *cause* of disease. This is where his concern was strongest and the field in which he worked in the long months after the first adjustment.

The extensive knowledge D.D. accumulated over the years now began to be its own reward. The strong convictions held by Palmer about the importance of his discovery apparently came soon after the first adjustment. D.D. quickly sought a name for his new health science. With the help of a patient and friend, the Reverend Samuel Weed, a word was coined. The "birth date" of the newly created word, *chiropractic,* was January 14, 1896.

A veteran of the Civil War, Reverend Weed had suffered some health problems as a soldier. One of his 11 children, a daughter, had gone to D.D. Palmer for magnetic healing treatments for a dislocated ankle in 1893. After her initial treatment at the hands of D.D., she returned home "carrying her crutches in her hands, walking on that sore foot."

In July 1894, prodded by his daughter, Reverend Weed went to D.D. for help. Weed continued to see D.D. Palmer both for magnetic healing and in 1895 for adjustments. D.D. told Weed he had discovered a new method of treatment for which he had no name. Reverend Weed, who had studied Hebrew and Greek and was something of a linguist, suggested three or four different names. Palmer looked them over and decided to use *chiropractic* from *cheir,* which means "hand" in Greek, and *praktos,* meaning "done."

D.D. Palmer's discovery was now named and a new era was born for the practitioner along the banks of the Mississippi. His golden decade was almost at an end as new challenges began to surface for the enigmatic healer.

EARLY CHIROPRACTIC PRACTICE

When D.D. Palmer founded chiropractic and began to practice and teach the fledgling art, he became embroiled in two major philosophical shifts, both of which originated in Germany. The Teutonic nation was determined to become the leader in all scientific pursuits, including medicine. The other area was in education; a rationale by which young people were taught to become more productive and useful citizens. These massive changes transpired in the latter half of the nineteenth century, and they were aggravating obstacles to Palmer's infant profession. The vigor of the Germans efficiently established them as leaders in science. In the ebb and flow between the schools of vitalistic and scientific thought, there was investigation into the sciences as the world had never seen before. Findings were promptly reported, and a scientific era was born at the very time D.D. Palmer could least afford it in terms of acceptance of his chiropractic profession.

D.D. Palmer was of the old school of teaching. During his era as a schoolmaster, it was his responsibility to teach children regardless of their ability to learn. His pupils, whether dullards or geniuses, were given the information with the expectation that information taught was education gained.

It was also customary of D.D.'s time that if a craft were taught, it would be offered without additional background or peripheral education. If a pupil studied to become a magnetic healer, for example, this is what was

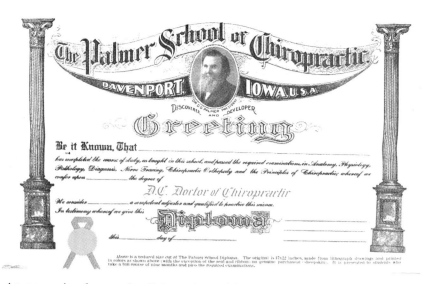

An example of an early diploma issued by D.D. while he was in Davenport.

Courtesy Palmer College of Chiropractic Archives, Davenport, Iowa.

taught. Nothing else was offered. A behavioral psychologist from Germany, Wilhelm Maximilian Wundt, changed this philosophy. Wundt believed that people are only what their experiences or stimuli allow them to be. His theories influenced John Dewey, a prominent American specialist in education. Dewey placed into practice three of the revolutionary beliefs he culled from the new psychology: to put children in possession of their fullest talents, education should be active rather than passive; to prepare children for a democratic society, schools should be social rather than individualistic; and to enable children to think creatively, experimentation rather than imitation should be encouraged.

Dewey's approach was in direct opposition to D.D. Palmer's background. No longer was it enough to just teach chiropractic. Now it became necessary to teach the subject with the support of other relevant topics.

As D.D. continued his work with chiropractic, he was extremely reluctant to share his discovery with others. But one day, an event took place that changed his mind about his healing discovery and who should practice it. In the *Adjustor*, D.D. wrote the following:

> Two years after the first adjustment was given I came near being killed at Clinton Junction, Illinois. I then determined to teach the science and art to some one as fast as it was unfolded. LeRoy Baker, of Fulton, Illinois, was my first student. He was not a graduate as represented by the "enveloper." If I had been snatched from earth-life it might have been a long time before the same combination of circumstances, combined with the same makeup of an individual, would evolve a science such as I saw in Chiropractic, therefore, I taught it as learned.

During this period, D.D. was optimistic and excited. He rewarded himself in 1897 with what proved to be among his proudest possessions, a matched team of Pinto ponies. A small surrey was made, and he raced up and down the streets and hills of Davenport behind the spirited team of Nip and Tuck. The combination of beautiful horses, a unique surrey, and Palmer was excellent promotion for his practice. Business continued to be good despite the encroachment of the medical establishment now dead set against "quacks" of any kind.

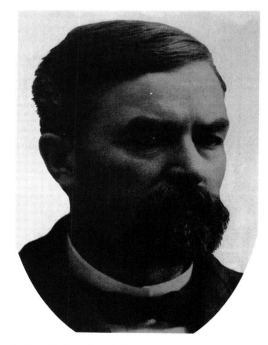

LeRoy Baker, D.D.'s first student, with whom D.D. decided to share his knowledge of chiropractic after he was involved in a near fatal accident.

Courtesy Palmer College of Chiropractic Archives, Davenport, Iowa.

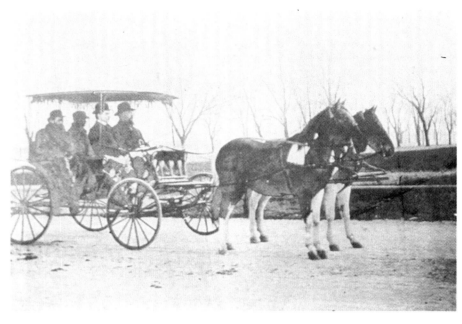

D.D. pictured with his matched pair of pinto ponies, Nip and Tuck.
Courtesy Palmer College of Chiropractic Archives, Davenport, Iowa.

D.D. Palmer did not practice in the morning. An account tells of 91 patients seated in the healer's reception room waiting for 1:00 PM, the appointed hour for D.D. to start his practice. As patients would come into his office, each would take a number from a hook. Later, as the matron would call out numbers, the patients would go into D.D.'s room for a chiropractic "treatment."

The patients were in the treatment room for only a brief period of time, usually about half a minute. This would indicate that Palmer no longer practiced magnetic healing. His charges were $10 a week for treatments. If continuing services were needed, charges were $5 a week.

THE BEGINNINGS OF CHIROPRACTIC EDUCATION

In January 1898, William A. Seeley became D.D. Palmer's first full-fledged student. The fee set by D.D. was $500. Initially, he wanted only two students to educate at a time. From a relatively small start, the educational process was underway at the Palmer School and Infirmary of Chiropractic at the corner of Second and Brady Streets in Davenport, Iowa.

The school at the foot of Brady Street had slow beginnings. Few students sought to embrace the new health science. D.D. Palmer once again began to write using the format that had served him so well in the past. As a result, these sometimes controversial publications spurred interest in the new healing art.

Because of his extensive background, D.D. was most capable of setting forth the premise that chiropractic was unique. In *The Chiropractic* published in 1899, D.D. was a mechanist. In extremely simple and effective language, he wrote the following:

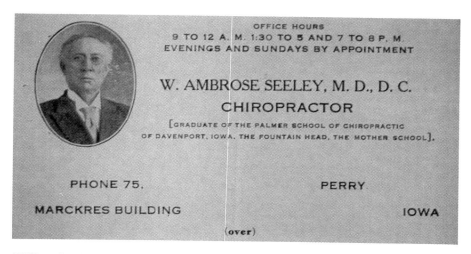

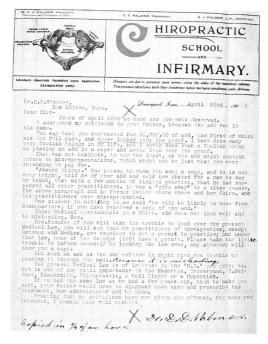

William Seeley, D.D.'s second student.
Courtesy Palmer College of Chiropractic Archives, Davenport, Iowa.

The 1902 letterhead of the Chiropractic School and Infirmary, with D.D.'s signature.
Courtesy Palmer College of Chiropractic Archives, Davenport, Iowa.

A human being is a human machine and like a machine, would run smoothly, without any friction, if every part was in its proper place. If every bone, every nerve and all the blood vessels, muscles, etc. were just right, there would be nothing wrong. . . .

Disease is the effect or result of some part of the body being disarranged. To put them in their proper place would give the diseased person ease and allow nature to rebuild without being obstructed.

We do not go the drug store nor ransack all creation to find a remedy. The remedy is in righting the wrong. The cause of the disease is in the sufferer, and the cause must be corrected. . . .

If every part of the human body was in its natural place there would be no friction, no inflammation, no fever, no weakness. . . . Why not remove the pressure, adjust the framework, and take the strain off those sensitive nerves?

As to the question, what is chiropractic healing? D.D. wrote the following:

It is a scientific method of treating diseases. It is a new and radical departure from all other known methods. Chiropractic healing uses no drugs or chemicals, no surgical operations. . . .

Chiropractic healers need a knowledge of the anatomical construction of the human body and the physiological laws governing the distributing of its vital fluids and forces.

Chiropractic healing simplifies the treatment of the most painful and prostrating forms of diseases. The human body is a very sensitive and delicately constructed piece of machinery. As the good book says: "We are fearfully and wonderfully made." There are numerous accidents which are liable to injure and misplace the various parts of this highly sensitive, nervous system. . . .

A pressure upon any one of the nerves causes such diseases as paralysis, rheumatism, neuralgia, asthma, female diseases and the numerous diseases of the stomach, liver and kidneys. All motor and sensory powers are derived through the nerves. How necessary then it is that they should be perfectly free to act. Strange but true, all the nerves of the body may be reached and acted upon by the hands.

Some years later, D.D. Palmer added concepts to his literature. The philosophical school of vitalism, so attractive to the metaphysical side of the healer, prompted him to write the following:

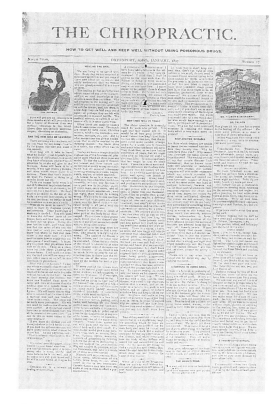

An issue of D.D.'s promotional journal, the Chiropractic, *which promised to inform the reader "How to Get Well and Keep Well Without Using Poisonous Drugs."*
Courtesy Palmer College of Chiropractic Archives, Davenport, Iowa.

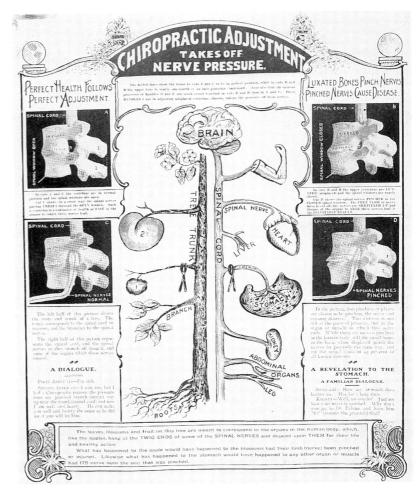

An early chart explaining chiropractic to the lay person.
From *Chiropractic Proofs* by B.J. Palmer, 1903.

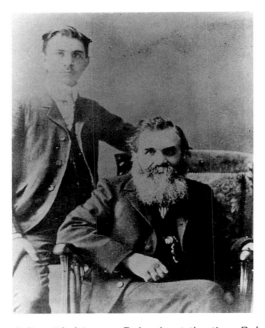

D.D. with his son, B.J., about the time B.J. earned his degree in chiropractic.
Courtesy Palmer College of Chiropractic Archives, Davenport, Iowa.

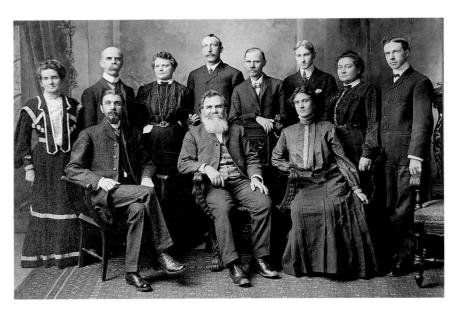

D.D., B.J., Mabel Health Palmer, and early graduates.
Courtesy Palmer College of Chiropractic Archives, Davenport, Iowa.

Man is a physical and spiritual epitome of the Universe. *The spiritual is the cause of action.* Action is life. The spiritual always did exist, always will. It is eternal, it is changeless. . . .

The linking together of the spiritual and physical, makes it *our duty to keep the corporal frame in proper alignment.* . . .

During this period, D.D. Palmer became belligerent in his writings toward osteopathy founded by A.T. Still and taught by his school in Kirksville, Missouri. A.T. Still and D.D. had many similarities. Both had been magnetic healers. Each sought religious comfort in spiritualism. Both had total confidence in their approaches to cure the ills of humanity. According to Still's biography, D.D. visited Still at his school in Missouri at least once.

In 1900, D.D. experienced his first setback as an educator. A student, H.H. Reiring of Chicago, filed suit against D.D. for misrepresenting his school. The plaintiff sought redress on the basis that the school did not offer what had been advertised. Reiring also maintained D.D. was "grossly ignorant of anatomy, physiology, therapeutics, pathology and true medicine and surgery." When Reiring suspected he was not getting anything of value from Palmer, he obtained the services of an attorney to get his tuition refunded. The case did not go to trial and was dismissed on the application of Reiring in 1901. There were similar cases in the future for Palmer's school, but most were resolved in favor of the educational institution, which slowly moved into Wundt's theory of learning.

On January 6, 1902, four students graduated as Doctors of Chiropractic. Among them was D.D.'s son Bartlett Joshua. Before attending his father's school, B.J. had been a sales clerk at St. Onge's Department Store, which operated on the ground level floor of the Ryan Building, and had practiced chiropractic without the benefit of formal schooling in Iowa, Michigan, and West Virginia.

After graduating, B.J. practiced in his father's school and infirmary. D.D. had added more students to the rolls and had a bustling set of offices seeing people from many parts of the country. The activity did not go unnoticed. On April 16, 1902, B.J. was indicted for publicly professing to cure and heal without having procured and filed a certificate with the board of medical examiners.

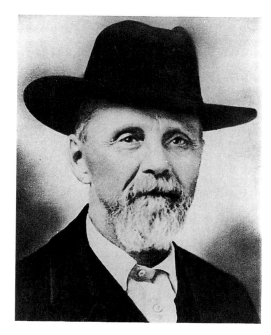

A.T. Still, the founder of osteopathy.
Courtesy Still National Museum of Osteopathy, Kirksville, Missouri.

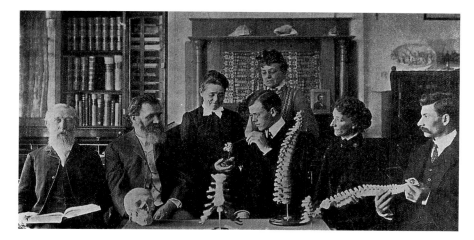

D.D. in the classroom, circa 1904.
Courtesy Palmer College of Chiropractic Archives, Davenport, Iowa.

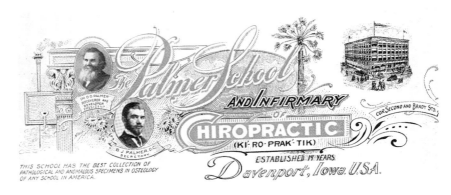

Letterhead of the Palmer School and Infirmary of Chiropractic.

Courtesy Palmer College of Chiropractic Archives, Davenport, Iowa.

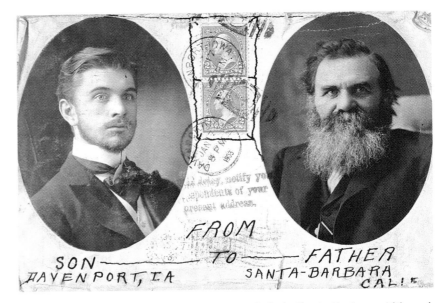

A 1903 postcard from B.J. in Davenport to D.D. in Santa Barbara. Although the postcard was returned for lack of an address, the Davenport Post Office knew to whom to return the card.

Courtesy Palmer College of Chiropractic Archives, Davenport, Iowa.

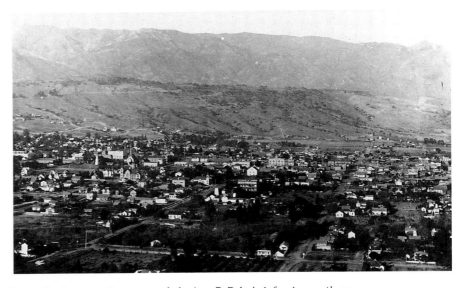

Santa Barbara as it appeared during D.D.'s brief sojourn there.

Courtesy Santa Barbara Public Library, Santa Barbara, Calif.

Although the trial was regularly delayed with no final disposition of the case, it may have been fear of similar legal maneuvers that prompted D.D. Palmer to make an inexplicable move. Without notice or explanation in late 1902, D.D. packed his household items from the many rooms of his infirmary and left Davenport. D.D. had received an urgent message from the family of Tom Storey, one of D.D.'s early graduates, telling him that Storey had disappeared suddenly and asking Palmer to help find him. D.D. found him in California and stayed to start a new school in Santa Barbara. Oakley Smith and Minora Paxson, the first woman chiropractor, joined him as faculty.

In the meantime, B.J., young and inexperienced, had taken over the bare facility, receiving financial support from L. Howard Nutting, Willard Carver's uncle. When D.D. returned to Davenport in late 1903, he and B.J. established an equal partnership that continued until May of 1906.

1905-1906—YEARS OF TURMOIL

In 1905, the Palmer Infirmary moved to 828 Brady Street. The property was a large Victorian house ideally suited to the purposes of the two Palmer families. B.J. and his bride lived in the house, which also accommodated the school's classrooms. D.D. and his wife resided nearby at 1518 Rock Island Street (now Pershing Avenue) in Davenport. In October 1905, D.D. was indicted for practicing medicine without a license. In November 1905, D.D.'s wife Villa died under tragic circumstances of an overdose of morphine. Villa Palmer had been in poor health for many years. She had sustained a fracture of the spine in a runaway accident while driving a team of ponies and frequently took morphine for the pain.

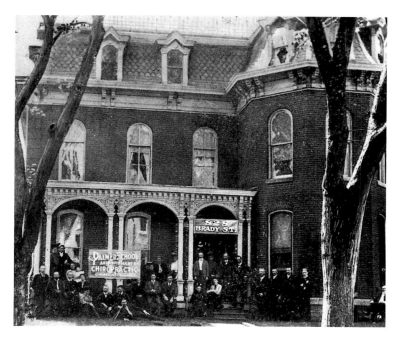

The Palmer School moved out of the Ryan Building and into this building at 828 Brady Street in late 1904.

Courtesy Palmer College of Chiropractic Archives, Davenport, Iowa.

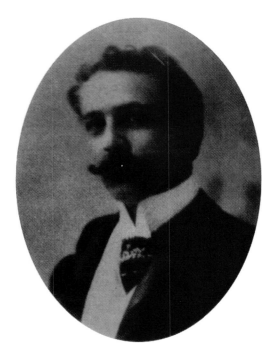

Solon Langworthy, a graduate of D.D.'s who started a chiropractic school in nearby Cedar Rapids, Iowa.

Courtesy Palmer College of Chiropractic Archives, Davenport, Iowa.

Also during 1905, two rival schools started nearby, one in Cedar Rapids, the American School of Chiropractic and Nature Cure, and the other in Ottumwa, Iowa, the Parker School of Chiropractic. The president of the Cedar Rapids school, Solon Langworthy, fostered a chiropractic law in Minnesota that annoyed D.D. Palmer because it liberally grandfathered untrained healers as chiropractors and allowed traction in chiropractic practice. D.D. made a hurried visit in 1906 to the governor of Minnesota and urged him to veto the bill, which the governor later did.

In January 1906, D.D. married his fifth wife, Mary Hudler. D.D.'s namesake grandson, Daniel David, was born to B.J. and Mabel. Although the year had begun auspiciously, the indictment for practicing medicine without a license was still hanging over D.D.'s head and would see him jailed before the summer was out.

The trial was brief. The jury was selected March 26, the state presented its case, and the case went to the jury at 12 PM March 27. The state used statements in *The Chiropractor* to claim that Palmer violated the law, and the jury quickly concurred. It was the first conviction in the county court on the charge of practicing medicine without a license. D.D. was fined $350. Had D.D. started his career as a magnetic healer in 1881, 5 years before he did in 1886, he would have been eligible for a certificate grandfathering him the legal right to practice.

D.D. was determined to serve out his sentence rather than pay his fine. When the judge asked D.D. if he had anything to say as to why he should not be sentenced, D.D. launched into a speech on the discovery and merits of chiropractic. After one particularly spirited declaration that the law had been made for the benefit of the doctors of medicine and was an infamous measure, the judge rebuked D.D. and ordered him to remain quiet the rest of the time he remained in the courtroom.

The Palmer trial and imprisonment received a lot of attention from the press. On April 2, the *Davenport Democrat and Leader* ran the following headlines:

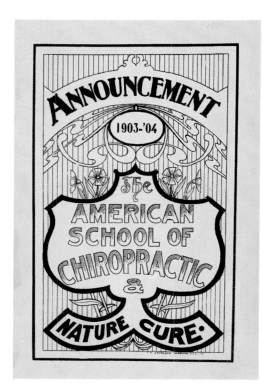

An announcement from Solon Langworthy's American School of Chiropractic, the first serious competitor to the Palmer school.

From American School of Chiropractic and Nature Cure: Announcement, 1903.

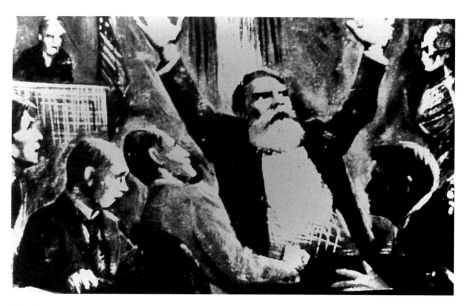

The drama of D.D.'s trial in 1906 for practicing medicine without a license.

From Maynard J: *Healing hands.*

Will Serve Out Entire Sen-
Tence Rather Than to
Pay Fine

Confined in a Cell 9 × 11 Feet in
Dimensions and Treated as Ordinary Prisoner

D.D. was allowed to set up his typewriter in his cell and produced over 40 column inches of newspaper copy under the heading of "Chiropractic Sunbeams." In it, he declared the following:

> The advancement of all sciences, especially when there has been such a radical change, have been attended with persecution. In fact it seems necessary in order to bring it to public attention. Thousands are now talking Chiropractic and its discoverer, who never knew of it before. The jailing of D.D. Palmer, a man who is ahead of the times, a man who dares to think, even in a cell, where the walls are iron and the floor of the best cement, will not check the onward march of the science he has discovered.

Evidently D.D. tired of his cell. He had turned 61 years old March 7, and the cell was obviously confining to his independent spirit. On April 20, Mrs. Palmer inquired about his release, and the newspaper carried these headlines the next day:

DR. D.D. PALMER
PAYS HIS FINE

Discoverer of Chiropractic
Released from Jail
Saturday

Striding out of the jail into the sunshine of freedom, D.D. walked out into a familiar world, however, a world which now had changed for him and never would be the same for the rest of his life.

D.D. LEAVES DAVENPORT

When D.D. had been indicted, B.J. had sent a telegram to Willard Carver urging him to come at once. Carver was in Ottumwa completing his course of chiropractic at the Parker School. The attorney and soon-to-be chiropractor met with D.D. in the jailhouse. He found D.D. very upset about the situation.

Carver made some recommendations to D.D. and his son: first, that the publications sent out from the Palmer School should be "edited" by a medical doctor and that the business affairs of the school should also be managed by someone who belonged to the American Medical Association. This was done with the use of M.P. Brown, M.D., D.C. Because of vulnerability to malpractice suits, other executions, and judgements, it was decided to transfer all property to Mabel H. Palmer, B.J.'s wife. Further, Willard Carver made an attempt to meet with the governor of Iowa to arrange a pardon for D.D. This mission apparently met with failure.

After D.D.'s release from confinement, he returned to the top of Brady Street Hill. On April 30, after lecturing at the school for a few days, D.D. sold his half of the school for $2196.79. D.D. had originally asked $3500 dollars for his interest in the school, and the final purchase price was decided with the help of a committee.

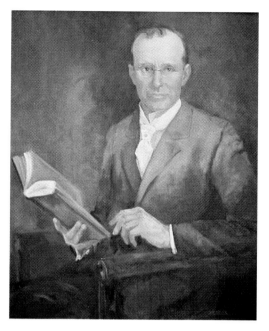

Willard Carver, once D.D.'s attorney, who became a chiropractor and rival schoolman.
Courtesy Texas College of Chiropractic, Pasadena, Texas.

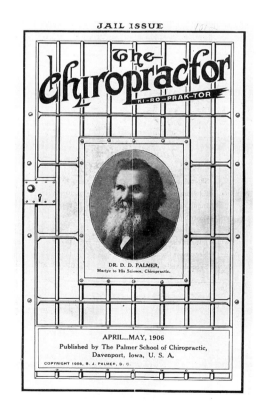

The cover of an issue of D.D.'s and B.J.'s journal the Chiropractor *while D.D. was in the Scott County jail.*
From *The Chiropractor* Apr-May 1906.

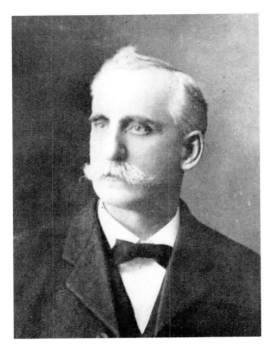

M.P. Brown, a medical doctor who was hired to act as a shield against charges of practicing medicine without a license.
Courtesy Palmer College of Chiropractic Archives, Davenport, Iowa.

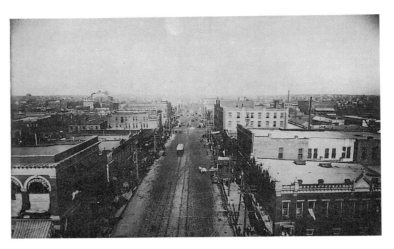

Oklahoma City circa 1907, about the time D.D. started his school there, the D.D. Palmer School of Chiropractic.
Courtesy Oklahoma City Public Library, Oklahoma City.

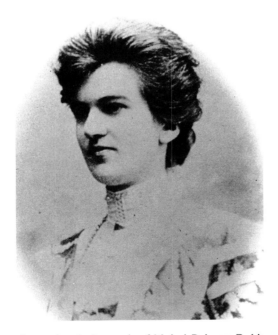

An early photograph of Mabel Palmer, B.J.'s wife and in whose name the school and its contents were registered.
Courtesy Palmer College of Chiropractic Archives, Davenport, Iowa.

After leaving Davenport, D.D. went to Medford, Oklahoma, where his brother Thomas J. was the publisher of the local newspaper. D.D. opened a grocery business, which was successful. Willard Carver, in conjunction with L.L. Denny, had opened a chiropractic school only a short distance away in Oklahoma City. Carver invited D.D. to come and lecture at his school, and D.D. did so after starting his own school with Alva Gregory, a recent graduate of Carver's school. The Palmer-Gregory affiliation lasted only 3 months, and D.D. was soon conducting his own separate institution in Oklahoma City, the D.D. Palmer School of Chiropractic. It is likely that D.D. also made a trip to Portland, Oregon, midyear and started a school there, the Gorby-Hinkley School. In October 1908, D.D. published the first issue of the *Chiropractic Adjustor.* The cover pictured Palmer and one of the more popular statements attributed to D.D.: "The most WONDERFUL study of mankind is man. Relieving human suffering and diffusing universal knowledge is humanitarian." A good portion of the brochure is devoted to an explanation of the words *fountain head.* He maintained that as the founder of chiropractic, wherever he chose to locate would become the fountain head.

Evidently the school in Oklahoma City did not last long, and in November 1908, D.D. went to Portland and started a school there, the D.D. Palmer College of Chiropractic. Palmer was its president and Leroy Gordon, a graduate of the original Palmer School in Iowa, soon became his partner. By 1909, John LaValley had replaced Gordon as manager of the college, and the institution had moved from the Oregonian Building to the fourth floor of the Drexel Building at Southwest Second Avenue and Yamhill.

Palmer initially proposed an 18-month curriculum including dissection, minor surgery, and obstetrics for a yearly tuition of $250. In November 1909 the first class graduated, so the course was likely 12 months rather than 18. When D.D. left Oregon in early 1910, his college ceased to operate, and the fate of his second class is unclear. Apparently the last issue of his journal the *Adjuster* was published in February 1910.

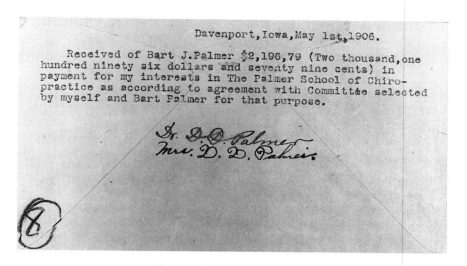

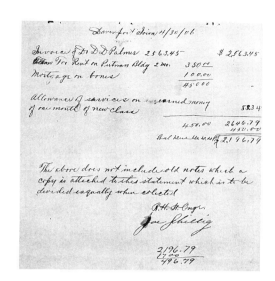

The purchase agreement whereby B.J. purchased D.D.'s half of the school for $2196.79.

Courtesy Palmer College of Chiropractic Archives, Davenport, Iowa.

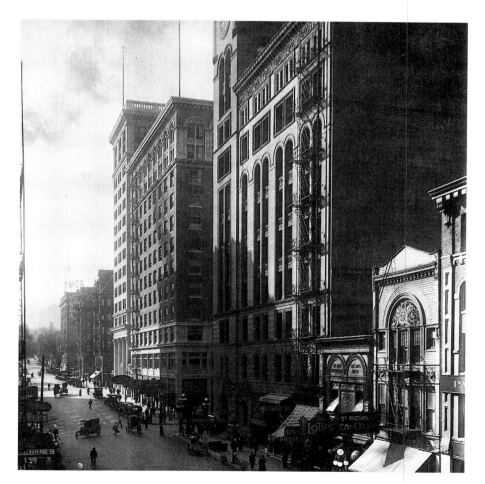

The Oregonian Building in Portland, Oregon, where D.D. had his offices in 1908 through 1909.

Courtesy Oregon Historical Society, Portland, Oregon.

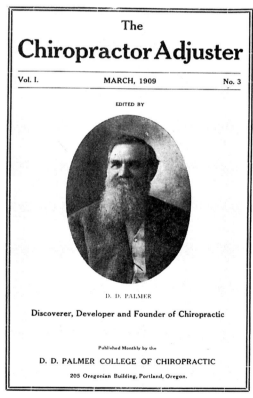

The cover of the third issue of the Chiropractic Adjuster, D.D.'s journal while he was in Portland, Oregon.

From Chiropractor Adjuster Mar 1909.

THE DEATH CERTIFICATE.

Form Health 47 B

HEALTH DEPARTMENT—CERTIFICATE OF DEATH

No. **B 1075**

Los Angeles, California, U. S. A. Feb. 17, 1914, **191**
Name **Daniel David Palmer.** Age of the Decedent **68 yrs. 7 mo. 14 days.** Nativity **Can.** Date of Death **Oct. 20, 1913.** Cause of Death **Typhoid fever.** Race **White.** Sex **Male.** Place of Death **Los Angeles, Cal.** Where Buried **Los Angeles, Crematory.** Physician in attendance **M. R. McBurney, M. D.** Issued at the request of **C. H. Murphy.** Fee received **50c.**

JNO. S. MYERE   **H. SIEP**
City Auditor.   Mortuary Clerk.

I CERTIFY that the above is a true abstract from the Records of Death in Health Office of the City of Los Angeles, California.

L. M. POWEST, M. D.
Health Commissioner.

I, **Chas. L. Wilde,** City Clerk of the City of Los Angeles, do hereby certify that **L. M. Powest, M. D.,** whose name is hereto attached, is the duly appointed, acting and qualified Health Commissioner of the City of Los Angeles.

IN WITNESS WHEREOF, I have hereunto set my hand and affixed the corporate seal of the City of Los Angeles, this **17th** day of **Feb., 1914.**

CHAS. C. WILDE, City Clerk.
R. DOMINQUEZ, Deputy.

The wording of D.D.'s death certificate, listing the cause of death as typhoid fever.

From Palmer BJ: *With malice aforethought,* 1915.

Very little is known about D.D. Palmer's activities after he left Portland. He did lecture extensively after the publication of his *Text-Book of the Science, Art and Philosophy of Chiropractic,* more popularly known as *The Chiropractor's Adjustor.* While in Portland, he had spent much time and effort compiling what was essentially an anthology of his previous writings. Additions discussed more contemporary issues on chiropractic and the personalities involved in the profession.

D.D. Palmer returned to Davenport only occasionally. He had not fully reconciled with B.J. and so aligned himself with the Universal Chiropractic College and Joy Loban.

In the spring of 1911, D.D. and his wife Mary took up residence at 42nd Street and Grand in Los Angeles. There he continued to lecture and write. D.D. taught at the Ratledge College of Chiropractic, which was also located in Los Angeles.

The founder of chiropractic died at 8:00 AM, Monday, October 20, 1913, at his home 420 West Vernon Avenue, Los Angeles. The cause of death was typhoid fever; he had been ill for 28 days. According to the death certificate, a "tendency for years to brain congestion" also contributed to his death. The effects of "brain congestion," a term no longer in common use, ran the gamut from ringing in the ears to arteriosclerosis to massive cerebral accidents. Because of this ambivalent definition, it is impossible to establish what health problems D.D. may have suffered in his later years. In retrospect, it may account for his occasional outbursts of extreme anger and actions not consistent with his early years.

D.D.'s remains were cremated and the ashes reposed in an urn placed for view in the plinth of his heroic-scaled bronze bust on the campus of Palmer College of Chiropractic. In the spring of 1981, to avoid desecration at the hands of vandals, the ashes were removed from the base of

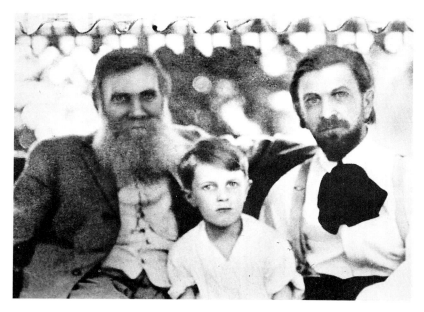

This photograph of the three generations of Palmers was taken in Davenport in the summer of 1913, shortly before D.D.'s death.

Courtesy Palmer College of Chiropractic Archives, Davenport, Iowa.

the statue and placed in the family crypt in the mausoleum of Oakdale Cemetery in Davenport.

D.D.'s last journey to the Tri-Cities had been in the previous summer of 1912, a visit that set the stage for bizarre allegations and bitter legal encounters. His return to the Midwest had been prompted by a desire to visit some friends in Rock Island. Frank Elliot, Palmer School registrar and night clinic director, discussed D.D.'s visit with B.J. and Mabel and

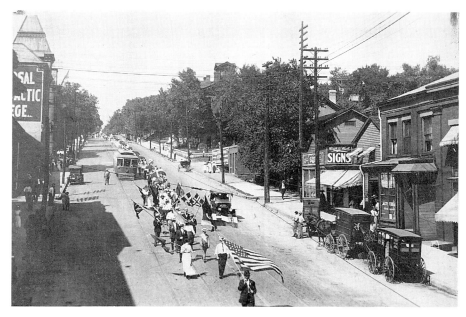

The 1913 Palmer lyceum parade in which D.D. allegedly was struck by B.J.'s car. The grand jury refused to indict B.J. and all charges were dropped.

Courtesy Palmer College of Chiropractic Archives, Davenport, Iowa.

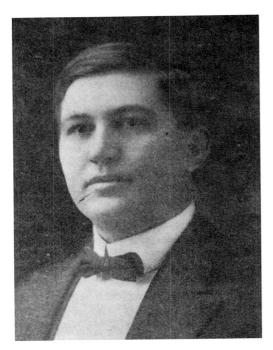

Frank Elliott, Mabel Palmer's cousin and manager of business affairs for the Palmer School for many years.

Courtesy Palmer College of Chiropractic Archives, Davenport, Iowa.

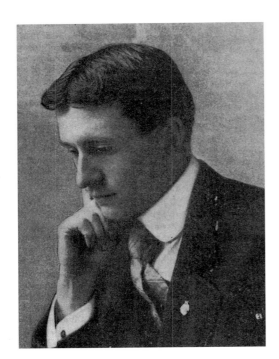

Joy Loban, President of Universal College of Chiropractic and executor of D.D.'s estate.

Courtesy Palmer College of Chiropractic Archives, Davenport, Iowa.

made the suggestion that D.D. take part in the annual lyceum that was about to occur on campus. Elliott, along with Cornelius Murphy, D.D.'s long-time friend and attorney, extended the invitation to D.D. in person. Along with the invitation to the lyceum, it was also offered that the elder Palmer was welcome as a house guest at B.J.'s home on 808 Brady Street.

D.D. accepted the invitation, and while on the campus of the school, he posed for a photograph that included the three generations of Palmers—D.D., B.J., and Dave—the only one of its kind.

As part of lyceum, a parade formed in front of the school. The head or starting point of procession was down the street at 8th and Brady. The American flag was to lead the parade, followed by a band, an open car in which D.D. was to ride with faculty, and another open vehicle with B.J. and Wisconsin Lieutenant Governor Thomas Morris.

It was a typical hot August day in Davenport. As most parades are inclined, this one must have appeared to D.D. as late in starting. He stepped out of his assigned car, strode to the person holding the flag in front of the band, and ordered the musical group to march. Elliot noticed the confusion and rushed to D.D.'s side, remonstrating with him to get back into his car. At this moment, B.J., who had seen what had taken place, drove his car out of the parade position and drew it to the east side of Brady Street where D.D. and Elliott were standing. Elliott was to comment later that B.J.'s car was close to D.D. and himself but did not touch either man.

In an effort to assist the elder Palmer, Elliott attempted to take D.D. by the arm to escort him to his automobile. D.D. rejected Elliott's assistance. He ran across the street and strode down Brady Street Hill.

The parade began, and as it passed in front of the Universal Chiropractic College, D.D. darted from the sidewalk to head the march. He did so for about a block until police took him out of the procession.

Universal College people had seen what had taken place and, after D.D.'s death, alleged that B.J. had struck his father with the automobile, which weakened D.D. to such an extent that he succumbed easily when afflicted with typhoid fever. Joy Loban, head of the Universal College and executor of D.D.'s estate, filed suit against B.J. Palmer on two counts and asked for damages amounting to $52,000.

Investigation to determine the possibility of criminal action on the part of B.J. went to several grand juries for consideration. The vicious struggle, which was costly and time consuming, came to an end on December 28, 1914, when Loban filed a petition to the district court dismissing his original action "without prejudice." Even in death, D.D. Palmer was to sleep restlessly.

A RETROSPECTIVE

A genius is often misunderstood, generally has few intimates, and has thoughts so keenly constructed as to defy easy translation. Who was D.D. Palmer? The question is difficult to answer because of the singleness of purpose toward which he dedicated his adult life. His quest for the cause of disease and the restoration of health led him into chiropractic, an all-consuming mistress. There was little time for typical socializing and friendships.

There were several contemporaries who seemed to know D.D. Palmer. They spoke at his memorial service held on Wednesday, October 23, 1913, at the Palmer School of Chiropractic. The first to present his verbal regards was long-time patient and confidant, the Reverend Samuel Weed:

> I think that I would not stand before you here today were it not for the science of Chiropractic. . . . I firmly believe that God raises up men for special purposes, and that he raised up D.D. Palmer for the purpose of giving to the world this science in its beginnings. . . .

L. Howard Nutting, uncle of Dr. Willard Carver and financial backer of B.J. in 1902, spoke next:

> He has gone—and gone forever. If he had faults, they are forgotten; if he squelched us at times with bitter sarcasm, they are forgiven. We and the world will remember Dr. Palmer for his indomitable courage and for the noble work he performed. For years he bore the scoffs, and scorns of his fellow man. He was not only sneered at as a faker, but was perse-cuted and finally arrested, tried and convicted and imprisoned for doing good, and through it all he wavered not, but conscious of right he stead-fastly trod the Chiropractic path and absolutely refused to be either led or driven aside. . . .

The final speaker at the memorial service was Cornelius H. Murphy, D.D.'s attorney, patient, and friend:

> We have not come here to palaver and say that Dr. Palmer was one of the greatest and wisest and best men that the world ever knew. I would not say that, because if I did, I would be lying in my own heart. . . . And when any one man, no matter how large or small he may be, can bring something good, that year after year brings the brainy young woman and the earnest, intelligent young men into a gathering like this that they ex-pect to learn and take out into the world with them that they may relieve the distresses of mankind, put an end to the miseries of a long suffering humanity, bring relief to the troubled minds of the sick, by the process of a Chiropractic adjustment: then I want to say that man that first invented or discovered that great movement is worthy of the highest respect that one man can give unto another. . . .

Gielow concluded the following:

> Because the three friends were of the same era as the man they hon-ored, they could not have known a greater accolade to extend to the founder of chiropractic. Only passage of years could determine the sig-nificance of a life.
>
> D.D. Palmer was a nineteenth century man. As a man representa-tive of that century, it was his responsibility to provide for himself and his family. If it became necessary to change locations to better himself, it was his solitary decision. As the head of the house, his word was pow-erful and the law. Discipline came swiftly with no relief.
>
> With singular leadership there came the respect of family members. As the man grew older, honor came in ever-widening circles from neigh-bors, friends, and associates. In his twilight years, a man's weaknesses were overlooked and forgotten because of the high esteem held for him and his accomplishments. It was expected of the younger to reverently address their elders.
>
> This honor born of another time came to Daniel David Palmer. Three words were used affectionately by those who knew him. D.D. thoroughly enjoyed and understood this grace of age. He wore his tribute well as only a nineteenth century man could—Old Dad Chiro.

The editors wish to acknowledge the seminal work on Daniel David Palmer done by Vern Gielow, which made the editing of this chapter possible.

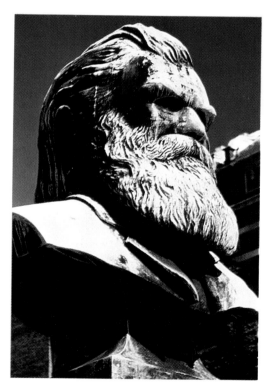

The bronze bust of D.D. on the Palmer College campus.

Courtesy Palmer College of Chiropractic Archives, Dav-enport, Iowa.

4

THE AGE OF WONDERMENT: CHIROPRACTIC IN THE EARLY TWENTIETH CENTURY

Health Care in the Midwest at the Turn of the Century

Joseph C. Keating Jr., Ph.D.

s the twentieth century dawned, health care in the Midwest included a wide variety of theories, methods, and practitioners. Many sources of health care were available, such as "regular," orthodox, or "allopathic" practitioners; physicians and surgeons; eclectic medical practitioners; homeopathic physicians; osteopaths; magnetic healers; nature cure practitioners; Christian Scientists and faith healers; patent medicine vendors; and self-health medical advice books. The Carnegie Foundation's precedent-setting Flexner Report on the deplorable state of medical education in the United States was still 10 years in the future. The Midwest, especially cities such as Chicago and Kansas City, was particularly noteworthy for the low standards of most medical schools, many of which amounted to little more than diploma mills. Although the growing European traditions of laboratory science, sanitation, and conservatism had begun to influence the content and quality of several university-based colleges of medicine along the Eastern seaboard (for example, Johns Hopkins University), such influences had not yet reached most practitioners along the Mississippi River. The gentler European alternatives to America's heroic medical methods were the province of the "irregulars." In many states, medical licensing laws, which had been repealed by public demand in the first 30 years of the nineteenth century, were reappearing, but were not yet so widely enforced that they prevented most irregulars from practicing their crafts at the turn of the century.

Many in society maintained the belief that health care should not be regulated or objected specifically to the licensing of one healing sect to the exclusion of any others. Their ideas can be traced to the views of Benjamin Rush, M.D., an eighteenth century regular physician and signer of the Declaration of Independence, who insisted that one group of doctors should exercise neither special privilege nor authority over any other group of health care providers. Ironically, Rush is also recalled as one of the major proponents of heroic medicine, and his philosophy permeated much of nineteenth century medical practice. Heroic medicine was a widely adopted school of thought among regular physicians in the early and middle 1800s. It held that the harshness of a medical remedy should be in proportion to the severity of the patient's condition. In other words, the sickest patients got the strongest doses of medicines, often with the result that the patient's natural recuperative powers were overwhelmed.

The available medicines and procedures at the time were a source of some serious concern. Mercurial preparations, cupping and counter-irritation, strong cathartics and emetics, and opiates were commonly prescribed and often in dosages that produced severe side effects. Bloodletting to purify the blood was still in vogue, and surgery was mainly limited to the extremities. The abdominal operations of the soon-to-be-famous

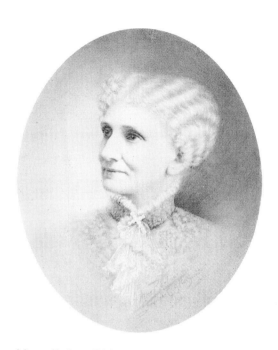

Mary Baker Eddy (1821-1910), founder of Christian Science. Portrait by Alice Barbour.
From *We Knew Mary Baker Eddy,* Boston, 1943, Christian Science Publishing Society.

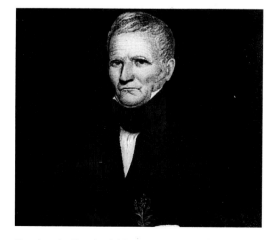

Benjamin Rush, M.D. (1746-1813).
Courtesy National Library of Medicine, Bethesda, Maryland.

91

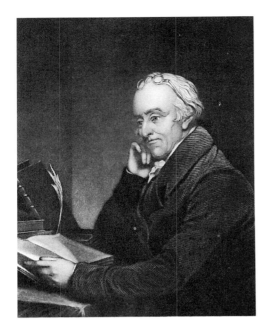

Samuel Thomson (1769-1843).
Courtesy National Library of Medicine, Bethesda, Maryland.

Mayo brothers of Rochester, Minnesota, were still in the experimental stages. There was little scientific justification for most medical methods of the day; much of what the doctor prescribed was based on either tradition or the physician's personal experience. There was little concern for the scientific validity of the methods doctors used, which was readily apparent, an idea that D.D. Palmer would later capture in the poem on p. 93.

Irregular healers offered a gentler alternative to the harshness of regular, heroic medicine. If the magnetic healer, homeopath, or osteopath did not help the patient, at least relatively little harm was done. The alternative practitioners of the day seemed to more closely approximate the hippocratic tradition: *first, do no harm.* Following the lead of Samuel Thomson, a nineteenth century advocate of self-care, many people would have nothing to do with any sort of doctoring, preferring instead to use their own home remedies and folk medicines and perhaps calling for a physician only at the extreme end stages of a serious illness. Doctors and more particularly hospitals were often considered a desperate last strategy and frequently signaled a loss of hope for recovery.

It was against this background of chaos in health care that Daniel David Palmer developed his preliminary theories of chiropractic. Like Christian Science's Mary Baker Eddy and osteopathy's Andrew Taylor Still, Palmer was influenced by the magnetic healing practices then popular in the Midwest. Magnetic healing had evolved from the work of Anton Mesmer, M.D., whose 1776 doctoral dissertation in medicine at the University of Vienna had been entitled "On the influence of the planets upon the human body by means of a magnetic force." Mesmer's theories were discredited by a prestigious panel of scientists, which included the then U.S. Ambassador to France, Benjamin Franklin. However, this did not discourage the enterprising physician. Mesmer's practice involved the "laying on of hands" and the use of magnetized iron rods to increase the vital forces believed to be depleted in the sick. His theories and methods were taken up and embellished by many subsequent "magnetics" and soon crossed the Atlantic to influence health care in America. ∾

MAGNETIC HEALING BECOMES CHIROPRACTIC

The father of chiropractic had begun his practice of magnetic healing in 1886 in Burlington, Iowa, but soon relocated to Davenport. In the advertising material he distributed throughout the Quad Cities region, he related that he had "taken lessons and studied...Christian Science, Faith Cure, Mind Cure, Metaphysics, Magnetic and Osteopathy." Palmer's decision to become a magnetic was probably influenced by the very successful magnetic healing infirmary established by the Caster family in Burlington. He believed that he had a special "gift for Magnetic Healing for 25 years" and with it the ability to pour his personal "life force" or "vital magnetism" into diseased tissue to effect a cure. D.D. Palmer believed that his particular variation of magnetic treatment was superior to that being practiced by other magnetics:

> Many so-called magnetics are massage healers. While the masseur is rubbing or slapping all over the body he is unconsciously throwing into his patient his vital force, with the disadvantage of a great waste of vitality because it is scattered over the whole body instead of into the organ or part diseased.

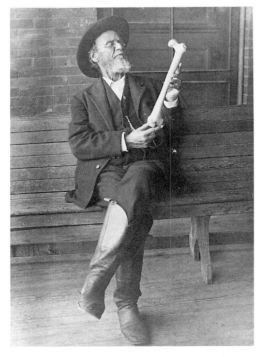

Dr. Andrew Taylor Still (1823-1917), the founder of osteopathy.
Courtesy Still National Museum of Osteopathy, Kirksville, Missouri.

THE PATH THE CALF MADE

One day through the Primeval wood,
A calf walked home as good calves should,
But made a trail all bent askew,
A crooked trail, as all calves do.

Since then two hundred years have fled,
And, I infer, the calf is dead;
But still, he left behind his trail,
And thereby hangs my moral tale.

The trail was taken up next day
By a lone dog that passed that way;
And then a wise bell-weather sheep
Pursued the trail o'er vale and steep.

And drew his flocks behind him, too,
As good bell-weathers always do.
And from that day, o'er hill and glade,
Through those old woods a path was made.

And many men wound in and out,
And dodged and turned and bent about,
But still they followed—do not laugh—
The first migrations of that calf;

And through the winding wood way stalked,
Because he wobbled when he walked.
This forest path became a land
That bent and turned and turned again;

This crooked lane became a road
Where many a poor horse with his load
Toiled on beneath the burning sun
And traveled some three miles in one.

And thus a century and a half,
They trod the footsteps of that calf.
The years passed on in swiftness fleet,
The road became a village street.

And this, before men were aware,
A city's crowded thoroughfare;
And soon the central street was this
Of a renowned metropolis.

And men two centuries and a half
Trod in the footsteps of that calf.
Each day a hundred thousand rout
Followed the zigzag calf about;

And o'er its crooked journey went
The traffic of a continent.
A hundred thousand men were led
By one calf near three centuries dead.

They followed still his crooked way.
And lost one hundred years a day.
For thus such reverence is lent
To well-established precedent.

A moral lesson this might teach
Were I ordained and called to preach,
For men are prone to go it blind
Along the calf paths of the mind;

They follow in the beaten track,
And out and in and forth and back,
And work away from sun to sun
To do what other men have done.

They go two miles instead of one,
To follow a path that was begun
By one lone calf; and to this day
They follow this old crooked way.

If each and every wise M.D.
The wisdom of these lines could see,
They would look back along their path,
And see the folly of the calf.

Years and years, o'er tortuous way,
They've given physic—made it pay,
And our straight Chiropractic plan
They laugh at, to a single man.

Their noxious drugs, no more we'll drink,
But think we are the ones to wink,
When viewing this devious path,
Made by some medicinal calf.

We hail with most sincere delight,
The dawn of scientific light,
That leads us from the old, old way
To this, our Chiropractic day.

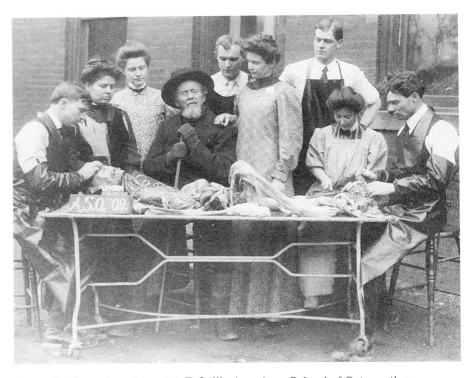

An early dissection class at A.T. Still's American School of Osteopathy.
Courtesy Still National Museum of Osteopathy, Kirksville, Missouri.

A homeopathic physician friend of Palmer's offered the following in support of D.D.'s improved methods of magnetic healing:

> He heals the sick, the halt, the lame, and those paralyzed, through the medium of his potent magnetic fingers placed upon the organ or organs diseased and not by rubbing or stroking, as other "magnetic curers" do. . . . Dr. Palmer seeks out the cause, the diseased organ upon which the disease depends, and treats that organ. Magnetics generally treat all cases alike, by general stroking, passes or rubbing. I think Dr. Palmer's plan is much more rational, and should be the most successful."

Palmer recognized that his methods had limitations, but the range of conditions he felt he could successfully treat by "animal magnetism" was broad:

> I treat successfully the following diseases:
> Rheumatism of any kind, neuralgia, the various kinds of stomach ailments, diseases of the liver, kidneys, bowels, bladder, spleen, heart, throat, and head, male and female diseases, periodical headaches, inflammation of the bowels or bladder, brain fever, lung fever, bronchitis, nervous diseases, shaking palsy, quinsy, running sores, abscesses of the lungs, liver or stomach, catarrh, pleurisy, sprains, lameness caused by injuries, asthma, malaria, dyspepsia, female weakness, diabetes, chronic diarrhoea, constipation, loss of strength and vitality, eczema, indigestion, erysipelas, dropsy, diphtheria, some diseases of the eye and ear, painful menstruation, piles, incontinence of urine or bed-wetting, consumption, lupus, cancers and tumors when not too far gone, and some cases of paralysis. I give no medicines, you do not have to wait months to see a change. Three to five treatments usually shows you what I can do. I treat causes, not effects. This Vital Magnetic Power of curing disease is sufficient to heal any disease when we know how.
> I do not claim to cure all diseases, but I now treat and cure many diseases which I had not thought of doing five years ago.

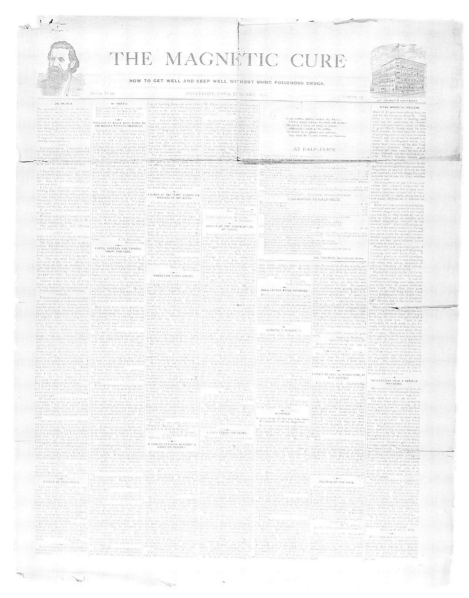

Masthead of The Magnetic Cure, *1896, published by D.D. Palmer.*
Courtesy Palmer College of Chiropractic Archives, Davenport, Iowa.

Medicine and medical doctors are necessary; we cannot get along without them. But they cannot cure everybody. Neither can I. I especially invite those who have tried all other remedies and have failed to find relief.

Palmer was a well-read, self-educated individual whose voracious appetite for books was sustained by his desire to find a rational, scientific explanation for the patient improvements he believed his magnetic methods were producing. His personal library is said to have encompassed much of what was then required reading for students at the University of Iowa's medical school, as well as many texts on spiritualism, theosophy, and the various alternative healing methods of his day. His studies had led him to the belief that by using his fingers, he could detect areas of inflamed tissue in his patients and that his personal magnetic force helped to cool these inflammations, thereby returning them to normal and producing a cure. For "Palmer the Magnetic," diagnosis meant the accurate

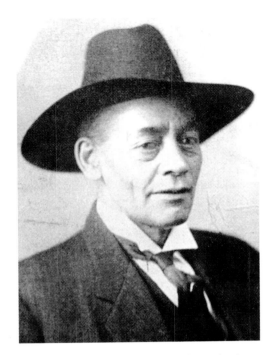

Harvey Lillard, first chiropractic patient.
Courtesy Palmer College of Chiropractic Archives, Davenport, Iowa.

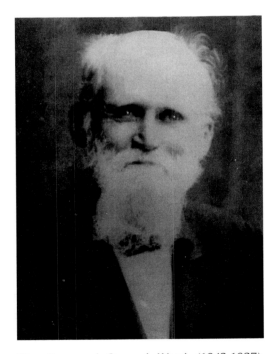

The Reverend Samuel Weed (1843-1927), who devised the name chiropractic.
Courtesy Palmer College of Chiropractic Archives, Davenport, Iowa.

identification of areas of inflammation. He recognized no beneficial effects of inflammation, a view disputed by modern biologists.

Palmer's magnetic methods and use of his hands to examine and treat his patients led him to wonder why he sometimes found "inflammation" or hot spots at places in the body remote from his patient's complaint. For example, he sometimes noted that patients with breast cancer also seemed to demonstrate inflamed tissue in the abdominal cavity. When his first chiropractic thrust into Harvey Lillard's midback apparently relieved the janitor of deafness, Palmer's theories became more systemic. He came to believe that dislocation of any part of the anatomy could produce friction and thereby dysfunction, much as a worn part in a watch causes other parts to malfunction. The first chiropractor reasoned that these distant effects were produced by pinching of arteries and nerves as they exited from the spinal column and other joints throughout the body. Early in 1896, with the assistance of his friend the Reverend Samuel Weed, Palmer named his new discovery *chiropractic,* from the Greek stems *chiro,* meaning "hand" and *praktikos,* meaning "to do." In July 1896, he chartered the Palmer School of Magnetic Cure to teach his improved methods of "magnetic manipulation" to others.

CHIROPRACTIC METAMORPHOSES

Palmer's practice and school provoked the ire of the osteopathic community, which had been growing steadily since 1892 when Andrew T. Still established his American School of Osteopathy in Kirksville, Missouri. The leading osteopathic journal claimed that Palmer had stolen osteopathy and renamed it chiropractic, which was understandable in light of the

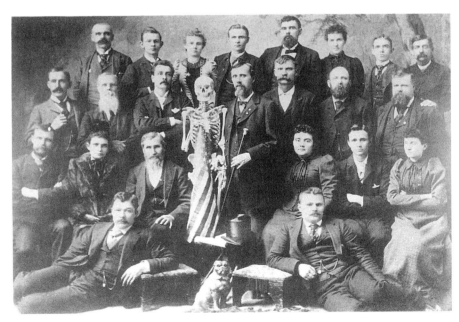

A.T. Still's first class (1892) at the American School of Osteopathy in Kirksville, Missouri.
Courtesy Still National Museum of Osteopathy, Kirksville, Missouri.

similar scope of practice advocated by both groups of healers. However, Palmer always contended that chiropractic differed significantly from osteopathy in both theory and technique. In part, Still taught that the brain was a sort of inborn drug store, capable of producing all the natural medicines necessary for the restoration of health. His manipulative methods were intended to reestablish normal arterial blood flow to and lymphaticovenous drainage of tissues to maintain good circulation from the brain to all parts of the body such that the brain's pharmacy could deliver those substances needed to heal diseased tissues and maintain wellness. Palmer's manual methods, on the other hand, were intended to replace inflammation-producing dislocations of the anatomy, thereby avoiding friction and the overheating of bodily tissues.

Palmer also noted that his methods of manipulation were decidedly different from those of the osteopaths. The father of chiropractic used his hands to deliver a short, sharp thrust into specific joints in contrast to the slower, "long-lever" techniques employed by Still and his followers. Old Dad Chiro believed that the specificity of his treatments, which were applied to individual joints rather than larger regions of the body, produced much quicker effects in patients. Palmer's advertising noted both the conceptual and technical differences between the two disciplines:

> The Osteopath and the Chiropractic both aim to put in place that which is out of place, to right that which is wrong; but the pathology, diagnosis, prognosis and movements are entirely different. The Chiro. is ten times more direct in the treatment and its efficiency, making cures in one-tenth of the time than an Osteo. usually does.

Such explanations did little to lessen the anger of the osteopaths, who continued to belittle the Davenport innovator. Attacks against Palmer continued in the osteopathic literature and probably prompted Old Dad Chiro to find additional differences between his chiropractic and Still's osteopathy. One important conceptual distinction came on July 1, 1903, when D.D., then teaching and practicing in Santa Barbara, California, "discovered that the body is heated by nerves, not by blood." The founder of chiropractic had decided that the nervous system alone was the primary mediator of disease, and from then on his exclusive concern was to maintain the optimal functioning of the nervous system. The osteopaths' "rule of the artery," that is, concern to maintain the unimpeded flow of the circulation, was thereafter eliminated for the most part, from the theoretical consideration of chiropractors.

D.D. Palmer's theories of chiropractic continued to evolve throughout the rest of his career. His notion of the "supremacy" of the nervous system involved a belief in the vibratory transmission of neural impulses. He believed that like the strings of a guitar, messages traveled along the nerves at greater or lesser rates depending on how tight the nerves were stretched. Although contemporary biologists would dispute this idea, at the turn of the century, vibrational transmission of neural impulses was one of several theories being explored. Moreover, vibrational theories of medical diagnosis and treatment were just becoming popular in the first decade of this century. Chiropractic historian Chittenden Turner noted the following in his 1931 volume, *The Rise of Chiropractic:*

> The publication of Dr. Albert Abrams' *Spondylotherapy* in 1910 brought the condemnation of the American Medical Association. This book advanced the theory that the organs of the body were governed by nerve centers in the spinal cord and could be made to dilate or contract by stimulating the nerve centers through the manipulation of the vertebrae.

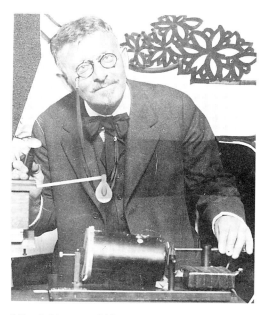

Albert Abrams, M.D., inventor of radionics.
Courtesy San Francisco Public Library, San Francisco, California.

Dr. Abrams was vice-president of the California State Medical Society, president of Emanuel Polyclinic, president of the San Francisco Medical-Chirurgical Society, professor of pathology at Cooper Medical College and professor at Leland Stanford University. He was graduated as a doctor of medicine at University of Heidelberg before he had reached the age of twenty. He studied in Berlin, Vienna, Paris and London, and for many years was regarded as one of the foremost minds in his profession.

Although Abrams would eventually earn the condemnation of organized medicine as an outrageous charlatan, his views were not dismissed at first. In the June 1911 issue of *Medical World,* the following notice appeared:

> The principles of spondylotherapy will form the subject of five clinics in San Francisco by that master of the subject, Dr. Albert Abrams, to be held on the five days following the Los Angeles session of the American Medical Association. All members of the association should write the Doctor at 246 Powell Street, San Francisco, California . . . it is realized that the valuable mechanical methods of treatment, wrongly labeled Osteopathy, originated with regular physicians in London as long ago as 1861, it is highly time for the profession to study them systematically
> . . . .

In somewhat similar fashion, Palmer, who refers to "friend Abrams" several times in his writings, thought of the nervous system as a meshwork strung across the skeletal frame of the body and believed that when the skeletal frame was out of kilter because of misalignment of one or more joints, the tension of the nerves was abnormally altered. Too little or too much tension in the nerves altered their vibrational frequency and thereby affected the functions of the end-organs the nerve served. Palmer believed further that the central nervous system, including the brain and spinal cord, controlled most if not all the functions of the body. Therefore if there were interference with transmission of the neural messages from the brain to the outer parts of the body, disease would result.

Old Dad Chiro's ideas about vibrational transmission of neural messages were consistent with his earlier theory that inflammation was at the core of most human illness. Excess vibration of the nerves, he thought, produced excess vibration in an end-organ. For example, an inflammation of the kidney or appendicitis was believed to be due to a "hot nerve," one that vibrated too quickly, causing friction and heat in the organ and thereby producing an inflamed condition. Palmer believed that he could trace the course of hot, vibrating nerves from their source in the spine to the malfunctioning end-organ or from the site of the inflammation to the spine; this technique was known as *nerve-tracing.* As a magnetic, he would then produce his cure by cooling this inflamed tissue with his vital energy; as a chiropractor, he adjusted the displaced bones of the joints so that restoration of the proper nerve tension prevented heat and inflammation in the tissues of the body. Excess heat in the body could be localized, as in inflammation, or systemwide, as in a generalized fever. Palmer also hypothesized that too little vibrational messages to an organ could produce cold, hard tumors. Clearly, the potential value of the chiropractor's methods of altering the skeletal frame were believed to have rather profound and far-reaching implications for health and disease.

The founder of chiropractic should also be remembered as the first "segmentalist" in the profession. Because the nerves exiting from the spinal cord had to pass between the joints of the spinal column, the spinal nerve roots were thought to be particularly susceptible to nerve interference. When another bone composing the spinal joints became misaligned, it could pinch or stretch the nerve. Moreover, because many of

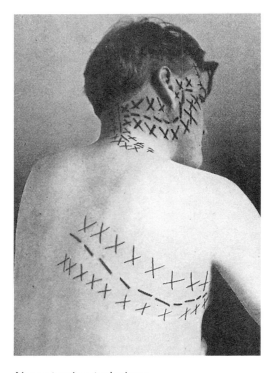

Nerve tracing technique.

From Gregory A: *Spinal treatment: auxillary methods of treatment,* 1912.

the controlling nerves of the body had to pass through these joints, it was believed that various diseases could be related to specific regions of the spinal column. Palmer believed that these misalignments occurred at individual segments of the spine, a "segment" being two adjacent spinal bones that together make up a joint. Later chiropractic theorists would suggest that a misalignment in one area of the spinal column necessarily causes misalignment elsewhere in the spine, but this idea apparently did not occur to the founder.

Palmer's first theories of chiropractic had made liberal use of machine metaphors to describe the nature of the chiropractic lesion and the chiropractor's role in resolving the lesion and helping the patient to gain health. For example, his earlier advertising had spoken of the operation of the body as similar to that of a fine watch. However, as the years wore on, the founder gradually returned to the more mystical constructs that had originally led him into magnetic healing. As his notions about the role of the nervous system evolved, he came to recognize the distinction between the voluntary nervous system, such as nerves controlling muscular contractions of the arms and legs, and the involuntary or autonomic nervous system, which regulates the internal organs of the body. By 1904, Palmer was referring to this distinction in terms of *educated* versus *innate* nerves but soon expanded these constructs into a theology of health and illness. He argued that the workings of human anatomy and physiology could not be adequately explained in terms of machine parts and their operation. Instead, he insisted, the regulation of human functioning was controlled by two minds within each person: Innate Intelligence and Educated Intelligence. Innate, he believed, was a fraction of Universal Intelligence or God and controlled human biology by directing signals through the nervous system to the various organs of the body. Educated Intelligence, on the other hand, was believed to be entirely mortal and corresponds loosely to human consciousness and its capacity to learn.

Palmer's introduction of this spiritual aspect added little to any scientific explanation of his theories of neural influence in health and illness and would attract considerable scorn to chiropractors. However, Palmer may have hoped to cloak his new profession in the guise of a religious movement to avoid the legal persecution of organized medicine. Many states had religious exemptions to their medical practice acts, and it was possible that unlicensed practice of chiropractic and other alternative healing arts could win in the courtroom by arguing that their methods and beliefs were protected under such exemptions. However, Palmer's writings also clearly suggest that he believed he had united the physical and spiritual under one theory. Nevertheless, he suggested that chiropractic could be practiced competently without knowledge of the spiritual aspects of his final theories. In later years, Palmer's son B.J. would make the spiritual aspects of D.D.'s chiropractic the centerpiece of his chiropractic writings. Innate Intelligence became B.J.'s emphasis in chiropractic and was offered as the explanation for all beneficial effects experienced by patients at the hands of the chiropractor. Many chiropractors, however, rejected the Innate construct as unscientific.

The founder's final written contributions to the chiropractic literature were created on the West Coast. D.D. Palmer arrived in Portland, Oregon, in the latter half of October 1908, and with Palmer-Davenport graduate Leroy M. Gordon, D.C., established his D.D. Palmer College of Chiropractic. This short-lived (1908-1910) institution offered a fairly broad curriculum that included obstetrics and minor surgery. Dr. Gordon was soon replaced as general manager of the school by John E. LaValley, D.C., who

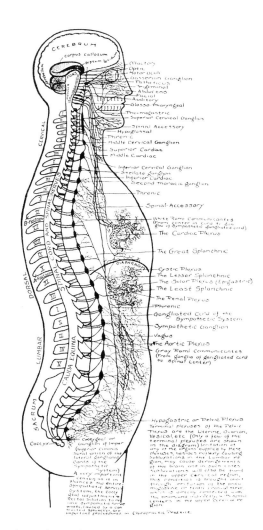

A traditional chiropractic illustration of neural innervation of the body.

From Riley JS: *Science and practice of chiropractic with allied sciences,* 1919.

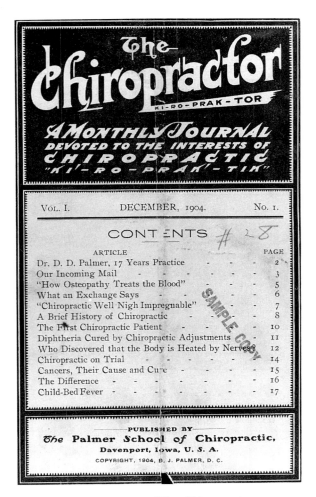

Cover of the first issue of The Chiropractor.

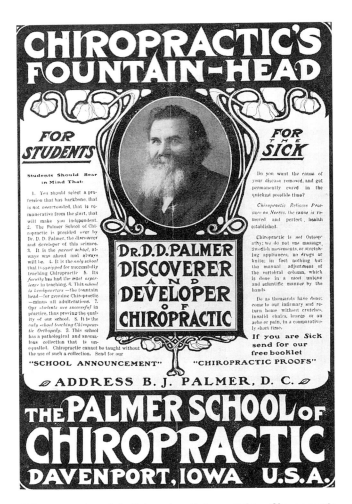

This example of D.D.'s advertising of his Chiropractic Fountain-Head was targeted for prospective students and patients.

would become owner and president of the facility following Old Dad Chiro's 1910 departure for Los Angeles. The journal published by D.D. and this college, the *Chiropractor Adjuster,* would form the bulk of the materials published in Palmer's classic 1910 book, *The Chiropractor's Adjuster: The Science, Art and Philosophy of Chiropractic.* The volume is not well organized for use as a textbook but clearly reveals the breadth of D.D.'s biological knowledge, his wit, and his concern that many of his followers had failed to grasp the nuances and significance of his various theories. A posthumously published second book, *The Chiropractor,* was released in 1914 by D.D.'s widow and provides a somewhat more reader-friendly presentation of the founder's final notions about chiropractic.

DISCIPLES AND HERETICS

The earliest students of the chiropractic profession earned their diplomas from Old Dad Chiro and went forth from Davenport, Iowa, with a missionary zeal for their new discipline. They considered themselves at

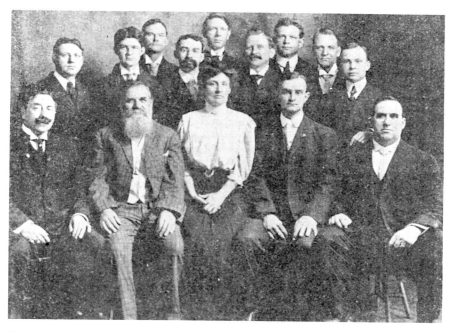

First class at the D.D. Palmer College of Chiropractic in Portland, Oregon on November 9, 1908.

From Palmer DD: *The chiropractor adjuster,* 1909.

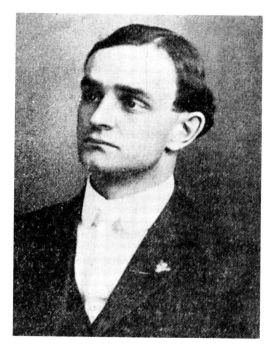

Leroy M. Gordon, D.C., first general manager of the D.D. Palmer College of Chiropractic of Portland, Oregon.

From Palmer DD: *The chiropractor adjuster,* 1909.

the cutting edge of health care technology. True to the teachings of D.D. Palmer, the earliest doctors of chiropractic (DCs) recognized few limitations to their new health service and were eager to apply the adjustive arts to all manner of illness and disease. In true experimental spirit, they felt that they could not know the boundaries of the chiropractic discovery without putting it to the test in the field. Although clearly grounded in the ancient art of manipulation, the chiropractic offered by Palmer held promise of an alternative to the harsh remedies of heroic medicine and the trial-and-error empiricism that prevailed in the Midwest at the end of the nineteenth century. There was no disease or pathology too extreme for DC's to try their methods on, and because regular medicine at the turn of the century often had little scientific merit with which to aid patients, a trial of chiropractic adjusting was considered a reasonable strategy by many in society.

The backgrounds of the earliest chiropractors were extremely varied, including those with relatively little education and others who held multiple doctorates in the healing arts. For example, Palmer's son B.J had no more than a tenth-grade education when he took his training in chiropractic at his father's school in 1901 through 1902. On the other hand, Andrew P. Davis, M.D., D.O., D.C., was an 1899 graduate of Palmer's School and held a homeopathic medical degree. Davis had also studied osteopathy under A.T. Still at the American School Of Osteopathy. Moreover, Davis had authored the first osteopathic textbook, *Osteopathy Illustrated,* in the same year that he took his chiropractic studies in Davenport under Old Dad Chiro. In later years a sworn affidavit from Davis, asserting the distinctiveness of chiropractic from osteopathy, would prove helpful to chiropractors who were prosecuted for unlicensed practice.

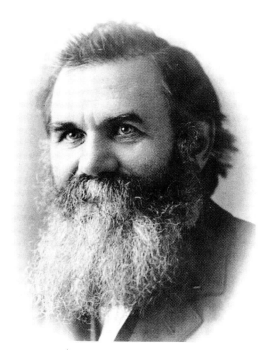

D.D. Palmer, the founder of chiropractic, circa 1900.

Courtesy Palmer College of Chiropractic Archives, Davenport, Iowa.

101

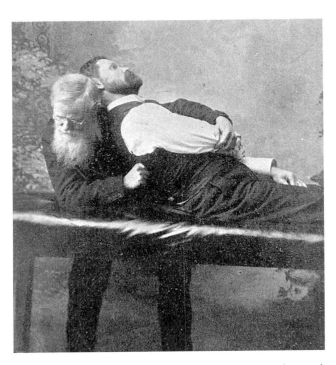

*A.P. Davis, M.D., D.O., D.C. (1835-1915), an early gradu-
ate of D.D.'s, performing an osteopathic manipulation.*

Courtesy A.T. Still Memorial Library Special Collections, Kirksville, Missouri.

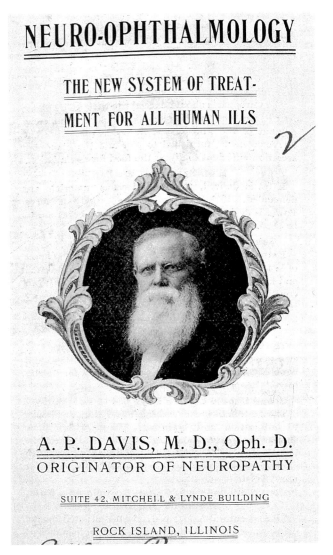

NEURO-OPHTHALMOLOGY

THE NEW SYSTEM OF TREAT-
MENT FOR ALL HUMAN ILLS

A. P. DAVIS, M. D., Oph. D.
ORIGINATOR OF NEUROPATHY

SUITE 42, MITCHELL & LYNDE BUILDING

ROCK ISLAND, ILLINOIS

*Advertising literature for Andrew P. Davis, M.D., D.O.,
D.C., an early graduate, who went on to develop his own
healing art named neuropathy.*

Courtesy Palmer College of Chiropractic Archives, Davenport, Iowa.

Davis freely mingled the many healing theories and methods he had
mastered, and from this mixture devised what he called a new science,
neuropathy. As a profession, neuropathy would never seriously rival chiropractic and osteopathy, but Davis would operate several schools of neuropathy in coming years. Although Palmer agreed with Davis that chiropractic and neuropathy were separate and distinct healing arts, Davis
would nonetheless earn Palmer's published criticisms for his apparent
misunderstanding of chiropractic methods. Old Dad Chiro insisted that
chiropractic should not be "mixed" with other healing strategies.

Solon Langworthy

Derivatives from Palmer's seminal theories and techniques were inevitable, and because of the authorization to "teach and practice" that
Palmer included on the first chiropractic diplomas he issued, the development of rival schools should not have been too surprising. However,
Palmer had not counted on competition in the school business from his
former pupils, and when 1901 graduate Solon M. Langworthy, D.C.,

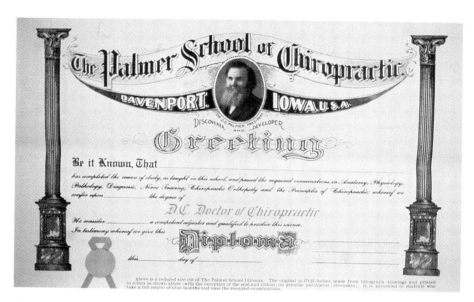

An example of D.D Palmer's early teach and practice diploma.
Courtesy Palmer College of Chiropractic Archives, Davenport, Iowa.

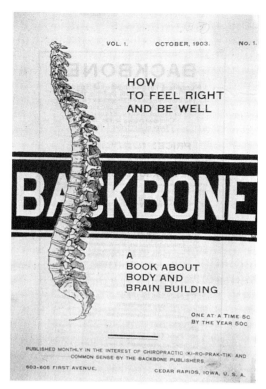

The cover of S.M. Langworthy's journal Backbone.
Courtesy Palmer College of Chiropractic Archives, Davenport, Iowa.

opened his American School of Chiropractic & Nature Cure in nearby Cedar Rapids, Iowa, circa 1903, D.D. was furious. Although Langworthy had suggested a partnership between himself and D.D., the founder would not hear of it. To make matters worse, Langworthy, who also held a degree from the American College of Manual Therapeutics in Kansas City, introduced several innovations that Palmer felt were outside the meaning of "done by hand." Among these were traction tables and methods borrowed from naturopathy. The American School of Chiropractic & Nature Cure also offered the first organized curriculum in the profession, which included instruction in obstetrics; Minora Paxson, D.C., another early graduate under D.D. Palmer, served as the chairperson of the school's department of obstetrics. Langworthy also proposed that the infirmities and enfeeblement of old age were due to narrowing of the spaces between the spinal joints as a consequence of degeneration of the disks. This narrowing was thought to squeeze the spinal nerve roots as they exited from the spinal cord; to remedy this, Langworthy recommended stretching the patient to open up the joint spaces, hence the use of traction tables.

Oakley Smith

Langworthy's dean at the American School of Chiropractic & Nature Cure was even more the heretic. An 1899 graduate of the Palmer School in Davenport and a former medical student at the University of Iowa, Oakley G. Smith, D.C., challenged D.D.'s ideas about the nature of the lesion that should be treated. Rather than the bone-pinching–nerve concept of Palmer's *subluxation,* Smith proposed that serious interference with the nervous system resulted from the cramping or strictures of connective tissues such as fascia and ligaments. Smith named his lesion the *ligatite* and, on the basis of his "discovery," eventually departed Langworthy's school for Chicago to establish the rival profession of naprapathy. However, during his tenure at the American School of Chiropractic & Nature Cure, Smith co-authored with Paxson and Langworthy the first textbook in the profession, *Modernized Chiropractic,* which was published by Langworthy. This book would later serve as the basis for one of the first courtroom victories for chiropractic. Although the extent of Smith's own re-

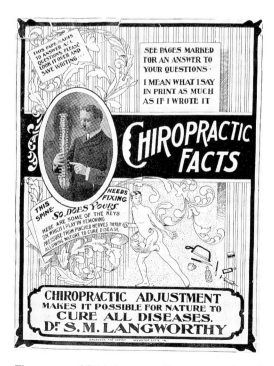

The cover of S.M. Langworthy's promotional piece Chiropractic Facts *circa 1902.*
Courtesy Palmer College of Chiropractic Archives, Davenport, Iowa.

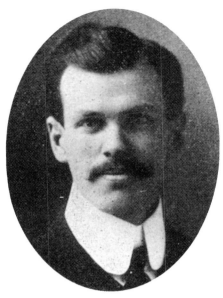

Oakley G. Smith, D.C. (1880-1967), an 1899 graduate under Old Dad Chiro, who served as dean of Langworthy's American School of Chiropractic & Nature Cure in Cedar Rapids, Iowa, in 1905. The following year, Smith co-authored with Solon Massey Langworthy, D.C., and Minora Paxson, D.C., the first text-book of chiropractic, Modernized Chiropractic. *Smith's lesion named the* ligatite *became the basis of his healing art naprapathy.*

Courtesy Palmer College of Chiropractic Archives, Davenport, Iowa.

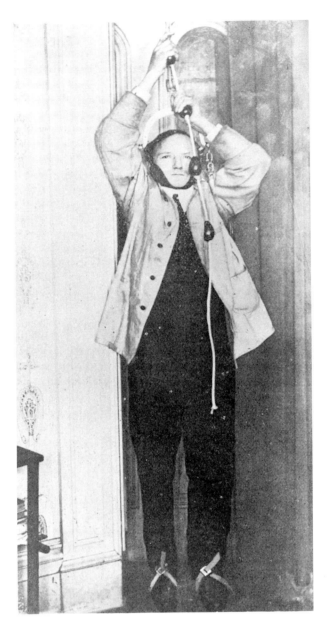

Joe Shelby Riley demonstrating a form of early cervical traction.

From Riley JS: *Science and practice of chiropractic with allied sciences,* 1919.

search is not known, his scholarly orientation apparently attracted the attention of a University of Chicago anatomist, Harold Swanberg, who acknowledged the young chiropractor as a stimulus for his anatomic studies of the spine in his 1914 volume, *The Intervertebral Foramen in Man.*

Thomas Storey

An early graduate who would expand the technique if not the theory of chiropractic was Thomas H. Storey, D.C. Storey had practiced as a "vitapathic physician" in Duluth, Minnesota, before he began his studies under D.D. in 1900 through 1901. After earning his D.C., Storey migrated from Davenport to the West Coast and soon began experimenting with the first adjusting instruments: a wooden chisel and mallet for tapping the processes of the spinal vertebrae. Palmer was intrigued with this idea and in later years may have experimented himself with a rubber mallet for

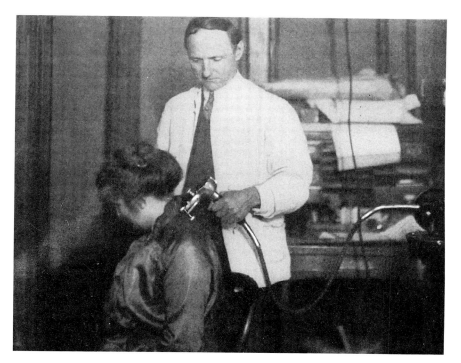

J.S. Riley, D.O., D.C., using a concussion instrument to make an adjustment.
From Riley JS: *Science and practice of chiropractic with allied sciences,* 1919.

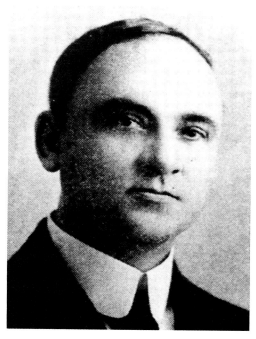

Charles A. Cale, N.D., D.C., circa 1922. Cale, a former schoolteacher, earned his chiropractic degree from Thomas Storey, a 1901 graduate of D.D. Palmer. Cale chartered the Los Angeles College of Chiropractic in 1911.
Courtesy Paul Smallie, Stockton, California.

adjusting the spine, but he also publicly disavowed these methods as beyond what he considered to be legitimately included in "done by hand." Storey's devices may be considered the forerunner of many similar instruments such as today's Activator instrument. Palmer also strenuously disapproved of his friend and former pupil's use of cervical traction (that is, suspension by the head) as a method of intervention but heartily approved of Storey's introduction of the bifid table. The bifid table refers to the nose hole common in most chiropractic tables and couches. Palmer's thrusts into patients backs had apparently bloodied a few noses before this innovation, and he approved of Storey's ingenuity.

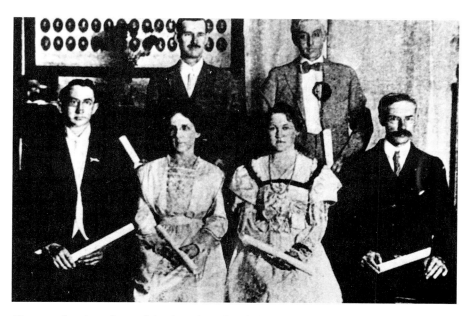

First graduating class of the Los Angeles College of Chiropractic, 1912.
Courtesy Los Angeles College of Chiropractic, Los Angeles, California.

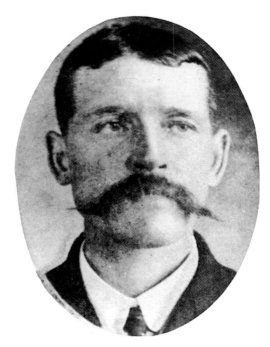

John F.A. Howard, D.C. (1876-1954), founder of the National School of Chiropractic, 1906.

From Palmer DD, Palmer BJ: *The Science of Chiropractic,* 1906.

Storey is also recalled as the mentor of Charles A. Cale, D.C., N.D., founder of the Los Angeles College of Chiropractic (LACC) in 1911. Over the years, Cale's school provided a strong naturopathic influence to chiropractic education, theory, and practice. Cale was licensed as a naturopath in 1910 on the basis of his diploma from Storey's Chiropractic School & Cure but would suspend operations of the LACC during 1914 while he and wife Linnie furthered their studies at the College of Osteopathic Physicians & Surgeons in Los Angeles. Their broad education in chiropractic, naturopathy, and osteopathy foreshadowed the broad-scope practice pursued by a majority of chiropractors in California for decades to come.

John Howard and William Schulze

Another prominent influence in chiropractic was John F. Howard, D.C. Howard had commenced his studies under D.D. Palmer in Davenport in 1905, but by the time he completed the 9-month curriculum in 1906, Old Dad Chiro had departed for Oklahoma after his conviction and jailing for unlicensed practice and son B.J.'s purchase of his half of the Palmer School. Some friction developed between B.J. and a number of students who felt that the younger Palmer's administration of the school did not provide sufficient scientific emphasis for the chiropractic art. With D.D.'s blessing, Howard and the dissident Palmer students organized the National School of Chiropractic in 1906 and thus began the tradition of "rational chiropractic." However, D.D. Palmer would later criticize his development of the Howard System of chiropractic, which combined elements of naturopathy and manipulative methods. In later years, Howard would recall the events that led to the formation of the National School:

> Students who had entered school to receive their instruction from the father (D.D. Palmer) became very much discontented, and the son with all his cleverness was unable to stem the tide of discontent . . . finally a delegation (of students) called upon me and implored me to organize a school and teach chiropractic *as it should be taught.*

The first home of this new institution was in the Ryan Building, the same building where D.D. Palmer had practiced as a magnetic 10 years before. However, Dr. Howard's desire to teach anatomy by dissection was hindered by restrictive laws that directed all human cadavers to the University of Iowa's medical school. Accordingly, Howard relocated the National School to Chicago in 1908 "to secure the clinical, laboratory, dissection, hospital and other facilities that were lacking in a small town." The school was also incorporated as a proprietary institution, which was the norm for chiropractic colleges in those days. The move to Chicago brought Howard in contact with eclectic, naturopathic, and other alternative healing arts that flourished in Chicago. Most significant among his new contacts were William Charles Schulze, M.D., a graduate of the University of Chicago's prestigious Rush Medical College, and Arthur L. Forster, M.D., a graduate of the medical department of the University of Illinois.

Schulze was born in Germany in 1870 and came to the United States in 1887. He earned his doctorate in 1897 and practiced for several years in Wisconsin before taking the position of medical director at the Zander Institute. Schulze was operating the Institute of Physiological Therapeutics in Chicago when Howard hired him as a faculty member at the Na-

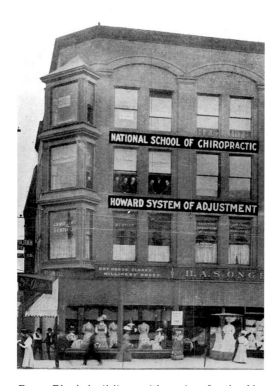

Ryan Block building with a sign for the National School of Chiropractic circa 1906.

Courtesy Palmer College of Chiropractic Archives, Davenport, Iowa.

John F. Howard
Davenport, Iowa

Kansas City, Mo.
May 28, 1906

Dear Sir and Friend:

You have been on my mind for several days, therefore I will write you a few lines.

Why should I not approve of your teaching the science of chiropractic; when I consider you a capable and qualified teacher. . . . In practice and as a teacher I consider you qualified. . . .

I cannot let your letter go until I tell you of the M.D.'s meeting yesterday. They have a county society which meets once each month. I attended. Did not do so at home (Davenport). A paper was read; each member discussed its merits. I asked to have a say. They reluctantly voted me 5 minutes. When the 5 minutes were up several said, on. So they voted me another 5 minutes. By that time all the rules were forgotten and I occupied most of the afternoon. . . . Dr. Martin said that he had a headache. I offered to cure it by one touch. He accepted. I seated him in front of the audience. He showed his surprise and admitted that the headache was gone. Several questions were asked for me to answer. Chiropractic captured the meeting. . . .

With best wishes,
D.D. Palmer

tional School of Chiropractic. Schulze and Forster pioneered physiological therapeutics within the chiropractic profession, including procedures involving light, heat, cold, electricity, water, nutritional interventions, and exercise regimens. The National School of Chiropractic offered coursework in the electrical modalities and naturopathic methods as early as 1912, a considerable time before the formation of the physical therapy profession. Schulze purchased the National School of Chiropractic from Howard circa 1918 and continued as its president until his death in 1936. Under Schulze's leadership and that of Arthur Forster, M.D., D.C., the National School of Chiropractic, renamed *National College of Chiropractic* in 1920, became a strong proponent for improvement in chiropractic and basic science instruction in the discipline. As an M.D. and D.C., Schulze was both respected and reviled by various elements in the profession. Forster, dean of the National College of Chiropractic under Schulze, was an instructor in anatomy, the editor of the journal published by the school in the early years, and the author of several texts, including *Principles and Practice of Spinal Adjustment* (1915), *Forster's System of Non-Medicinal Therapy* (1919), and *The White Mark* (1921).

Lee Edwards

Another important allopathic physician-turned-chiropractor in the early years of the century was Lee W. Edwards, an 1893 graduate of the medical department of the University of Nebraska. Inspired by his own recovery under chiropractic care from an injury that had caused semiparalysis of his arms, Edwards enrolled at the Palmer School of Chiropractic and graduated in 1911. His Omaha-based practice eventually became

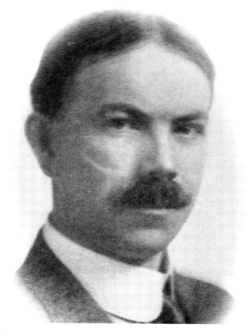

William C. Schulze, M.D., D.C. (1870-1936), president and owner of the National College of Chiropractic from 1916 to 1936.

Courtesy National College of Chiropractic, Chicago.

107

exclusively devoted to chiropractic, and he was very active in supporting chiropractic legislation in Nebraska. His dual credentials in medicine and chiropractic placed him in great demand as an expert witness on behalf of chiropractors arrested for unlicensed practice in the early decades, and it is said that he testified in more trials of chiropractors than any other person. On behalf of the Universal Chiropractors Association, Edwards also presented the chiropractors' case for separate licensing laws before most of the state and provincial legislatures in North America. He served as the last president of the Universal Chiropractors Association before its 1930 merger with the American Chiropractic Association to form the National Chiropractic Association.

Joy Loban

Several other early students and acquaintances of D.D. Palmer influenced chiropractic theory, technique, and education. Exemplary was Joy Loban, D.C., who began his studies at Davenport before the founder's conviction, incarceration, and departure for Oklahoma. He continued at the Palmer School of Chiropractic as a member of the faculty under B.J., and earned his glowing endorsement as a "philosopher of chiropractic." In April 1910, however, Loban and a number of dissidents walked out of B.J.'s lecture, marched down Brady Street Hill, and formed the rival Universal Chiropractic College. The nature of the dispute between Palmer and Loban and associates is not entirely clear but may have involved B.J.'s introduction of the new technology of x-ray examination at the Palmer School of Chiropractic. Loban reputedly objected to this new assessment strategy because it went beyond the meaning of chiropractic "done by hand" and therefore constituted an inappropriate mixing of chiropractic with other methods. This twentieth century marvel of science, which permitted the first practical internal view of the human body, would have profound effect on the theory of chiropractic. X-ray technology shifted the chiropractor's attention from the nervous system via nerve tracing and palpation toward the skeletal structure as seen on x-ray films. Ironically, Loban and other faculty at the Universal Chiropractic College developed

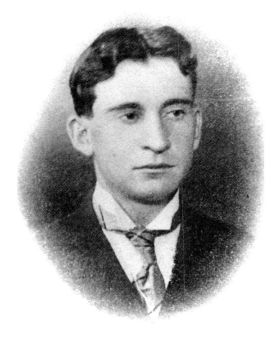

Joy Loban, D.C., founder of the Universal Chiropractic College.
Courtesy Palmer College of Chiropractic Archives, Davenport, Iowa.

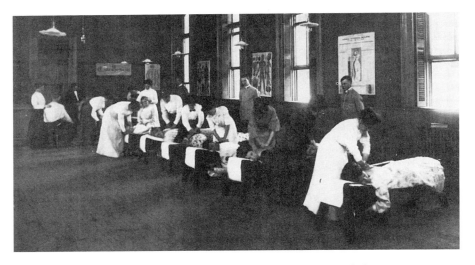

An adjusting class at Universal Chiropractic College, circa 1912.
From Mawhiney R: *Chiropractic in Wisconsin* 1984, Wisconsin Chiropractic Association.

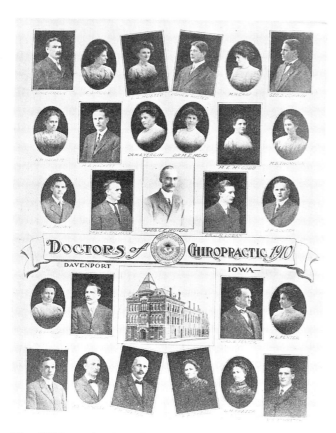

The 1910 graduating class of the Universal Chiropractic College.

Courtesy Palmer College of Chiropractic Archives, Davenport, Iowa.

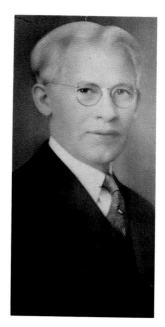

Hugh B. Logan, D.C., 1915 graduate of the Universal Chiropractic College and founder (in 1935) of the Logan Basic College of Chiropractic of St. Louis.

Courtesy Logan College of Chiropractic Archives, Chesterfield, Missouri.

full-spine x-ray techniques in later years. Loban was involved in four schools in three cities—Universal Chiropractic College in Davenport, the Washington School of Chiropractic in the District of Columbia, and the Pittsburgh College of Chiropractic (later the Universal Chiropractic College of Pittsburgh). His influence also included a number of written contributions, including *Technique and Practice of Chiropractic* (1912), *Diet and Exercise* (1928), and *Textbook of Neurology* (1929), which were considered rather scholarly in their day. His successor as dean at the Universal College of Chiropractic, Leo J. Steinbach, D.C., earned a reputation as an early clinical researcher. In 1935, graduates Hugh B. Logan, D.C., and son Vinton F. Logan, D.C., established the St. Louis college that bears their name today.

Willard Carver

Willard Carver was one of the most influential chiropractors in the first half of the century. Although a 1906 graduate of the Charles Ray Parker School of Chiropractic in Ottumwa, Iowa, rather than D.D. Palmer's Davenport institution, Carver always described himself as the "oldest chiropractic student," apparently on the grounds that as D.D.'s confidente and attorney in the mid-1890s, he had one been one of the first to be privy to

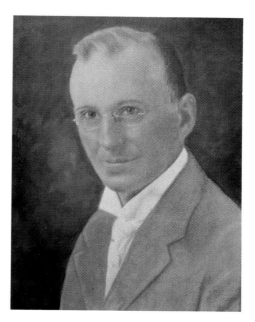

Willard Carver, LL.B., D.C. (1866-1943), founder of the Carver-Denny School of Chiropractic in 1906.

Courtesy Mel Rosenthal, New Castle, Delaware.

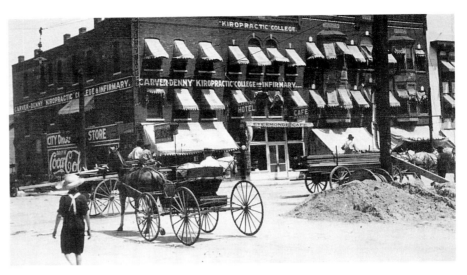

Exterior view of the Carver-Denny School of Chiropractic, circa 1910.
Courtesy Robert Jackson, Jones, Oklahoma.

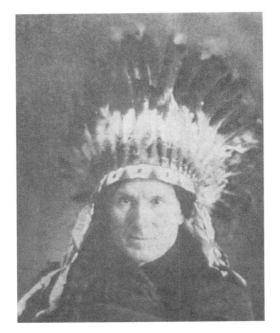

Willard Carver, LL.B., D.C. in Indian head-dress.
From *Scientific Head News,* 1917. Courtesy Mel Rosenthal, New Castle, Delaware.

Palmer's burgeoning ideas. Carver, who had graduated from Drake University School of Law in Des Moines, Iowa, brought a distinctly different perspective from that of the formally uneducated Palmers and the early physician-chiropractors such as Davis, Gregory, Schulze, and Forster. Carver's "structural approach," which first emerged circa 1910, adopted a perspective that may be labeled a "systems theory" of subluxations. Carver believed that many disrelations of spinal joints were compensatory, that is, were adaptations produced by other subluxations. Like B.J. and most of D.D. Palmer's earliest students, Carver adhered to the founder's preliminary ideas about "obstructive nerve pressure" rather than the nerve-stretching concepts Old Dad Chiro proposed in the final years of his life. Carver was also a strong advocate of suggestive therapeutics such as psychotherapy. Carver seems to have been as comfortable with the broad-scope members of the American Chiropractic Association (ACA) as he was with B.J. Palmer's organizations. He claimed to have been the first to introduce minor surgery to the chiropractic curriculum in 1906.

Carver, who characterized himself as the "Constructor" of chiropractic in contrast to B.J.'s self-designation as the "developer," influenced the profession in the first part of the century through his colleges, his writings, his legal and political activities, and his many presentations. The attorney-chiropractor established chiropractic schools in Oklahoma City, Washington, D.C., New York, and Denver. Although none of these have survived, the Oklahoma and Denver institutions were prominent for decades. In addition to his Oklahoma college's journal, the *Scientific Head News* (in contrast to B.J.'s *Fountain Head News*), Carver authored 18 books dealing with chiropractic and biopsychology, most notably *Carver's Chiropractic Analysis,* first published in 1909. He was also instrumental in establishing some of the early licensing laws for chiropractors, although his home state of Oklahoma did not pass such legislation until 1921. Several of Carver's early graduates also had significant effects on the evolution of the young profession, most especially Alva Gregory M.D, D.C., and Tullius deFlorence Ratledge, D.C.

Tullius deFlorence Ratledge

T.F. Ratledge was born to itinerant school teacher parents in 1881 and attended Central State College in Edmond, Oklahoma, before enrolling at Carver Chiropractic College in 1907. During his studies at Carver's institution, he also attended lectures given by D.D. Palmer in Oklahoma City. Ratledge developed a deep respect for both his mentors but leaned toward the orientation of the founder. Under Carver's supervision, he operated a "free adjustery" for members of Oklahoma's first state legislature. Ratledge also successfully treated the Oklahoma Secretary of State for what had been medically diagnosed as appendicitis.

Ratledge established the first several of his Ratledge System of Chiropractic Schools in Guthrie, Oklahoma, Arkansas City, Kansas, and Topeka. He was instrumental in having the first law in the nation to license chiropractors passed in Kansas in 1913, although by this time he had relocated to Los Angeles. T.F. chartered his fourth or fifth college in southern California in 1911, just a few months before Charles Cale, D.C., incorporated the LACC. He and Cale feuded over the scope of chiropractic practice for more than a decade. However, they also collaborated during 1920 to 1922 to win the state law to license chiropractors in California. This law, which was unique in that it was passed by popular vote of the people rather than by the legislature, was positively influenced by Ratledge going to jail for his beliefs, which garnered positive press for chiropractic. Arrested in 1914 and convicted in 1916 for unlicensed practice, Ratledge appealed to the governor for a pardon on the grounds that his chiropractic practice had "done only good" for society. Governor Johnson offered to pardon Ratledge if he would accept a license as a "drugless healer" from the board of medical examiners. Ratledge was outraged because he considered the medical board unqualified to judge his competence as a chiropractor. To accept such a license, he replied, would be "fraud against the people."

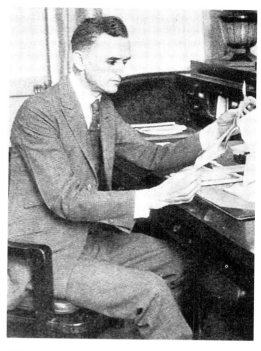

T.F. Ratledge, D.C. (1881-1967), founder of the Ratledge Chiropractic College in Los Angeles (1911).

Courtesy Paul Smallie, Stockton, California.

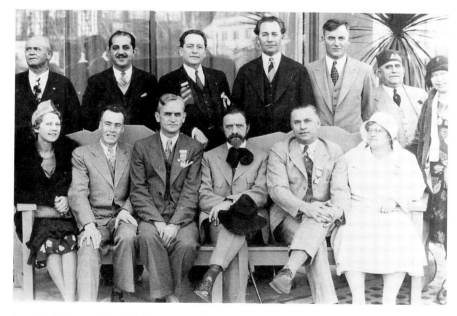

T.F. Ratledge with B.J. Palmer and members of the California Chiropractic Association in 1931.

Courtesy Palmer College of Chiropractic Archives, Davenport, Iowa.

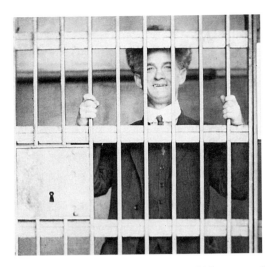

Linden McCash, D.C., circa 1920, one of many D.C.s jailed in California for unlicensed practice.

From *California Chiropractic Association Bulletin* 1(4), 1932.

Ratledge's self-martyrdom captured the imagination of the press, and after his release from 90 days in Los Angeles County Jail, many other California chiropractors accepted his "go to jail for chiropractic" policy. It was rumored that at one time the Los Angeles County Sheriff's Office had more chiropractic adjusting tables in its possession than all the chiropractors in the state because the tables were usually confiscated when the chiropractor was arrested. Legend also holds that the policy of the state medical board before passage of the 1922 Chiropractic Act was that at least one chiropractor should be kept in jail in each county in the state at all times to set an example. Many chiropractors set up practices within the jails and won the support of fellow prisoners and their jailers. Others made their incarcerations into potent political statements when their patients came to the jails for their adjustments.

After California's chiropractic law was passed by popular vote in 1922, T.F. Ratledge continued to influence the profession in California and throughout the country as president of his Los Angeles institution, an active participant in the state's chiropractic politics, a voice in the continuing disagreements among straight and mixer practitioners, and a leader among Universal Chiropractors Association's straight chiropractic college leaders. In 1951, Ratledge sold his school to Carl S. Cleveland Sr., D.C. Today's Cleveland Chiropractic College of Los Angeles is the continuation of the Ratledge College.

Alva Gregory

Carver College graduate Alva Gregory, M.D., D.C., received his medical training at the University of Texas and enrolled at the original Carver-Denny School of Chiropractic in Oklahoma City in 1906. When D.D. Palmer arrived in the Indian Territory (soon to become the state of Oklahoma), Willard Carver invited the founder to consider a faculty position or partnership at Carver College. Instead, Palmer encountered Gregory and went into competition with Carver as the Palmer-Gregory School of Chiropractic in Oklahoma City. This partnership continued for only a short time, and D.D. soon departed for Portland, Oregon. Physician-chiropractor Gregory continued to operate the Palmer-Gregory School for a number of years, thereby earning the founder's further ire.

Part of the disagreement between Gregory and Palmer revolved around theoretical considerations of the lesions that chiropractors adjusted. Although Palmer held that the correction of subluxations was the exclusive concern of the chiropractor, Gregory allowed that thrusting into or percussion of various spinal segments could have therapeutic value by influencing end-organ activity regardless of whether a subluxation was detected. Palmer considered this "medical" thinking and would have none of it; he objected further to Gregory's use of various percussive devices. Gregory denigrated Palmer as an uneducated practitioner who understood little of modern biology but who had stumbled upon the broadly useful health care method of adjusting.

Gregory's influence on chiropractic theory and practice continued for many years. His college merged with the St. Louis School of Chiropractic in Missouri in 1913 but not before he had trained a number of chiropractors who would also leave their mark on the young profession. Among these were Edward L. Cooley, N.D., D.C., Oph.D. and son C. Sterling Cooley, D.C., of Enid, Oklahoma, who worked with Gregory to form the American Chiropractic Association, which sought to organize chiroprac-

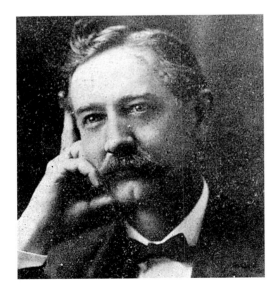

Edward L. Cooley, N.D., D.C., Oph.D., graduate of the Palmer-Gregory School of Chiropractic.

From *The American Drugless Healer* 1(2), 1911.

tors nationally. This association is not related to today's American Chiropractic Association. In the 1930s and 1940s, C.S. Cooley served as the third president and for many years as a member of the board of directors of the National Chiropractic Association, a true forerunner of today's American Chiropractic Association. Albert W. Richardson, D.C., also took his training under Gregory in Los Angeles. In 1913, Richardson founded the first of his California Chiropractic Colleges, institutions that promoted very broad-scope chiropractic practice for decades and that eventually merged with the modern LACC.

Gregory's influence was derived from not only his Palmer-Gregory school and numerous seminars held throughout the United States but also his many writings. For several years, he edited *The American Drugless Healer,* the official publication of the Oklahoma-based American Chiropractic Association, and authored several significant early textbooks, including *Spinal Adjustment* (1910), *Spinal Treatment* (1912), and *Rational Therapy* (1913).

His attitude of eclecticism in health care struck a responsive chord among many chiropractors and drugless healers of the day. This attitude was well captured in the subtitle to his 1912 volume: *Spinal Treatment: The True Principle of Progress in the Healing Art, Namely, Try All Things With an Open Mind, and Hold Fast to That Which is Found to Be Good.*

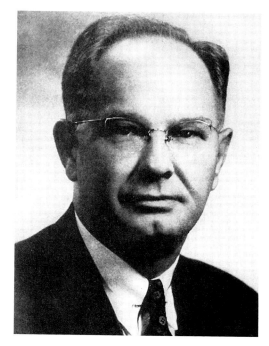

C. Sterling Cooley, D.C. (1890-1965), president of the National Chiropractic Association in 1934 and 1935.

Courtesy Palmer College of Chiropractic Archives, Davenport, Iowa.

Joe Shelby Riley

Another graduate of the Palmer-Gregory School was Joe Shelby Riley, M.D., M.S., Ph.D., D.M.T., D.P., D.O., D.C., Ph.C., who served as Vice-President, Professor of Anatomy, and Clinic Director of the Palmer-Gregory School after his graduation circa 1908. Riley was also active in Gregory's Oklahoma-based American Chiropractic Association and was a frequent contributor to the association's journal. It is not known from where most of the degrees Riley claimed to have were acquired, nor which of the many may have been spurious. However, over the years, Riley's many publications confirmed his status as a scholar and a prodigious writer on alternative therapies. Among these works were *Science and Practice of Chiropractic with Allied Sciences* (1919) and *Zone Reflex* (1942).

In 1912, Riley arrived in Boston and established the New England College of Chiropractic, which offered an 18-month curriculum in broad-scope chiropractic. He was soon challenged by the medical community in Massachusetts and was fined in April 1914 for offering the "Doctor of Chiropractic" degree without authorization from the state. Riley appealed this ruling to the state's Supreme Court, which upheld an earlier Massachusetts ruling that the practice of chiropractic, whether couched in terms of spinal analysis and adjusting or diagnosis and treatment, was legally the practice of medicine. This ruling outlawed chiropractic in the state until 1966 when a chiropractic law was finally passed. This ruling was also used as a precedent in legal efforts to bar chiropractors from practice in many court cases in other states. Riley, whose enthusiasm for the healing arts was matched by his many extravagant claims, earned the scorn of the state's Palmer-straight D.C.s. Riley relocated to Washington, D.C., around 1915, where he established the Washington School of Chiropractic. For several decades, he continued to operate on the fringes of the chiropractic profession and was associated with the American Drugless Association and the American Naturopathic Association and its lu-

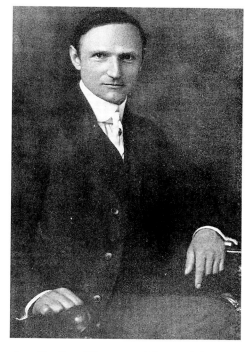

Joe Shelby Riley, president of the broad-scope New England College of Chiropractic and the Washington School of Chiropractic.

From Riley JS: *Science and practice of chiropractic with allied sciences,* 1919.

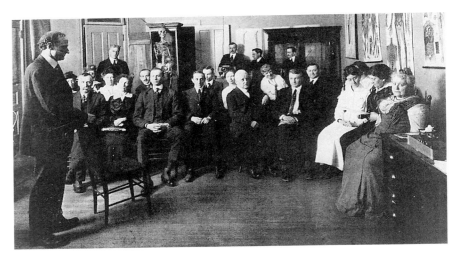

J.S. Riley lecturing at his Washington School of Chiropractic.

From Riley JS: *Science and practice of chiropractic with allied sciences*, 1919.

minaries, Benedict Lust, M.D., N.D., considered the "father of naturopathy in America"; Alva Gregory, M.D., D.C.; and Fred W. Collins, D.O., D.C., dean of the Mecca College of Chiropractic in Newark, New Jersey. Like Thomas Storey and Alva Gregory, he was a strong advocate of adjustive and concussive instruments and of Gregory's and Albert Abrams' "spondylotherapeutic" methods of conservative spinal care. Riley and associates were characterized as arch villains in B.J. Palmer's repeated diatribes against "mixer" chiropractic.

B.J. PALMER, THE "DEVELOPER"

The son of D.D. Palmer may be considered both a disciple of and a heretic relative to his father's teachings and, after the founder, is undoubtedly the single most influential individual in the profession's history. B.J. Palmer was born in 1882 in What Cheer, Iowa, and grew up in Davenport, Iowa, where D.D. had moved his magnetic practice. His influence in the early years of the profession dates to 1902, just shortly after he earned his chiropractic diploma, at which time he took over the operation of the Palmer School and Cure during his father's first sojourns on the West Coast. In those very earliest years, B.J. was a follower of his father's theories, which at that time still considered the value of chiropractic treatments to free up pinched arteries and nerves. Although he was initially willing to consider rival school leader Solon Langworthy's proposition for a combined teaching venture and the inclusion of naturopathic methods in the chiropractic curriculum, he rejected Langworthy's offer when his father rejected it and argued against the mixing of chiropractic methods with other healing arts. For the rest of his career and especially after his father's death in 1913, B.J. became the undisputed champion of "pure, straight and unadulterated chiropractic."

The developer of chiropractic continued as the secretary of the Palmer School of Chiropractic until shortly after D.D. Palmer's conviction and jailing for unlicensed practice in Scott County, Iowa, in 1906. Old Dad Chiro had signed over his ownership of the school to B.J.'s wife, Mabel Heath

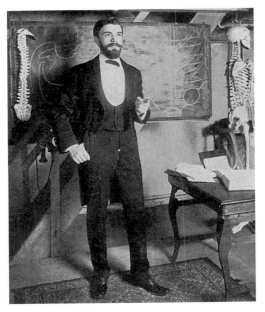

B.J. Palmer (1882-1961) delivering lectures in the lecture hall of the Palmer School of Chiropractic.

From Palmer BJ: *The science of chiropractic*, 1907.

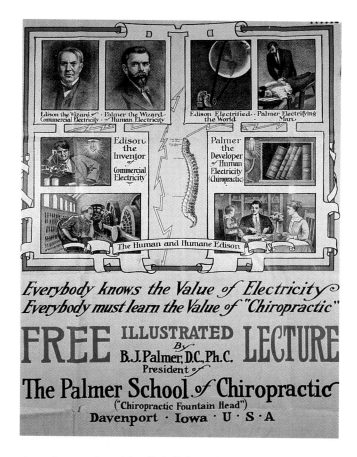

A poster produced by B.J. Palmer in which he compares himself to Thomas Edison.

Courtesy Palmer College of Chiropractic Archives, Davenport, Iowa.

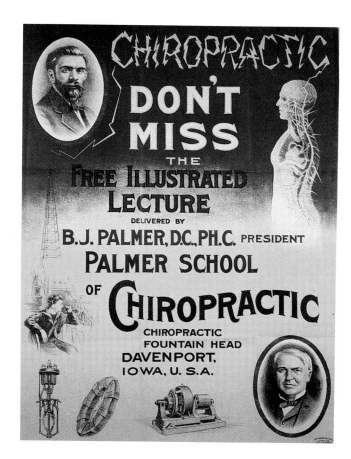

A poster advertising B.J. Palmer's lecture on chiropractic.

Courtesy Palmer College of Chiropractic Archives, Davenport, Iowa.

Palmer D.C., to avoid its confiscation in any legal judgments. After D.D.'s release from jail, he sold his share in the school to B.J. From then until his death in 1961, B.J. functioned as president of the school. As the senior Palmer began his wanderings through Oklahoma, Oregon, and California, B.J. began to expand the school and its many related activities, such as advertising; a correspondence program; publication of two regular magazines, *Fountain Head News* and *The Chiropractor;* and the introduction of new technologies. B.J. brought the first x-ray machine to Davenport in 1909. By 1916 the Palmer School of Chiropractic offered a course leading to a special diploma in this new medium.

This early introduction of x-ray technology, discovered by Wilhelm Roentgen in 1895, had a subtle but significant effect on chiropractic theory. Although D.D. Palmer focused most of his attention on the function of the nervous system and had relied predominantly on nerve tracing as a means of identifying dysfunctional organs and corresponding subluxations, the use of roentgenology redirected chiropractors' attention toward the skeletal structure. The bones could be seen on x-ray films; the nervous system could not. Several oblique comments published by the founder suggest that he disdained this deviation from his "done by hand" notion of chiropractic. The possibility that x-ray technology prompted Joy Loban to depart the Palmer School of Chiropractic and to found the Universal Chiropractic College has already been noted. However, the new technology lent an air of science and technology to the budding profession, and B.J. encouraged chiropractors to advertise their

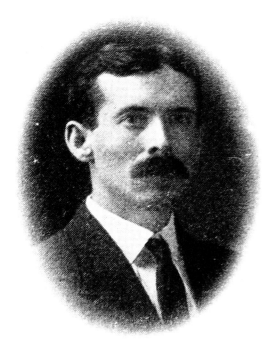

James F. McGinnis, D.C., Palmer School spinographer and photographer, circa 1910.

Courtesy Palmer College of Chiropractic Archives, Davenport, Iowa.

x-ray services in marketing their practices. Meanwhile, nerve tracing began to fade from prominence among the chiropractors' assessment methods; with the introduction of B.J.'s heat-sensing instrumentation the neurocalometer in 1924, the manual methods of neurological diagnosis used by Old Dad Chiro nearly disappeared.

Like his father, B.J. may be grouped among the "segmental" theorists in the early years of chiropractic. Misalignments of spinal bones were thought to occur individually, that is, without causing subluxations elsewhere. Although the developer would later posit the existence of major and minor subluxations in every spine, he initially leaned heavily on what has come to be known as the *Meric theory* of subluxation. The Meric system focused on the presumed relation between dysfunctions at particular spinal joints and specific diseases of particular organs. B.J. never adopted his father's idea of nerve stretching, preferring instead to focus on the idea that chiropractors relieved the pinching of nerves as they exited the spine. Early promotional material warned the reader to "Get off the hose!" meaning that the chiropractor sought free flow of nerve force through the nerves by realigning the spinal bones that pinched them. X-ray technology seems to have encouraged this idea, and oversized pictures of the spinal column and pinched nerves became common in informational materials from The Fountain Head.

The younger Palmer's influence was also derived from his phenomenal success in expanding the student body. The Palmer School of Chiropractic grew to several hundred students by 1915, which was far more

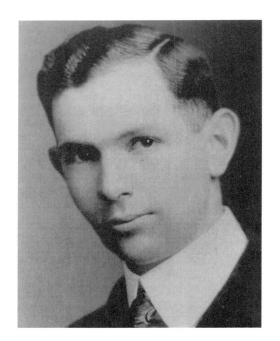

E.A. Thompson, D.C. (1891-1976), first chair of the Spinography Department at the Palmer School.

Courtesy Palmer College of Chiropractic Archives, Davenport, Iowa.

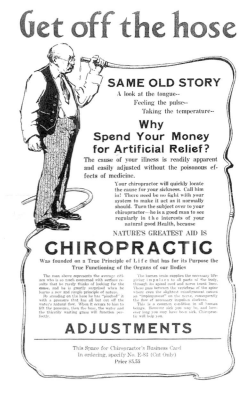

Early promotional material from the PSC warning the reader to "GET OFF THE HOSE!", meaning they should have their spines checked by a chiropractor who would relieve nerves being affected by the spine.

Courtesy Palmer College of Chiropractic, Davenport, Iowa.

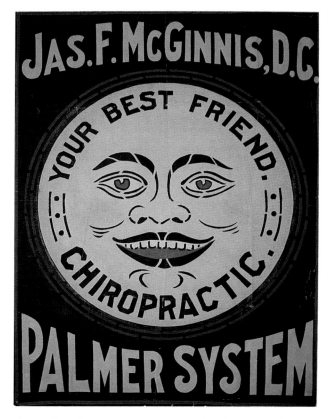

An early advertising poster done by James McGinnis.

Courtesy Palmer College of Chiropractic Archives, Davenport, Iowa.

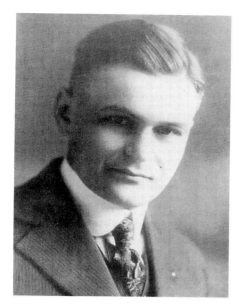

Stephen J. Burich, B.S., D.C. (1887-1946), early faculty member at the Palmer School of Chiropractic.

Courtesy Palmer College of Chiropractic Archives, Davenport, Iowa.

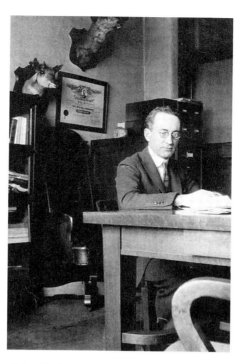

John H. Craven, B.A., D.C., early faculty member at the Palmer School of Chiropractic.

Courtesy Palmer College of Chiropractic Archives, Davenport, Iowa.

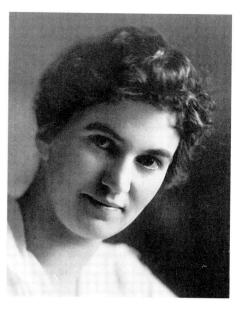

Mabel Heath Palmer, D.C. (1881-1949), B.J.'s wife and secretary of the Palmer School of Chiropractic. "Mabel" also taught anatomy for more than 40 years.

Courtesy Palmer College of Chiropractic Archives, Davenport, Iowa.

than any other chiropractic training institution at the time. Indeed, by the early 1920s the Palmer School could boast of over 1000 future doctors in training, and for many decades to come, the city of Davenport could justly proclaim that the majority of chiropractors in the world were Palmer graduates. Moreover, the Palmer curriculum and its faculty became models for other schools to emulate. Although organized medicine's criticisms in this early period emphasized the poor quality of chiropractic training, chiropractic students, and their instructors, the Palmer School of Chiropractic counted a number of liberal arts college graduates as teachers. Stephen J. Burich, B.S., D.C., for example, graduated from Beloit College and taught chemistry in the Milwaukee public schools before earning his doctorate and joining the Palmer faculty in 1913. Dr. Burich became an instructor in neurology and authored a textbook in chemistry. Similarly, John H. Craven, B.A., D.C., an ordained Methodist minister, earned his baccalaureate degree from Kansas Wesleyan University before commencing his studies at Palmer. He joined the faculty in 1913 and authored and co-authored a number of books over the years, including *The Science of Chiropractic* (1920), *A Textbook on Chiropractic Orthopedy* (1921), and *Hygiene and Pediatrics* (1924). Mabel Heath Palmer, D.C., who had married B.J. in 1904, studied at Augustana College before earning her chiropractic diploma in 1903. She reputedly studied anatomy at a Chicago medical school circa 1906, authored *Chiropractic Anatomy* in 1918, and taught anatomy for decades at Palmer. In ad-

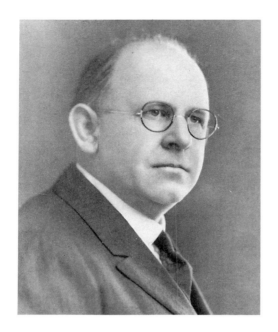

A.B. Hender, M.D., D.C. (1874-1943), dean of the Palmer School of Chiropractic from 1912 to 1943.

Courtesy Palmer College of Chiropractic Archives, Davenport, Iowa.

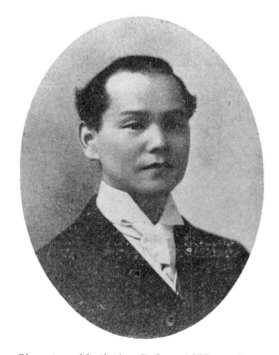

Shegataro Morikubo, D.C., a 1903 graduate of D.D. Palmer's. This Japanese chiropractor was successfully defended against the charge of practicing osteopathy without a license in LaCrosse, Wisconsin.

Courtesy Palmer College of Chiropractic Archives, Davenport, Iowa.

dition, at least one medical physician was always included on the Palmer faculty. A.B. Hender, M.D., D.C., earned his medical degree from Iowa in 1901 and served as a part-time lecturer at the Palmer School of Chiropractic from 1905 to 1910, at which time he accepted B.J.'s appointment as chairman of the Department of Obstetrics. By 1912, he had become dean of the Palmer School of Chiropractic, a position he held for more than 30 years. Hender never severed his ties with medicine but instead maintained his surgical privileges at area hospitals and became a well-known obstetrician in the Quad Cities. He also served as an expert witness in the chiropractors' many early courtroom battles against charges of unlicensed medical practice. A.B. Hender's son, Herbert, earned his D.C. from the Palmer School of Chiropractic and succeeded his father as dean of his alma mater for many years.

B.J.'s educational progeny, including those who idolized B.J. and those who rejected him, would together lead in the development of a chiropractic organization, "separate and distinct" legislation for doctors of chiropractic, and the growth of adherents and patients. Most of the early political activity originated from the Palmer School of Chiropractic and the national organization that B.J. and several of his graduates founded in Davenport in 1906. The Universal Chiropractors' Association was established primarily for the purpose of providing legal protection for chiropractors prosecuted for unlicensed practice. Old Dad Chiro's conviction and jailing in Scott County in 1906 undoubtedly provided much of the impetus for the association's formation, although competition from the earliest known American Chiropractic Association, organized by rival school leader Solon Langworthy, D.C., in 1905, was also a stimulus. Among the Universal Chiropractors' Association's first actions was a condemnation of the broad-scope, mixer policies of Langworthy's American Chiropractic Association.

CHIROPRACTIC THEORY AND PRACTICE POLITICS

The Universal Chiropractor's Association's first legal challenge, one that would exert a profound effect on the profession's future, came in 1907 when Shegataro Morikubo, D.C., a 1901 graduate under D.D. Palmer, was arrested in LaCrosse, Wisconsin, at the request of the state medical board's osteopathic member for unlicensed practice of medicine, surgery, and osteopathy. Morikubo was a member of the Univeral Chiropractors' Association and was among the Palmer graduates who had organized the protective association in Davenport the previous year. B.J. Palmer, secretary of the association, rushed to LaCrosse, Wisconsin, at Morikubo's request, where he engaged the services of lawyer and state senator Tom Morris to defend the chiropractor. Morris appealed to the prosecuting attorney to drop the charges of practicing medicine and surgery without a license, since Dr. Morikubo had used only his hands in attempting to heal the sick. When the prosecutor agreed, the chiropractor was brought to trial on the reduced charge of the unlicensed practice of osteopathy. Morris' legal task was to make a case that chiropractic was distinctly different from osteopathy and that Morikubo was therefore not guilty of practicing osteopathy when he used chiropractic theories and techniques to help his patients.

To establish this distinction between the two forms of "bonesetting," Morris relied heavily on the first textbook of chiropractic, *Modernized Chi-*

ropractic, which had been co-produced the year before by Oakley Smith, D.C., Minora Paxson, D.C., and Solon Langworthy, D.C., at the American School of Chiropractic & Nature Cure in Cedar Rapids, Iowa. *Modernized Chiropractic* proclaimed that chiropractic had a separate and distinct philosophy and practice that was unlike any other healing method. To bolster this contention, Morris called several expert witnesses who held degrees in both osteopathy and chiropractic. The jury deliberated less than 30 minutes before returning a verdict of not guilty for the young chiropractor.

This first courtroom victory for chiropractic was a turning point for several reasons. The defense counsel's winning contention that chiropractic theory and practice constituted a separate and distinct healing art became the basis of legal arguments and acquittals in the thousands of prosecutions that chiropractors would undergo in the next several decades (an estimated 15,000 by 1930). Moreover, the separate and distinct character of chiropractic would also form the basis for successful appeal to state legislatures for separate licensing laws and examining boards for those seeking licensure. Chiropractors could argue credibly that medical practice acts and boards of medical examiners were not qualified to encompass or judge the competence of the practitioners of chiropractic. Even those chiropractors with little or no respect for the flamboyant B.J. and his association took notice of the success in the Morikubo case and subsequently patterned their legal and political strategies after attorney Morris' winning contention.

The LaCrosse trial also brought Tom Morris to the attention of the profession, and he served as chief legal counsel for the Univeral Chiropractors' Association until his death in 1928. Although he served a term as Lieutenant Governor of Wisconsin and made an unsuccessful gubernatorial run, the last two decades of his life were primarily devoted to the Universal Chiropractors' Association and its defense of chiropractors. Morris has been credited as the architect of "chiropractic philosophy" because it was he who showed how to use chiropractic theories legally. B.J. Palmer was greatly impressed with Morris' use of philosophy to keep chiropractors out of jail. Soon after the trial, he had the Palmer faculty award him the first Ph.C. (Philosopher of Chiropractic) degree, and while Morris became chief legal counsel to the association, B.J. became the "philosophical counsel" to the organization. For the next several years, most of the textbooks authored by B.J. included the term *philosophy* in their titles, for example, *The Science, Art and Philosophy of Nerve Tracing.* "Separate and distinct" philosophy would become a central feature of chiropractic rhetoric.

Attorney Morris' courtroom use of Smith, Paxson, and Langworthy's *Modernized Chiropractic* also had a lasting influence on chiropractic theories. Although D.D. Palmer had abandoned his interest in the circulatory system, arteries, and veins after his 1903 decision that the "body is heated by nerves and not by blood," many of his earliest graduates had not. With the Morikubo victory, chiropractors had compelling legal reasons to leave the "rule of the artery" to the osteopaths and to focus their chiropractic concerns exclusively on the nervous system. Moreover, Morris' adoption of Smith, Paxson, and Langworthy's theories of subluxation (spinal bones pinching nerves) overshadowed D.D. Palmer's later theory that misaligned spinal bones stretched nerves, thereby increasing their vibrational frequency and causing inflamed tissues and organs. In this way, the courtroom experience of the young profession became a powerful determinant of its theories, and Old Dad Chiro's later hypotheses were never seriously adopted by chiropractors.

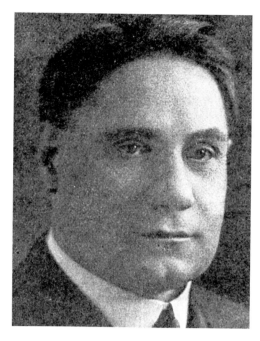

Tom Morris, chief legal counsel to the Universal Chiropractors' Association from 1906 to 1928.

From *The Chiropractor,* Sept 1928.

119

OTHER PIONEER FAMILIES

During the early period in chiropractic history from 1900 to 1915, several significant family traditions began within the profession. One example is Almeda Haldeman, D.C., a 1905 graduate of the short-lived Chiropractic School & Cure operated by E.W. Lynch, D.C., of Minneapolis. Like so many of the earliest chiropractors, Mrs. Haldeman was inspired to study the new healing art after her husband recovered from a then medically unmanageable condition—diabetes—while under chiropractic care. Lynch's recommendation that her husband move to a drier climate prompted the couple to relocate to Herbert, Saskatchewan; Almeda thereby became the first chiropractor to practice in Canada in 1906. Her son Joshua Norman Haldeman graduated from the Palmer School of Chiropractic in 1926, played an active role in chiropractic politics in the province of Saskatchewan, and was a co-founder of the Canadian Memorial Chiropractic College in Toronto in 1945. In the early 1950s, Joshua and his family emigrated to South Africa, where he developed one of the largest chiropractic clinics on that continent. The family's influence on the profession continues by virtue of Almeda's grandson and Joshua's son, Scott Haldeman, D.C., Ph.D., M.D., a Palmer graduate who also holds diplomas in neurophysiology and neurology and who has been a major stimulus in the development of scientific research in the profession during recent years.

Three generations of the Schillig family, five chiropractors in all, have contributed to the chiropractic saga. Most significant among these were

Joshua Norman Haldeman, son of the first chiropractor to practice in Canada, Almeda Haldeman, D.C.

Courtesy Scott Haldeman, Santa Anna, California.

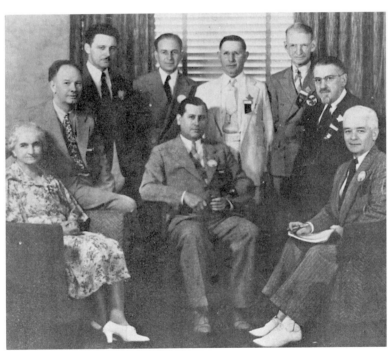

Charles E. Schillig, D.C. (1881-1960), president of the Universal Chiropractors' Association (1926-1930) and cofounder of the National Chiropractic Association, is second from the right in this 1938 photo of executives of the associations. Lillard T. Marshall is seated in the center; left to right are Sylva Ashworth (seated), C. Sterling Cooley, Gordon M. Goodfellow, F. Lorne Wheaton, O.L. Brown, A.B. Cochrane, C.E. Schillig and Harry K. McIlroy (seated).

From *The Chiropractic Journal* Sept 1938.

Joseph Schillig, D.C., who had been a friend of D.D. Palmer since the 1880s when both were living in What Cheer, Iowa, and son Charles Elmer Schillig. Joseph Schillig, a 1912 graduate of the Palmer school, was one of the first chiropractors to practice in Ohio. Joseph's son Charles followed his father and elder brother to the Palmer school, where he also received his doctorate in 1914. His arrest, conviction, and fining for unlicensed practice prompted his participation in the formation and governance of the Ohio Chiropractic Association. When re-arrested and convicted on this charge in 1923, Charles Schillig opted for 6 months imprisonment rather than pay a fine. From his jail cell, he organized a drive to legalize the practice of chiropractic, which attracted 100,000 petitions and the attention of many newspapers nationwide. Charles Schillig served as president of the Universal Chiropractors' Association from 1926 and worked diligently behind the scenes in collaboration with the ACA's past president, Frank R. Margetts, LL.B., D.C., to bring about the association's merger with the American Chiropractic Association. The National Chiropractic Association was born of a September 1930 meeting in Louisville, Kentucky, among Schillig, Margetts, and soon-to-be first president T. Marshall, D.C. In later years, Charles Schillig served as a consultant and spokesperson for Anabolic Foods, Inc. in southern California.

Another multigenerational pioneer family's story began in 1907, when Sylva L. Ashworth, a single parent of four children in rural eastern Nebraska, developed diabetic gangrene in one leg and was rejected as a surgical candidate because her physicians did not expect her to survive. On advice of her sister, she sought the services of Dr. Olson, presumably a Palmer school graduate, who taught her to monitor her urine chemistries and provided her with twice-daily adjustments of her lower spine. Sylva watched as the condition of her lower limb gradually improved and her urinalyses became more normal. Inspired by her thorough recovery, she mortgaged her farm and moved her family to Davenport, Iowa, to enroll at the Palmer school. Mrs. Ashworth completed the 12-month program in May 1910 and returned to Nebraska to establish a private practice that lasted for 46 years.

Sylva quickly became a successful practitioner, and her winning ways and enthusiasm for chiropractic won her many loyal patients; her practice was considered one of the largest in the country. She also soon became involved in chiropractic politics in Nebraska, and after the passage of the twentieth amendment to the U.S. Constitution, which granted women the right to vote, she became very active in Democratic party politics. She was one of the first women to serve as a state delegate to the Democratic National Convention in New York City in 1924 and became a close confidante of many public officials in Nebraska, including Governor Charles Bryan, brother of William Jennings Bryan. In 1926, Dr. Ashworth served briefly as president of the Universal Chiropractors' Association, the only woman ever to preside over a national chiropractic professional association in the United States. Despite her personal friendship with straight chiropractor B.J. Palmer, Sylva was a founding member of the National Chiropractic Association, predecessor of today's American Chiropractic Association. In 1944, Dr. Ashworth helped to organize the Chiropractic Research Foundation, a nonprofit organization that would evolve into the largest funding agency for chiropractic scientific studies.

Dr. Ashworth's commitment to chiropractic was astounding and was matched only by her concern for her patients. It is recalled that she regularly made charity visits to prisoners and condemned men at the Nebraska Penitentiary and that no one was ever turned away from her clinic

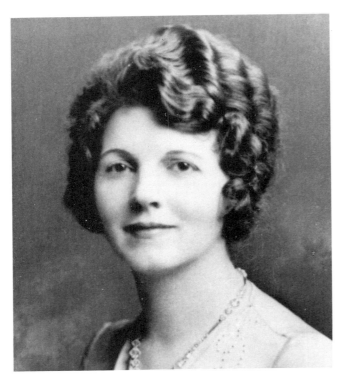

Ruth Ashworth Cleveland (1895-1975), D.C., circa 1940.
Courtesy Cleveland College of Chiropractic, Kansas City, Missouri.

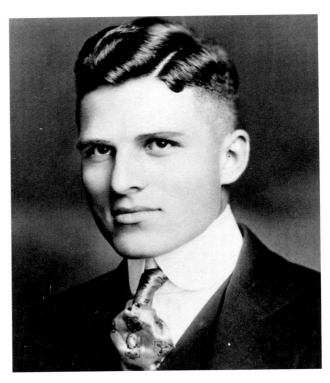

Carl S. Cleveland, Sr., D.C., circa 1917.
Courtesy Cleveland College of Chiropractic, Kansas City, Missouri.

for their inability to pay. When she learned of cancer victims who had been given up as incurable or who could not afford medical care, she would pay their train fare to Lincoln, Nebraska, and lodge them in her home while she provided free chiropractic care. At one time an "Ashworth Special" train ran between Omaha and Lincoln to bring patients to her clinic. She is remembered as the "Grand Old Lady of Chiropractic."

Sylva's devotion to chiropractic inspired her daughter Ruth to follow in her footsteps. While studying at the Palmer school from 1916 to 1917, Ruth Ashworth met the school's baseball star, Carl S. Cleveland. The couple were married in the Palmer mansion in 1917, and B.J. gave the bride away. After practicing briefly in Webster City, Iowa, the Clevelands relocated to Kansas City, Missouri, where they founded the Cleveland Chiropractic College in 1922. Their only child, Carl S. Cleveland, Jr., was born in 1918 and is now chancellor of the Cleveland Colleges in Kansas City and Los Angeles, and his son, Carl S. Cleveland, III, is president of the colleges. Sylva Ashworth's great-great-granddaughter, Ashley Cleveland, daughter of Carl III, is currently a doctoral student at Cleveland College in Kansas City.

SPIRIT OF THE TIME

The first several decades of the chiropractic story were a period of struggle and perseverance in the face of tremendous odds. The early pioneers built a profession from scratch despite the enormous barriers erected by established health care interests. The dogged determination of the early chiropractors and their success in defending and propagating the profession may be attributed to many factors, but perhaps chief among these was the raw courage of their conviction that the chiropractic art had something very valuable to offer to society. It was an age of wonderment, and if those early pioneers were guilty of naiveté in scientific matters, this was balanced by their genuine concern for their patients and their passion to explore the limits of the new theories and methods. As they left those early schools with diplomas in hand, their imaginations soared as they contemplated the range of health problems to which they would apply their new skills. Given the limited knowledge of cause and cure available for most health problems at that time, a visit to the chiropractor was probably a wise choice. Like the magnetic, homeopath, and osteopath, the chiropractor offered a conservative alternative to the lingering heroic medical traditions of the Midwest, and if the chiropractor failed to benefit the patient, great harm was also unlikely.

Although many early chiropractors restricted their treatments to chiropractic adjustments, a number quickly became involved in providing other "drugless" methods, and the self-defined scope of chiropractic care rapidly expanded. Doctors of chiropractic soon became entangled in the struggle for control of health care that had begun in the late nineteenth century as medical licensing laws were gradually reintroduced in most states. This entanglement created a siege mentality that persists to the present and that has significantly shaped the character of the chiropractic profession. The age of wonderment gave rise to an age of turbulence in which chiropractors battled organized medicine for the right to exist and fought among themselves over the nature of chiropractic.

Preparation of this paper was supported by the National Institute of Chiropractic and the Palmer College Archives in Davenport, Iowa.

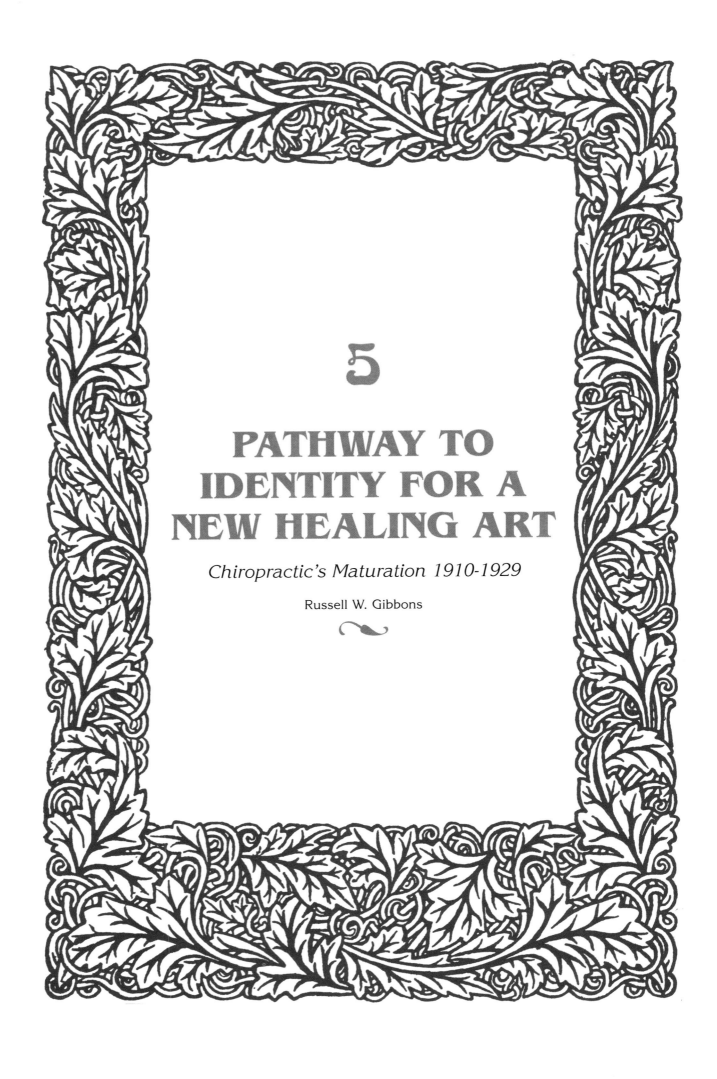

5

PATHWAY TO IDENTITY FOR A NEW HEALING ART

Chiropractic's Maturation 1910-1929

Russell W. Gibbons

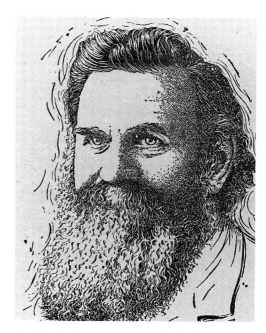

An illustration portraying D.D. Palmer, done in the style favored by Elbert Hubbard, founder of the Arts and Crafts community known as the Roycrofters.

Courtesy Palmer College of Chiropractic Archives, Davenport, Iowa.

The Golden Age of Technology held sway at the start of the second decade of the new century. Thomas Alva Edison, the "Wizard of Menlo Park," was at work in perfecting concepts of motion pictures. Henry Ford was in Detroit, researching and developing what would be the first radical change in transportation in this century—the assembly line for the Model T. Wilbur and Oliver Wright saw their primitive, fixed, heavier-than-air flight become the symbolic industry of twentieth century progress.

In Davenport, the Palmers, father and son, also dreamed. They saw the technological marvels that were taking place around them as just part of the great new body of knowledge that was to be released to the world. Their contribution to this new knowledge would be toward solving the age-old illness of the human body. Although the relationships between Daniel David (D.D.) Palmer and Bartlett Joshua (B.J.) Palmer had chilled to the point that the senior Palmer only visited Davenport a few weeks at a time from his new West Coast homes in Oregon and California, there still existed elements of mutual respect and even admiration.

D.D. Palmer had departed from the city where he launched his new dissenting school 11 years previously and had abdicated titular leadership to his son, whose Van Dyke beard and newly acquired prosperity had placed him in the center of the chiropractic universe. Indeed, a Palmer School of Chiropractic reproduction circa 1911 had B.J. as the center of the world, warding off spectors labeled *disease* and *death* and the medical nemesis. For those not sure, Davenport was shown to be the center of the world and the heroic Greeklike figure with a loincloth was marked "B.J.P."

Palmer hegemony by the son appeared to be all encompassing in every area. The Palmer School advertised in popular home magazines and medical remedy journals, and its designation as "The Fountainhead of Chiropractic" repeated the well-themed advertising message that if it was chiropractic and it was good, then it had to come from Davenport. The struggle for absolute control in the emerging profession by the younger Palmer took place at a time when a similar sea change of activity was affecting traditional medicine.

Paul Starr, a medical sociologist and author of *The Social Transformation of American Medicine,* described the period as a consolidation phase following the profession's own "civil war and reconstruction" period of the late nineteenth century.

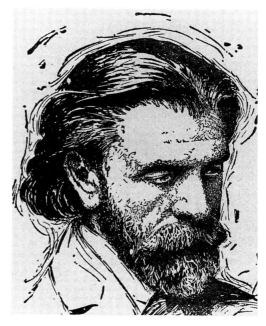

An illustration of B.J. Palmer done in the style used by the Roycrofters. B.J. was a friend and admirer of Elbert Hubbard, the founder of the Roycroft community.

Courtesy Palmer College of Chiropractic Archives, Davenport, Iowa.

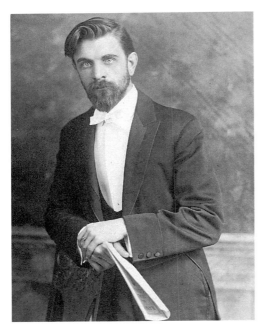

A formal photograph of B.J. circa 1910.

Courtesy Palmer College of Chiropractic Archives, Davenport, Iowa.

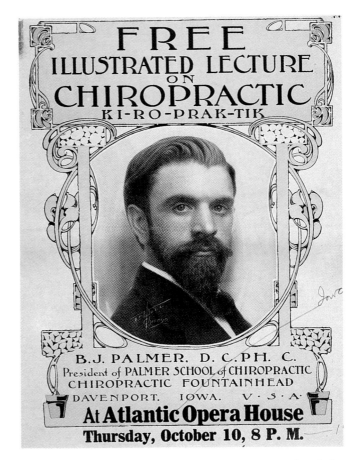

A poster advertising a lecture on chiropractic by B.J. Palmer, circa 1910.

Courtesy Palmer College of Chiropractic Archives, Davenport, Iowa.

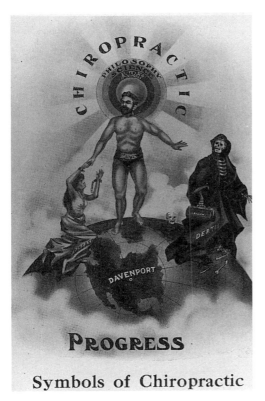

A Palmer broadside circa 1911 with B.J., representing chiropractic, warding off disease and death.

Courtesy Palmer College of Chiropractic Archives, Davenport, Iowa.

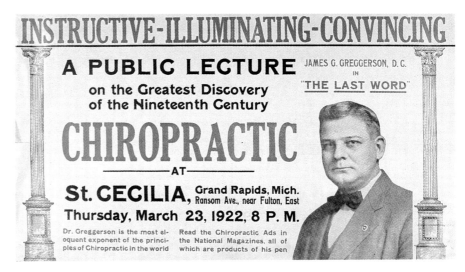

A poster advertising a lecture by James Greggerson, who was employed by the Universal Chiropractors Association to publicize chiropractic.

Courtesy Palmer College of Chiropractic Archives, Davenport, Iowa.

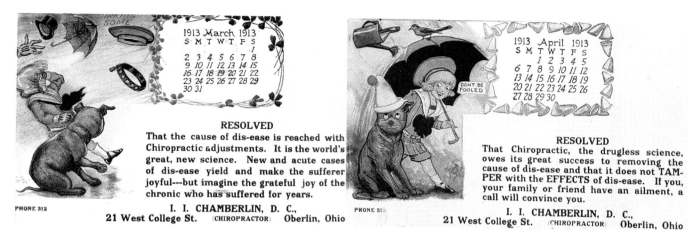

An enterprising chiropractor sent these colorful postcard calenders to prospective patients in 1913.
Courtesy Palmer College of Chiropractic Archives, Davenport, Iowa.

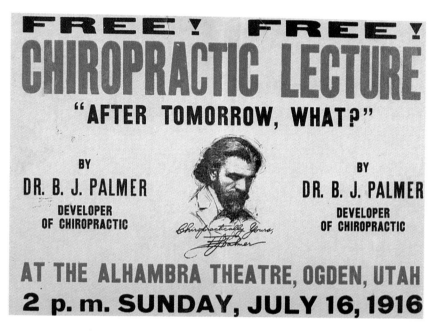

A poster advertising a 1916 lecture by B.J. Palmer.
Courtesy Palmer College of Chiropractic Archives, Davenport, Iowa.

EVOLUTION OF MEDICAL EDUCATION

Americans had consistently expressed disdain for organized medical services and institutions through most of the first 100 years of the new republic. During the middle third of the nineteenth century when America's urban centers were growing and Jacksonian Democracy was at its height, newly practicing doctors found that society's most influential elements did not look with favor on either professions or callings whose members sought self-regulation of their occupations. Such attempts were beat back as antidemocratic efforts to enact "licensed monopolies."

BOOM YEARS AT THE PSC

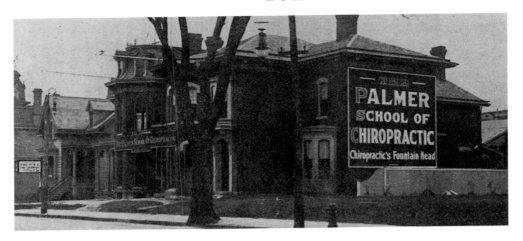

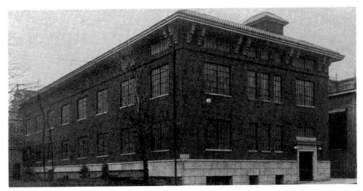

"Watch Us Grow" said a headline in B.J.'s Fountainhead News *in 1915, as the Palmer School began a 6-year capital building project which expanded the original facility at 828 Brady Street and adjacent buildings* (above) *with the D.D. Palmer Memorial Building* (right), *the printing plant* (below), *and later the administration building and the clinic-classroom building, which was dedicated in 1921.*

Courtesy Palmer College of Chiropractic Archives, Davenport, Iowa.

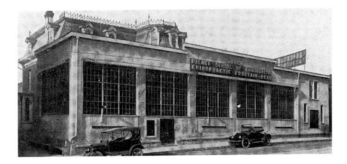

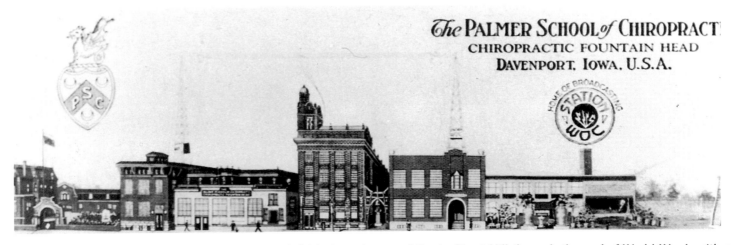

The "Mother School of Chiropractic" occupied a full block at the top of Brady Street Hill through the end of World War I, with a student population estimated at 3100 in attendance during 1921. The physical plant was dominated by "Up E Nuf" and the towers of radio station WOC ("Wonders of Chiropractic").

Courtesy Palmer College of Chiropractic Archives, Davenport, Iowa.

1913—HOMECOMING PARADE AND FALSE CHARGES

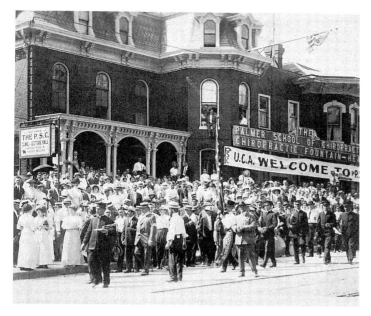

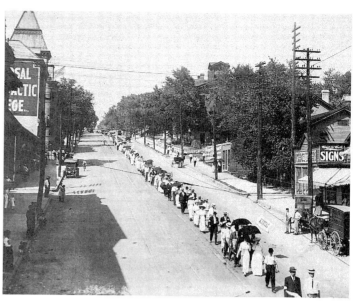

August 27, 1913 about noon. The PSC band assembles in front of the school buildings at the top of Brady Street hill. It was standing-room only on campus as hundreds of students, chiropractors, patients, and their families waited for the parade to begin.

Evidence of the torrid Davenport August is apparent with the number of umbrellas in the line of march as the parade passes Sixth at Brady. Most of this delegation of students and practitioners were behind the Kansas sign.

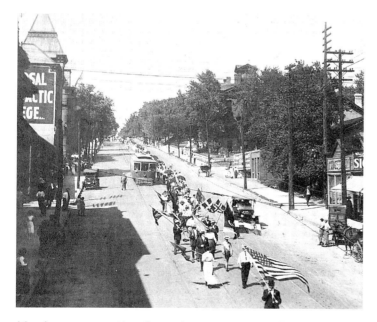

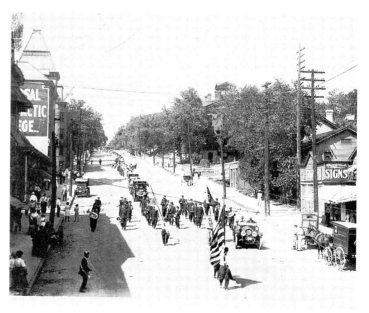

Marchers representing the various countries in the PSC student body, just behind the lead party and the band. Flags represent Norway, Sweden, Denmark, Great Britain, and possibly France.

The critical picture: was this just after the incident involving "Old Dad Chiro"? B.J. can be seen in the open car with the U.C.A. attorney Tom Morris. Notice part of the sign of Universal College at left.

The controversy that continued to plague B.J. Palmer for much of a generation had its origins on August 27, 1913. Allegations that the son had knocked his father to the curb during the homecoming parade proved to be without foundation, despite attempts by rival Universal College school owners and association officials to obtain an indictment with the Scott County Jury. B.J. provided full details in publications issued in 1914, 1939, and 1949 to respond to the false and vicious charges of "patricide."

Courtesy Palmer College of Chiropractic Archives, Davenport, Iowa.

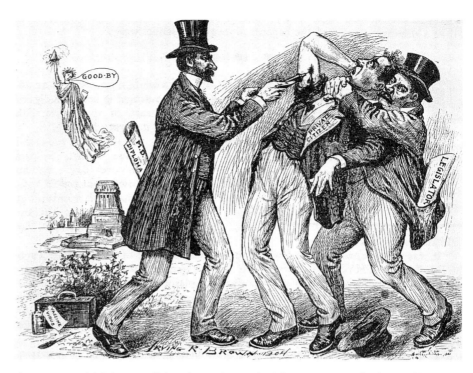

A cartoon criticizing medicine for trying to legislate a monopoly for itself.
Courtesy Palmer College of Chiropractic Archives, Davenport, Iowa.

The so-called regulars, medical practitioners who followed acceptable healing dogma passed along by the physicians of the colonial era and who taught in pioneer medical schools such as Harvard and Yale, found a public as wary of medical authority as it was of political or religious institutionalism. Thus began an era of evolution and transformation in medicine, which later would include a sort of itinerant medical entrepreneurism among some of the sects rivaling the old school physicians.

By the 1890s, medical schools had proliferated dramatically, thus correspondingly was the supply of generally ill-prepared physicians. One writer notes that "the immediate beneficiaries of this expansion in supply were the proprietors and professors of the medical schools."

Reform was clearly necessary. The clarion call can be traced to 1870, the early years of a period of rapid urban population growth, when Har-

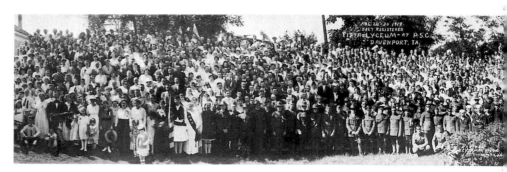

The PSC's Fifth Annual Lyceum, August 1918. Notice the large number of men in uniform.
Courtesy Palmer College of Chiropractic Archives, Davenport, Iowa.

vard President Charles Elliott declared that "the ignorance and general incompetency of the average graduate of American medical schools, at the time when he receives the degree which turns him loose upon the community, is something horrible to contemplate."

Medical education's foremost critic was Abraham Flexner, a nonphysician commissioned by the Carnegie Foundation for the Advancement of Teaching to survey all medical schools during 1909 to 1910. The resulting study, known as the *Flexner Report,* is a landmark work that directly led to the reformation of medical education in the United States. In the *Report,* Flexner essentially condemned the state of medical education as "deplorable and wretched."

Indeed, medical education in the first decade of this century was a proprietary money-making business. Flexner surveyed 155 schools and fully 80%, or 122 institutions, were for-profit concerns. Most of the revenue, principally from student tuition and fees and occasionally from clinics of associated hospitals, went into what Flexner derided as "professional pockets."

The country was well into the Reform period, and for many the state of American education was an obvious target. The injunction of the president of the Carnegie Foundation in 1910 laid the basis for Flexner's sweeping, if not revolutionary, recommendations deploring the situation in which "American youth, too often the prey of commercial advertising methods, is steered into the practice of medicine with almost no opportunity to learn the difference between an efficient medical school and a hopelessly inadequate one." Henry S. Pritchert, the Carnegie Foundation head, warned that "such a boy falls an easy victim to the commercial medical school, whether operating under name of a university or college, or alone."

Visiting the University of Pittsburgh's medical school in February 1910, Flexner observed that "a more thorough piece of house-cleaning within so short a period is hardly credible," saying that only a year before "the so-called laboratories were dirty and disorderly beyond description." Flexner tended to go overboard in his condemnation, each institution seemingly a candidate for "the worst" school, including the alma mater of brother Seimon Flexner, who became research director for the Rockefeller Foundation. The medical program at Pittsburgh was no exception. Before the university's takeover of the proprietary medical program, it "was a highly prosperous concern to its managers; nowhere in the country were worse conditions found."

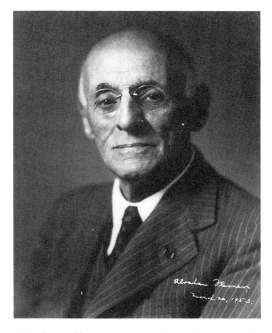

Abraham Flexner, a non-physician commissioned by the Carnegie Foundation to survey medical schools during 1909-1910. His study led to the reformation of medical education in the United States.

Courtesy National Library of Medicine, Bethesda, Maryland.

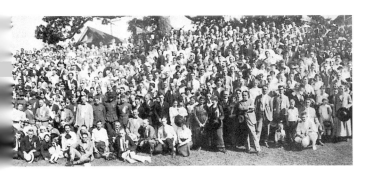

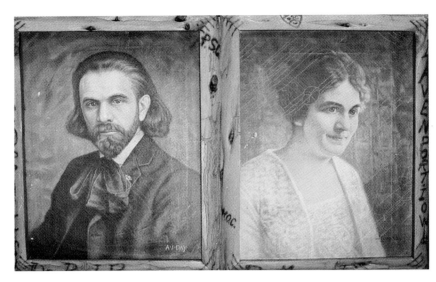

B.J. and Mabel Palmer, by artist J. Day. These reproductions of oil portraits were given to friends of the PSC during the 1920s when they sent a student to the "Fountainhead."
Courtesy Texas Chiropractic College, Pasadena, Texas.

CHIROPRACTIC EDUCATION: THE PSC

It was in this environment that early chiropractic education began to flourish. The Palmer School of Chiropractic (PSC), prompted by its first rivalry with educator and organizational promoter Solon Massey Langworthy of Cedar Rapids, Iowa, extended the basic course to 12 months and then to 18 months. By 1910, B.J. had not only assumed the title of President of the PSC, he was slowly expanding his activities to assume the leadership of virtually every aspect of chiropractic: he was chiropractic's maximum promoter and advocate. He installed a printing house and bindery within PSC's Brady Street complex. He also began mailing tens of thousands of advertisements, flyers, and brochures to prospective patients and students, as well as to other chiropractors.

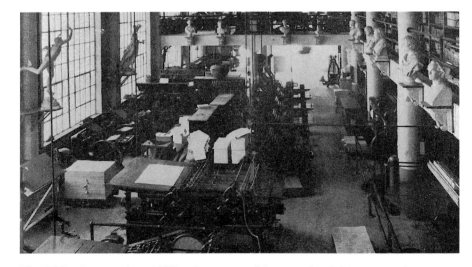

The PSC printery, circa 1925, where tens of thousands of chiropractic flyers, pamphlets, and brochures were sent to chiropractors and prospective students.
Courtesy Palmer College of Chiropractic Archives, Davenport, Iowa.

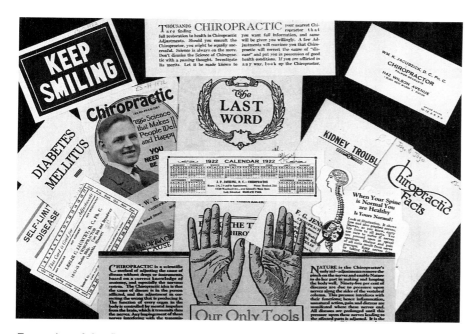

Examples of the flyers, pamphlets and brochures printed at the Palmer School.
Courtesy Palmer College of Chiropractic Archives, Davenport, Iowa.

B.J. had launched his own personal commentary to the profession, *The Fountainhead News,* in which missives "by B.J. Himself" would fuel the personal loyalty that held sway in Davenport for much of the century. *The Chiropractor,* the monthly journal launched by father and son in late 1904, now became the voice of the PSC, the Universal Chiropractors Association (UCA), and B.J. The UCA, begun at the PSC during December 1906, would become chiropractic's leading "protective" and professional association, not to be seriously challenged until B.J. had a falling out with the association almost 2 decades later. Attorneys Tom Morris and Fred Hartwell became PSC and UCA counsel and travelled to defend chiropractors in the courts. Thus in education, organization, public relations, and litigation, the PSC became the center for chiropractic leadership for much of 1910 to 1930.

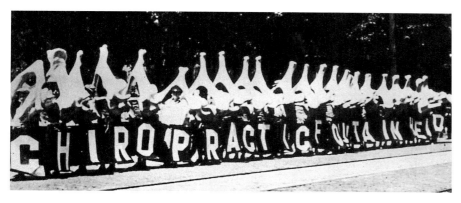

A PSC Lyceum parade down Brady Street featuring a spine spelling "Chiropractic Fountainhead," circa 1916.
Courtesy Palmer College of Chiropractic Archives, Davenport, Iowa.

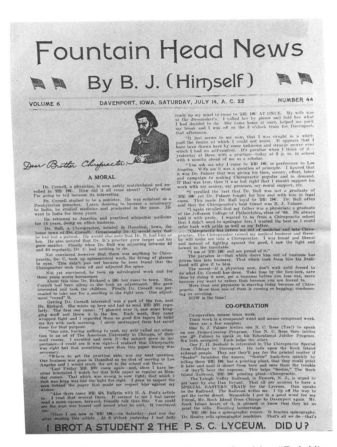

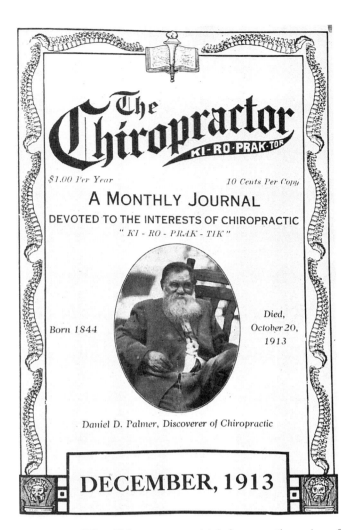

An issue of the Fountain Head News *edited by "B.J. Himself."*
Courtesy Palmer College of Chiropractic Archives, Davenport, Iowa.

An issue of *The Chiropractor, which became the voice of the PSC and the Universal Chiropractors Association.*
Courtesy Palmer College of Chiropractic Archives, Davenport, Iowa.

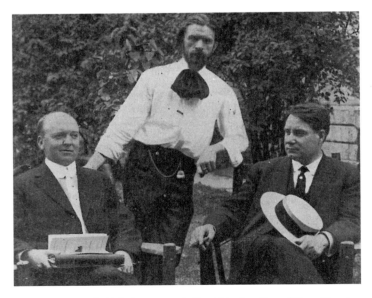

B.J. Palmer with U.C.A. counsel, Fred Hartwell and Tom Morris.
Courtesy Palmer College of Chiropractic Archives, Davenport, Iowa.

RIVAL SCHOOLS: NATIONAL AND UNIVERSAL

Challenges to Palmer's chiropractic leadership first surfaced with the founding of Solon Langworthy's American School of Chiropractic in Cedar Rapids, Iowa in 1904. Dr. Langworthy had also established the first of several organizations to be called the American Chiropractic Association (ACA). He was also among the first in the early quixotic effort to achieve chiropractic legislative recognition when he worked to pass legislation in Minnesota in 1905.

The next year, 1906, John A. Howard who, according to his accounts, was rebuffed by B.J. over any serious concerns for human dissection at the PSC, led a group of PSC students to the same Ryan Building where D.D. had his early offices to begin the National School of Chiropractic. Two years later he moved his school to the Flatiron Building in southwest Chicago and developed what would be the true rival to the Palmer's leadership and philosophy in the first third of this century.

National School of Chiropractic

John Howard and his "mixer" institution would become anathema to B.J. Palmer and the "straight" chiropractors. Howard would always claim an apostolic line of succession from D.D. Palmer, the Discoverer, and widely disseminated an endorsement of his National School of Chiropractic from the senior Palmer. In one of these most-often quoted communications, D.D. Palmer wrote Howard about a medical reception that the father of chiropractic claimed he had received in Kansas City in May 1906. It was at this meeting that D.D. said "chiropractic captured the meeting".

By the time Howard left the National School in 1916, the faculty boasted six doctors of medicine who also listed the D.C. degree. The dean

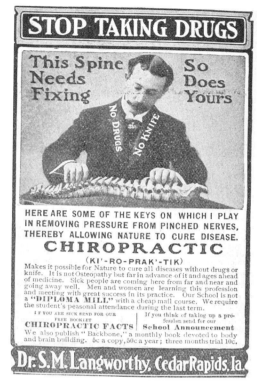

An advertisement featuring Solon Massey Langworthy, circa 1909.

Courtesy Palmer College of Chiropractic Archives, Davenport, Iowa.

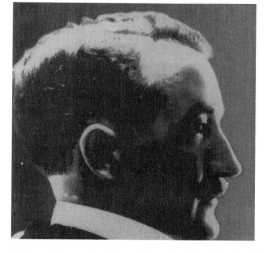

John Howard, Founder of the National School of Chiropractic.

Courtesy National College of Chiropractic, Lombard, Illinois.

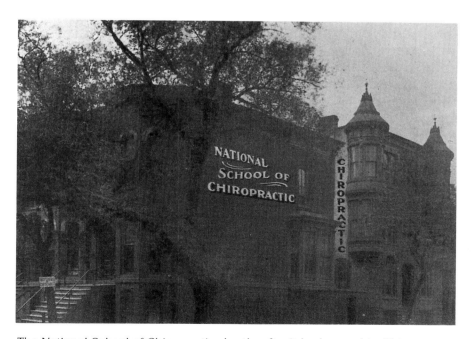

The National School of Chiropractic shortly after it had moved to Chicago.

Courtesy Palmer College of Chiropractic Archives, Davenport, Iowa.

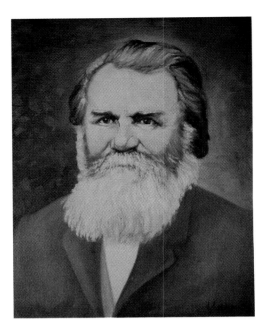

An oil portrait of D.D. Palmer.
Courtesy Texas Chiropractic College, Pasadena, Texas.

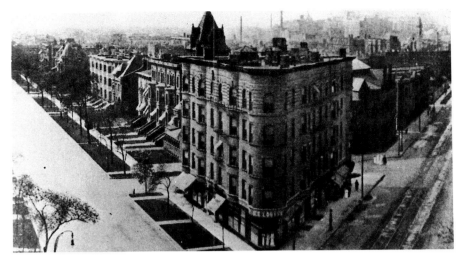

The Flatiron Building in southwest Chicago where the National School moved in 1908.
Courtesy National College of Chiropractic, Lombard, Illinois.

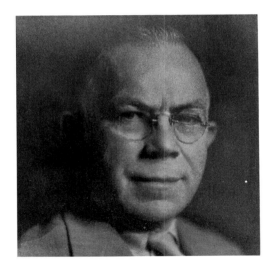

William C. Schulze, an 1897 graduate of Rush Medical College, joined the National faculty in 1910 and later became its President and owner.
Courtesy National College of Chiropractic, Lombard, Illinois.

of the faculty was an 1897 graduate of Rush Medical College, William C. Schulze. A native of Germany, he graduated from a small liberal arts college in Missouri before entering Rush, the medical department of the University of Chicago. After practicing in Wisconsin and after 5 years as medical director of the Chicago Zander Institute, Schulze joined the National faculty in 1910, taking the chairs of Obstetrics and Gynecology. His publications included *A Textbook of the Diseases of Women.*

Arthur L. Forster, who taught diagnosis, wrote one of the first texts for the school, *Principles and Practices of Spinal Adjustment.* His degree was from the medical department of the University of Illinois. The other M.D.s listed on the National School of Chiropractic faculty in 1915 included graduates of Northwestern University Medical School, Bennett, Loyola, Chicago Hospital, and the Chicago College of Medicine and Surgery. Running from the top of Flexner's curve line, Rush was among the better medical schools in the country, while at the bottom was Bennett, which Flexner had declared to be "wretched."

Forster, in the introduction to his text, recognized that he and his medical colleagues in chiropractic were regarded as little better than professional pariahs by the mainstream of orthodoxy. Forster may have expressed the reservations of those medical defectors who had joined this new army of irregulars:

> Palmer, however, fell into one serious error. He did as so many before him have done. He became overzealous. He claimed that all disease is due to subluxations of the vertebrae and that all diseases could be eradicated by adjustment of the vertebrae. Naturally, such views could not be subscribed to by anyone with a liberal training in the sciences underlying the art of healing, and especially, one with a knowledge of pathology.

The Schulze-Forster administration at the National College was to produce one of the more remarkable instances of a chiropractic intrusion into traditional orthodox territory. While neither the lost nor strayed repositories of records have yet to reveal the connection, apparently from 1908 to 1924 there was an arrangement for students at the National School (after 1920 the National College of Chiropractic was located in a

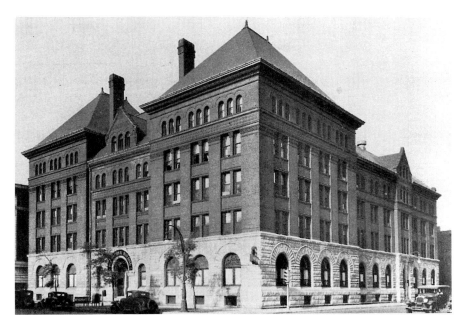

The massive stone structure on Ashland Avenue where National College was located.

Courtesy National College of Chiropractic, Lombard, Illinois.

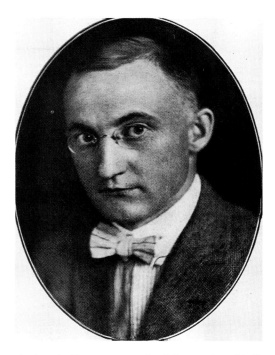

Arthur L. Forster, a medical doctor, taught diagnosis at the National School of Chiropractic.

Courtesy National College of Chiropractic, Lombard, Illinois.

massive stone structure on Ashland Avenue) to visit the wards of Cook County Hospital. The connection could have been any one of the six M.D.s who were listed as professors in the school catalogue for those years. However, considering that the majority of the 11 Illinois schools surveyed by Flexner in 1910 had either similar formal or informal arrangements at Cook County—and that Flexner recommended the closing of all but three—the relationship may not have been so surprising.

In any event, the arrangement appears to have ended after complaints from operating surgeons at Cook County who reported that the overzealous students of Forster and Schulze would on occasion, shout from the surgical amphitheater balcony, "Have you tried chiropractic?" Whatever credence may be placed in this account, it recalls Flexner's dry commentary on the purported claims of a Philadelphia osteopathic institution, whose catalogue boasted of privileges for witnessing operations at the University Hospital and Jefferson Hospital: "This is not the case. These students are intruders, without either rights or privileges of any description whatever."

It should be observed that in this period the leading chiropractic schools, Palmer, National and smaller institutions located in St. Louis, Oklahoma City, Los Angeles, Portland, Oregon, and San Antonio, Texas, had administrators who claimed M.D. designations. The 1918 bulletin of the Pacific College of Chiropractic, the successor to an institution operated by D.D. Palmer in Portland a decade earlier, listed two Doctors of Medicine as faculty members and boasted that "unlike any other chiropractic college in America, we have access to the surgeries of the leading hospitals."

However, with the exception of the Palmer and National schools, the physical plants, laboratory facilities, clinics, and faculties of the smaller schools might have been comparable to the worst of the medical schools visited by Flexner. They were in the phrase that repeatedly appeared

137

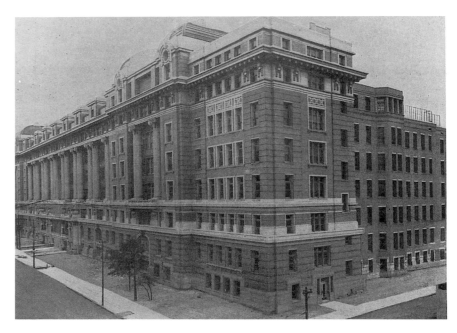

Cook County Hospital, where National College had an arrangement where their students were allowed to view surgeries.
Courtesy National College of Chiropractic, Lombard, Illinois.

throughout his classic report "inexpressively bad." Flexner's descriptions of the majority of the institutions on which he reported in 1909 to 1910 could be applied to any chiropractic institution for the next two decades: ". . . the schools were essentially private ventures, money-making in spirit and object. A school that began in October would graduate a class the next spring—it mattered not that the course of study was 2 or 3 years; immigration recruited a senior class at the start."

Yet in 1927, the Council on Medical Education and Hospitals of the American Medical Association (AMA) would damn with faint praise some aspects of Palmer's Fountainhead of "P.S. & U. chiropractic," a B.J. euphemism for "Pure, Straight and Unadulterated" chiropractic. The same was true of National School of Chiropractic, the bastion of "mixer chiropractic" in Chicago, where obstetrics, gynecology, proctology, the coagu-

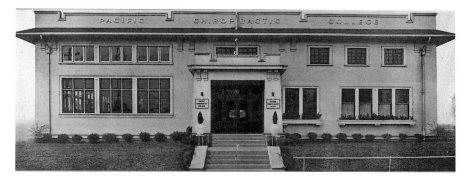

Pacific College of Chiropractic was the successor to the institution operated by D.D. Palmer in Portland a decade earlier.
Courtesy Palmer College of Chiropractic Archives, Davenport, Iowa.

lation of tonsils, and diathermy competed with the essential "chiropractic thrust" in the curriculum.

Following a visit to PSC, the Council investigators acknowledged that the school's osteological museum was "without doubt, the best collection of human spines in existence." The National School of Chiropractic laboratories and roentgenological facilities got high marks, but the four physicians on the faculty in 1927 were noted "not to have any standing in the organized medical profession of America," which may have meant they did not belong to the AMA.

Whatever his standing, Schulze presided over the National School of Chiropractic in Chicago for 21 years. He is credited with emphasizing the inclusion of both diagnosis and physical therapy in the curriculum. Upon his death in 1936, the college journal noted "that many will recall occasions when Dr. Schulze was almost thrown out of conventions for suggesting diagnostic methods other than palpation." His leadership gave some promise for achieving minimal standards, despite the unreserved hostility of the Chicago medical community.

Universal Chiropractic College

If B.J. Palmer was a ubiquitous figure on the early chiropractic landscape, then Joy Loban was an uncharacteristically low profile personality who for a short tenure was B.J.'s designated "philosophical heir." B.J. praised Loban "as a companion (who) gives backbone to my research and to me personally and professionally." Responded Loban in *The Chiropractor*, "never have I met such a man (B.J.) who possessed this faculty for original philosophical thought . . . " The mutual admiration soon turned. Loban left the Palmer School of Chiropractic faculty, went into private practice and returned to Davenport in early 1910, where he associated himself with a group of dissident students. It was this group who formed the nucleus of a rival school just a few blocks down the hill from the Fountainhead.

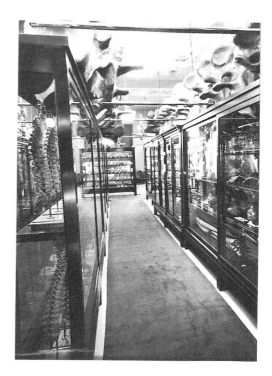

The Palmer School of Chiropractic Osteological collection was acknowledged in 1927 by an inspection team of the Council on Medical Education to be "without doubt, the best collection of human spines in existence."

Courtesy Palmer College of Chiropractic Archives, Davenport, Iowa.

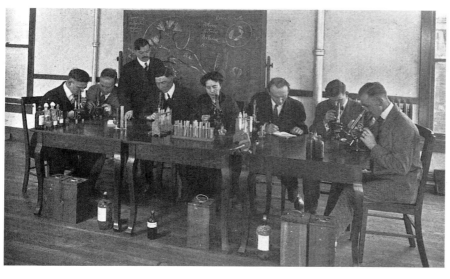

A National College laboratory got high marks in the 1927 inspection by the Council on Medical Education.

Courtesy National College of Chiropractic, Lombard, Illinois.

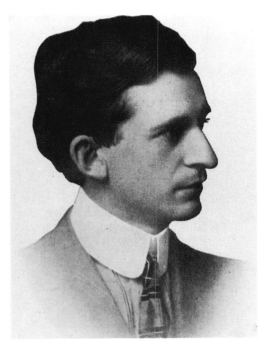

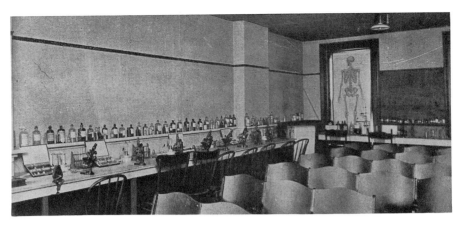

Another chiropractic school laboratory, circa 1920.
Courtesy Palmer College of Chiropractic Archives, Davenport, Iowa.

Joy Loban was instrumental in forming the Universal Chiropractic College.
Courtesy Palmer College of Chiropractic Archives, Davenport, Iowa.

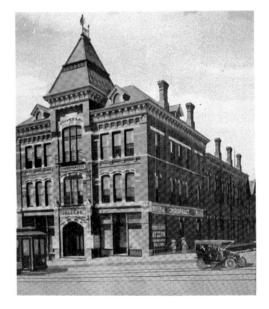

The Davenport location of the Universal Chiropractic College, circa 1911.
Courtesy Palmer College of Chiropractic Archives, Davenport, Iowa.

In one of the more romantic myths associated with early chiropractic, accounts of the Palmer walkout report that a sizeable number of students stood up in B.J.'s philosophy class at a prearranged command, exited the classroom, and marched down the Brady Street hill to a building on the corner of Sixth and Brady Streets. There under the direction of Loban and an associate named George Otto they formed the Universal Chiropractic College. Whether this break was over B.J. Palmer's philosophy or his forceful leadership style is arguable. B.J. had by this time offended a number of students who considered his lectures both coarse and flamboyant.

There are many stories about the 9 years of the Universal Chiropractic College's operation on Brady Street that have become part of chiropractic lore. The most frequently told story revolves around the encounters between Universal Chiropractic College and PSC student recruiters at the Davenport train station, which was down the hill just blocks

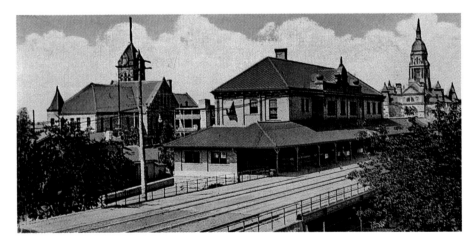

The Davenport train station, where Universal College would greet students recruited by the PSC and take them to "the chiropractic college."
Courtesy Palmer College of Chiropractic Archives, Davenport, Iowa.

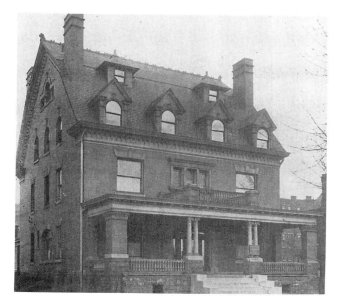

The building in Pittsburgh where the Universal Chiropractic College relocated in 1918.
Courtesy Palmer College of Chiropractic Archives, Davenport, Iowa.

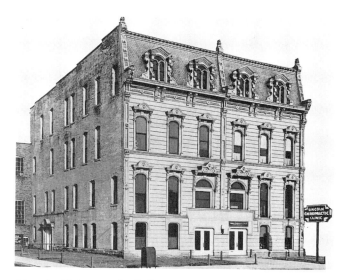

Lincoln Chiropractic College, which absorbed the Universal College in 1944, then became part of the National College of Chiropractic in 1967.
Courtesy Palmer College of Chiropractic Archives, Davenport, Iowa.

from the two schools. Arriving students, most of whom were attracted to PSC through the school's marketing campaigns, would often be met by Universal Chiropractic College teams ready to take them to "the chiropractic college." Physical encounters between the two student bodies and those of another rival institution, the Davenport School of Chiropractic, which had a briefer tenure in a former church on Tenth and Brady Streets, made good copy for the Davenport newspapers during that decade.

Interestingly, in 1914, students from all three institutions met for an Independence Day picnic on Davenport's Credit Island, an island in the middle of the Mississippi River. There they founded Delta Sigma Chi, the first chiropractic fraternity, which survives to this day. Interestingly also is survival of the Universal Chiropractic College building at Sixth and Brady Streets. Part of the UCC sign painted on the building facing south toward the river is still visible on the bricks. But both Universal and Davenport schools went the way of the dozens of early institutions that sought to challenge the PSC for chiropractic leadership.

In 1918, Loban was part of a buyout plan that transferred the name and the few assets of Universal Chiropractic College, which was close to bankruptcy, to Pittsburgh, where it merged with the Pittsburgh College of Chiropractic. There, the Universal College produced a generation of solid chiropractors. In 1944, Universal College moved to Indianapolis, merging with Lincoln Chiropractic College. In 1967, Lincoln Chiropractic College ceased operation and became a part of the multicollege lineal heritage of National College of Chiropractic in Chicago.

If Howard and Loban were to be the initial challengers to the leadership of D.D. and B.J., the Founder and the Developer, then "The Four Horsemen" of 1925 to 1926 were to be a group of strong-willed challengers to Palmer's dominance regarding the profession's educational leadership. A smoldering dispute among the PSC faculty took place at a time

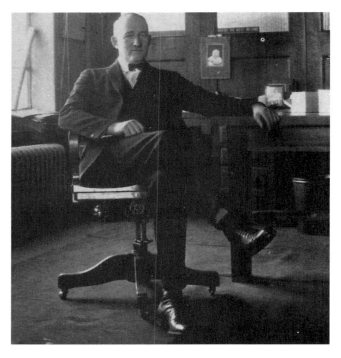

James Firth, one of the profession's most respected diagnosticians, left PSC in 1926 to start the Lincoln Chiropractic College.

Courtesy Palmer College of Chiropractic Archives, Davenport, Iowa.

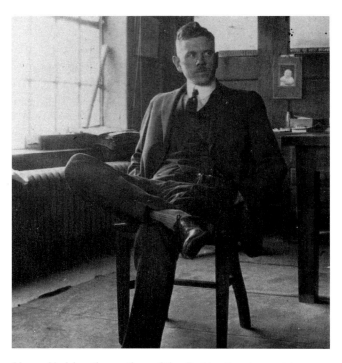

Harry Vedder, the author of the first textbook on chiropractic gynecology, also left PSC to help form Lincoln College.

Courtesy Palmer College of Chiropractic Archives, Davenport, Iowa.

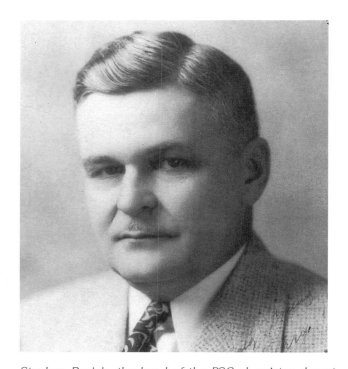

Stephen Burich, the head of the PSC chemistry department, also left to start Lincoln Chiropractic College .

Courtesy Palmer College of Chiropractic Archives, Davenport, Iowa.

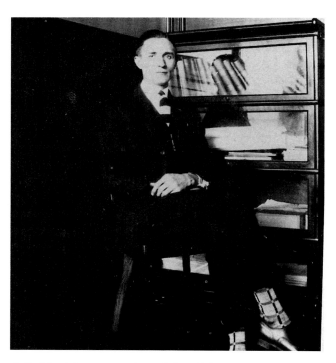

A.G. Hinrichs, a member of the PSC clinical department, was one of the Lincoln "Four Horsemen."

Courtesy Palmer College of Chiropractic Archives, Davenport, Iowa.

when B.J. was at the apex of his leadership in the profession. The curriculum changes instituted by B.J. centered around his insistence on the theory that the atlas subluxation automatically eliminated the need for undue emphasis on the basic sciences. In 1926, several of the faculty trained in other disciplines before they took up chiropractic disagreed with B.J.'s emphasis. It was during this year that James Firth, Harry Vedder, Stephen Burich, and A.G. Hinrichs left the PSC and started the Lincoln Chiropractic College in Indianapolis.

CHIROPRACTIC IN THE COURTS

The 1920s also consolidated legislative gains for the profession. Chiropractic historian William Rehm said that

> Tom Morris won the Morikubo case which established for the first time that chiropractic was indeed a separate and distinct school of healing. And while his defense was considered brilliant in a purist sense, it had the effect of both opening up and controlling chiropractic for years to come.

The "philosophy" of chiropractic was now established. B.J. Palmer had begun to use the term in his writings by 1908, and in 1911 revised his first book, *The Science of Chiropractic* (1906), under the title *The Science and Philosophy of Chiropractic*.

After the Morikubo victory in La Crosse, Wisconsin, a consolidation of sorts took place with Tom Morris and his partner Fred Hartwell, acting as counsel to the newly formed UCA. The Morris and Hartwell team came to the defense of thousands of chiropractors—and established a network of regional attorneys who served as local counsel when chiropractors were arrested.

In 1926, a legal defense group succeeded Morris and Hartwell. The Chiropractic Health Bureau took up the cause of militant courtroom defense, urging new chiropractors to enroll as members:

> In time of peace prepare for war. Membership in the CHB denotes the highest degree of preparation and intelligent action. Be prepared for war. The CHB never advises its members to enter pleas of guilty in criminal actions and OF COURSE it never advises the settlement of a civil action out of court.

The prosecutions continued in the states where chiropractic legislation was not enacted in the first period of licensure (1913 to 1926) and were especially vehement in California and Texas, populous states that attracted a substantial supply of chiropractors. A Texas chiropractor described his early encounter with the law as such:

> In 1918 they sent the deputy sheriff to Van Alstyne from Sherman to my office. He took me to Sherman and I promised that I would quit charging my patients and they let me go. The patients would just leave their money on a table when they were ready to leave my office. Then the grand jury called me. I went before the grand jury three times. The last time I got up and made a little talk. I stood up and pointed my finger at the men around me. I told them that this was my state the same as it was theirs and if they did take me out of the state I was coming back. So they never did bother me about that any more.

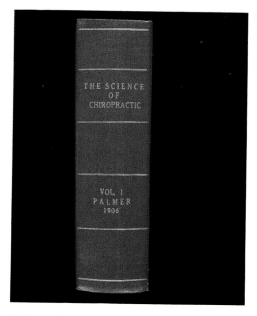

D.D. and B.J. Palmer's first book, The Science of Chiropractic, *1906.*

Courtesy Palmer College of Chiropractic Archives, Davenport, Iowa.

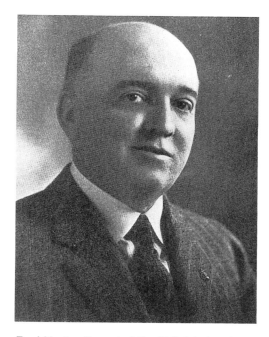

Fred Hartwell, part of the U.C.A.'s legal team that came to the defense of thousands of chiropractors accused of practicing medicine without a license.

Courtesy Palmer College of Chiropractic Archives, Davenport, Iowa.

Advertisements for the Chiropractic Health Bureau, which succeeded the U.C.A. and took up the cause of chiropractors' courtroom defense.
Courtesy Palmer College of Chiropractic Archives, Davenport, Iowa.

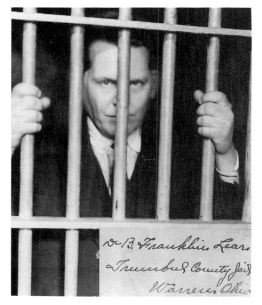

Dr. B. Franklin Lear, of Warren, Ohio, who served time for practicing medicine without a license.
Courtesy Palmer College of Chiropractic Archives, Davenport, Iowa.

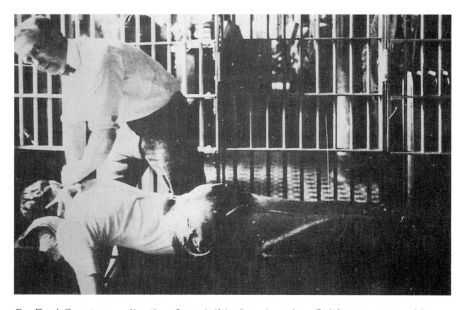

Dr. Fred Courtney adjusting from jail in Los Angeles, California, circa 1921.
From *Fountainhead News* 10(26), 1921.

California: The "Round-Ups"

Prosecutions and persecutions were part of the occupational career outlook for newly graduated chiropractors in years before World War I. The process of legislative action was slow but relentless with successful efforts in the various states, beginning with Kansas in 1913. By far the most dramatic instances of prosecutions took place in California, which had seen chiropractors on that mixed healing landscape as early as 1902 when D.D. Palmer practiced in Pasadena and later Santa Barbara. In fact, D.D. Palmer was arrested in 1902, but the complaint was dismissed after a brief hearing in a local court.

For better than a decade, culminating in a referendum in 1922 that established and regulated the practice of chiropractic, California became

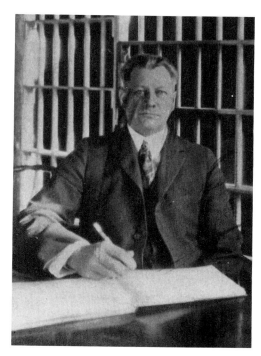

California chiropractor D.S. Tracy, serving time in the Los Angeles County jail for practicing medicine without a license.

Courtesy Palmer College of Chiropractic Archives, Davenport, Iowa.

The Campaign Bulletin

Published in the interest of the Chiropractic Initiative and for its successful enactment on November the 7th, 1922

Vol. I.　　　　FEBRUARY, 15, 1922.　　　　No. 2.

The California Situation
By R. A. RATLEDGE

To defeat the Chiropractic Initiative Measure in November, cleverly designed propaganda by the Medical Board is being heralded throughout the length and breadth of California at this time.

On the 11th of this month there will be held an examination in Los Angeles for licensing drugless practitioners who pass (?) the Board. According to press reports of interviews with Charles B. Pinkham, Secretary, the State Medical Board has adopted a "new and liberal" policy which will simplify and facilitate the entire matter to be heard at that time.

So far as we are able to ascertain at this time, the chiropractors have completely ignored this ruse to ensnare the chiropractic profession; and it is to be hoped that no chiropractor will apply to the Medical Board for examination and compromise and embarass the chiropractic profession in its campaign for a law.

We must look this situation squarely in the face. It is no time to sidestep and avoid the issue. The character of chiropractic schools and colleges, and the chiropractic quality of instruction given therein, has undergone no such readjustment as would meet the requirements of the Medical Board. There has not been any modification of Chiropractic Philosophy.

Chiropractic schools and colleges of California, and elsewhere, are not now equipped to better teach chiropractic, and are not now entitled to recognition and approval by the Medical Board any more than in former years; and the chiropractor is today not any more nearly qualified for medical examination and license than in the years 1921, 1920, 1919, 1918, 1917, here in California.

Do you believe that the welfare of chiropractic, and your practice as well, will be best served by this act of the Medical Board? Is the adoption of this new and liberal policy by this Board really an evidence of a change of heart? Or shall we see, are under stand it in its true light, a political necessity to confuse the mind of the voter and cause him to vote against the Chiropractic Initiative Bill.

For the purpose of meeting and overcoming the obstacles of the emergency, the situation demanded some effective blow be struck. No more strategic and telling thing could have done than for the Medical Board at this time to open wide the gates to examination and license, appearing, for the purpose of this examination on the 14th instant, all schools and colleges that graduates might qualify as applicants.

Public opinion is both for us and with us here in California; and will support us in our campaign as long as it believes in us. That our position is correct, and that our honesty of purpose is unquestioned, is the voice of the people as expressed through the ballot upon the Chiropractic Bill in 1920. Break faith with the public by applying to the Medical Board for examination and license and you destroy that confidence upon the strength of which we should have ridden to victory. Keep faith with the public, do not abandon the Chiropractic Banner, and victory is ours next November.

You studied long and hard preparing for a proper practice of Chiropractic. Measured in dollars and cents, it has cost you thousands of dollars. It is a noble inspiration that determined finally for you a chiropractic career. You are practicing today, not because of the Medical Board, but on account of the helpfulness of the thing you are doing and the indisputable confidence in your ability to achieve.

Your financial and moral investment in chiropractic is sufficiently insignificant to permit you to cast it aside and enter other lines of service, well and good; we have not one penny to ask of you; but if your interest in the profession is just that great that you can not afford to get out of the work, then know that it is your duty to yourself and to Chiropractic to financially support our campaign, and give to the Campaign Committee your moral, active and cheerful support.

The campaign for the Chiropractic Initiative Bill is the biggest event of your professional career, comprehending or encompassing every element of your life. It is not possible for you to make too great a sacrifice in the achievement of success at the polls next November.

The fight for chiropractic legislation in California provoked a spirited defense in several journals of that time.

Courtesy Palmer of Chiropractic Archives, Davenport, Iowa.

the battleground. "Nowhere was the conflict with medical authorities more intense, nor the prosecution of chiropractors pursued with a more relentless policy" wrote early historian Chittenden Turner in 1931, adding with this flourish: "It is a tale of stratagems and spoils, of political intrigue and reprisals. Attacked on all sides, weakened by defection within the ranks and with hundreds sent to prison, only an appeal to the public through the launching of an initiative petition finally won success. Then began a new battle."

As arrests continued, fighting spirits rose. Among the more sensational cases was that of J.E. and Reba I. Willis of Porterville. On December 8, 1920, "their office was ransacked by two investigators and their patients insulted," according to Turner, and they themselves were placed under arrest. The local magistrate released them under bond to appear in the superior court for the arraignment on January 24, when they were sentenced to 100 days in jail or the payment of $200. The Willises chose imprisonment and said goodbye to their 3-year-old twin girls at the jail door. It was the first time a mother had been incarcerated and much indignant comment was voiced. Letters came to the jail from foreign countries, "and all told, more than 100,000 pieces of mail are said to have been received by the imprisoned couple," Turner concluded.

In the late fall of 1920, five chiropractors at Long Beach were arrested in one day. So aroused were citizens of the community that 1200 assembled at a mass meeting.

In other parts of the state the "round-up" continued. Fresno and Bakersfield were scenes of numerous arrests. A judge in Bakersfield refused to issue a warrant authorizing the search of chiropractors' offices in Taft and arraigned at Bakersfield. When the judge asked the sheriff why there were so few witnesses, in view of the many subpoenas issued, the sheriff said:

> Your Honor, the sheriff's office has been unable to catch the witnesses. They hide under beds and run out the back doors. They won't testify against these chiropractors. The sheriff's office has a lot of important business, so if you want these witnesses you'll have to catch them yourself."

The case was dismissed for lack of evidence.

New York and Massachusetts

If California and Texas were formidable bastions of medical opposition, it remained for New York and Massachusetts to be the bearers of the torch of orthodoxy. The medical and hospital centers of Boston and New York would be understandable sources of hostility. Long-established lobbies in the state capitals would become the frontline in what amounted to trench warfare for the chiropractors in those two northeastern states.

Lyndon Lee, a one-time Amherst student, took up chiropractic at the PSC and graduated in 1915. He would be the antithesis of the medical establishment's stereotype of ex-baggage handlers or barbers as their chiropractic opponents. When Dr. Lee entered the legislative fray he not only held his own but demolished fuming opponents from the medical lobby. This exchange in Albany in 1926 reflected his wit and fervor in defending chiropractic:

> A medical society spokesman snarled at Lee: "Yes, we are against you. We are against chiropractic and all other fakers. If this legislature will give us this bill, we will drive you and your ilk out of this state! What do you think about that?"
> "First, sir," Lee responded, "I'd like to see your driver's license."

The 1920s produced two towering political figures in the Democratic party who would have disappointing roles for organized chiropractic and its efforts to seek legislation. Al Smith, the 1928 Democratic presidential candidate, and Franklin D. Roosevelt, who would win the 1932 election and usher in the New Deal decades, were both New York governors in the critical 1920s when chiropractors almost obtained status in the Empire State. Historian J. Stuart Moore found the following:

> In 1924, the State Chiropractic Society had purposely avoided taking sides in the Democratic gubernatorial race between Franklin Roosevelt and Al Smith because they believed that chiropractic influence could not alter the result and would only make an enemy of the candidate they opposed. The Society had expected that Roosevelt's prior Assembly record against chiropractic legislation would mean that chances with Smith 'would be much better' than with Roosevelt. Smith instead became a sore disappointment.

In 1926, Smith vetoed the first successful chiropractic bill to pass the legislature. A Roosevelt administration also brought disappointment, as expected. During FDR's term as governor from 1929 to 1933, chiropractic bills failed each year except 1932 when for the first time since the legislative attempt began in 1913, no bill was introduced. Chiropractors in the state also met an intensified effort at courtroom prosecution during the late twenties and early thirties. It would be a half-century struggle, with the first chiropractic law in New York not signed until 1963.

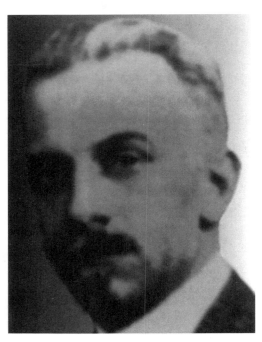

Lyndon Lee, a one-time Amherst student and 1915 graduate of the PSC. He was instrumental in the fight for chiropractic legislation in the state of New York.

Courtesy Palmer College of Chiropractic Archives, Davenport, Iowa.

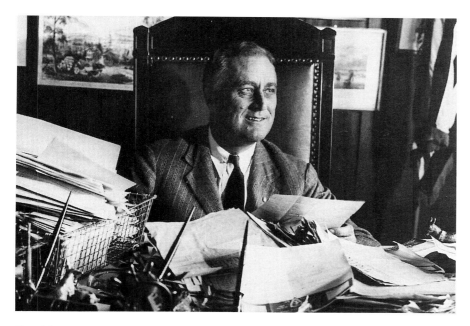

Franklin D. Roosevelt, governor of New York, was opposed to chiropractic legislation, and chiropractic bills failed in that state every year they were introduced, until 1963, when the chiropractic law was signed by Nelson Rockefeller.

Courtesy Franklin D. Roosevelt Library, Hyde Park, New York.

The all-time record for arrests—66—was held by Charles C. Lemly (1892-1970), a former pharmacist and co-owner with his brother of a chiropractic sanitarium in Waco, Texas. After his fellow Texan, Paul Meyers of Wichita Falls, was arrested for the tenth time, a parade with a band, many chiropractors, "patients and friends, and local celebrities," arranged in honor of his release, so impressed the authorities that "he was never bothered again."

As with so many other movements that flourished outside of the mainstream of the American social fabric, chiropractors found that their role as an underdog brought them favor with large constituencies of "common people" outside of the establishment layers of political, government, academic, and medical authority. The populist strain of distrust of many of these forms of authority were evident in the years of chiropractic survival and growth, which paralleled the first third of this century.

Tolerance and mild acceptance would come only after federal agencies acknowledged chiropractic as a reality in the health care field and recognized chiropractic educational institutions. That acceptance, however, was not to come until the doors of countless jailhouses, county lockups, and prison farms were to close on these practitioners.

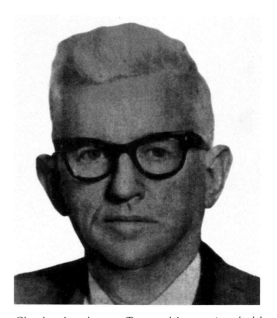

Charles Lemley, a Texas chiropractor, held the record for the most arrests for practicing medicine without a license—66.

Courtesy Palmer College of Chiropractic Archives, Davenport, Iowa.

THE DECLINE OF B.J. PALMER'S INFLUENCE

The 1920s were a fateful transition decade for most Americans. America was emerging from participation in a world war, struggling with the turmoil that came with the retooling of the national industrial engine, the flight from the farm to the cities, a financial boom that turned to a bust, and the depression that began in 1929. Chiropractic did not escape

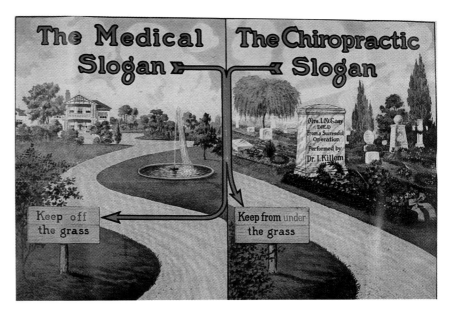

A cartoon that compares medicine's territorial claims with chiropractic's concerns for the patient's health.
Courtesy Palmer College of Chiropractic Archives, Davenport, Iowa.

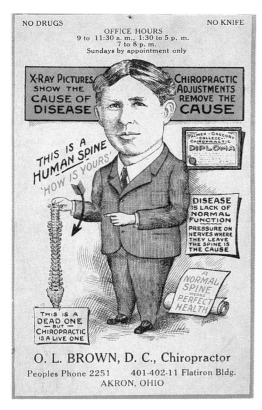

This chiropractor's card distributed in the 1920's advertised "No drugs, no knife."
Courtesy Palmer College of Chiropractic Archives, Davenport, Iowa.

the economic tailspin that consumed almost a third of the workforce by 1930 to 1939 and moved the financial centers to a crisis mode.

In Davenport it was the end of a decade that had begun with such bright prospects for the Palmers and their school. PSC had the largest enrollment ever, surpassing by hundreds any medical school in North America; a successful marketing image that included the acquisition and building of the nation's second commercial radio station WOC, "Wonders of Chiropractic"; and legislative successes in a majority of the states. Yet B.J.'s penchant for Barnum-style promotion proved to be the

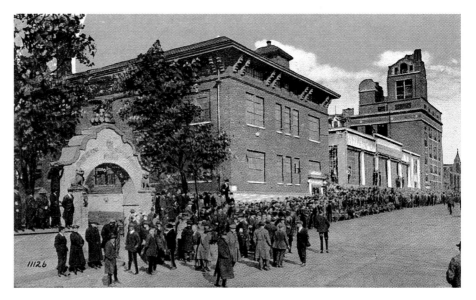

The Palmer School in the early 1920s.
Courtesy Palmer College of Chiropractic Archives, Davenport, Iowa.

148

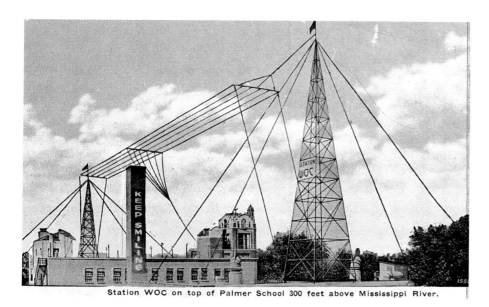

Station WOC on top of Palmer School 300 feet above Mississippi River.

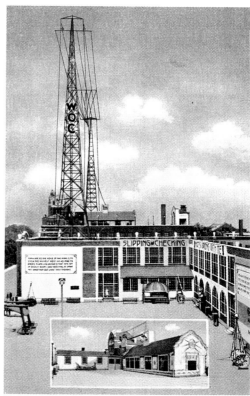

The transmission towers of WOC, the second commercial radio station established west of the Mississippi River, topping the buildings of the PSC.

Courtesy Palmer College of Chiropractic Archives, Davenport, Iowa.

unravelling of the "Golden Age," as Mabel Palmer referred to the early 1920s. "I will sell chiropractic, serve chiropractic, and save chiropractic if it will take me twenty lifetimes to do it," B.J. would write. The PSC "gave birth to Specific, Pure and Unadulterated Chiropractic," and B.J. set forth to sell, serve, and save in the best of the Barnum tradition.

Introduction of the Neurocalometer

In August 1924, under the tent that was erected on the east end of the campus, B.J. unveiled the neurocalometer, a pioneer heat-sensing device that was a double-pronged instrument to determine the existence of a subluxation.

B.J.'s Lyceum address was given an advance billing as "The Hour Has Struck," and chiropractors who came by the thousands were led to believe that the very future of the profession would be decided at this historic occasion. A critical view agreed that it was historic, but only in that it marked the beginning of the decline of B.J.'s unquestioned leadership. Said New York chiropractor Ben Saur:

> Who shall forget that torrid night under the tent when BJ spoke . . . in that philippic he maligned chiropractic . . . said many ugly things to the field. It was the hour that nearly rimracked and slaughtered and destroyed chiropractic.

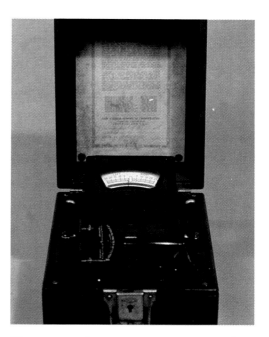

The neurocalometer was a pioneer heat-sensing device that was a dual-probed instrument used to determine the location of a subluxation.

Courtesy Palmer College of Chiropractic Archives, Davenport, Iowa.

149

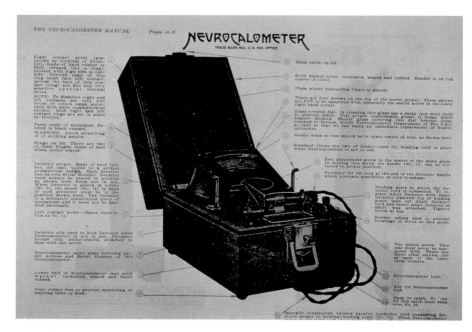

An advertisement describing the features of the neurocalometer.
Courtesy Palmer College of Chiropractic Archives, Davenport, Iowa.

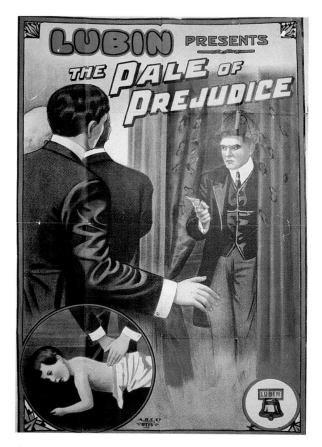

A poster used to promote the movie The Pale of Prejudice, *which featured chiropractic* (insert).
Courtesy Palmer College of Chiropractic Archives, Davenport, Iowa.

A massive wave of defections of purist followers came after the 1924 Lyceum, although a hard core of believers would hold to B.J.'s assertion that "no chiropractor can practice chiropractic without an NCM (neurocalometer), no chiropractor can render efficient, competent or honest service without the NCM."

The "neurocalometer debacle" would effectively split the profession, for it gave reason for the "mixers" who had derided the "SPU" extremes of Palmer chiropractic to form their rival constituencies into groups that would in the next decade revise the agenda of the profession. The UCA began to have its own factions that were critical of B.J., finally leading to his 1926 resignation as secretary-treasurer.

This, coupled with the Lincoln Chiropractic College formation as a result of the defection by Firth and his colleagues, the unity meetings between anti–Palmer-UCA leaders and the ACA, set the stage for a significant organizational structure to challenge B.J. Palmer. By 1929, the outline of the new National Chiropractic Association (NCA) would take shape.

If the 1920s were chiropractic's "growing up years," then there was plenty of professional adolescence to deal with. The insularity that came with evolution of a health occupation outside the medical and health care mainstream would stay with its practitioners for much of another 30 years. Governmental agencies looked on it as marginal at best, and the academic establishment relegated its schools to technical institutions or trade schools. The teachers at its larger schools had little if no intercourse with universities, laboratories, or hospitals. Indeed, most data from these years survives only on the rolls of state registrations where licensure was obtained.

The depression took a terrible toll on chiropractors and chiropractic students. The student population at the PSC took a dramatic plunge from more than 3100 in 1922 to just over 300 students in 1929. David Daniel Palmer, the son of "The Developer" and the grandson of the profession's founder, returned from graduation at the University of Pennsylvania that year to find the school in receivership by the Davenport National Bank. The huge classroom building became the temporary location of a mop-handle facility. The glory years had been replaced with a reality check that made many wonder if chiropractic would indeed survive the next decade.

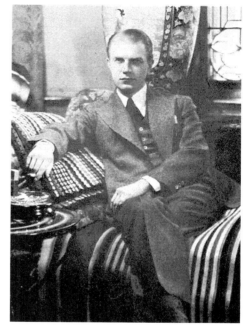

Young David Palmer returned from college at the University of Pennsylvania's Wharton School of Business in 1929 to find PSC in receivership.

Courtesy Palmer College of Chiropractic Archives, Davenport, Iowa.

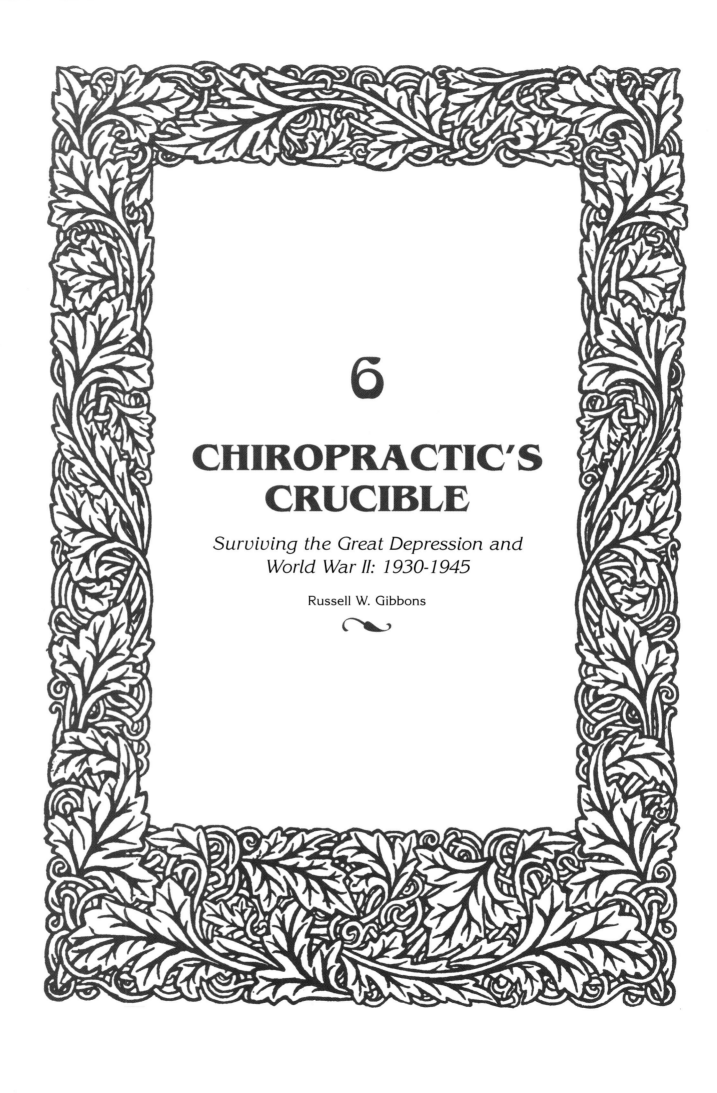

6

CHIROPRACTIC'S CRUCIBLE

Surviving the Great Depression and
World War II: 1930-1945

Russell W. Gibbons

T1930s proved to be an ominous decade for most Americans; the "Great Crash" on Wall Street in the last weeks of 1929 projected the virtual collapse of the economic system that had sustained them after the first war. Daily grim statistics mounted—by the last months of the Hoover administration over 14,000,000 Americans would be unemployed. Bread and soup lines and apple sellers in business suits became common street scenes.

While unemployment hit the ranks of factory workers, farmers, and the unskilled hardest, it also took its toll among those who had always held jobs and even attained some status in society. Diminished incomes and loss of position were to visit the ranks of bankers, storekeepers, and businessmen and would even touch those who offered health care as their profession.

Economic ruin and bankruptcy were common in the small towns and the cities of the Midwest, where chiropractors became a significant demographic factor in the "Golden Age" that Mabel Palmer had characterized of 1920s chiropractic. These failures would have their impact on chiropractic's ranks, which by some analysts had already swelled beyond the market for the young alternative profession during the years of Palmer consolidation.

The receivership of the Palmer School of Chiropractic just a few years after B.J. returned from one of his world tours collecting memorabilia suggested the contradiction of the era: the excesses of the "flapper" generation amidst the growing underclass who had lost homes and even the ability to feed their families. Graduates of the Palmer School and other surviving institutions of chiropractic of that period were facing the reality of not only a diminished market for alternative healers, but also a diminished purchasing power among those who might seek out their services.

How many chiropractors actually failed in this period may be conjecture, but there is circumstantial evidence that as many as a quarter of the graduates of the Palmer School, the National School, the Los Angeles School, and the other larger schools would not survive in practice. Many others chose to practice part-time, in the evenings, or on weekends while sustaining themselves and their families with other employment.

The 1930s were the crucible for chiropractic. There was within the profession both organizational and educational dissent at every level; the tolerance of public officials and the courts was growing thin. Chiropractic took a surprising turn during this time toward true reform of its training institutions and began to make changes within its professional organizational structure that would eventually bring it standing as a true profession rather than as a marginal occupational calling. ∽

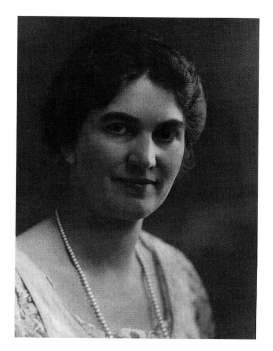

Mabel Heath Palmer, circa 1920, the first lady of chiropractic.
Courtesy Palmer College of Chiropractic Archives, Davenport, Iowa.

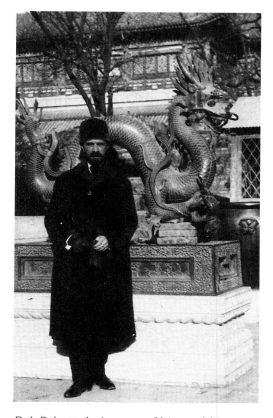

B.J. Palmer during one of his world tours.
Courtesy Palmer College of Chiropractic Archives, Davenport, Iowa.

CHIROPRACTIC RETRENCHMENT

Isolated from the mainstream of education and science, the owners and faculties of chiropractic schools resided in a world in which external hostility and internal controversies were common. Resentment toward the influence of the "schoolmen" into chiropractic politics and legislative battles was evident. Rivalries and intense debate raged, costing many schools support within the profession and the public.

This climate, coupled with the economic depression that affected all nonpublic educational activities from 1929 through 1941, reduced the number of schools by more than 50% during the 1925 to 1935 decade. It was literally a period of survival for chiropractic with many leaders of the profession predicting an ominous future. The records of the number of schools in existence in the various years of this period are reflected from lists supplied by the Universal Chiropractors Association (UCA) and later the National Chiropractic Association (NCA). Ironically, the Council on Medical Education and Hospitals of the American Medical Association (AMA) provided some of the most authoritative data.

The Council's annual report to the AMA in 1928 declared that there were 79 chiropractic schools in 1920. By 1927, their number had been reduced to 40 with a total student population of 2000—less than that enrolled at just the Palmer School in 1922. Seven years later, the Committee on the Costs of Medical Care at the University of Chicago made a survey of chiropractic schools and found 21, which was possibly fewer than actually existed.

The Committee, whose report was published in 1930 as part of a book by medical sociologist Louis A. Reed, *The Healing Cults,* was harsh in its indictment of chiropractic schools "as business institutions run for the profit of their owners. Most of them fairly reek of commercialism . . ." The proprietors themselves, however, must have many times questioned their business acumen in this period, especially the decade of the 1930s.

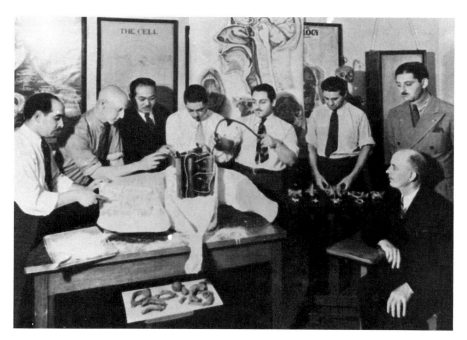

Standard School of Chiropractic, New York City, circa 1937.
From *What Chiropractic Is Doing,* 1938, Indianapolis, Burton Shields.

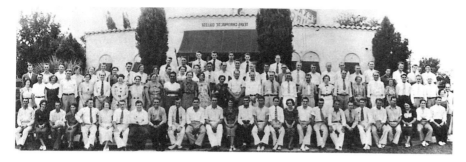

Texas Chiropractic College, San Antonio, Texas, circa 1937. During the hard times of the 1930s, its student body numbered no more than 70.

From *What Chiropractic Is Doing*, 1938, Indianapolis, Burton Shields.

A history of one of the oldest schools, the Texas Chiropractic College founded in 1908, observed that there was only a single graduate during a 1-year period and that "the school averaged only 60 to 70 students annually in the best of the years before World War II." Its corporate owners deferred any administrative or teaching salaries in this period. Similar financial horror stories are related by graduates of other institutions that survived this long night in chiropractic.

It may be surprising then to note the first non-profit and professionally owned institutions came into being during this same period. This would have been a full decade or more before the chiropractic's educational reform movement, which sought to eliminate the proprietary ownership of schools.

The Columbia Institute of Chiropractic in the 1920s and the Logan (Basic) College of Chiropractic in St. Louis in 1935 were among the first

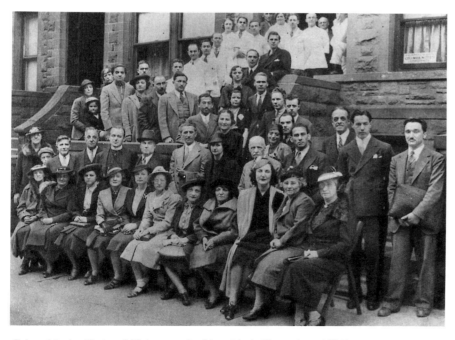

Columbia Institute of Chiropractic, New York City, circa 1937, was one of the first non-profit chiropractic colleges.

From *What Chiropractic Is Doing*, 1938, Indianapolis, Burton Shields.

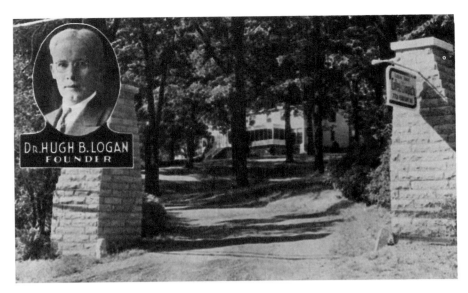

Logan Basic College of Chiropractic, St. Louis, circa 1937, was a non-profit institution founded by Hugh Logan in 1935.

From *What Chiropractic Is Doing*, 1938, Indianapolis, Burton Shields.

non-profit and professionally owned institutions. This list also included the College of Chiropractic Physicians and Surgeons in Los Angeles, formed in 1930, and the Western States Chiropractic College as reorganized in 1932 by W. A. Budden. These institutions, along with the National College of Chiropractic, which was proprietary until 1945, were to establish a 4-year course because of a legislative situation that had all but required most schools to offer the option of the collegiate length course by the end of the 1930s. The evolution of the length of study developed from 12 months in 1909 to 18 months by 1916 to 24-, 27-, and 30-months' offerings by various institutions until standardization became a viable factor.

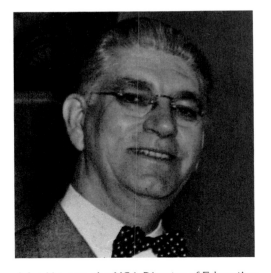

John Nugent, the NCA Director of Education, carried the unpopular message that all institutions must become non-profit, professionally owned with standardized curriculums.

From *NCA Journal*, January 1942.

EDUCATIONAL REFORMS AND JOHN NUGENT

In 1935, the NCA, the broad-scope organization that had absorbed the UCA and had become the dominant organization after the decline of B.J. Palmer's influence, created a Committee on Educational Standards. Named as NCA Director of Education was John J. Nugent. Nugent was destined to change the course of chiropractic education in the next 3 decades.

Like B.J., John Nugent was persuasive and articulate, had great political instincts, but possessed the ability to communicate with intellectual sectors who had consigned chiropractic as nothing but a distasteful cultist experience. Yet to many within the profession he appeared arrogant with a condescending air that seemed at times little more than a constant diatribe against anything and everything Palmer. Nugent had been "expelled" from the Palmer School of Chiropractic by B.J. in 1922 "for disloyalty, disrespect and insult to the President" but was reinstated by faculty action 3 weeks later.

John Nugent put his classical studies training at the National University of Dublin and the United States Military Academy at West Point into good service for chiropractic, testifying before countless legislative committees and meeting with educators who felt that he had the hopeless task of elevating "trade schools" to a professional status. He visited virtually every chiropractic school head during the 1935 to 1960 period. He carried his equally unpopular message that smaller schools must merge; all schools must teach "4 years of 9"; all institutions must become non-profit and professionally owned with standardized curriculums; faculties should be strengthened; and clinical opportunities expanded.

Nugent, one chiropractic lobbyist offered in the late 1950s "had become the most hated name in chiropractic." One school head reportedly warned Nugent off his property with a gun. He was an anathema to readers of the *Fountainhead News* and many a mixer school owner had even less reason to like him. Yet 13 years after the NCA had called its first meeting to discuss methods of raising educational standards, the results of Nugent's persistence began to unfold. By that time, the NCA reported, "46 of the 51 private school owners had surrendered their equities in 19 schools, upon mutually satisfactory terms negotiated by the Director of Education. Some of these 19 schools were closed and others merged to form eight, non-profit (NCA) accredited schools."

The surviving institutions located in Los Angeles, New York, Indianapolis, and Chicago allied themselves with Texas Chiropractic College, Western States College of Chiropractic, and Northwestern College of Chiropractic. NCA and broad scope-oriented schools in Colorado, Missouri, Ohio, Kansas, and California gave up their charters and merged. The influx of "GI Bill" students following World War II gave a surge to the curve graph of chiropractic student population and with it an inevitable crop of

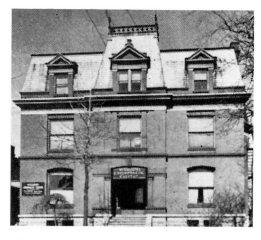

Missouri Chiropractic College, St. Louis, was one of the schools to give up its charter as a result of Nugent's push for educational reform, circa 1937.

From *What Chiropractic Is Doing,* 1938, Indianapolis, Burton Shields.

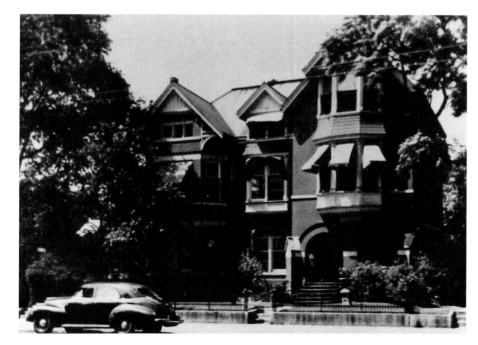

Canadian Memorial Chiropractic College, Toronto, Ontario, shortly after it was founded in 1945.

Courtesy Canadian Memorial Chiropractic College, Toronto, Ontario.

157

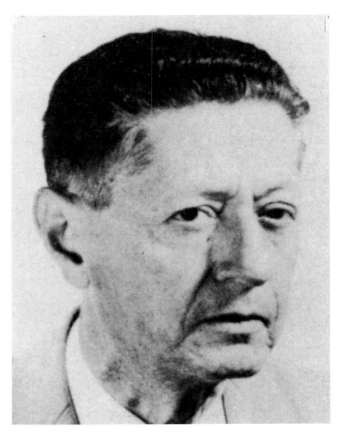

George Haynes, long-time faculty member and administrator at Los Angeles College of Chiropractic.

Courtesy Los Angeles College of Chiropractic, Los Angeles.

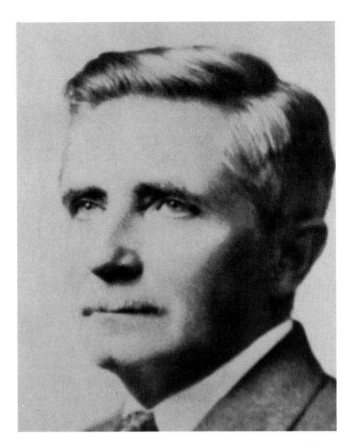

Frank Dean, president of the Columbia Institute of Chiropractic from 1919 to 1959.

Courtesy Palmer College of Chiropractic Archives, Davenport, Iowa.

new schools. However, most succumbed to the merger cycle by the end of the 1950s. John Nugent retired in 1961, not receiving fully the acknowledgment of a profession that he almost singularly bootstrapped into educational maturity. He died in late 1979 in the Bahamas largely forgotten. Not honored in his lifetime, he may yet gain posthumous recognition for his contributions. This role may earn him the distinction of being the Abraham Flexner of chiropractic educational reform.

The founding of the professionally owned Canadian Memorial Chiropractic College on the 50th anniversary of the first adjustment in 1945 marked the first nonproprietary school in Canada. Supported by the profession since its inception, the college later built a modern facility adjacent to York University in Toronto. The Ontario Council of Health in 1978 had recommended that Canadian Memorial Chiropractic College become a part of the provincial university system. Yet it was another university in Montreal that would make that breakthrough in 1993.

The story of chiropractic survival through the end of World War II is one of countless and largely unrecorded acts of individual sacrifice and dedication. The story of its schools parallel that odyssey. Many times it was only through the very unassuming yet costly sacrifices of individuals such as Wilbur Budden, George Haynes, Frank Dean, Thure Peterson, Hugh Logan, Carl S. Cleveland, Sr, Joseph Janse, David D. Palmer, Ernest Napolitano, James Firth, and many others that the difference between keeping academic doors open and the closing of many of their schools was effected.

CHIROPRACTIC LEGISLATIVE TRAVAILS

If the 1930s were the beginning of chiropractic educational reform, then those years proved to be a watershed of sorts in state legislation. An increasing presence was a tactic encouraged by the medical lobby and initiated as early as 1925. This tactic had the disastrous consequences of closing as many as a dozen key states to new chiropractors for most of four decades: the so-called basic science laws.

The initial surge of chiropractic regulation in the states began with the death of D.D. Palmer. From 1913 to the end of World War I, 14 states passed chiropractic legislation. Through the 1920s, chiropractic legislation was passed in 26 states, more than half of the total states. By the end of the 1920s the passage of this legislation gave the upstart profession a status unequalled by any other dissenting school of health care in medicine. Of the 48 jurisdictions (including the Territory of Hawaii), 40 had granted recognition. During the 1930s only South Carolina, Michigan, Delaware, and the Territory of Alaska were added.

Still there were the "open" states in which prosecutions would take place through mid-century. These states included New York and Texas, which at times might have accounted for more than 10% of all chiropractors in the United States. Other "open" states such as Pennsylvania and Alabama regulated chiropractors under licenses granted by older sections of the Medical Practice laws. Solitary chiropractors sat on medical boards at different times in Virginia, Indiana, New Jersey, Ohio, and other states.

Compromise legislation, which resulted in chiropractors in the minority on the Board or establishing entrance requirements beyond the minimum secondary school graduation and with the professional course longer than the "three of nine" or 18-month Palmer standard, had its own effect of limiting licensed practitioners. In 1925 the first basic science laws

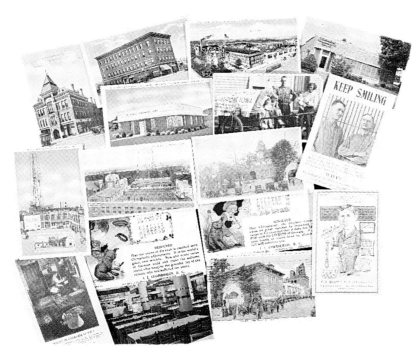

A selection of postcards with a chiropractic connection.
Courtesy Palmer College of Chiropractic Archives, Davenport, Iowa.

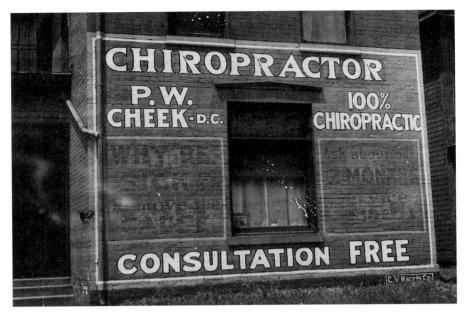

A chiropractor's advertisement, larger than life. Date and location unknown.
Courtesy Palmer College of Chiropractic Archives, Davenport, Iowa.

were passed; applicants of all "healing" professions—medicine, osteopathy, chiropractic, and naturopathy—were required to pass tests in physiology, pathology, chemistry, and in some cases bacteriology, toxicology, and diagnosis.

During the next 16 years more than a third of the states, as well as Alaska and Hawaii, passed such basic science legislation, which many chiropractic leaders saw as the death knell for the profession. The states where chiropractic enjoyed significant numbers and patient populations and which were most severely affected were Connecticut, Iowa, Minnesota, Nebraska, Washington, and Wisconsin. The grim statistics—which the representatives of the National Federation of Medical Licensing Boards reported with particular triumph—were evident in states such as Nebraska.

This farm-belt state, which had been among the first to license chiropractic in 1915 and had been a popular intake from the graduates of the nearby Palmer School, was virtually closed to chiropractic for over 4 decades. Not a single D.C. applicant sitting for the basic science board between 1929 and 1950 was able to pass the examinations and the state Board of Chiropractic Examiners could only record 70 licensed practitioners in 1945.

The statistics were equally disappointing with pass/fail figures revealed by the various basic science states and compiled by the Federation of Medical Licensing Boards in 1944. From 1927 until 1944 the Federation said that 87% of some 20,000 medical students, or 17,400 medical applicants, passed the examinations. Only 367 chiropractic students attempted the examinations with a dismal 28%, or 93 chiropractors, passing.

Considering that the major chiropractic institutions of the 1930s had only a few dozen university trained instructors, it may be more amazing that the pass percentage in difficult subjects such as physiology, chemistry, and pathology was even 28%. Only chiropractors taught these subjects in many of the schools, leading to the allegation in the *Illinois Medical Journal* that chiropractic faculties were constituted of "the ignorant instructing the uneducated."

NATIONAL CHIROPRACTIC ASSOCIATION

The first year of the new decade would bring consolidation of the new organizational presence in chiropractic, the NCA. Its evolution was the result of discontent of B.J. Palmer's Palmer School of Chiropractic alumni and the growing number of non-Palmer graduates who resented his dominant leadership of everything chiropractic. Keating and Rehm, who have done the definitive history of the NCA, reported that "a ferment of dissension" within B.J.'s UCA had resulted from his neurocalometer marketing and led to his resignation as the secretary-treasurer of the UCA in 1925.

Craig Kightlinger, a Palmer School of Chiropractic and university graduate, reflected the "proverbial last straw" of many chiropractors in their reaction to the neurocalometer. In 1926 he resigned from the UCA to join efforts with other "progressives" in the American Chiropractic Association (ACA), founded in 1922, to create a greater united front of disgruntled UCA members and "straights" with the largely "mixer" ACA ranks. Cutting the cord, Kightlinger paid cognizance to B.J. Palmer in his letter of resignation:

> We cannot forget the many trying times that The Developer of our science went through to keep and to bring it to a point where it could stand on its feet. To him we owe more than we can ever repay and to him is due the fact that the Science of Chiropractic is where it is today. He took us through the Dark Ages of the development, but now the time has come when once again the Natural Law must be taken into account and the leader of old must either sit at the council table and consult with the minds of the many or take his place on the side lines and let the march of Progress pass. We need him but we need as much and more the ideas that result from the clear thinking of the interested members of our profession.

Kightlinger, president of the Eastern Chiropractic Institute, which was one of three private New York institutions that would survive the Great Depression and World War II to form the non-profit Chiropractic Institute of New York in 1944, said what many practitioners felt: "there is nothing the matter with chiropractic. There is a great deal the matter with chiro-

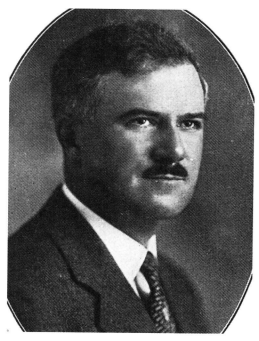

Craig Kightlinger, president of the Eastern Chiropractic Institute, circa 1938.

From *What Chiropractic Is Doing,* 1938, Indianapolis, Burton Shields.

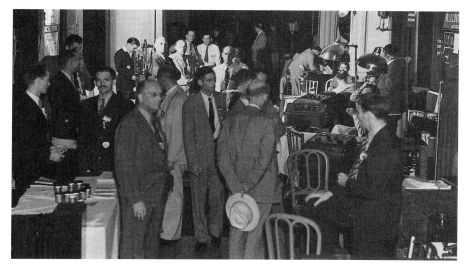

The exhibit area of a National Chiropractic Association convention, circa 1940.
Courtesy American Chiropractic Association, Arlington, Virginia.

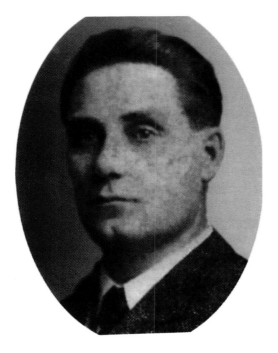

Tom Morris. His offices in LaCrosse, Wisconsin housed the Universal Chiropractor's Association after its split with B.J. Palmer.
From *The Chiropractor*, Sept/Oct 1910.

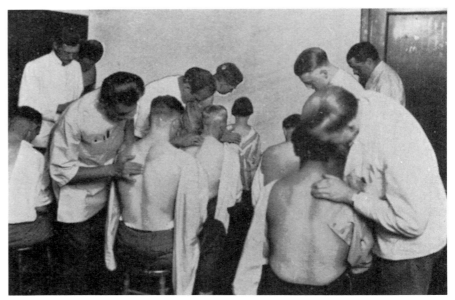

A classroom scene from the Eastern Chiropractic Institute, circa 1930.
From *Annual Catalogue, Eastern Chiropractic Institute*.

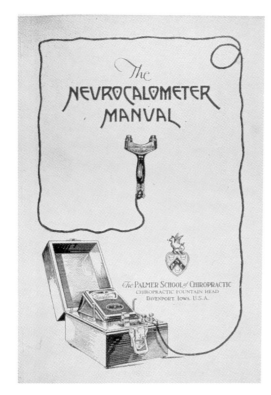

The neurocalometer, a heat sensing device which B.J. insisted was necessary for the detection of a subluxation.
Courtesy Palmer College of Chiropractic Archives, Davenport, Iowa.

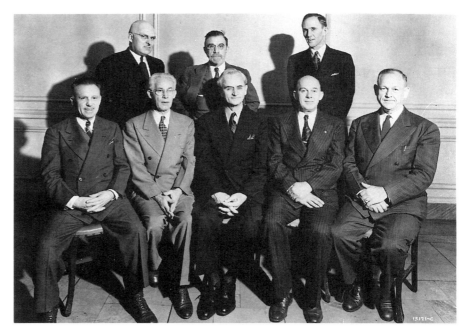

A meeting of school presidents to arrive at a common definition of chiropractic in Kansas City, Missouri, 1939. Standing left to right are Carl Cleveland, Sr., Cleveland Chiropractic College; B.J. Palmer, Palmer College of Chiropractic; and Home Beatty, University of Natural Healing Arts. Seated left to right are Dr. O'Neil O'Neil-Ross College of Chiropractic, Fort Wayne, Indiana; Hugh Logan, Logan College of Chiropractic; T.F. Ratledge, Ratledge College of Chiropractic, Los Angeles; H.C. Harring, Missouri Chiropractic College; and James Drain, Texas Chiropractic College.

practors. They have never been used to thinking for themselves. . ." Indeed, there would be an ingathering of chiropractors "who could think for themselves" at the UCA's 1925 convention in Chicago, described as "tempestuous" by Turner:

> (Tom) Morris said the (NCM) could be made for $30.00, could not be forced upon the profession at a figure so exorbitant as to be commensurate with an interest of 7,000 percent . . . Morris addressed the delegates, enunciated again the principles which condemned the nerve-tester, and tendered his resignation as chief consul of the association. Dr. Palmer followed with his resignation as secretary . . . Morris was reinstated. The office of the association was moved from Palmer School to the suite occupied by the Universal Chiropractors Association attorney in LaCrosse, Wisconsin.

The next year, some of B.J.'s UCA followers sought a restoration, and after failure joined him in a new "purist" grouping, the Chiropractic Health Bureau, a protective association on the original UCA model, which claimed about a third of the strength of the post-Palmer UCA-ACA opposition. It was inevitable that these two organizations would merge, which Keating and Rehm said occurred only after the death of Tom Morris and the reconciliation of personalities that had resided in both organizations. Not until November of 1930 was the NCA born.

By the mid-1930s, the profession—at least that part which had decided that a long-term separation if not a divorce was necessary from B.J. Palmer's leadership—took stock of its situation. The structure of the NCA had evolved to the degree that it embraced affiliates in the major states with a concentration of practice and had begun the public relations war that many had advocated. While B.J. had always advanced the "selling of chiropractic" and was as flamboyant in advertising as he was in his philosophy of the practice of chiropractic, others sought to portray a profession in a less cultish manner and with an acknowledgment of the public welfare.

Thus the NCA, following B.J.'s chiropractic advocacy model, began a campaign of providing "boilerplate" advertisements that local members could use with their names in local newspapers, radio "spots" that could be sold locally, and the first of many "Posture Queen" and "Beautiful Back" contests that were always good copy and even gained the attention of the producers of the news clips by RKO and Paramount used in tens of thousands of local theaters preceding the latest movie. Nugent's Committee on Educational Standards sent signals to the profession and to the world outside chiropractic that standards would have to be raised if survival were to take place.

Essentially, what happened to chiropractors, the students who enrolled in the remaining colleges, and much of the chiropractic patient constituency in this decade was the creation of a circled-wagon mentality, a "them and us" psychology. Circled-wagon mentality doctrines were simple enough and familiar to other minorities in American society: the members of the profession were in a constant state of friction—a sometimes hot but more often cold war in which chiropractors became a despised group of "outsiders" in conflict with medicine and seemingly much of the public sector.

The "medical lobby" became an all-important, larger-than-life force behind most of the toil and turmoil experienced by chiropractors and their followers. There was enough truth in this assertion to give it credence for

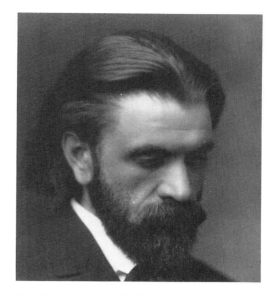

B.J. Palmer, circa 1925.
Courtesy Palmer College of Chiropractic Archives, Dav-

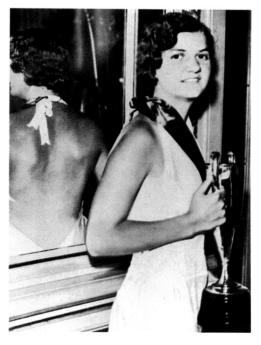

"Perfect Back" and "Posture Queen" contests made good copy. The contestants' spines were x-rayed.
From *What Chiropractic Is Doing,* 1938, Indianapolis, Burton Shields.

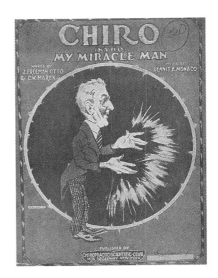
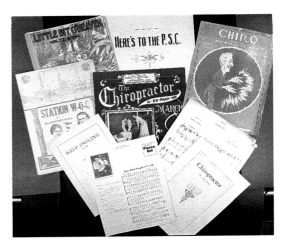
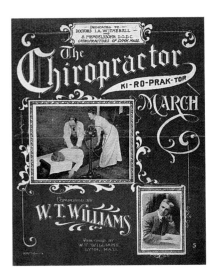

Chiropractic has inspired several song writers.
Courtesy Palmer College of Chiropractic Archives, Davenport, Iowa.

indeed there were operatives in the AMA and its larger state societies who sought the literal eradication of chiropractic from the health care scene. While the legislative wars had been reduced to a half-dozen jurisdictions, there was enough evidence that a policy of exclusion, ridicule, and out-right condemnation was being followed.

Morris Fishbein, the long-time editor of the *Journal of the American Medical Association* led the assault, contrasting osteopathy "as a method of entering medicine by the back door (while) chiropractic is an attempt to arrive through the cellar." The Department of Investigation of the AMA was not formalized until after World War II, but there always had been a large repository of "anti-quackery" materials in the Chicago AMA head-

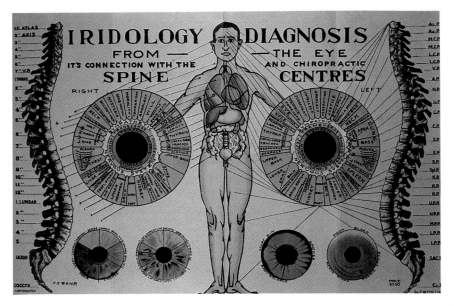

Though not chiropractic, some broad-scope chiropractors used iridology, the diagnosis by studying the eye's iris.
Courtesy Palmer College of Chiropractic Archives, Davenport, Iowa.

quarters with quantities of reprints warning of the dangers of chiropractors circulated freely by state medical society affiliates.

Indeed, there was enough to be cautious about in the nether world of sectarian medicine. It may have been inevitable that a good part of the profession would reside in this subculture of alternative healing, which through the quirks of legislative enactments or "other healer" provisions of the medical practice acts had given additional opportunity for broader practice and the inevitable intrusion into "allopathic" domains of medication, surgery, and obstetrics. The literature of "drugless" associations and journals in the 1930s and of those colleges who offered dual degrees in chiropractic and naturopathy (National College of Chiropractic, Los Angeles College of Chiropractic, and Western States College of Chiropractic were the most prominent) suggests that it was widespread enough to attract remnants of the branches of the medical tree that had all but died: homeopathy and the eclectics.

The last homeopathic college closed in 1922. The final eclectic medical class was graduated in 1939 in Cincinnati, Ohio. Yet their adherents, along with assorted hydropaths, mechanotherapists, "sanipractors" (the Washington state designation for naturopaths), naprapaths, and others could be found at annual conclaves of drugless physician groups. Many of them also held either chiropractic degrees or licenses, as well as utter contempt for the Palmer adherents of straight practice. In the 1940s an umbrella group called the *National Medical Society* embraced all of these groups, as well as some allopaths.

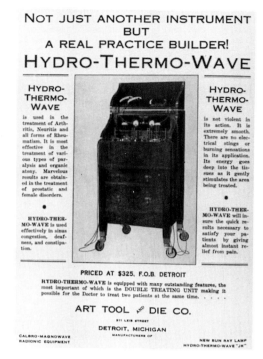

An electrotherapy machine, used by some broad scope chiropractors in their patients' care.

Courtesy Logan College of Chiropractic, Chesterfield, Missouri.

ECLECTIC CHIROPRACTIC

B.J. Palmer was convinced in the 1930s that the NCA was to be the advance guard of "medical mongrelization" that would dilute the principles of The Founder. Some of the "murky modalities" that found an audience in chiropractic were the electronic medical gadgets of San Francisco physician Albert Abrams, "the King of Quacks," according to one

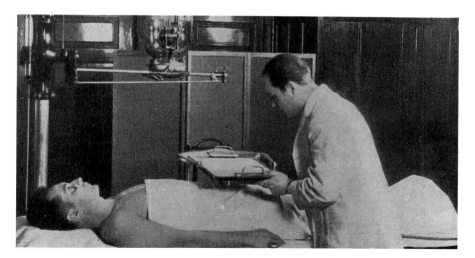

The physiological therapeutics introduced at the National School of Chiropractic included colonic therapy.

Courtesy National College of Chiropractic, Lombard, Illinois.

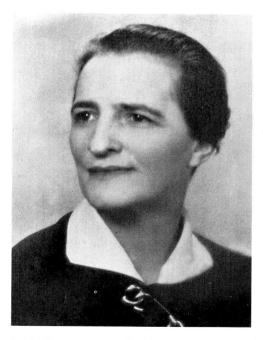

Ruth Drown, who developed a radiovision instrument used by some chiropractors.

From Drown R: *The Theory and Technique of the Drown H.V.R. and Radio-Vision Instruments*, London, 1939, Hatchhand.

prominent medical historian. Similarly, the "black box" of California chiropractor Ruth Drown was another popular gadget. Less known but fascinating for its acceptance in "mainstream" chiropractic was the Kolar school of "bloodless surgery."

Many of those who advocated the "physiological therapeutics" were introduced by the early National School of Chiropractic leadership of A.L. Forster and W.C. Schultze. Both had elevated "heat, light, water, and color," to acceptable modalities for "mixer chiropractors."

The dissolution of the old UCA and its merger with the ACA in 1930 brought greater acceptance to this broad scope school of practice. The new post-1930 NCA provided a forum for newer modalities. The 1932 convention of the NCA in Wichita, Kansas was the initial demonstration of what proved to be a remarkable flirtation of chiropractors with "bloodless surgery" and a nonmedical form of anesthesia, termed *chromotherapy*.

Kolar Bloodless Surgery

Francis Kolar came to Kansas in January 1932 from California. The several accounts found about Kolar do not identify his chiropractic training, but he is supposed to have studied with Adolf Lorenz, a Vienna orthopedist who popularized bloodless surgery at the turn of the century and who lectured in the United States. D.D. Palmer heard him lecture in Chicago. Joining two Kansas chiropractors, he established the Kolar Health Clinic on North Market Street in Wichita. A history of chiropractic in Kansas published in 1965 reported on his practice:

> Because the Kansas law permitted the replacement of any body tissues, he did not restrict his work to the spine. He had studied under a Viennese orthopedist, in Europe, to care for stubborn cases. Through the use of special lenses over the patient's eyes, he directed a beam of light through them to effect the thalamus, a sensory switchboard of the brain. This means was used to replace the anesthetics of the medical profession in surgery, by which means his "bloodless surgery" was done by hands only, to remove tumors, goiters, adhesions, cysts and replace prolapsed organs, and no pain was felt.

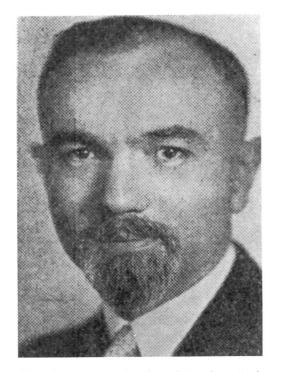

Francis Kolar practiced and taught a technique of "bloodless surgery."
From *The Chiropractic Journal*, June 1934.

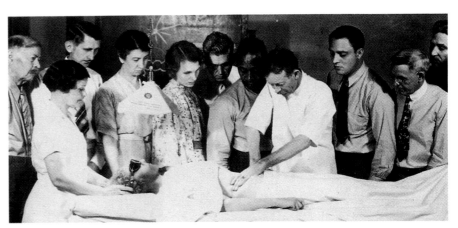

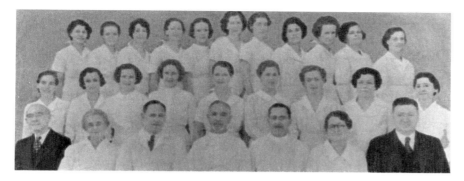

Francis Kolar (middle front row) *and the staff of the Kolar Health Clinic, circa 1937.*
From *What Chiropractic Is Doing,* 1938, Indianapolis, Burton Shields.

Kolar permitted as many chiropractors at the conventions as could get into a room to see such an operation. He was also on Kansas convention programs to explain his work in 1933 and 1934. In 1937 he was appointed to the State Board of Examiners, eventually returning to California.

The *Journal of the National Chiropractic Association* described a "Kolar operation" in May 1935:

> One operation was for cataracts (a patient from California) and the other abdominal conditions (a Kansas patient). Before proceeding with his work, Dr. Kolar gave a short sketch of his method, stated the conditions which affected the patients, outlined his procedure in correcting those conditions and gave the prognosis in each case. He then began the operation and as he worked he explained what he was doing and stated the reasons why each step was taken. At the end of the operations he asked the patients to state whether or not they felt any pain. They both replied, with voices loud and clear, that they had felt no pain whatever.

Spears Chiropractic Hospital

If the Kolar therapy was an aberration in chiropractic, then its acceptance in the "mainline" was not. Others who were featured on the NCA programs in the 1930s included Denver's Dr. Leo Spears, who matched B.J. in flamboyance, innovation, and marketing acumen. The classic Southern "poor boy" who supposedly attended his classes at the Palmer School of Chiropractic in his World War I uniform because he could not afford other clothes, Dr. Spears captured notice in the "mile high" Colorado city with his "painless adjustment" advertising and his "free clinics for poor children" offered in a mobile trailer.

The latter led to his incorporation of the name that would constitute his "impossible dream"—which came true during the unlikely tenure of World War II—the Spears Hospital and Free Clinic for Poor Children. A shrewd land speculator, as well as a direct mail advertising advocate, Spears purchased several acres near what would become Stapleton Airport and reinvested in the property that would house Spears Hospital. When building materials and supplies were restricted because of the war, he began construction of his first hospital unit in 1943, naming it after Willard Carver.

Reportedly, B.J. had rebuffed him in his request to name it after The

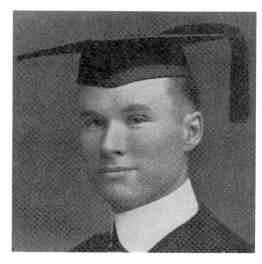

Leo Spears, who began construction of his Spears Hospital in 1943.
Courtesy Palmer College of Chiropractic Archives. Davenport, Iowa.

167

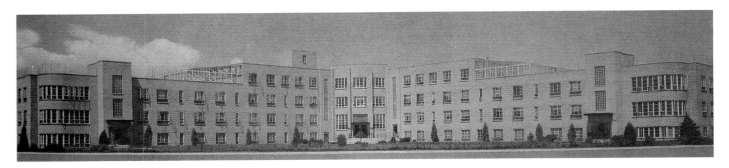

Spears Chiropractic Hospital, Denver, Colorado.
Courtesy Palmer College of Chiropractic Archives, Davenport, Iowa.

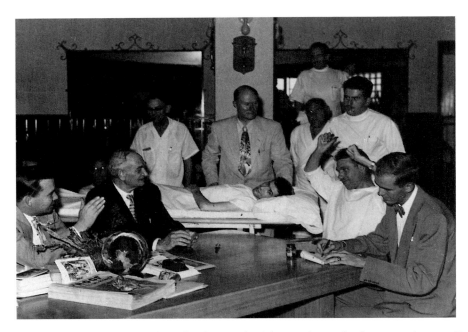

Leo Spears and patients from his hospital with members of a Senate subcommittee investigating charges of medical monopoly in the Veteran's Administration.
Courtesy Russell Gibbons, Pittsburgh, Pennsylvania.

Discoverer, because Palmer had authorized an effort to build on top of the B.J. Palmer Clinic and open the facility as a chiropractic hospital. Solicitation of funds for this purpose had actually netted several thousand dollars. That one of his former students would actually accomplish what Palmer had proposed did not set well with B.J.. Carver died a few months after the 230-bed facility named after him was opened. It received the first inpatients in the summer of 1943.

College of Chiropractic Physicians and Surgeons

As evidence of the parameters of broad practices that many in the profession had achieved in the third decade of its existence, the rather remarkable example of the College of Chiropractic Physicians and Surgeons may be offered. Founded in 1931, it operated for 15 years on West Ninth Street in Los Angeles and then merged with the present Los Angeles College of Chiropractic.

The College of Chiropractic Physicians and Surgeons was non-profit and professionally owned, but what made it unique despite its name was its stress on general practice and specialties, which have all but disappeared from the chiropractic scene today. The college announcements for 1933 under "Physicians and Surgeons Post Graduate Course," offered:

> Advanced course in medicine and surgery extending over a period of two years open and to graduate chiropractors, who desire to increase their knowledge of therapeutics and who can present to the College Credential Committee proper credentials of having completed a one-year course of college grade in physics, chemistry, and biology. At the completion of this course, the chiropractor is in a position to intelligently give advice when called upon to do so. Surgery and surgical specialties are taught in such a manner that the student learns to distinguish between cases which do and do not require surgical care. The general management of surgical cases with the possibilities and disadvantages of surgical methods are made clear.

While the college qualifies that those chiropractors granted its "Physicians and Surgeons Certificate" would not be expected to become general practitioners, it did offer a course in "Chiropractic Surgery." The clinical experience was not limited to the two outpatient facilities associated with the College of Chiropractic Physicians and Surgeons, but through an inpatient teaching arrangement with an affiliated hospital:

> Through the facilities of the Bellevue Hospital, a 60 bed general hospital owned and operated by the chiropractic profession, the student receives direct instruction by the attending staff in the care of surgical and obstetrical cases, together with a wide variety of acute and chronic diseases. This is in addition to the practical work which the student secures in the college clinic.

Bellevue Chiropractic Hospital

Bellevue, one of half a dozen chiropractic hospitals in Los Angeles that long ago succumbed to the undertow of private hospitalization, was known as a maternity facility. The Obstetrical Department at the College of Chiropractic Physicians and Surgeons included a service in the college clinic, a department in Bellevue, and a service for home maternity cases. The announcement stressed the emphasis on this specialty:

> There is also established the obstetrical clinic in the college where the pre-natal examination of the patient is conducted by the student under the supervision, at all times, of one of the instructors of the department. The treatment prescribed is given by the student and the general welfare of the patient is closely watched so that a normal completion of the term of pregnancy may be expected.

Chiropractic obstetrics, which survives today within the legal scope of practice only in Oregon but is generally not practiced, once enjoyed a chiropractic specialty status in California and half a dozen other states, notably Oklahoma.

In a seeming contradiction of the professional evolution of chiropractic, with educational standards yet to be elevated and legislative battles still to be fought, there were instances of broad practice rights enjoyed by individual chiropractors and advocated by "specialty" societies in several states throughout the 1930s and to the end of World War II. In addition to obstetrics and minor surgery, some states allowed procedures that might be considered within the orthopedic sphere, such as casting and splinting. California and Oregon had chiropractors who "specialized" in gynecology and proctology. Adverse court and examining board decisions and the complexities of malpractice insurance eliminated most of them in the decade following World War II.

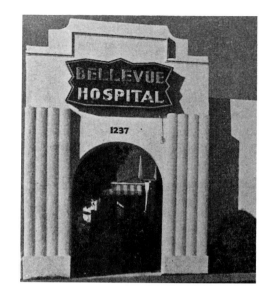

Bellevue Hospital, Los Angeles, California, was owned and operated by the chiropractic profession.

From *The Scientific Chiropractor,* May 1937.

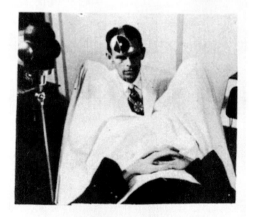

FRANK B. HAMILTON, B.Sc., D.C.
Chairman Dept. Obstetrics & Gynecology
De Landas Univ., Western States Univ.
Col. Chiropractic Physicians & Surgeons
Lecturer Col. Chiropractic Physicians & Surgeons
Grad. School, LACC Member, NCA, CCA,
Delta Phi Psi
Obstetrical & Gynecological Soc.

Chiropractor Frank Hamilton, Chairman of the Department of Obstetrics and Gynecology at the College of Chiropractic Physicians and Surgeons.

From *Chiropractic History* 2(1), 1982.

169

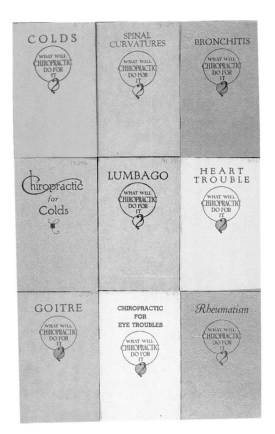

These pamphlets were used by some chiropractors during the 1930s to educate the public about the benefits of chiropractic.

Courtesy Palmer College of Chiropractic Archives, Davenport, Iowa.

B.J. PALMER CHIROPRACTIC RESEARCH CLINIC

Following the Palmer School of Chiropractic's Lyceum during the Summer of 1935, B.J. opened the B.J. Palmer Chiropractic Research Clinic. The continuing controversies between the broad-scope and narrow-scope advocates within the profession moved each of two factions toward trying to scientifically prove the claims of one approach was more efficacious than the other, whether it was the upper cervical subluxation complex of B.J.'s or the modality approaches of Schultz and National College.

The Palmer School had always had a patient clinic on campus with faculty both teaching and practicing. Many chiropractors had wanted to send their patients to B.J. in Davenport when they had failed to relieve their patients of pain or suffering, but B.J. had not openly accepted such referrals. It was with the establishment of the research clinic that he openly began to seek out, diagnose, adjust when necessary, and systematically record the findings of these problem cases using a variety of medical and scientific measures.

When the B.J. Palmer Chiropractic Research Clinic was established it was

> . . . dedicated to finding scientific constants in cases. To establish *before adjustment constants,* we have not less than 30 different records made and interpreted. This number grows as we eliminate variables. Many of these are checked against (the) case weekly. All of them repeat when case leaves our Clinic, that we may establish *after adjustment constants.*

The chiropractic research clinic was organized with two divisions, a Medical Division and a Chiropractic Division. The Medical Division was staffed by medically trained doctors and support staff to administer a battery of medical tests. The medical laboratory contained all the standard diagnostic equipment of the day to administer medical tests to establish a "medical diagnosis" of the patient's condition. The Medical Division even maintained an ambulance service for the transportation of patients to and from the Clinic.

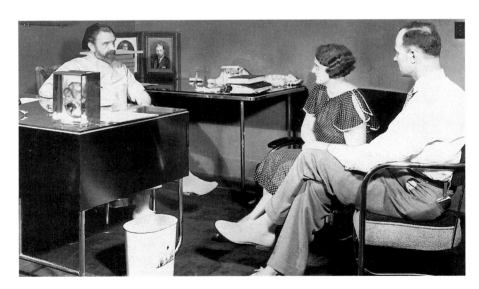

Herb Hender, doing a physical examination in the B.J. Palmer Clinic, circa 1945.

Courtesy Palmer College of Chiropractic Archives, Davenport, Iowa.

B.J. Palmer consulting with patients in the B.J. Palmer Clinic, a clinic to which chiropractors in the field were encouraged to send patients who were not responding to normal care.

Courtesy Palmer College of Chiropractic Archives, Davenport, Iowa.

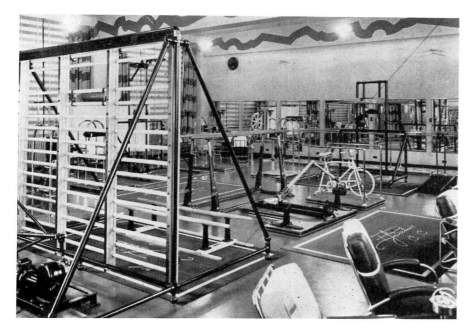

The B.J. Palmer Clinic rehabilitation lab, circa 1945.
Courtesy Palmer College of Chiropractic Archives, Davenport, Iowa.

The second laboratory was the Chiropractic Division. The Chiropractic Laboratory included not only the standard chiropractic office equipment and analysis equipment of the day, but also a number of specifically designed research equipment pieces to graphically record and document information about the chiropractic adjustment's effects to the body. There was a specifically designed spinograph, a radiographic machine designed to shoot full spine radiographs; a neurocalograph, a recording machine used in conjunction with a neurocalometer, used to record temperature variances along the spine; a conturographometer, which recorded the curvature variations of the spine; a Keeler polygraph, which was more popularly known as a lie-detector machine, to record pulse and respiratory responses; and the electroencephaloneuromentimpograph, a pioneering diagnostic predecessor of today's electromyography diagnostic machine.

The results and findings of these patient cases were published in B.J.'s writings over the next 30 years, including a number of special research publications that outlined the cases, the findings, and results of care. The B.J. Palmer Chiropractic Research Clinic operated on campus until B.J.'s death in 1961.

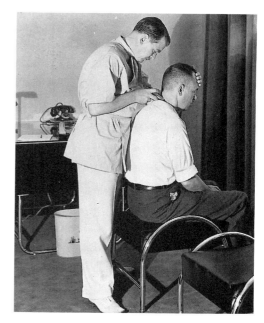

Lyle Sherman, Director of the B.J. Palmer Clinic, performing an NCM reading on a patient.
Courtesy Palmer College of Chiropractic Archives, Davenport, Iowa.

SOCIAL CHANGE AND POLICIES—THE NEW DEAL

Franklin D. Roosevelt and the New Deal policies expanded the role of government into virtually every sector of society and dominated this time line of chiropractic. He came into office in early 1932 and died weeks before the end of the war in Europe. The consequences of new social policy and federal activism designed to pull the country from the despair of depression—and later to marshall its resources toward the victory over the Axis powers and consolidation of the United States as the world's leading power—characterized this period.

As players in the field of health care, however small and lacking in respect, chiropractors were to evolve with the New Deal and the Recovery and later as part of the home front against fascism. The *National Chiropractic Journal* in the 1930s would play a role in the "Blue Eagle" campaigns of the National Recovery Administration (NRA), one of the support organizations enlisted for that purpose. Individual practitioners were urged to display the Blue Eagle in their offices and at state society conventions.

The other New Deal attraction was the proposed Professional Code relating to labor services under NRA, which NCA leader L.M. Rogers and others saw as an opportunity to enter the ranks of other professions and gain public respect and official recognition at the same time.

The Denver convention of the NCA advocated the Code and named its first full-time Director of Public Relations. The adoption of the chiropractic emblem came at the 1934 convention in Pittsburgh, and a year later at the historic Los Angeles convention the formal structure for educational reform was authorized with the Committee on Educational Standards. These efforts of the NCA in this period were a major step in the maturation of the chiropractic profession. If the early 1920s were the "Golden Age" of Palmer influence within chiropractic, then the later 1930s and the war years would be a similar period of activism and increasing influence for the NCA leadership.

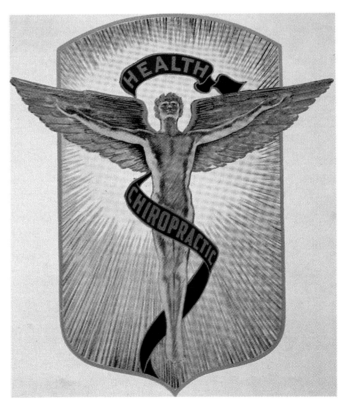

The chiropractic emblem was adopted at the 1934 NCA convention in Pittsburgh.

From *What Chiropractic Is Doing,* 1938, Indianapolis, Burton Shields.

The crossroads convention that established the start of the "classic reformation" period in chiropractic education could well have had its symbolic occurrence during the depths of the depression when chiropractic was buffeted by the economic decline, as well as its assault by medicine, repressive "basic science" legislation, and internal fratricide in the "mixer-straight" wars.

The Fortieth Anniversary Convention of the broad-scope NCA was held in Los Angeles in hospitable "mixer" territory, with an impressive 2000 chiropractors, family, and friends gathering for sessions that reflected the myriad kaleidoscope of the profession. NCA past-president Arthur W. Schweitert reported that the president of the Nebraska Board of Chiropractic Examiners had written him that the profession was slowly dying in that state:

> . . . the basic science law in Nebraska has been very detrimental to chiropractic. We have not had a single new Chiropractor in the state since the basic science law went into effect. There have been five applicants for admission, but all failed . . ..

The "Chiropractic Special" was a special train package of Midwestern and Eastern chiropractors who took their families to the first Western convention of a national association, picking up chiropractors in Nebraska, Wyoming, Utah, and Nevada and converging on the convention site—the Hollywood Roosevelt Hotel. The leadership of the NCA was taking strength from an exceptional increase of 51% over membership from the preceding year, attesting to the publicity conscious efforts directed by L.M. Rogers from the NCA headquarters in Webster City, Iowa.

The NCA's leadership had also committed itself to true educational reform, choosing the 1935 convention to announce the Committee on Educational Standards which John Nugent had carefully constructed in previous undertakings and school visitations. Walter Wardwell would recount his 1948 Nugent interview decades later, in which "chiropractic's

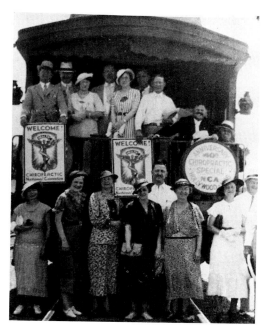

Chiropractors on their way to an NCA convention, circa 1935.

Courtesy American Chiropractic Association, Arlington, Virginia.

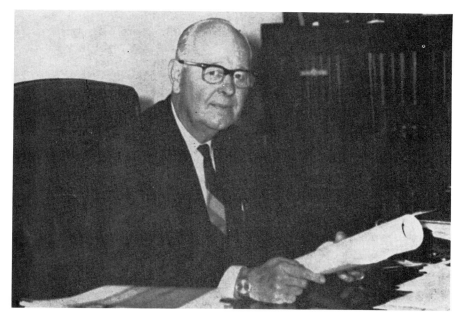

Loran Rogers, executive director of the National Chiropractic Association and the American Chiropractic Association, from 1932-1972.

Courtesy American Chiropractic Association, Arlington, Virginia.

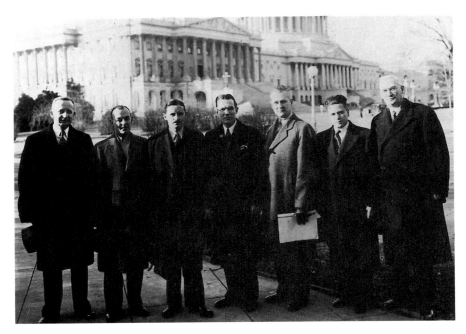

Emmett Murphy, lobbyist and Labor Relations Director for the NCA (fourth from left) *standing with* (left to right) *Wayne Crider, Lawrence J. Mills Jr., Melvin Smith, G.W Will, Cash Asher, and E.M. Gustafson in front of the Capitol after a hearing before the Farm Security Administration.*

Courtesy American Chiropractic Association, Arlington, Virginia.

Abraham Flexner" declared that "In 1935 we called a meeting in Hollywood, California, to which 19 state examining boards sent representatives. Initially we sought to raise chiropractic standards through uniform examinations, but soon saw that this would not work."

The deep rift between the proprietary school owners and the NCA's education committee over what they considered an invasion of their turf, as well as a forced acceptance of an offensive "mixer" ideology, was best reflected by the reply of T.F. Ratledge, a California "straight" school president, to the NCA's Rogers:

> On July 9th, we notified Dr. Crider that we would not consent to any classification whatsoever by the National Chiropractic Association or any of its affiliates and definitely warned that in case he or the Council does attempt to so classify our institution among Chiropractic teaching institutions we will resort to the courts to recover any damages which we believe to have resulted to said Ratledge Chiropractic College by such classification.

It was amazing that at the time when the profession was at its low ebb in practitioners, its schools in a survival mode, and many chiropractors failing in their practice, the NCA was able to gather 2000 adherents in a convention that would mark significant and even fundamental changes in the course of the profession. C. Sterling Cooley, whose father had studied under "Old Dad Chiro" in Oklahoma, took the podium at the convention to suggest that it was the best and worst of times for chiropractic and urged his listeners "not to choose the path of another 40 years of wandering the wilderness of uncertainty, persecution and chaos."

Organizationally, Rogers and a succession of strong NCA presidents and executive committee members would strive to make the NCA a broad-based professional organization. Chiropractors who sustained themselves with their practices but who gave more and more time to specialized assignments began to make a difference. Nugent gained the title as Director of Education in 1941 but had been virtually the NCA's minister of education without portfolio for 6 years. Emmett J. Murphy, a handsome and articulate glad-hander in Washington, D.C., began to spend more time on Capitol Hill than in his practice. He was a regular feature at Democratic National Conventions and had access to various congressional offices, becoming the NCA's Washington, D.C., lobbyist at the same time.

The Rogers-Nugent-Murphy triumvirate would become the political center of the NCA and in many ways chiropractic for the next 3 decades. As with B.J. in an earlier survival and growth period, they provided the organizational, educational, and political glue to sustain the profession in dark economic times and the war years.

Chiropractic was essentially in a no-growth valley during the 1941 to 1945 years of emergency and war effort. Younger chiropractors answered the call to arms or were drafted, and soon a regular column about chiropractors in the service began to appear. The handful of commissioned chiropractors gave some measure of prestige to those left at the home front, but the vast number of enlisted men were noncommissioned pharmacist's mates, medical corpsmen, and x-ray technicians. Many were in front-line combat units.

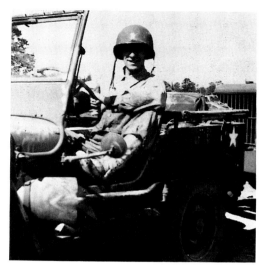

Many younger chiropractors answered the call to arms or were drafted during World War II serving as technicians or medical corpsmen.

From *NCA Journal* February 1944.

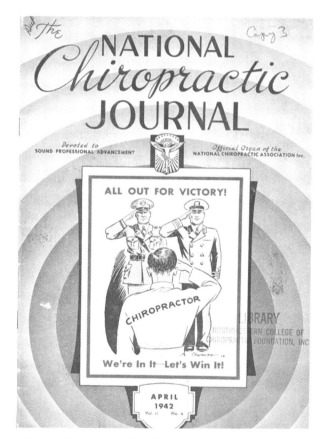

A journal cover inspired by the patriotic fervor of a nation at war.

From *National Chiropractic Journal* April 1942.

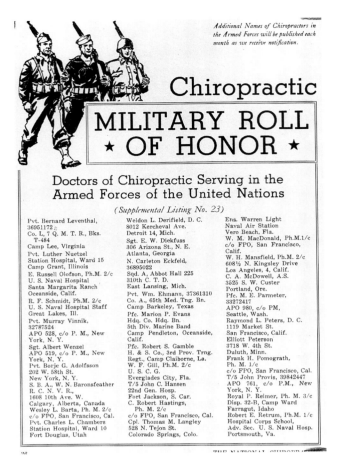

A list of chiropractors serving in World War II was published monthly in the National Chiropractic Journal.

From *National Chiropractic Journal* May 1944.

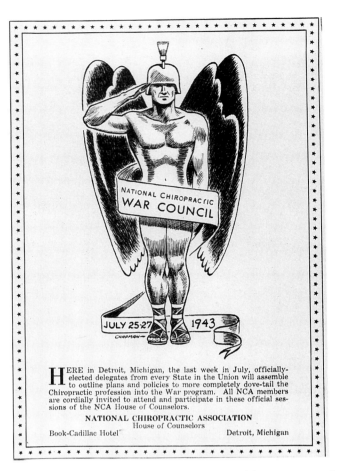

A militant version of the chiropractic emblem, prompted by World War II, appeared in the National Chiropractic Journal.

From *National Chiropractic Journal* April 1942.

An outgrowth of this wartime experience was the American Society of Military Chiropractors, which became a recognized NCA Council and served to cement the linkage between the profession and those from its ranks in service. The window emblems that were proudly displayed in millions of American homes and apartments, telling of a family member at war, now were visible in the reception rooms of the chiropractic colleges.

CHIROPRACTIC HEALTH BUREAU AND THE INTERNATIONAL CHIROPRACTORS ASSOCIATION

By 1926, chiropractic was still a young profession—only 30 years old and still struggling over its identity as either a narrow-scope or broad-scope health care art. Beginning in the mid-1920s the UCA, which until this time was predominantly a narrow-scope organization, began absorbing more liberal-oriented and broad-scope chiropractors into its membership. With this came the subsequent debates about the proper scope-of-practice orientation of the profession. Following the introduction of the neurocalometer, B.J. Palmer resigned as the secretary-treasurer of the UCA in 1926. During 1926, B.J. and other more narrow-scope oriented chiropractors organized the Chiropractic Health Bureau. The Chiropractic Health Bureau was created as a "protective" organization and its mission was outlined in its constitution:

> The organization shall aim by research, publicity, combative and defensive legislation, lawful legal protection, cooperation, and in every legitimate and ethical way, to promote and advance the Philosophy, Science and Art of Chiropractic and the professional welfare of its members to the end that every locality shall have knowledge of chiropractic and have unhampered right and opportunity of obtaining the services of chiropractors . . . this organization without reservation affirming its belief in the justice of the principle of allowing the sick to seek and obtain the services of practitioners of their own choice, of whatever calling, or school; and this bureau to undertake to attempt everything that it can legally and lawfully do in the defense of this principle.

Through its membership assessments, the Chiropractic Health Bureau established a legal counsel program that agreed to help defend any member chiropractor who was accused of practicing medicine, osteopathy, or surgery without a license; help defend member chiropractors against malpractice suits and judgment expenses; and help defend member chiropractors against any other offenses including criminal charges of either first-degree murder or manslaughter (since chiropractors were sometimes charged if a patient died). The lawyers hired by the Chiropractic Health Bureaus traveled tens of thousands of miles across the country performing their duties. The Bureau's General Counsel George Rinier reported in 1931 that during the past year he had traveled 32,004 miles at an expense of $1,765.78 defending member chiropractors.

In 1932 the Chiropractic Health Bureau created a public relations department called the *Chiropractic Health Bureau's Layman Division*. The Layman's Division included in its membership laymen interested in furthering "the philosophy, science, and art of chiropractic" and to "promote and preserve the inherent rights of all free people" to receive "the service of any health method that has proven its worth and merit." One such project was a chiropractic rally held at Madison Square Garden on January 23, 1932, which was attended by 16,500 supporters of chiropractic. With the establishment of other layman's units around the country, officials from the Bureau were traveling through the country meeting and educating such support groups and lobbying for chiropractic legislative support in the states.

Given the overall decline in the number of chiropractors educated dur-

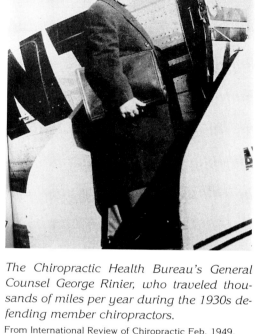

The Chiropractic Health Bureau's General Counsel George Rinier, who traveled thousands of miles per year during the 1930s defending member chiropractors.
From International Review of Chiropractic Feb. 1949.

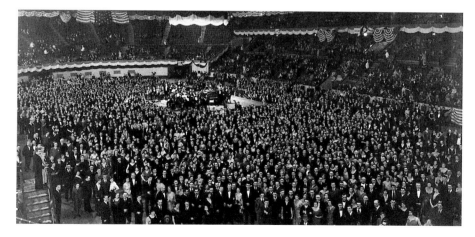

More than 16,500 chiropractic supporters attended a rally held by the American Bureau of Chiropractic in Madison Square Garden on January 23, 1932.
Courtesy Russell Gibbons, Pittsburgh, Pennsylvania.

ing the 1930s primarily because of the whole economic downturn of the decade and with the subsequent Bureau's decline in membership, another attempt at strengthening the profession by improving the relationship between its two national organizations was initiated in 1940 by B.J. and Willard Carver and centered on establishing a defined chiropractic curriculum.

At the 1939 NCA conference, an Allied Chiropractic Education Institution was formed by the college heads who allied themselves with John Nugent and the NCA. B.J. proposed a meeting of all the non-NCA college heads that would affirm their commitment to the preservation of chiropractic "in its simplicity and purity" and that all would agree "that chiropractic educational institutions shall teach and maintain only a specific course in chiropractic education. . . ."

Although the meeting between the two national organizations' educational affiliates did not take place, one of the results of the meeting with the college heads affiliated with the Chiropractic Health Bureau was several recommendations on the rechartering of the organization. Among the changes made in 1941 was the creation of a cabinet of advisors to the President that was composed of a representative and/or the head of the affiliated chiropractic educational organization. The other noteworthy change was the renaming of the organization. Carver suggested the International Chiropractic Health Society, which was adjusted to the International Chiropractors Association.

WORLD WAR II'S EFFECT ON CHIROPRACTIC

Student populations declined dramatically during World War II, as did the elevation of the average age of the remaining male students who were exempt from military service. Even the citadels of chiropractic education in Davenport, Chicago, and Los Angeles could claim no more than 250 or 300 students each in the best of the 1942 to 1944 war years. According to the research of Wiese and Ferguson, at least a dozen schools closed or merged in the period ending in 1945, including four smaller institutions in California and others in Kansas, Michigan, Tennessee, and Texas. Three long-time Manhattan schools were consolidated into the Chiropractic Institute of New York in 1944.

It was during 1944 that Congress authorized the legislation that would effectively rejuvenate chiropractic education and the profession itself through the next decade. The GI Bill of Rights, which brought an economically level playing field and access to higher education to millions of Americans who previously had been in a cultural and economic divide that separated them from that opportunity, literally opened the doors of America's colleges to millions of returning veterans. The remaining doors of the some 17 chiropractic schools would soon bulge with the sons and daughters of the Doughboys who had gone to Davenport and other schools a generation earlier.

Their numbers would inflate the schools and lead to the first modest expansion programs on the Palmer campus and the other surviving institutions, most of whom had accepted NCA affiliation. Unsuccessful petitions to the War Manpower Commission and other government agencies during the war had not removed chiropractic from its limbo in an occupational nether land. Unlike the osteopaths, their manipulative cousins who had long since joined the allopaths in abandoning drugless therapy chiropractors survived the war years without either the prestige or prac-

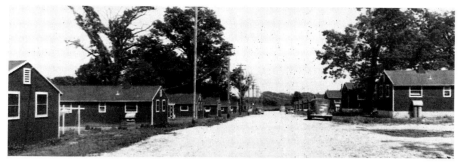

To handle housing for its students after World War II, the Palmer School of Chiropractic erected these trailers in an area known as Palmerton.
Courtesy Palmer College of Chiropractic Archives, Davenport, Iowa.

tical advantages of the gasoline stickers "necessary to the war effort," although in some instances they too filled the void created by absent family doctors off to war from the rural landscape.

The end of the war would also begin to change the face of chiropractic with a small but growing presence of women and blacks within the ranks of the profession. Women had always been a factor, providing early leadership in state societies and even colleges, three of D.D. Palmer's first 15 "disciples" were women, including a textbook co-author and school official. With Mabel Palmer as a significant role model, an influx of women entered the profession in the 1920s. The opportunities of World War II—and the GI Bill—were an impetus for the second wave, and also for the first numbers of black students in three or four institutions founded after World War II in Ohio and Kansas.

The post-World War II presence of women has grown. Today's chiropractic student population is approximately 20% women and with it a steady increase of women practitioners. Blacks are still a decided minority within a minority health care profession but a growing factor that is mirrored in professional association leadership and activity. That it began in these dismal years of the Great Depression and World War II is a reflection of the capacity for regeneration within chiropractic. By the end of World War II, Davenport would no longer be the profession's focus of attention, but in time neither would Webster City, Iowa, home of the National Chiropractic Association. Chiropractic practitioners, students, and its other adherents would share the passion and action of the times.

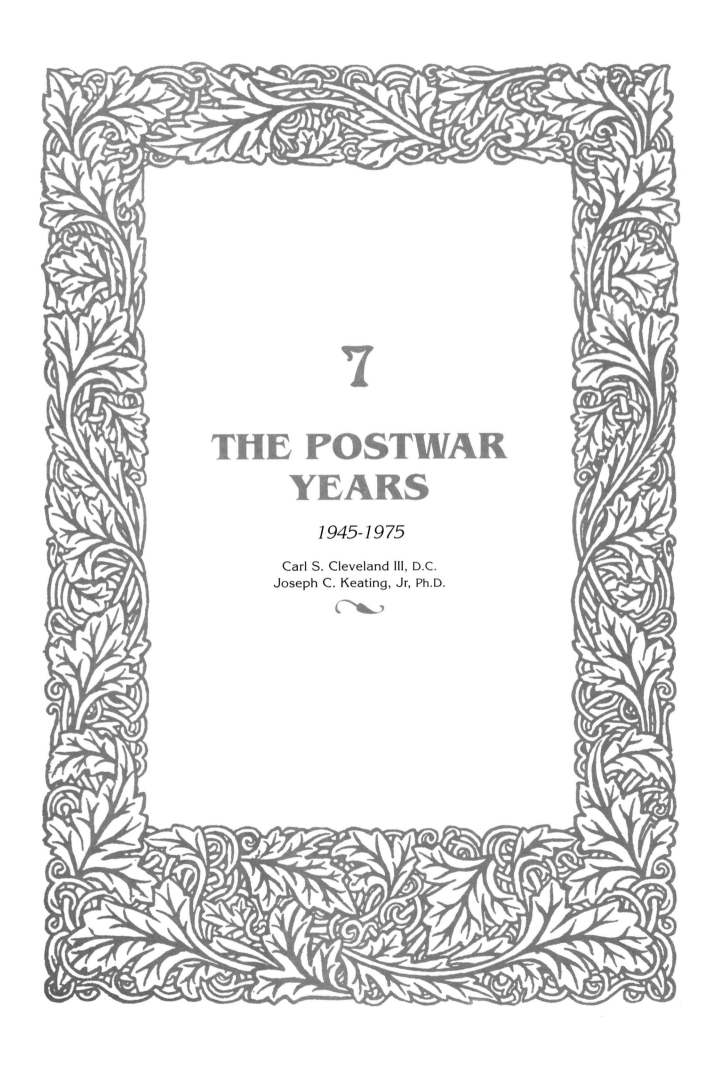

7

THE POSTWAR YEARS

1945-1975

Carl S. Cleveland III, D.C.
Joseph C. Keating, Jr, Ph.D.

The 30 years after World War II were a time of achievement and progress in chiropractic. It was an era characterized by a "can-do" attitude and a commitment to strengthening and improving the profession from within. Efforts to set professional and educational standards provided an early path toward integration with mainstream health care. By the middle of the war, 43 of the then 48 states had implemented chiropractic laws, and by 1950, census records indicated that 13,084 doctors of chiropractic were practicing in the United States. Chiropractic was positioned for another major phase in its development.

Throughout this postwar period, chiropractors battled not only the medical community but themselves. The major antagonists were the members of the International Chiropractors Association (ICA) and the National Chiropractic Association (NCA), which in 1963 would become the American Chiropractic Association (ACA). The ICA, concerned especially with maintaining the profession's "separate and distinct" identity and distinction from medicine, advocated a "hands-only," "straight chiropractic" scope of practice. The NCA promoted a "mixer" concept of the chiropractor's role and prerogatives and encouraged a wider range of therapeutics (in addition to adjusting) for the practitioner and student. The ICA practitioners looked askance at this "mixing" of therapies and "true" chiropractic. The NCA adherents felt that historically chiropractic legitimately included a broad range of chiropractic therapeutics and common domain clinical procedures. Much of this dispute had waned by the end of the postwar era, and by the mid-1970s, representatives from the straight and mixer movements would come together for the sake of achieving federally recognized accreditation of chiropractic education. A modicum of unity from within was apparent.

During the war the military draft drastically affected student enrollments at all the nation's colleges and professional schools. Subsequently, for chiropractic education the resultant enrollment declines became critical, and many institutions were forced to close for lack of students. World War II's end brought an upturn in students for all institutions of higher education and bright prospects for expansion. Medical education benefited from federal funding during the New Deal, and with the 1946 Hill-Burton Act, teaching hospitals received millions of government dollars for construction and development. However, there was no comparable public-sector funding for chiropractic colleges. Although ex-servicemen were able to use their GI benefits to pay tuition at chiropractic school, tuition continued to be the nearly exclusive source of operating funds for chiropractic education.

The Chiropractic Research Foundation (CRF), created by leaders of the National Chiropractic Association in 1944, was an early attempt to

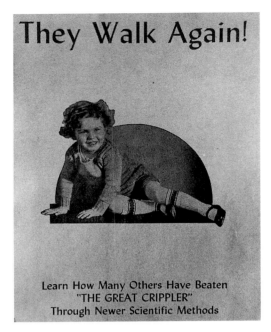

They Walk Again!

**Learn How Many Others Have Beaten
"THE GREAT CRIPPLER"
Through Newer Scientific Methods**

The polio epidemic of the 1940s and 1950s demanded chiropractic's attention, as it did the rest of the health care industry.
From *They Walk Again,* circa 1950.

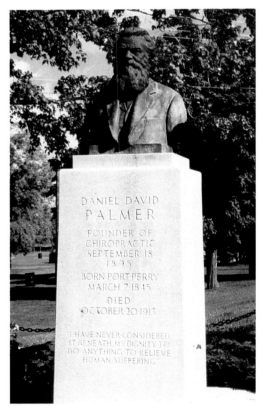

This tribute to D.D. Palmer was erected by the NCA in Port Perry, Ontario, to celebrate chiropractic's Golden Jubilee.
Courtesy Herbert Lee, Toronto, Ontario.

promote educational reform, research, public relations, fundraising, and hospital development, and would play a central role in a number of developments in the next 30 years. Fundraising and the inclusion of chiropractic in government-sponsored research became much-publicized issues, but another 40 years would pass before any federal funds for chiropractic scientific investigations would be realized. In the decade immediately following the war's end, chiropractic care for veterans and the rehabilitation of polio victims were popular issues.

A first order of business after the war was to celebrate the *Golden Jubilee* of Chiropractic. Plans to celebrate the fiftieth year of chiropractic in the founder's native country in September 1945 had to be postponed because of the Canadian government's wartime ban on convention travel. Accordingly, during August 12 to 16, 1946 the NCA held a convention at the Royal York Hotel in Toronto, and the conventioneers traveled to Port Perry, Ontario to dedicate a monument to D.D. Palmer in the town of his birth. It was a very happy moment.

The early postwar period was a time of expansion at Spears Chiropractic Sanitarium and Hospital in Denver. Leo L. Spears, D.C., was a former World War I marine and 1921 graduate of the Palmer School of Chiropractic. Dr. Spears had earned a nationwide reputation between the world wars for his efforts to have the federal government provide chiropractic services to veterans and to have D.C.s commissioned in the medical corps of the armed forces. During 1928, he had struggled with the state's medical board to maintain his chiropractic license, which was revoked after his advertisement in a Denver newspaper charged that the Veterans' Bureau was responsibile for the death of an ex-serviceman. Outspoken and litigious, Spears would do battle in courtrooms many times.

The combative chiropractor had his own vision of chiropractic and had opened the doors to a 236-bed inpatient facility on May 1, 1943. At the end of World War II, he began construction on a second building, which when opened in 1949 brought the total capacity of the institution to 600 beds. It was an achievement for chiropractic hospitals that has never been

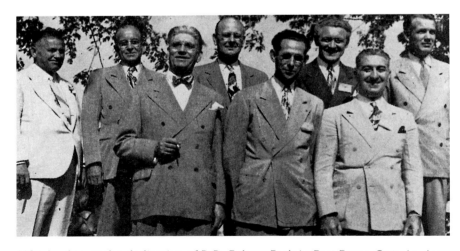

NCA leaders at the dedication of D.D. Palmer Park in Port Perry, Ontario, August 1946. Front row, left to right, *John Nugent, Floyd Cregger, George Hariman. Back row,* left to right, *Frank Logic, F. Lorne Wheaton, L.M. Rogers, Gordon Goodfellow, and Emmett Murphy.*
From *The National Chiropractic Journal,* September 1946.

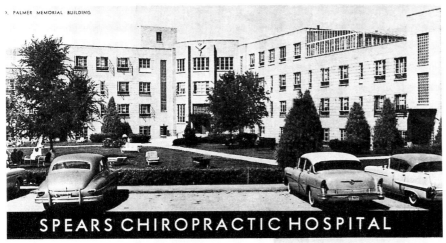

SPEARS CHIROPRACTIC HOSPITAL

rld's Largest Chiropractic Hospital
DENVER, COLORADO

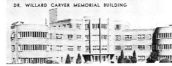

The cover of an informational booklet on Spears Hospital in Denver, Colorado,
which had 600 beds in 1949. The hospital, which provided neither drugs nor
surgery, closed in 1984.
From *The Spears Chiropractic Hospital*, circa 1950.

equaled. Spears' ambitions for his hospital soon ran up against an already
outraged medical community, who found his methods, advertising, and
claims concerning chiropractic care for the relief of nearly all forms of
human illness to be spurious. When Spears failed to receive a permanent
state license to operate his facility, he charged that a conspiracy between
the Colorado State Board of Health and the Denver Medical Society was
in force and brought suit against them. The Colorado Supreme Court
ruled in Spears' favor on July 1, 1950, licensed the hospital retroactively
to its original date of application in 1943, and found that: "It (chiropractic) may not be arbitrarily limited or discriminated against, and its advocates may lawfully erect and operate buildings and facilities for the treatment, according to its tenets, of patients seeking its aid . . ."

Leo Spears briefly toyed with the idea of turning his hospital over to
the Chiropractic Research Foundation (CRF), which was interested in developing hospital experience for chiropractors and in establishing a national center for chiropractic research. However, the Colorado chiropractor could not fully accept loss of control of his hospital, and this arrangement fell through. Nevertheless, the Denver facility did operate a postgraduate internship for D.C.s, one of the few such experiences open to
chiropractors in the 1940s and 1950s. One former intern recalls that
"there were so many patients that they occupied beds in the halls of both
the Palmer and Carver buildings. . . . The pediatrics ward always had a
waiting list."

In accordance with its license, and Dr. Leo's commitment to "natural
healing," Spears Hospital provided neither drugs nor surgery. Its hard-won
authorization from the State Board of Health also disallowed maternity
cases, and patients with infectious and contagious disorders were not admitted. By 1975, an estimated 250 chiropractors had gained an inpatient
experience at Spears hospital. After Leo Spears death in 1956, the hospital continued operation under nephews Don and Howard Spears into
the early 1980s.

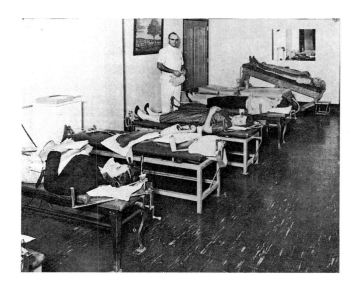
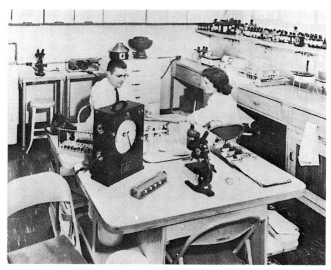
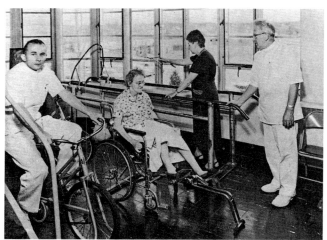
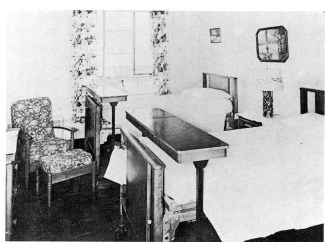

Interior photographs of the Spears Hospital, circa 1950, showing the women's adjusting room, the diagnostic and research laboratory, the physiotherapy room, and a patient's room.

From *The Spears Chiropractic Hospital*, circa 1950.

EDUCATIONAL REFORM

The influx of ex-GI students at the end of the war was like a tidal wave on arid shores. Chiropractic schools that had clung to survival during the lean war years suddenly found their pared-down institutions inadequate for the surge of new students whose veterans' benefits included tuition support. A number of colleges began expansion programs, and several new schools were launched. The first to be developed outside the United States was the Canadian Memorial Chiropractic College (CMCC), where classes began on September 18, 1945, the fiftieth anniversary of the birth of chiropractic.

The profession's efforts to bring about a consistent chiropractic training program can be traced to at least 1917, when an International Association of Chiropractic Schools and Colleges (IACSC) was formed at the annual lyceum of the Palmer School of Chiropractic to standardize the educational requirements of various state licensing laws (see table on p. 185). The IACSC lasted only a few years, owing partly to the unwilling-

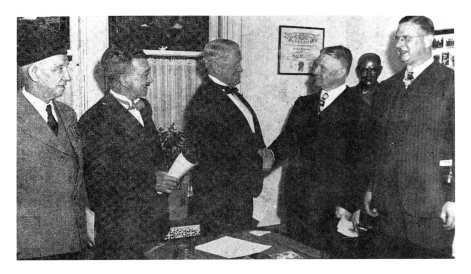

Speakers at the dedication of the Canadian Memorial Chiropractic College, September 1947. Left to right, *W.A. Caswell, C.A. Cameron, Honorable Russell Kelley, Alderman J.A. Wilson, and V.C. Knowles.*
From *The National Chiropractic Journal,* November 1947.

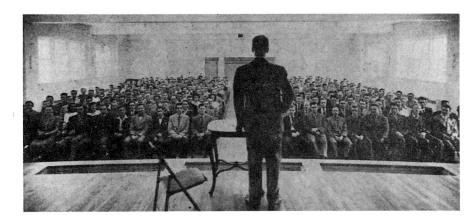

Dean R.O. Mueller addressing the Canadian Memorial Chiropractic College student body in 1947.
From *The National Chiropractic Journal,* November 1947.

FOUNDING MEMBERS OF THE INTERNATIONAL ASSOCIATION OF CHIROPRACTIC SCHOOLS AND COLLEGES

Name	Position	School
Ernest Duval, D.C.	President	Canadian Chiropractic College, Hamilton, Ontario
N.C. Ross, D.C.	President	Ross College of Chiropractic, Fort Wayne, Indiana
B.J. Palmer, D.C.	President	Palmer School of Chiropractic, Davenport, Iowa
Frank W. Elliott, D.C.	Registrar	Palmer School of Chiropractic, Davenport, Iowa
Willard Carver, LL.B., D.C.	President	Carver Chiropractic College, Oklahoma City, Oklahoma
L.W. Ray, M.D., D.C.	President	St. Louis Chiropractic College, St. Louis, Missouri
R. Trumand Smith, D.C.	President	Davenport School of Chiropractic, Davenport, Iowa
W.C. Schulze, M.D., D.C.	President	National School of Chiropractic, Chicago, Illinois
A.L. Forster, M.D., D.C.	Secretary	National School of Chiropractic, Chicago, Illinois
W.F. Ruehlmann, D.C., M.C.	President	Universal Chiropractic College, Davenport, Iowa
George Otto, D.C.	Secretary	Universal Chiropractic College, Davenport, Iowa
Andrew C. Foy, D.C.	President	Kansas Chiropractic College, Topeka, Kansas
Tom Morris, LL.B.	Chairman	LaCrosse, Wisconsin

From *Fountainhead News* 7(1-2): 1-2, 1917.

EVOLUTION OF "NARROW-SCOPE/STRAIGHT AND BROAD-SCOPE/MIXER" EDUCATIONAL ORGANIZATIONS ⌒

Straight	Mixer
1938 Associated Chiropractic Colleges of America	1935 NCA Committee on Education
1940 Allied Chiropractic Educational Institutions	1935 Affiliated Universities of Natural Healing
circa 1952 North American Association of Chiropractic Schools & Colleges	1938 NCA Committee on Educational Standards & Colleges
circa 1955 ICA Chiropractic Educational Commission	1947 NCA Council on Education
1968 Association of Chiropractic Colleges	1971 Council on Chiropractic Education

ness of the owners of many for-profit schools to agree to any outside regulation of their business, and partly to the perception that control of the IACSC was vested in B.J. Palmer and the Palmer School. Additionally, many in chiropractic feared that anything that interfered with the ability to build the profession by producing larger numbers of chiropractors would be deleterious; raising standards created the risk that few students would enroll in chiropractic schools.

Attempts to develop an accrediting body that could achieve recognition by the federal government dated to at least 1935 when the NCA had organized its Committee on Education. However, disputes among chiropractic colleges and between the two major professional associations, the NCA and the Chiropractic Health Bureau, had impeded unified action toward federal recognition for decades. Over the years each camp developed a number of educational organizations (see table above).

Before World War II, several straight chiropractic colleges, including Cleveland in Kansas City, Palmer in Davenport, Eastern Chiropractic Institute in New York City, and the Ratledge Chiropractic College in Los Angeles, established the Associated Chiropractic Colleges of America (ACCA) as an alternative to the NCA's Committee on Education. Following the 1935 convention of the NCA in Hollywood, California, at which time the NCA disavowed the use of electrical modalities as alternatives to surgical interventions (e.g., for hemorrhoids and tonsillitis) several of the more liberal chiropractic schools felt compelled to organize their own educational accrediting body, the Affiliated Universities of Natural Healing. This organization has long been forgotten, but its "straight" chiropractic rival, the ACCA, has not. This body became incensed at the NCA's plan to introduce instruction in diagnosis and physical therapy and was further angered by the NCA Committee on Educational Standards' intention to inspect and accredit colleges with or without the colleges' consent.

The ACCA evolved into the Allied Chiropractic Education Institutions (ACEI); the ACEI let it be known that it would not tolerate NCA's efforts to "medicalize" chiropractic. While the NCA and its Committee on Educational Standards developed its standards for broad-scope education and practice and hired John J. Nugent, D.C., to supervise the college improvement and standardization process, the ACEI affiliated with the ICA.

The later activities of the ACEI are not known; it may have discontinued operations during World War II. During the early 1950s a number of colleges, including several within the NCA's orbit, organized the North American Association of Chiropractic Schools and Colleges (NAACSC). Although this body's formation produced great consternation within the ranks of the NCA's Council on Education, NAACSC functioned as a forum for chiropractic school leaders to discuss mutual problems rather than as an accrediting body at least initially.

MEMBERS OF THE ICA'S CHIROPRACTIC EDUCATION COMMISSION IN 1956

Name	City
Clarence J. Yocum, D.C.	Allentown, Pennsylvania
Leonard K. Griffin, D.C.	Fort Worth, Texas
Carl S. Cleveland, Sr., D.C., Ph.C.	Los Angeles, California
William Coggins, B.S., Ph.D., D.C.	St. Louis, Missouri
Hugh E. Chance, B.A., J.D.	Davenport, Iowa
O.D. Adams, M.S., Ed.D.	San Francisco, California

Of more realistic concern for NCA was the organization of the ICA's Chiropractic Education Commission (CEC). In 1949 the ICA had commissioned a study of the college accreditation process per se. O.D. Adams, Ed.D., Assistant Superintendent of Schools for the City of San Francisco, was recruited as an educational consultant. In 1952 the ICA Board of Control voted to establish the CEC. Dr. Adams was hired as Education Director to visit all chiropractic colleges and to assist in developing accreditation standards (see tables). The standards of the CEC did not require non-profit status, and emphasized the ability of instructors to present materials from a chiropractic orientation. Based on Adams' inspection, a list of colleges meeting the ICA Commission's standards and desiring accreditation by the ICA was released.

With increased GI enrollment, a sudden spurt in tuition revenues created a propitious moment for Nugent, the NCA's Director of Education. Nugent was the prime mover in the NCA's efforts to reform chiropractic training through negotiated mergers of smaller, private proprietary schools into larger, financially sounder, non-profit, and professionally controlled colleges. During 1939 and 1940 he had inspected most chiropractic schools and wrote the first college accreditation standards adopted by the NCA. In 1944 he negotiated the merger of the Universal Chiropractic College of Pittsburgh and the Lincoln Chiropractic College of Indianapolis, the first of many amalgamations. The following year, Nugent was influential in the creation of the Chiropractic Institute of New York by amalgamation of the former Eastern Institute of Chiropractic, the Standard College of Chiropractic, and the New York School of Chiropractic.

With the assistance of the CRF, Nugent next set his sights on California, where more chiropractors practiced than anywhere else. In the Golden State there had long been a desire among broad-scope practitioners to consolidate chiropractic education, to eliminate proprietary

COLLEGES ACCREDITED BY THE ICA'S CHIROPRACTIC EDUCATION COMMISSION IN 1956

School	President or Dean
Atlantic States Chiropractic Institute, Brooklyn, New York	Martin I. Phillips, D.C.
Carver Chiropractic College, Oklahoma City, Oklahoma	Paul O. Parr, D.C.
Cleveland Chiropractic College, Kansas City, Missouri	Carl S. Cleveland, Jr., D.C.
Cleveland Chiropractic College, Los Angeles, California	Carl S. Cleveland, Sr., D.C.
Columbia Institute of Chiropractic, New York, New York	Frank E. Dean, M.B, D.C.
International Chiropractic College, Dayton, Ohio	A.M. Valdiserri, D.C., D.M.
Logan Basic College of Chiropractic, St. Louis, Missouri	Vinton F. Logan, D.C.
Palmer School of Chiropractic, Davenport, Iowa	B.J. Palmer, D.C., Ph.C.

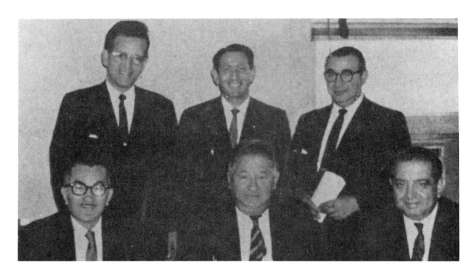

Participating in the formalities of the merger of Atlantic States and Columbia Institute of Chiropractic in 1964 were (standing, left to right): Ernest Napolitano, Charles Krasner, and Anthony Aragona; and (sitting, left to right) Hyman Hammer, Martin Phillips, and Robert Limber.

From *The ACA Journal of Chiropractic*, November 1964.

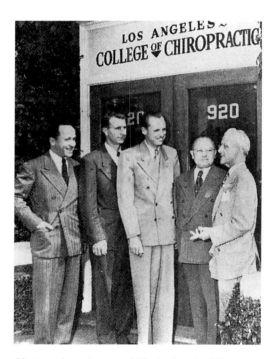

Photo taken (circa 1950) in front of the new Glendale campus of the Los Angeles College of Chiropractic, which had merged with Southern California College of Chiropractic in 1947. From left to right, Harry Scott, business manager of LACC; Ralph Martin, president; Raymond Houser, dean; Lee Norcross, graduate school dean; and Harry Bybee, president of the NCA.

From *Journal of the National Chiropractic Association,* August 1950.

schools, and to place all chiropractic education under professional control. The Southern California College of Chiropractic (SCCC) (no relation to the current school in Pico Rivera by the same name) was originally founded in 1925 by Charles A. Cale, D.C., N.D. as the Cale College of Chiropractic. During 1929, SCCC was reincorporated by Cale as a non-profit institution. The SCCC, which had long been influential in intraprofessional politics in California, was allied with the state's broad-scope professional group, the California Chiropractic Association, and with the predominantly "mixer" members of the California Board of Chiropractic Examiners. The SCCC's leaders allied themselves with Nugent in seeking amalgamation with the state's largest institution, the Los Angeles College of Chiropractic (LACC), a for-profit, privately owned enterprise. This merger was finalized in May 1947. The California branch of the CRF helped fund the purchase of the LACC; CRF appointees served on the Board of Regents of the resulting institution, which today is the non-profit LACC. Ralph J. Martin, D.C., N.D., the last president of the SCCC, served as the first president of the consolidated, non-profit LACC. Martin would be a leader in broad-scope chiropractic education for the next several decades.

The merger of the LACC and the SCCC encouraged a number of other consolidations in California and helped to legitimize and add credibility to Nugent's efforts elsewhere in the nation. The NCA education director would often be vilified, since many chiropractors continued to view the push for higher standards as a misguided force that would tend to "medicalize" chiropractic and inhibit the growth in the number of chiropractors. On August 4, 1947, under Nugent's direction, the NCA created its Council on Education, which would henceforth assume total responsibility within the broad-scope community for accreditation matters. It would be this Council in 1974 that would achieve federal recognition as an accrediting body for professional training and would thereby bring a modicum of unity to chiropractic in terms of education standards, preadmission requirements, program length, and basic curriculum content. In 1959, after 18 years on the job, Nugent reported to the NCA that:

Of 51 private chiropractic school owners, 46 had surrendered their equities in 19 schools upon mutually satisfactory terms negotiated by the Director of Education. Some of these 19 schools were closed and others merged to form eight non-profit, accredited schools.

At this early stage in 1947, however, unity within the profession around educational issues was still far in the future, and college leaders from opposing narrow-scope and broad-scope camps encountered one another mainly on their lecture tours. The ACEI, formed in the early 1940s by B.J. Palmer, Carl S. Cleveland, Sr., and other narrow-scope chiropractic college leaders, resisted the changes urged by the NCA. Straight chiropractors maintained that chiropractors should confine their practices to the detection and adjustment of subluxations only. The "straights" argued that state licensure for chiropractors was predicated on the idea that chiropractic was distinctly different from the medical practice acts. Straight chiropractic educators argued that inclusion of physical therapies and naturopathic procedures in the chiropractic curriculum were clinically indefensible and that use of such broad therapies would subject the practitioner to arrest and incarceration for unlicensed medical practice. Consistent with his legal and political strategy, B.J. Palmer suggested that

> Chiropractic differs fundamentally and absolutely from any other method of getting sick well. If this were not true, there would be no reason for asking state legislatures for recognition as a separate and distinct science. To justify the claim for recognition we should differ from other methods, and for this reason most chiropractors scorn the use of any method used by others.

Broad-scope or "mixer" chiropractors, on the other hand, believed that chiropractors should not only detect and remove subluxations but should also make diagnoses of disease states and should use a broad range of "natural," conservative remedies, including dietary recommendations, prescription of vitamins, nutritional supplements and naturopathic remedies, employ colonic irrigation and physiotherapy devices

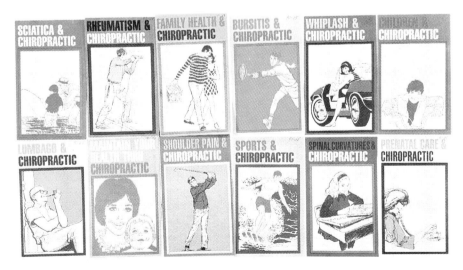

In an effort to educate the layperson about what chiropractic could do, chiropractors would often display pamphlets like these in their office waiting rooms.
Courtesy Palmer College of Chiropractic Archives, Davenport, Iowa.

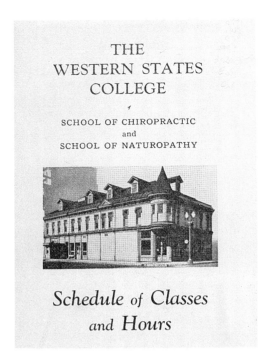

THE
WESTERN STATES
COLLEGE

SCHOOL OF CHIROPRACTIC
and
SCHOOL OF NATUROPATHY

*Schedule of Classes
and Hours*

The NCA sought to distance chiropractors from other drugless healers, eventually dissuading colleges like Western States from offering a naturopathic degree.

From Western States College School of Chiropractic and School of Naturopathy Catalog, circa 1935.

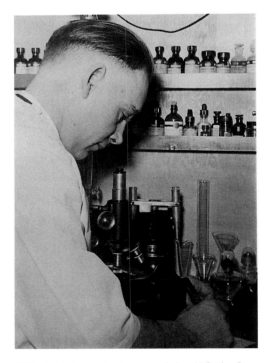

C.O. Watkins, chairman of the NCA's Committee on Research in the early 1950's, was a vocal advocate of clinical research by chiropractors.

Courtesy Joseph C. Keating, Jr, Whittier, California.

(such as electrical stimulation, heat lamps), and in some cases (such as at Western States College, School of Chiropractic and Naturopathy), advocated minor surgery and obstetrics in the chiropractic curriculum. The broad-scope chiropractic community believed that the role of the chiropractor should be that of a conservative, general practioner who used a wide range of "natural" remedies.

The NCA's educational reformers were also advocates of longer chiropractic college training programs and more in-depth study of the basic sciences, so to make the chiropractor a more competent general diagnostician and to increase graduates' chances of passing the dreaded basic science examinations. At the same time, however, the NCA and its Director of Education moved to distance the chiropractic profession from other drugless healers. By 1940 the NCA had begun to urge and eventually mandated that NCA-affiliated colleges cease to issue naturopathic degrees, and college administrators were expected to discontinue listing of their naturopathic credentials (N.D.). This move may have been intended partly to placate the "straight" community but was also designed to prevent criticism that chiropractors earned two doctorates for one course of study. This NCA policy would be a source of some divisiveness within its own ranks; college leaders such as Budden of Western States College School of Chiropractic and School of Naturopathy, although a stalwart supporter of improved basic science instruction, resisted NCA's attempts to have his school discontinue naturopathic training and credentialing. The naturopathic division of the Western States College would not separate from the chiropractic division until after Budden's death in 1954. By 1960, however, most if not all chiropractic colleges came into compliance with this NCA stipulation and dropped their naturopathic programs.

A few chiropractors believed that reconciliation among the various factions within the profession was not realistic, not so much because of straight/mixer differences in scope of practice, but because of differences in their philosophical orientations to science and in their belief in the value of clinical research to the practice of chiropractic. C.O. Watkins, D.C., who had originally proposed in 1935 the NCA Committee on Education, suggested that the fundamental bases for chiropractic held by various members of the profession were diametrically opposed and admitted of no compromise. Watkins became a vocal advocate of clinical research by chiropractors and served as chairman of the NCA's Committee on Research in the early 1950s. Although both he and W.A. Budden, D.C., N.D., President of the Western States College, were central players in the NCA's early educational reforms in basic science training and standardization of the curriculum, Budden opposed Watkins' proposal that training in clinical research should become a routine course offering in chiropractic colleges.

Despite differences of opinion about the proper scope of chiropractic practice and despite the profession's lack of consensus about the content of chiropractic education, external forces were operating that would mandate change. Since the early 1920s, organized medicine had been increasingly successful in enacting basic science laws in the various states. Basic science laws required that chiropractors, osteopaths, and medical physicians pass tests in subjects such as anatomy, physiology, pathology, and diagnosis before taking the examination in their particular professional field. Leaders of the National College of Chiropractic and the Western States College had long suggested that the only way to overcome the "basic science barrier" was to intensify instruction in the basic science subjects. Some eighteen states had passed basic science legis-

REVOCATION OF BASIC SCIENCE LEGISLATION IN THE UNITED STATES, 1967-1979

Date of Revocation	Jurisdiction
1967	Florida
1968	Arizona
1968	New Mexico
1969	Kansas
1970	Alaska
1971	Rhode Island
1972	Michigan
1973	Iowa
1973	Oklahoma
1973	Oregon
1974	Minnesota
1975	Alabama
1975	Connecticut
1975	Nebraska
1975	Nevada
1975	South Dakota
1975	Wisconsin
1976	Colorado
1976	Tennessee
1977	Arkansas
1978	District of Columbia
1979	Texas
1979	Utah
1979	Washington

lation by the end of World War II, and an additional six states (Alaska, Texas, Nevada, Kansas, Utah, and Alabama) passed similar laws between 1946 and 1959. Although the basic science barrier would begin to reverse toward the end of the postwar period (Florida was the first state [1967] to repeal its basic science regulations; see table), this development was not expected. By 1975, chiropractors had grown increasingly successful in passing the basic science examinations, but the primary impetus for the repeal of basic science laws would come from the medical community, which increasingly found such examinations troublesome for their own graduates.

The NCA's standards-raising campaign in the postwar period had a direct influence on the viability of many chiropractic institutions. In Los Angeles the oldest surviving chiropractic school in the state, the Ratledge Chiropractic College, was unwilling to meet the increased requirements for curriculum length (from the previous 2400 hours to 4000+ hours), basic science instruction, and training in physiotherapy. T.F. Ratledge, D.C., founder and president of the school since 1911, had resisted the broad-scope chiropractors' efforts to "medicalize, druglessize, and naturopathicize" chiropractic education and practice. As a consequence, the Ratledge College lost its contract with the Veterans Administration to train returning GIs. The lean war years were consequently followed by equally lean postwar years, and while other schools, most notably Ratledge's competitor, the LACC, enjoyed an infusion of new student tuition dollars, the Ratledge College was forced to temporarily close its doors in 1949. Demoralized, Ratledge negotiated with Carl S. Cleveland, Sr., for sale of the 40-year-old institution. The college operated as the "Ratledge Chiropractic College under Cleveland management" from 1951 until 1955

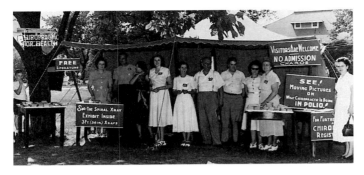

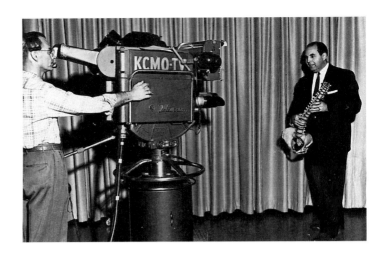

Chiropractors tried to "get the word out" in many different ways. Left, *The Missouri State Chiropractors Association staffed a booth at the 1949 Missouri State Fair.* Right, *Carl Cleveland, Jr, appeared on the weekly TV show "So You May Know" in Kansas City, 1955.*

Courtesy Cleveland College of Chiropractic, Kansas City, Missouri.

when a sale price of $40,000 closed the transaction, and the Cleveland board took possession of the one-building campus, its 17 students, and minimal equipment. The institution eventually became today's non-profit Cleveland Chiropractic College of Los Angeles.

The North American Association of Chiropractic Schools and Colleges (NAACSC) was the successor to the ACEI, and served as an accrediting body for chiropractic schools outside the NCA's orbit during the 1950s and 1960s. Originally intended to constitute an educational accrediting body that would be independent of the national professional association, the NAACSC became an alternative to the NCA's Council on Education (see Tables). The NAACSC became affiliated with the ICA, and its functions were taken over by the ICA's Chiropractic Education Commission. Member institutions included the Cleveland Chiropractic Colleges of Kansas City and Los Angeles, the Palmer School, Logan Basic College of Chiropractic in St. Louis, the Columbia Institute of Chiropractic in New York City, and the Texas Chiropractic College in San Antonio. Although the ICA was the smaller of the two national professional associations in chiropractic, the NAACSC and the Chiropractic Education Commission could justifiably claim to represent the largest body of students in the profession.

MEMBER INSTITUTIONS OF THE NCA'S COUNCIL ON EDUCATION IN 1952

College	President (or Dean)
Canadian Memorial Chiropractic College, Toronto, Ontario	Rudy O. Mueller, D.C.
Carver Chiropractic College, Oklahoma City, Oklahoma	Paul O. Parr, D.C.
Chiropractic Institute of New York, New York, New York	Thure C. Peterson, D.C.*
Lincoln Chiropractic College, Indianapolis, Indiana	James N. Firth, D.C.
Logan Basic College of Chiropractic, St. Louis, Missouri	William N. Coggins, D.C.
Los Angeles College of Chiropractic, Glendale, California	Raymond H. Houser, D.C., N.D.
Missouri Chiropractic College, St. Louis, Missouri	Henry C. Harring, D.C., M.D.
National College of Chiropractic, Chicago, Illinois	Joseph Janse, D.D.T., D.C., N.D.
Western States College School of Chiropractic and School of Naturopathy, Portland, Oregon	William A. Budden, D.C., N.D.

*Dr. Peterson served as President of the National Chiropractic Association's Council during 1952.

MEMBER INSTITUTIONS OF THE NORTH AMERICAN ASSOCIATION OF CHIROPRACTIC SCHOOLS & COLLEGES ⌒

College	President (or Dean)
Cleveland Chiropractic College, Kansas City, Missouri	Carl S. Cleveland, Jr., D.C.
Cleveland Chiropractic College, Los Angeles	Carl S. Cleveland, Sr., D.C.
Columbia Institute of Chiropractic, New York, New York	Frank Dean, M.B., D.C.
Logan Basic College of Chiropractic, St. Louis, Missouri	Vinton Logan, D.C.
Palmer School of Chiropractic, Davenport, Iowa	B.J. Palmer, D.C., Ph.C.
Texas Chiropractic College, San Antonio, Texas	James R. Drain, D.C., Ph.C.

CAMPAIGN BY AMA TO CONTAIN AND ELIMINATE CHIROPRACTIC

Despite the inclusion of chiropractic education as a legitimate educational benefit for returning GIs, President Truman's 1951 executive order exempting chiropractors from the military draft, and in spite of success in garnering the support of the American Legion for chiropractic services in the rehabilitation of veterans, the profession was unsuccessful in having chiropractic care made available to those who had served their country. The chiropractic graduate could *not* expect a commission in the armed forces' medical corps on the basis of the chiropractic degree. Although the NCA and ICA had supervised and accredited a number of schools since the 1940s, this professional recognition had no federal standing in higher education. Credit for courses taken in chiropractic institutions would ordinarily not transfer to other colleges and universities.

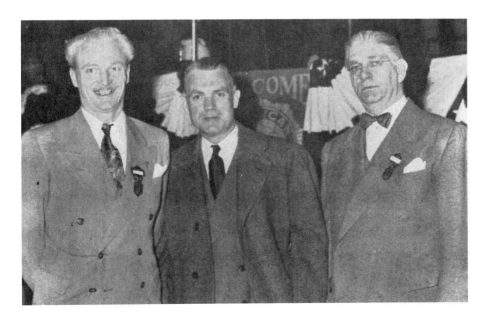

Senator Neal Bishop, Emmett Murphy, and John Nugent at a 1945 American Legion convention. Despite the American Legion's endorsement, the profession was unsuccessful in obtaining federal reimbursement of chiropractic care for veterans. From *The National Chiropractic Journal,* December 1945.

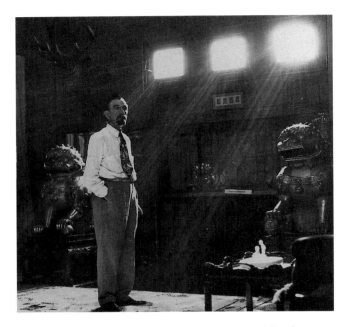

An elderly B.J. Palmer in the dining area of his home at 808 Brady St., Davenport, Iowa.

Courtesy Palmer College of Chiropractic Archives, Davenport, Iowa.

Organized medicine's continuing campaign to impede chiropractic legitimacy was in many respects successful.

The multiple school closures in the several decades after the war came during a period of renewed attack by organized medicine. Although Morris Fishbein, M.D., the chiropractors' arch-nemesis since 1924, was relieved of his duties as editor of the *Journal of the American Medical Association* in 1949, his policies toward chiropractors seem to have found renewed vigor within the AMA. At the end of World War II, political medicine's 1930s prediction that chiropractic was a "doomed sect" had still not been realized, and only a few states (Louisiana, Massachusetts, Mississippi, and New York) had not enacted some form of chiropractic legislation. Despite the imposition of the basic science barriers to chiropractic licensure in many states, the continued divisiveness among chiropractors, the closure of many chiropractic schools in the postwar era, and the increasingly spectacular success of scientific medicine and its "wonder drugs" (penicillin was introduced during the war), the chiropractic challenge to medicine's authority had not "withered on the vine" as expected. To the consternation of the medical establishment, D.D. Palmer's resistance to allopathic hegemony was now more than 50 years old and in the wake of World War II seemed to be thriving. The ranks of the chiropractors were swelling from the infusion of ex-servicemen. Organized medicine decided that a new assault on chiropractic was necessary.

The renewed campaign to "contain and eliminate" chiropractic began in November 1963, when the AMA formed a Committee on Quackery. The committee was influential in having the AMA adopt an "ethical guideline" for its members that forbade any sort of professional interaction been M.D.s and chiropractors. This ban on interprofessional cooperation meant that AMA members were not free to exercise their own judgment about whether chiropractic care might be in the best interests of any particular patient, M.D.s could not teach in chiropractic schools or lecture at chiropractic conventions, and M.D.s could not even accept a patient on referral from a chiropractor. Many medical physicians who might have considered it appropriate to interact with members of the chiropractic profession had to reconsider in light of this threatened ostracism, which could have grave personal consequences including loss of hospital privileges.

The AMA also orchestrated a nationwide, anti-chiropractic publicity campaign, and in the late 1960s funded author Ralph Lee Smith to write a scathing indictment of chiropractic, *At Your Own Risk: The Case Against Chiropractic.* High school and college guidance counselors and instructors were contacted and "10,000 pieces of AMA propaganda" were distributed. The Committee on Quackery reported to the AMA Board of Trustees that: "The Committee was instrumental in blocking the inclusion of a chiropractic chapter in a *Health Careers Guidebook* being prepared by the United States Department of Labor for distribution to guidance counselors and others throughout the country." A variety of organizations allied or affiliated with the AMA cooperated in the boycott and would eventually be sued in 1976 for violation of antitrust laws.

In 1967 the US Congress considered the desirability and feasibility of including the services of licensed, nonmedical health care providers within the Medicare program. The Secretary of the Department of Health, Education, and Welfare (HEW), Wilbur J. Cohen, was directed to prepare a report concerning alternative and supplementary providers such as chiropractors, naturopaths, podiatrists, psychologists, and other professionals. The Secretary commissioned the Surgeon General of the United States Public Health Service (USPHS), rather than an independent outside agency, to prepare the report, which was entitled *Independent Practitioners under Medicare.* "Expert" review committees were established to consider the merits of each practitioner group. Peculiarly, the USPHS did not include chiropractors on the review committee established to consider chiropractic but did include five M.D.s and three Ph.D.s, one of whom was employed by the University of Texas Medical School at Galveston. Although this committee of "independent" experts met several times to review and discuss a considerable volume of information about the chiropractic profession largely provided by AMA, much of the final report on chiropractic and inclusion in Medicare had actually already *been* prepared by USPHS staff before any review committee meetings took place.

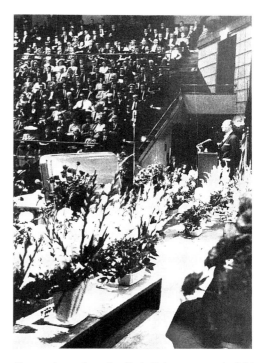

Funeral services for B.J. Palmer were held in Davenport's Masonic Temple, May 31, 1961, to accommodate the thousands of well-wishers who came to pay their last respects to the "Developer" of chiropractic.
Courtesy Palmer College of Chiropractic Archives, Davenport, Iowa.

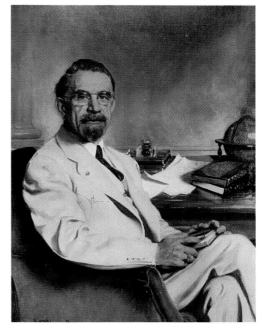

B.J. Palmer, 1882-1961.
Courtesy Palmer College of Chiropractic Archives, Davenport, Iowa.

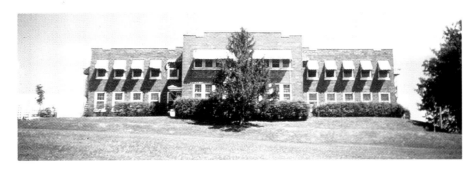

Clearview Sanitarium, an in-patient chiropractic psychiatric facility that operated in Davenport, Iowa from 1926 to 1961
Courtesy Palmer College of Chiropractic Archives, Davenport, Iowa.

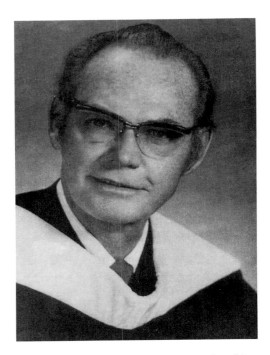

William Quigley Heath, who served as Director of the Clearview Sanitarium, Administrator of Palmer College, and President of Los Angeles College of Chiropractic (1976-1979).
Courtesy Palmer College of Chiropractic, Davenport, Iowa.

In short, the AMA had gotten to the USPHS first. The AMA had contacted the Stanford Research Institute to arrange for an "independent" study of chiropractic for HEW Secretary Cohen modeled after Stanford's negative evaluation of *Chiropractic in California* in 1960. When the pressure of time disallowed an external investigation of chiropractic, H. Doyl Taylor, LL.B., who chaired the AMA's Bureau of Investigation, and Joseph Sabatier, M.D., chairman of AMA's Committee on Quackery, supplied the USPHS staff with the raw materials for use in their finished product. Next, the AMA brought considerable pressure to bear on members of the Expert Review Committee to assure a report that would be unfavorable to chiropractic. When Secretary Cohen finally reported back to Congress, his recommendations were predictable: "Chiropractic theory and practice are not based on the body of basic knowledge related to health, disease, and health care that has been widely accepted by the scientific community." Moreover, irrespective of its theory, the scope and quality of chiropractic education did not prepare the practitioner to make an adequate diagnosis and provide appropriate treatment.

The HEW's supposedly "independent, unbiased study of chiropractic" effectively delayed chiropractic's inclusion in Medicare for another 5 years, but in other ways was a boon to the profession. Although relations between the "straights" and "mixers" had been rather strained since the 1963 formation of the ACA, through the joining of the old NCA and a splinter group from the ICA, now the common foe of organized medicine and the prospect of continued exclusion from the Medicare program brought these old antagonists together in a common purpose. A *White Paper on Health, Education and Welfare Secretary's Report* was jointly issued by ACA and ICA in 1969, and a grass roots political campaign was launched that produced 12 million letters to Congress in 1970 in support of chiropractic inclusion in Medicare. Federal lawmakers reversed themselves in 1972, and Medicare reimbursement for chiropractors commenced in 1973.

The developments in college accreditation, scholarship, and science, which appeared on the chiropractic scene in the early 1970s, occurred despite the continuing and strenuous opposition of organized medicine. As detailed in a landmark federal antitrust court case brought by chiropractors in 1976 against the AMA and fourteen co-conspirators, political medicine worked feverishly to block the accreditation of chiropractic schools by the United States Office of Education, sought to discredit chiropractic as a legitimate career choice among students in liberal arts colleges and universities, prevented the collaboration of medical and chiropractic physicians in patient care and education, blocked hospital privileges for doctors of chiropractic, encouraged insurance companies to disallow chiropractic claims for reimbursement, suppressed legitimate data concerning the effectiveness of chiropractic care, and rigged a federal study of chiropractic authorized by the United States Congress to show that there was no merit in chiropractic.

STATE LICENSURE: THE FINAL STRUGGLE

The final struggle for licensure between the chiropractors and the medical community occurred after World War II. Efforts to secure independent licensing boards for doctors of chiropractic had begun early in

A CHRONOLOGY OF CHIROPRACTIC LICENSING IN THE UNITED STATES

1913
Kansas
North Dakota

1915
Arkansas
Ohio
Oregon

1916
Nebraska

1917
Connecticut
North Carolina

1918
Montana

1919
Florida
Idaho
Minnesota
Vermont
Washington

1921
Arizona
Georgia
Iowa
New Hampshire
New Mexico
Oklahoma
South Dakota

1922
California

1923
Illinois
Nevada
Rhode Island
Tennessee
Utah

1924
Maine

1925
Hawaii
West Virginia
Wisconsin

1927
Indiana
Missouri

1928
Kentucky

1929
District of Columbia
Maryland
Wyoming

1932
South Carolina

1933
Colorado
Michigan

1937
Delaware

1939
Alaska

1944
Virginia

1949
Texas

1951
Pennsylvania

1953
New Jersey

1959
Alabama

1963
New York

1973
Mississippi

1974
Louisiana

From Wardwell W: *Chiropractic: History and Evolution of a New Profession,* 1992, St Louis, Mosby.

the century when Solon M. Langworthy, D.C., and Dan Reisland, D.C., had a bill introduced in the Minnesota legislature. This early attempt was defeated in 1905 when D.D. Palmer urged the governor to veto the bill. Kansas was the first state to pass a chiropractic law in 1913, although Arkansas issued the first chiropractic license in 1915. Organized medicine had been stunned by the early success of the chiropractors' legislative initiatives: two dozen states had licensed these new practitioners by the mid-1920s. Forty-three states had chiropractic legislation by midcentury. However, it would be several more decades before the last jurisdiction granted practice privileges to the profession.

Licensing laws provided for a self-sustaining board of chiropractic examiners or a board of healing arts. In Kansas, for example, a healing arts board was comprised of chiropractors, medical doctors, dentists, and other licensed health care professionals. Many states authorized the board of chiropractic examiners to review and approve or reject the educational programs offered by license applicants' schools, which inevitably brought some state boards into conflict with some chiropractic colleges. The 1978-1979 annual report of the California Board of Chiropractic Examiners listed over 150 chiropractic schools from which California chiropractors had graduated. Although most of these schools were no longer in existence at the time of publication, their number provides an indication of the extensiveness of chiropractic institutions in the first eight decades

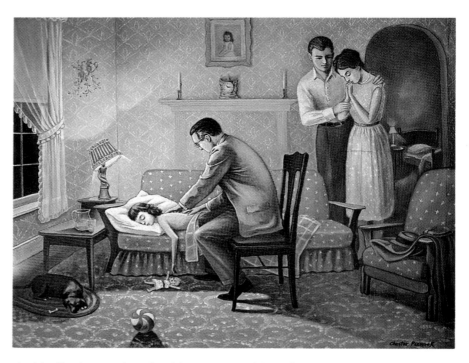

An idealized recreation of a chiropractor making a house call titled In Good Hands *by Chester Paciorek.*

Courtesy Chiropractic Chart Publishers, Niagara Falls, New York.

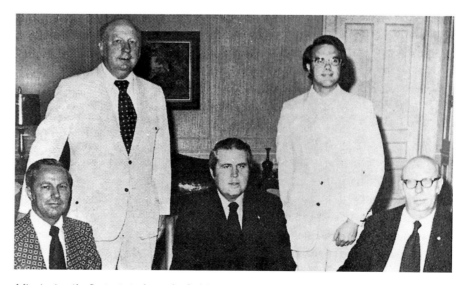

Mississippi's first state board of chiropractic examiners, 1973. Left to right, *Hubert Smith, B.F. Simmons, Governor Bill Waller, Tom Morgan, J.T. Grantham.*

From The ACA Journal of Chiropractic, June 1973.

of the century. Twenty schools are in operation on the North American continent at the time of this writing.

The examining boards were authorized to award, suspend, or revoke individual licenses; to examine the qualifications of applicants for licensure; to create administrative rules; and to ensure that licensed providers observed all state and municipal health regulations. State boards were also expected to review applicants' prechiropractic educational preparation, and in some jurisdictions, by legislation or administrative ruling, to inspect individual chiropractic schools and to mandate specific courses, course content, and/or the number of hours of instruction to be taught by an approved chiropractic college.

Licensure provided more than the mere legal protection from prosecution for unlicensed practice. Laws regulating chiropractic also offered legitimacy, legal standing, and a defined scope of practice. However, each American state and Canadian province exercised its prerogative to define for itself what chiropractic practice would and would not include, and the result was a great diversity in legally acceptable practices. In some states, chiropractors were limited to the adjustment of spinal vertebrae, while in others they were permitted to manipulate any part of the body. Some jurisdictions, for example, Illinois and Ontario, did not license chiropractors per se but provided for the licensure of drugless healers who were not permitted to administer medications or to perform major surgery. In states where "mixers" predominated, chiropractic laws provided that licentiates "may practice as taught in chiropractic schools or colleges," a strategy which served to maintain the influence of educational leaders. Alternatively, in many jurisdictions the orientation (straight versus mixer) of the majority of the chiropractic board determined the content of the curricula of schools within the state or province and influenced the instruction of schools located elsewhere that wished to prepare students for licensure in the intended jurisdiction. State board majority sometimes resulted in the approval of only those schools affiliated with one versus another national professional association, for example, NCA/ACA versus CHB/ICA, although most states examined graduates approved by either national association, and such partisan politics were the exception rather than the rule for boards of chiropractic examiners.

Coursework and required hours were often established based on comparison with medical school curricula. Similarities in basic science instruction between chiropractic and medical institutions were often presented to legislators and public health officials both to attest to the quality and intensity of chiropractic education and as a strategy for preventing passage of basic science legislation. The latter strategy had been helpful in preventing passage of a basic science bill in California in 1942, although it was not until 1948 that the required course of instruction in that state was raised to a minimum of 4000 hours.

In those few states that still did not license chiropractors, organized medicine worked arduously to prevent such legislation. In New York State their efforts after 48 years of legislative and judicial struggle against the chiropractors were finally lost in 1963, when Governor Nelson A. Rockefeller signed a chiropractic bill into law. This bill provided "grandfather" licenses to those chiropractors who had practiced in the state for some time, but permitted future licenses to be granted only to chiropractors who had graduated from colleges accredited by the New York State Department of Education. Since there were no chiropractic institutions with this sort of recognition in 1963, the law threatened to stifle further licensing in the Empire State.

Comparison Subjects and Class Hours
Johns Hopkins Medical School
The Palmer School of Chiropractic

Subject	Johns Hopkins Class Hours	Johns Hopkins % of Total	P.S.C. Class Hours	Palmer School % of Total
Anatomy	508	15.0	520	11.6
Physiology	256	7.3	520	11.6
Pathology	401	11.8	195	4.4
Chemistry	200	5.9	325	7.2
Bacteriology	114	3.4	130	3.0
Diagnosis	224	6.6	520	11.6
Neurology	112	3.3	130	3.0
X-Ray	48	1.4	292	6.5
Psychiatry	144	4.3	65	1.4
Obstetrics and Gynecology	198	5.8	65	1.4
Pharmacology	80	2.4	0	
Psychology	16	.5	0	
Medicine	656	19.3	0	
Pediatrics	72	2.1	0	
Surgery	352	10.4	0	
Therapeutics	16	.5	0	
Clinic	0		585	13.0
Hygiene	0		65	1.4
Chiropractic Technic	0		553	12.3
Chiropractic Philosophy	0		195	4.4
Public Speaking	0		65	1.4
NCM and NCGH	0		65	1.4
Principle and Practice	0		130	3.0
Ethics and Jurisprudence	0		65	1.4
TOTAL	3397	100%	4485	100%

Comparisons of course work and required hours were often presented to legislators and public health officials to attest to the quality and intensity of chiropractic education.

From *Comparison Between Class Hours Approved Medical School and the Palmer School of Chiropractic*, Palmer School of Chiropractic, circa 1950.

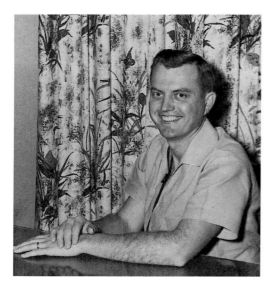

Jerry England's defeat in a Louisiana court-room provided the final impetus for chiropractic educational institutions to pursue federally recognized accreditation.

Courtesy Jerry England, Theodore, Alabama.

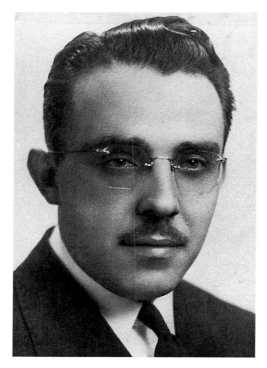

Joe Janse, a 1938 graduate of National College of Chiropractic, served in various administrative and teaching roles at his alma mater until 1945, when he was appointed president of National. During the next 4 decades, Janse was a vocal advocate of educational improvement throughout the profession.

Courtesy National College of Chiropractic, Lombard, Illinois.

Another classic example of the reinvigorated struggle between organized medicine and chiropractic was the case of Jerry England, D.C., and a number of additional chiropractors in Louisiana, where political medicine had successfully resisted passage of a chiropractic law. The England case had begun in the late 1950s and involved a test of chiropractors' right to practice their clinical art without first having graduated from medical school. Legal maneuvering continued for 8 years and included a challenge to the state's constitutional right to license health care providers, which the chiropractors lost. When the case proper came to trial in 1965, educators Joseph Janse, D.C., N.D., president of the National College of Chiropractic, and William D. Harper, D.C., president of the Texas Chiropractic College and author of the textbook, *Anything Can Cause Anything,* took the stand on behalf of plaintiff chiropractors. Their defense of the rational basis of chiropractic practice was remembered by one attorney as "the most dramatic courtroom scene he had ever witnessed." However, the case was lost, and it would be another 9 years before Louisiana passed a chiropractic law, the fiftieth and final U.S. state to do so.

It is said that Dr. Janse's experience on the witness stand in Louisiana's England case provided him with the impetus for the final push towards accreditation by his alma mater, the National College of Chiropractic. Attorneys for the medical lobby hammered away at the lack of federally recognized accreditation for chiropractic colleges. One chiropractor observer of the period recalled that:

> The usefulness of chiropractic was the central issue in the case. The corollary issue of equal importance was whether or not the requirement, that chiropractors possess a diploma from an accredited medical school teaching materia medica, theory and practice of medicine and surgery, and successfully stand an examination in these subjects was constitutionally permissible, as a condition precedent to allowing chiropractors to practice in Louisiana. The England case involves a constitutional attack against the Louisiana statute making such a requirement necessary . . .
>
> Dr. Janse was our chief witness and occupied the stand most of Monday. . . . Accreditation of colleges prompted several questions. Etiology, diagnosis and treatment of most every disease problem came into the picture. Specific emphasis was placed on infectious and fatal disease processes, particularly those of great notoriety and fear-instilling quality, e.g., tetanus, polio, typhoid, cancer, etc. The subject of immunization was not ignored. Dr. Janse maintained his composure, forthrightness and dignity. We think his testimony was indeed an outstanding contribution.

Another historian of the period recalls of Janse's testimony in U.S. District Court in Louisiana on March 22, 1965 that Janse

> . . . was appalled when confronted with legal testimony on radical chiropractic literature dating back to the 30's and 40's and frequent legal references to the fact that chiropractic colleges were not accredited, neither regionally nor professionally, by any government recognized agency. He vowed that he would correct this fault . . . "or leave the profession."

The England case was a short-term defeat for chiropractors. From this defeat though, it became clear that the time for chiropractic education to establish its credibility within the higher education community was long overdue. The AMA had consistently blocked the listing of the two competing agencies (Council on Chiropractic Education and Association of Chiropractic Colleges) then vying for federal authority to act as the accrediting body for chiropractic professional education by the United States Office of Education. Janse's National College of Chiropractic was determined to break the accreditation barrier as an individual institution and looked to the ACA, successor of the NCA, for assistance. With funding from the ACA's grant-making arm, the Foundation for Chiropractic Education and Research (FCER) the descendant of the NCA's Chiropractic Research Foundation, the National College struggled to develop its operations to conform to the accreditation requirements of the New York State Department of Education (NYSDE).

The NYSDE was unique among state education departments in that it had received authorization from the USOE to act as a regional accreditor of the colleges comprising the New York State University system, founded in 1948. If the National College could meet the accreditation requirements of NYSDE, it would become the first chiropractic school to achieve federally recognized accreditation. Such recognition would also help to establish the legitimacy of chiropractic in higher education circles, and thereby facilitate USOE endorsement of a chiropractic accrediting agency. Accreditation by NYSDE would also meet the provisions of New York's 1963 licensing law, thereby making National College graduates eligible to be licensed in the state, a status not then achieved even by the chiropractic schools within New York.

The National College's improvements were multifaceted and due in no small measure to ACA/FCER's short-term infusion of significant funds, which provoked considerable criticism from other ACA schools. National's improvements included an increase in the faculty/student ratio, growth in the number of faculty with master's and doctoral degrees in the basic sciences, recruitment of clinical instructors who were alumni of other chiropractic schools, quadrupling the number of books in the library and employment of a full-time professional librarian, expanded laboratory facilities, and elaboration of the administrative and academic departmental structures within the institution. In 1971 the National College was approved by New York State, and thereby became the first federally recognized chiropractic college. Three years later, National received "accredited" status from the North Central Association of Schools and Colleges and received "full accreditation" in 1981. Cleveland Chiropractic College of Kansas City and Palmer College in Davenport achieved NCA "full accreditation" status soon thereafter.

By 1943, some 43 states had some type of licensure provisions for chiropractors. Certain states recognized chiropractic separately from the medical profession and separately licensed chiropractors. Many states, however, lumped chiropractors, physicians, and osteopaths together and required them to be examined by the same composite boards of examiners comprised of members of the various healing arts. In those states without licensure for chiropractors the unlicensed practitioner was subject to arrest and incarceration. In 1949, Katherine (Kitty) and Mack Scallon of Manhattan, New York, a husband and wife chiropractic team, were sent to jail for refusing to tell the *court* that they would "desist in the practice of medicine without a license." Mack Scallon, whose patients included the late Ambassador Joseph Kennedy, was confined at the maximum security jail on Harts Island. Kitty Scallon, D.C., was sent to the Women's House of Detention. While in jail Kitty wrote the following letter to a friend:

> Being here is something like a bad dream when you think of it being for nothing but doing good . . . I felt downhearted when the news came that Mabel (Palmer) died, but I would always perk up when I thought of chiropractic and the many people that it had helped . . . and then I throw my shoulders back and be ready and willing to make any sacrifice to help free our beloved science.

The Scallons are noteworthy for the number of times that they were

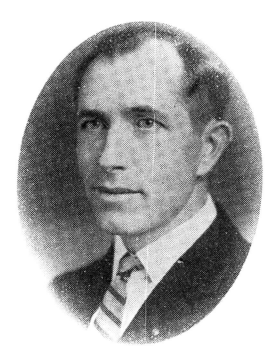

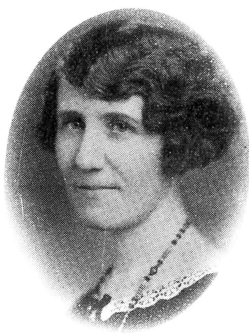

Mack and Kitty Scallon, a husband and wife chiropractic team, received the first "Chiropractor of the Year" award by the ICA in recognition for the many times they were arrested and jailed for "practicing medicine without a license."

From *The Recoil*, Palmer School of Chiropractic, October 1926.

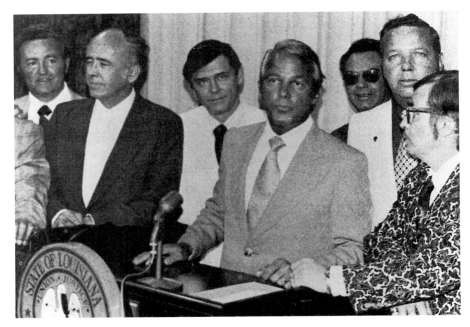

Louisiana Governor Edwin Edwards (center, at podium) just before signing the chiropractic bill into law in 1974. From left, Edward Mernin, vice-president of the Chiropractic Association of Louisiana; John Flynn, President of the Chiropractic Association of Louisiana; Representative J. Richard Breaux. From far right, James Parker, representing the Parker Foundation, which contributed nearly $24,000 to the Louisiana licensing cause.

From *Digest of Chiropractic Economics,* July/August 1973.

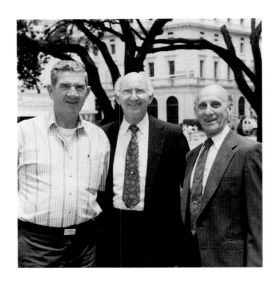

Caddo Parish Chief Deputy Michael Sullivan (left), B.D. Mooring (center), and E.J. Nosser (right), reunited in 1994 in front of the courthouse 20 years after Mr. Sullivan arrested Drs. Mooring and Nosser for practicing chiropractic. Mr. Sullivan was then and still is a patient of Dr. Nosser's.

Courtesy B.D. Mooring, Idabel, Oklahoma.

arrested and jailed for practicing without a license. In honor of their sacrifices, the first "Chiropractor of the Year" awarded by the ICA went jointly to the Scallons in 1950.

In a final irony to the seven-decade struggle for chiropractic licensure in America, two Louisiana chiropractors went to jail 6 months after Governor Edwards had signed that state's first chiropractic legislation in 1974. Brutus D. Mooring, D.C., and Ellis J. Nosser, D.C., of Caddo Parish had been arrested for unlicensed medical practice before the enactment of the chiropractic law, and Judge Jack Fant had issued an order forbidding them to practice chiropractic while they awaited trial. As had been the custom throughout the chiropractic century, the doctors immediately returned to practice in defiance of Judge Fant's ruling. Although it had been expected that all pending prosecutions for unlicensed practice would be dropped once the Louisiana chiropractic act passed, the judge insisted on punishment for defiance of his restraining order. Dr. Mooring, who had served 10 days in jail in 1955 for unlicensed practice was considered a "repeat offender" and was fined $500 and sentenced to 30 days incarceration; Dr. Nosser received a $500 fine and a 15-day jail sentence. Like so many chiropractors behind bars in past years, they developed a clientele within the jail from among the sheriff's deputies. Moreover, as if to further reenact the history of chiropractic struggles of the previous 70 years, the judge was forced to reconsider his treatment of the errant doctors when the sheriff's office switchboard was jammed by sympathetic patients calling in to see about the welfare of the doctors. The local press "went wild" over this final martyrdom in the last state to license chiropractors, and Drs. Mooring and Nosser were released after serving only 3 days of their sentences.

FEDERATION OF CHIROPRACTIC LICENSING BOARDS

The earliest ancestor of the Federation of Chiropractic Licensing Boards (FCLB) was the International Congress of Chiropractic Examining Boards, organized in September 1926 at a meeting of various state examining board members in Memphis. From this Congress evolved the Council of State Chiropractic Examining Boards (CSCEB) in 1933. At first the CSCEB was loosely affiliated with the NCA, but by 1947, although formally identified as the National Council of Chiropractic Examining Boards, this body endeavored to remain independent from the influence of either national professional association. The Council was incorporated in Wyoming in 1968 and received federal tax-exempt status.

Renamed the Federation of Chiropractic Licensing Boards in 1974, the organization's mission was the following:

a. To promote unified standards in the operation of all chiropractic licensing boards

b. To aid in problems confronting individual chiropractic licensing boards

c. To promote and aid in cooperation between chiropractic licensing boards

d. To disseminate information of mutual interest to various chiropractic licensing boards, and

e. To encourage uniformity of educational standards in colleges teaching chiropractic.

Recognizing that state boards often lacked both the funding and the qualified personnel to conduct proper inspections of chiropractic colleges, the Federation of Chiropractic Licensing Boards leadership pushed strongly for the accrediting bodies of the ACA and ICA to combine their efforts and to form an independent accreditation agency that would make a unified application for recognition to the United States Office of Education. In 1968 the ICA organized the Association of Chiropractic Colleges (ACC) with the intent of establishing it as an agency recognized by the USOE. The ACC should not be confused with the present Association of Chiropractic Colleges (ACC), an organization of chiropractic college presidents.

The first ACC became the most serious competitor to the Council on Chiropractic Education, and its member institutions accounted for 75% of all chiropractic students. The Council on Chiropractic Education, which had been established in 1947 as the NCA Council on Education, became the independently incorporated Council on Chiropractic Education in 1971. The seemingly irreconcilable differences between the two agencies eventually prompted the Federation of Chiropractic Licensing Boards to insist on binding arbitration; the Federation of Chiropractic Licensing Boards's influence in this respect derived from its ability to make recommendations to individual state licensing boards about which college accreditor best represented the educational enterprise within the profession. Although the ACC agreed to binding arbitration and prepared to send representatives to work out their disagreements with the Council on Chiropractic Education, the Council on Chiropractic Education independently and without informing the Federation of Chiropractic Licensing Boards and the Association of Chiropractic Colleges, pursued its petition to the United States Office of Education for accreditation. With the imminent likelihood of federal recognition of the Council on Chiropractic Education and in view of the implausibility of approval for two chiropractic accrediting agencies, the Federation of Chiropractic Licensing Boards subsequently withdrew its insistence upon arbitration and backed the Council on Chiropractic Education's government petition.

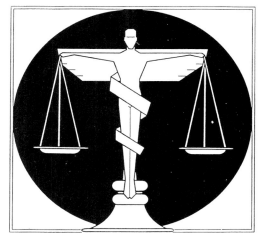

The FCLB was formed in 1974 to promote cooperation and uniformity of standards among state chiropractic licensing boards.

From Federation of Chiropractic Licensing Boards, Greeley, Colorado.

NATIONAL BOARD OF CHIROPRACTIC EXAMINERS

Organized chiropractic had made two unsuccessful attempts to establish a national board of chiropractic examiners during the first half of the chiropractic century: the first circa 1919 by the Universal Chiropractors' Association was an effort to establish reciprocity among state boards, and then a latter effort by the NCA. In 1962, Joseph Janse, D.C., proposed that an agency comparable to those being established by organized medicine, dentistry, and osteopathy be considered. Such boards were introduced in part to wrest basic science examinations from the control of various state boards of basic science and to place them under the control of the respective disciplines. This movement would reach its culmination during 1967-1979, when all states having basic science examinations repealed their basic science laws (see table on p. 191). The existence of national boards of examiners in the various health care disciplines provided part of the justification for the revocation of the basic science boards.

With support from the ICA and NCA, an organizational meeting was held in Detroit on July 26, 1962. The National Board of Chiropractic Examiners was incorporated in Texas on June 19, 1963, and the first meeting of the board was held in Chicago. Edward M. Saunders, D.C., of Florida served as the first president of the National Board of Chiropractic Examiners and directed a staff of clerical and support personnel. Question pools were created by soliciting multiple-choice questions and answers from various department heads at the chiropractic colleges. In 1965 some 1200 students were tested during the first examinations, which included questions in twelve basic and clinical science areas plus an optional test in physiotherapy to satisfy those states that required examination in this area. Five examination sites were selected: Los Angeles, Chicago, Indianapolis, New York City, and Davenport, Iowa. Applicants' answers were graded by the Department of Testing and Measurement of the University of Missouri at Kansas City under the direction of Harrison Godfrey, Ph.D.

The concept of the National Board of Chiropractic Examiners met with early resistance from state examining boards. The program was seen as an attempt to usurp the state examining board's authority. However, by the early 1970s the National Board of Chiropractic Examiners was recognized by 29 states and 37 licensing boards, including the basic science boards of Kansas, Michigan, Nevada, South Dakota, and Washington, who accepted National Board of Chiropractic Examiners test scores in lieu of their own examinations. The National Board of Chiropractic Examiners at first operated out of Edward M. Saunders', D.C., private office, but in 1969 a headquarters was established in Cheyenne, Wyoming.

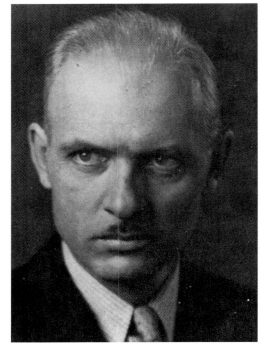

Major Bertrand DeJarnette, D.O., D.C., author, publisher, lecturer, founder of the sacro-occipital technique, and co-incorporator of the National Board of Chiropractic Examiners in 1963.

Courtesy Palmer College of Chiropractic Archives, Davenport, Iowa.

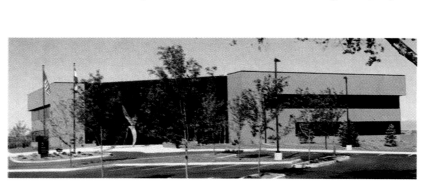

Headquarters of the National Board of Chiropractic Examiners, Greeley, Colorado, circa 1990.

Courtesy National Board of Chiropractic Examiners, Greeley, Colorado.

The Board entered into an agreement with the University of Northern Colorado in nearby Greeley, Colorado to score National Board of Chiropractic Examiners examinations, and the headquarters was later moved to its present site in Greeley to centralize all aspects of operations and to facilitate access to the University's computer services.

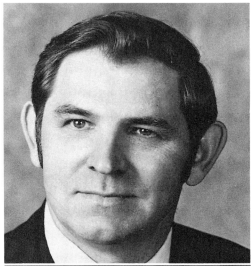

COUNCIL ON CHIROPRACTIC EDUCATION AND THE USOE

On August 26, 1974, United States Commissioner of Education T.H. Bell informed the Council on Chiropractic Education of its listing as a "Nationally Recognized Accrediting Agency"; it was a truly landmark event in the profession's history. Federal recognition of Council on Chiropractic Education opened many doors previously closed to chiropractors. Among the new opportunities were eligibility for federal educational and research grants, student eligibility for federal loans, and greatly enhanced legitimacy for the profession overall. Principally responsible for this achievement were attorney-chiropractor, Orval Hidde and four broad-scope college administrators: Joseph Janse, D.C., N.D., and Leonard Fay, D.C., N.D., of National College; George Haynes, D.C., N.D., M.S., of the Los Angeles College; and John B. Wolfe, D.C., of Northwestern College of Chiropractic.

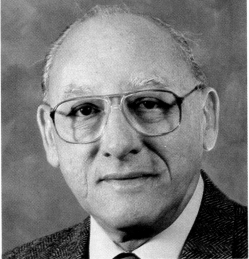

Several broad-scope schools had moved to raise preprofessional requirements for admission to chiropractic colleges as early as 1953, but falling enrollments had required a relaxation of these standards. In the late 1960s as the Council on Chiropractic Education moved closer to submitting its petition to United States Office of Education, increased prerequisites of 1 and then 2 years of prechiropractic college training were again introduced. National College of Chiropractic first required the 2-year prerequisite in 1967 and all Council on Chiropractic Education-aligned schools followed in 1968. Administrative structures were also revamped at several schools to more closely meet the expectations of higher education. The federal approval of the Council on Chiropractic Education put Association of Chiropractic Colleges-accredited colleges at a competitive disadvantage with respect to federal student loans. Additionally, many state boards, on recommendation of the Federation of Chiropractic Licensing Boards, revised their educational standards for licensure to require graduation from a chiropractic college accredited by a federally recognized agency, and in some states the Council on Chiropractic Education was specifically named. With these pressures and realities, within 2 years the former Association of Chiropractic Colleges-accredited institutions would apply for Council on Chiropractic Education recognition.

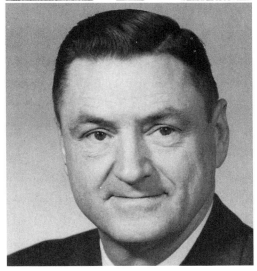

Attorney chiropractor Orval Hidde (top), *Joseph Janse and Leonard Fay* (middle), *and George Haynes and John Wolfe* (bottom) *were largely responsible for the recognition of the Council on Chiropractic Education by the United States Office of Education.*

Courtesy Orval Hidde, Watertown, Wisconsin; National College of Chiropractic, Lombard, Illinois; Northwestern Chiropractic College, Bloomington, Minnesota.

SCHOLARSHIP AND RESEARCH

The profession's 41-year climb from proprietary training to federally accredited colleges would have been much lengthier if not impossible without the assistance rendered by the CRF, which was reorganized in 1958 as the Foundation for Accredited Chiropractic Education (FACE).

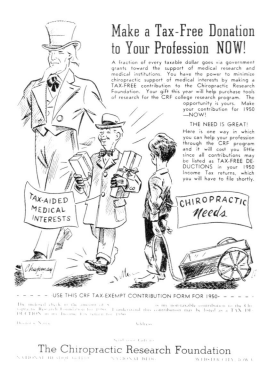

Make a Tax-Free Donation to Your Profession NOW!

A fraction of every taxable dollar goes via government grants toward the support of medical research and medical institutions. You have the power to minimize chiropractic support of medical interests by making a TAX-FREE contribution to the Chiropractic Research Foundation. Your gift this year will help purchase tools of research for the CRF college research program. The opportunity is yours. Make your contribution for 1950 —NOW!

THE NEED IS GREAT!

Here is one way in which you can help your profession through the CRF program and it will cost you little since all contributions may be listed as TAX-FREE DEDUCTIONS in your 1950 Income Tax returns, which you will have to file shortly.

– – – – USE THIS CRF TAX-EXEMPT CONTRIBUTION FORM FOR 1950 – – – –

The Chiropractic Research Foundation

This 1950 plea for funds for chiropractic research from the Chiropractic Research Foundation went largely unheeded.

From *The Journal of the National Chiropractic Association,* November 1950.

In operation since 1944 but largely inactive since the early 1950s owing to its striking lack of success in raising funds from the public for chiropractic research, the CRF/FACE's reemphasized educational mission gave it a purpose that paralleled the colleges' desperate needs. Over the next decade the FACE pumped hundreds of thousands of dollars, largely raised through dues assessments from the membership of the NCA and subsequently the ACA, into those schools affiliated with the broad-scope professional organization. These educational block grants and matching funds went for capital developments such as new college-campus acquisitions, new classroom buildings and laboratories, purchase of instructional and laboratory equipment, and the recruitment of more and better credentialed basic science instructors, for a more favorable faculty/student ratio. When federal recognition was finally achieved, the Foundation, now renamed the Foundation for Chiropractic Education and Research (FCER), returned to its original mission of encouraging scientific investigations within the profession.

Research had not been an entirely neglected area for the CRF/FACE. For instance, FACE had contributed significant dollars in 1959 and later to underwrite the investigations of Henry G. Higley, D.C., N.D., M.S, Director of Research at the Los Angeles College of Chiropractic, whose studies focused on the "Intervertebral Disc Syndrome." Higley had worked with C.O. Watkins, D.C.; George Haynes, D.C., M.A.; and John B. Wolfe, D.C., on the NCA's Committee on Clinical Research in the early 1950s. In 1965, Higley commenced an investigation "Study, Analysis and Evaluation of Chiropractic Education in the United States" with funds contributed by FACE. Following the CRF's disastrous attempts at fundraising in the late 1940s, research had come to be viewed suspiciously in the profession, and the non-profit corporation attempted to regroup and to place the Foundation on sounder fiscal ground. Continuing interest in clinical science investigations came to rest in Watkins' committee and in the

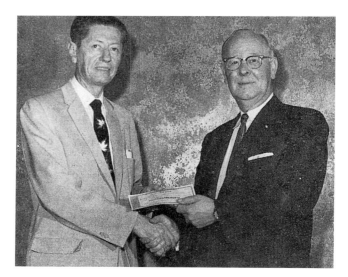

Loran Rogers (right), *NCA Executive Secretary, presenting George Haynes, dean, Los Angeles College of Chiropractic, a grant from the FACE in 1959. FACE was to pump hundreds of thousands of dollars into broad-scope schools over the next decade.*

From *Journal of the National Chiropractic Association* Jun 1959.

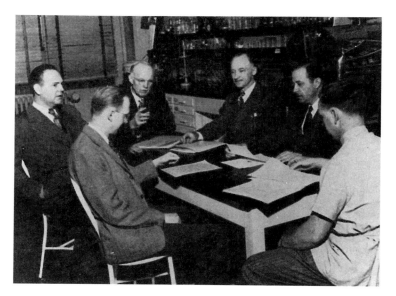

The ICA's research committee, circa 1949. Shown are C.F. Aumann, at the head of the table, and left to right, W.S. Brown, Raymond Johnston, W.W. Coulter, Lyle Sherman, and George Huff.

From *International Review of Chiropractic,* April 1949.

NCA's Council on Public Health and Research. Earl Rich's, D.C., techno-logical developments in cineroentgenography during the 1960s at the Lincoln Chiropractic College in Indianapolis were pursued in collaboration with the Picker X-ray Company and were funded in part by the FACE. When Rich died in 1967, continued funding was solicited from the FCER and the ACA by Joseph Howe, D.C., D.A.C.B.R.

Dr. Higley's investigations were somewhat more successful than his efforts to interest the NCA's, and later the ACA's, leadership in developing research programs in the colleges and the field. In sympathy with the NCA Research Committee chairman, C.O. Watkins, D.C., Higley believed that the schools should do more to develop research skills among the rank and file of the profession. His "Proposal for the establishment of research in the chiropractic colleges," presented to the profession at the NCA's 1953 convention in Los Angeles, called for the recruitment of honors students at the colleges who would work under research faculty supervision to analyze field data contributed by practitioners. The proposal apparently generated little interest.

Similarly, little interest in scientific publishing was apparent in the 1960s and 1970s, although several worthy exceptions deserve mention. The *Journal of Clinical Chiropractic (JCC)* was established in 1968 "to present basic research, educational information, scientific and techno-logical data, and relevant tangential materials to the chiropractic profession. The *JCC* has no social or political design whatsoever. . . . " Independence from the warring political factions, as reflected in an editorial board drawn from the various political camps within the profession, was considered an important characteristic, since it often determined who would subscribe to a periodical. The *JCC* continued publishing until 1981.

From 1960 until the mid-1980s, the *Annals of the Swiss Chiropractors Association* provided an early scholarly model for later scientific periodicals in the profession. In describing the journal's objective, founding editor Walter Bollier suggested that "The Swiss Chiropractors' Association would see its ultimate goal realized if medical researchers, working on problems of vertebral diseases, could receive stimulations for further work from its publication." The *Swiss Annals* was able to attract quantitative data from original clinical and basic science investigations conducted by its members and occasionally contributed by medical physicians.

The *Swiss Annals*, although eclipsed by the *Journal of Manipulative & Physiological Therapeutics (JMPT)* in the early 1980s, had served a valuable function by maintaining high standards for scientific publishing in chiropractic. Also noteworthy was the International Chiropractors' Association's short-lived *Science Review of Chiropractic;* an example of studies published by this periodical was Carl S. Cleveland, Jr.'s, 1965 manuscript, "Researching the subluxation in the domestic rabbit," which involved an effort to create an animal analogue of human spinal lesions.

Unfortunately, none of the profession's scientific periodicals were accessible through standard biomedical indexes, which prevented the information collected in their pages from being accessed by the worldwide health science community. This limited accessibility would continue until 1982, when the *JMPT* was accepted for indexing by *Index Medicus,* a publication of the National Library of Medicine.

In the early 1970s the ICA's efforts in scientific development became linked with the biomechanical investigations of Chung-Ha Suh, Ph.D., Professor and Chairman of the Department of Engineering Design and Economic Evaluation at the University of Colorado at Boulder. Dr. Suh, a

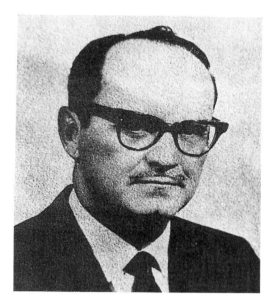

Earl Rich's technological developments in cineroentgenography during the 1960s at the Lincoln Chiropractic College in Indianapolis were funded in part by the FACE.
Courtesy William Rehm, Baltimore, Maryland.

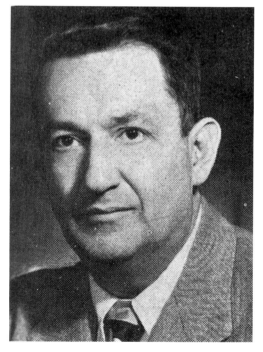

Henry Higley, Director of Research for FACE and Professor at Los Angeles College of Chiropractic.
From *The ACA Journal of Chiropractic,* November 1964.

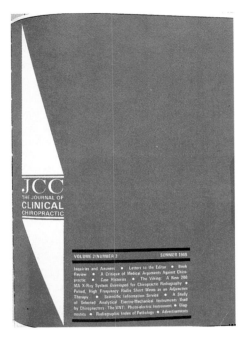

ANNALS

of the Swiss Chiropractors' Association

1971

Editor: Epifanio Valentini, Montreux

Owned and published by the Swiss Chiropractors'
Association as its official journal.
All copyrights reserved.

Print: Imprimeries Populaires, Geneva

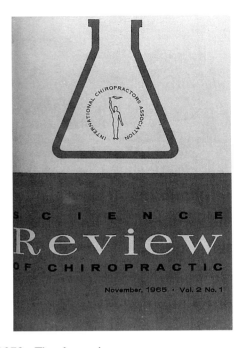

This trio of scientific journals appeared during the 1960s and 1970s. The Journal of Clinical Chiropractic (JCC) *was established in 1968;* The Annals of the Swiss Chiropractors' Association *appeared in 1960; and the short-lived* Science Review of Chiropractic *in 1965.*

From *The Journal of Clinical Chiropractic,* Summer 1969, *The Annals of the Swiss Chiropractors' Association,* volume 7, 1981; *The Science Review of Chiropractic,* February 1965..

University of California/Berkeley trained engineer, had been approached by several Colorado chiropractors who were interested in the testing and development of instrumentation for upper cervical spinal adjusting. The chiropractors' interests prompted the Korean-born scientist to explore the theories and procedures of chiropractic, among which he found considerable basis for legitimate scientific inquiry. Among the hypotheses that intrigued him were those related to the effects that altered spinal biomechanics may have in creating slight compression of spinal nerve roots and the potential effects on nerve conduction that compression may cause.

With seed money from the International Chiropractors' Association, Dr. Suh began a series of pilot investigations that culminated in several proposals to the National Institutes of Health. Although the researcher's grant applications were judged to have scientific merit, funding was denied, ostensibly owing to low-priority ratings for this work. Dr Suh, who had previously established a respectable track record in attracting federal support for his work, was informed in confidential communications from National Institutes of Health staff that his work would not be funded so long as the term *chiropractic* appeared in his proposals.

Dr. Suh did not relent. With the assistance of ICA President William Day, D.C., a former Washington state legislator, and ICA's Legislative Representative, former Brigadier General Joseph P. Adams, they took their case to US Congress. On May 18, 1973, Drs. Suh and Day addressed the House Appropriations Committee, Subcommittee on Labor, Health, Education and Welfare and argued that the government and the people of the United States needed the benefits of chiropractic research. A simi-

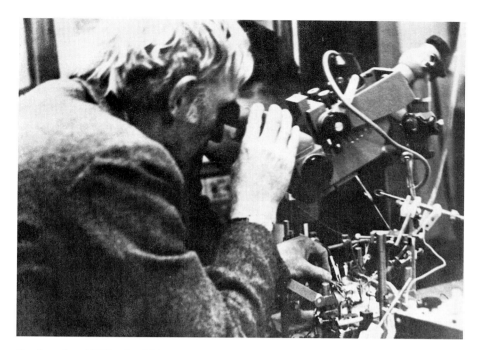

During the 1970s the ICA sponsored research by Dr. Chung-Ha Suh, Professor and Chairman of the Department of Engineering Design and Economic Evaluation at the University of Colorado at Boulder. Here Dr. Seth Sharpless studies nerve roots under compression.

From *The International Review of Chiropractic,* July 1973.

lar message was delivered on July 26, 1973, to Senator Warren Magnuson's Appropriations Subcommittee on Labor, Health and Welfare. The final report of the House Appropriations Subcommittee indicated:

> The committee believes that in view of the recent inclusion of chiropractic services under Medicare, this would be an opportune time for an independent, unbiased study of the fundamentals of the chiropractic profession. Such studies should be high among the priorities of the NINDS and a budget of as much as $2 million should be earmarked for this study and chiropractic research to be conducted by chiropractors . . .

This $2 million Congressional appropriation would have profound effects for chiropractic. The funds were directed to the National Institute of Neurological Disorders and Stroke (NINDS), which awarded Dr. Suh a total of $238,000 in research funds for his studies. The NINDS' Associate Director, Murray Goldstein, D.O., M.P.H., an osteopathic physician and clinical scientist, decided that a portion of the $2 million would be well spent by convening a conference to study the available scientific literature bearing on chiropractic. However, to encourage participation by all persons interested in manual methods and to avoid the possibility of boycott by those who would have nothing to do with chiropractors, the meeting was promoted as an interdisciplinary conference on spinal manipulative therapy (SMT), rather than one on chiropractic exclusively. Held at the National Institutes of Health in Bethesda, Maryland during February 2 to 4, 1975, the NINDS conference attracted practitioners, scientists, and others from chiropractic, medicine, osteopathy, and sociology. The available basic and clinical science knowledge related to SMT was laid out for all to discuss, and a consensus was reached that there was inadequate scientific data available from which to draw a conclusion

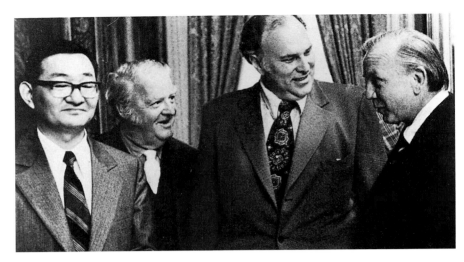

Research Director Suh, Brigadier General Joseph P. Adams, ICA President William Day, and Board of Control member Dr. Grady Lake lobbied in 1973 for federal funds for chiropractic research. As a result of their efforts, the NINDS conference was funded.

From *Vision to action: a history of ICA, the first 60 years, 1926-1986, Internation Review of Chiropractic,* 1986.

about the effectiveness of manipulative methods. The NINDS produced a compilation of the conference proceedings entitled "The Research Status of Spinal Manipulative Therapy," which would serve as a starting point for the research investigations on SMT that have been conducted since.

The NINDS conference was an important turning point in the history of chiropractic. In addition to being the first federally sponsored convening of those interested in SMT, the meeting was also the first time that an interdisciplinary group of practitioners of manipulation had ever come together to share terminology, definitions, scientific data, and to acknowledge in a frank manner the deficiencies in the knowledge base related to SMT. The conference had tremendous political import, for it implicitly acknowledged that there was a potential scientific basis for the practice of SMT and chiropractic. Moreover, chiropractors, osteopaths, and medical practitioners of manipulation discovered that not only were there important differences in their approaches to patient care but also that there were many similarities.

Historians have since suggested that the 1975 NINDS conference marks the birth of chiropractic's phase of research development. That same year the president of the ACA called for controlled clinical trials of chiropractic methods, a first in the organization's history. Two years later chiropractor Alan Breen broke the science journal "ice" when he published a demographic study of British chiropractors, their patients and clinical practices in the prestigious periodical *Rheumatology & Rehabilitation.* Four years later the ICA sponsored the first of its series of International Conferences on the Spine (ICS). The proceedings of the initial ICS resulted in the first scholarly work on chiropractic to be released by a medical publishing house, *Modern Developments in the Principles and Practice of Chiropractic* in 1980. The NINDS conference also provided an opportunity for interaction between the National Institutes and the chiropractic colleges. Conference organizer, Murray Goldstein, D.O., M.P.H., influenced the funding priorities of the FCER by emphasizing the importance of developing research programs within the chiropractic colleges to improve their "scientific climates"; this in contrast to the notion of funding studies such as those of Dr. Suh at nonchiropractic institutions. Dr.

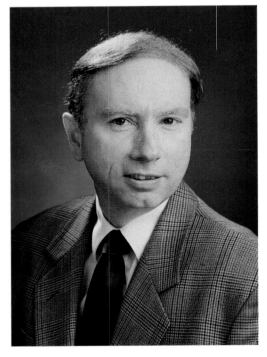

Alan Breen, director of research at Anglo-European College of Chiropractic, broke the barrier to publication in science journals when his study of British chiropractors was published in the prestigious periodical Rheumatology & Rehabilitation.

Courtesy Alan Breen, Bournemouth, England.

Goldstein's suggestions were reiterated by the USDE the following year, when it was suggested that the Council on Chiropractic Education must encourage scientific development within its accredited schools.

The NINDS conference also produced a valuable research tool for chiropractic investigators and others interested in the scientific basis of manipulation. In preparation for the NINDS meeting faculty members at the Canadian Memorial Chiropractic College had prepared an extensive bibliography of chiropractic, osteopathic, and medical literature bearing on manipulation. This bibliography, which initially included several thousand references to worldwide health science literature, has been periodically updated since 1975 and is known as the *Chiropractic Research Archives Collection (CRAC)*. The *CRAC* index facilitates scholarly reviews of the literature on SMT and thereby provides an initial search strategy for anyone interested in investigating manual therapies.

Simultaneous with the ICA's development of research programs at the University of Colorado, the ACA's research funding arm, FCER, developed a program to increase research skills among chiropractors. Funding for fellowships to train chiropractors in university based science departments awarding advanced degrees (M.S. and Ph.D.) became available; noteworthy among the early recipients of these awards have been Scott Haldeman, Reed Phillips, and John Triano, each of whom has since completed graduate programs in the basic or social sciences and have made significant contributions to research in chiropractic.

Also, at about the same time (1970-1973) the government of the Canadian province of Ontario authorized a series of Royal Commissions and an Ontario Task Force Investigation into the scope of practice of chiropractic. This experience prompted a number of Canadian chiropractors to make concerted efforts to develop chiropractic scientist-teachers to populate the faculties of the colleges. Their effort produced the College of Chiropractic Science (Canada) in 1975, which established a certification program for its members through the Canadian Memorial Chiropractic College (CMCC). Fellows of the College of Chiropractic Science (Canada), designated F.C.C.S.(C), have since been among the most active members of the profession in scholarly and scientific endeavors. In 1977 the first resident completed a CMCC-based CCS program, including a thesis involving original research, and in later years a research-oriented training program in orthopedics at the teaching hospital of the University of Saskatchewan would be established. This early initiative accounts in part for the significant leadership that the Canadian branch of the profession has shown in research and scholarship.

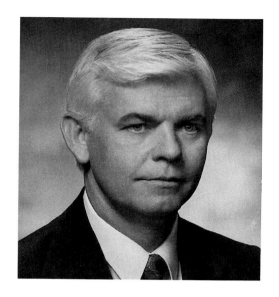

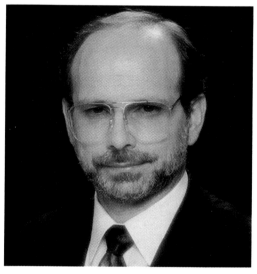

Reed Phillips (top), *Scott Haldeman, and John Triano* (bottom) *were among the first recipients of the ACA's research funding arm, FCER.*

Courtesy Reed Phillips, Whittier, California, and John Triano, Plano, Texas.

SUMMARY

The profession moved from the fighting 1940s to an increased respect and credibility among its patient base in the 1950s, increased its power and political influence in the late 1960s, and ultimately broke new ground with research by the mid-1970s. In the mid-1970s, the profession grew to 23,000 practitioners, efforts were made to standardize chiropractic education to include the requirement that faculty in basic sciences hold M.S. and Ph.D. degrees, a two-year pre-professional requirement was established, and the academic programs were upgraded. No longer could medicine claim that chiropractors were ignorant of the basic sciences.

By 1974, chiropractic education had received federally recognized accreditation, and doctors of chiropractic were licensed in all 50 states as independent portal of entry practitioners and their services were widely reimbursed through the third party payer systems. By the close of 1975, federal recognition of the Council on Chiropractic Education resulted in standardization of chiropractic professional education, eligibility for federal student loans, and an increased respect and prestige for chiropractic educational institutions and the profession. Federal recognition of the Council on Chiropractic Education also provided an annual forum for the leadership from many factions within the profession, including the colleges, the national professional associations, and the Federation of Chiropractic Licensing Boards. By the end of 1975 the seeds of scientific investigation within the profession were apparent, including the birth of peer-reviewed journals, intraprofessional funding for chiropractic research, and the development of instructional programs in research methodology at the colleges. The profession also gained eligibility for reimbursement through the Medicare Act by mobilizing patients and members of the profession in an effective grass-roots political lobby.

These accomplishments occurred despite the AMA's long-standing campaign to contain and eliminate the chiropractic profession. As the postwar period ended, chiropractors began to take the initiative to challenge organized medicine's illegal efforts and in the hard-won victory of the 14-year-long Wilk versus AMA lawsuit would find greater opportunities to serve the public through better integration in the health care system.

We wish to thank Fred H. Barge, D.C., Ph.D.; William S. Rehm, D.C.; the Council on Chiropractic Education; the Federation of Chiropractic Licensing Boards; and the Palmer College Archives for their assistance in locating source works and Leonard Fay, D.C., N.D. for his critical review of the manuscript. They are not responsible for the finished product. This work was made possible by the financial support of the National Institute of Chiropractic Research and the Cleveland Chiropractic Colleges.

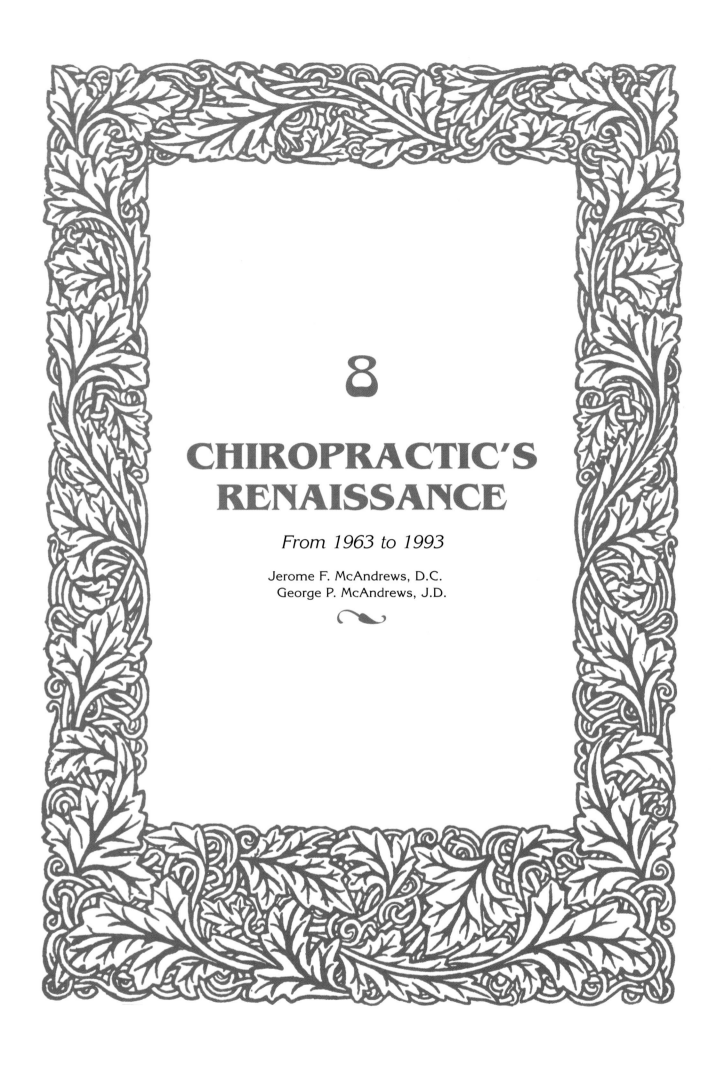

8

CHIROPRACTIC'S RENAISSANCE

From 1963 to 1993

Jerome F. McAndrews, D.C.
George P. McAndrews, J.D.

The last 20 to 30 years might best be characterized as a period of agony and ecstasy for the chiropractic profession. Chiropractic entered this period as a predominantly patient-driven profession, but as the 1970s and 1980s progressed, it shifted to a patient-and-science–driven profession.

It is difficult to contain one's enthusiasm when writing about chiropractic's advances and disappointments over the past 30 years. Starting in the 1970s, chiropractic was accepted within and began to be a more active partner in the federal health care system. On both federal and state levels, lawmakers legislated their support of chiropractic as never before. There are a record number of chiropractors licensed and practicing today and with the solidification of chiropractic education, there are more students in the classrooms than ever. The pursuit of the scientific underpinning of chiropractic and the building of chiropractic's knowledge base is proceeding at an incredible pace. To single out and touch on just a few of these exciting advances is to invariably leave out yet another important piece of chiropractic's story.

While chiropractic has reached many milestones, these advances have been paralleled by critical negative episodes in the field. During the 1960s, turmoil within the medical profession was created partially by the question of what new direction health care delivery would go in the United States. The political upheaval from the creation of President Johnson's "Great Society" also placed chiropractic squarely into organized medicine's focus as an unwanted competitor and resulted in the 1965 Medicare law that excluded chiropractic. There were resounding promises that new breakthroughs in medicine would solve all of the nation's health care problems without having to resort to nontraditional providers of health care such as chiropractors. States became more restrictive in their licensure of chiropractic while chiropractic health care services increased in popularity. This discrepancy between supply and demand placed an unfair burden on licensed providers and put the profession at grave risk. Despite the fact that chiropractic was decidedly being left out of the nation's mainstream health care system, the profession continued to develop and grow.

As the chiropractic profession approaches its centennial celebration during the summer of 1995, health care provision in the United States is changing again. With this uncertainty comes a concern over how chiropractic's second century of service will be shaped.

The word *perseverance* is an excellent description of chiropractic from its beginning and throughout its history. Perseverance is also the reason chiropractic's second century of service and the approaching revolutionary changes in health care legislation in the United States should be approached calmly and with determination. In the words of W. McCune, "If a person has any brains at all, let them hold on to his or her calling and, in the grand sweep of things, their turn will come at last."

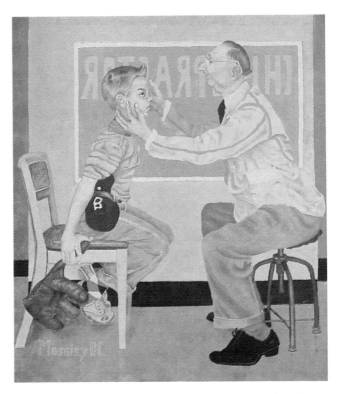

The Adjustment, *a skillful and witty parody of a Norman Rockwell illustration, done by chiropractor/artist Mark Mosely.*

Courtesy Mark Mosely, Burbank, California.

A RENEWED CHIROPRACTIC EDUCATION AND MANPOWER ERA

As the 1960s drew to a close, the "Baby Boomer" generation had a profound effect on not only the mood and state of our nation but also on the chiropractic profession. More students were seeking postsecondary schooling in college and professional schools than at any other point in history. Alternative lifestyles and thinking were being explored. This search for alternatives also included health care as patients became more interested in natural, conservative, and holistic approaches to health.

Chiropractic's ranks began to grow during the 1950s and 1960s as Korean and Vietnam veterans used the G.I. Bill to finance their chiropractic education. As with previous wars, the end of the Korean and Vietnam wars brought with them an influx of students. There were an estimated 17,559 licensed doctors of chiropractic in the United States in 1974; 17,895 in 1976; 23,000 in 1979; 28,000 in 1981; 34,000 in 1984; and 45,000 licensed doctors of chiropractic in the United States in 1993.

Chiropractic education achieved several great milestones in recent years. The first was the formal recognition of the Council on Chiropractic Education by the United States Office of Education as the profession's college accrediting agency. The Council's application was approved and became effective in August 1974. With the recognition of the

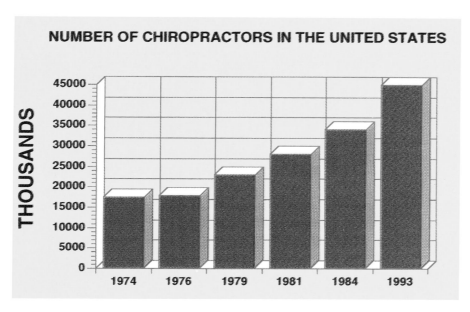

NUMBER OF CHIROPRACTORS IN THE UNITED STATES

During the 20 years between 1974 and 1993, the number of licensed chiropractors increased from 17,559 to 45,000.

Courtesy Instructional Media Services, Palmer College of Chiropractic, Davenport, Iowa.

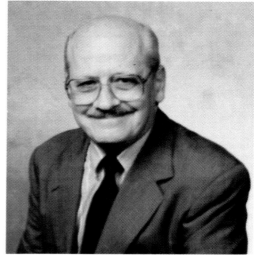

Council on Chiropractic Education, many opportunities for federal support became available, such as additional federal student loan support.

Another milestone reached by chiropractic education was the overall increase of the number of students in the country during this time. From a relatively low number of student enrollments during the 1950s and 1960s, chiropractic college enrollments doubled during the 1973 to 1974 period. It is likely that much of this increase was tied to the changing public image of chiropractic. The profession was now included in Medicare coverage and accredited educational programs were available.

In 1978, the United States Congress authorized $250,000 for a Health Manpower Study to examine the demand for chiropractic services, the cost of chiropractic education, and the supply of chiropractors to meet

William Rehm, a National College graduate helped organize the Association for the History of Chiropractic in Denver, Colorado in 1979. He served as its Executive Director for 12 years.

Courtesy William Rehm, Baltimore, Maryland.

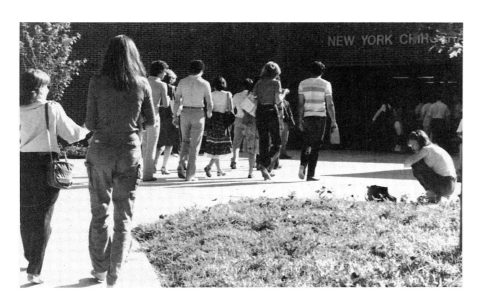

The Old Brookville Long Island campus of New York Chiropractic College, circa 1974.

Courtesy New York Chiropractic College, Seneca Falls, New York.

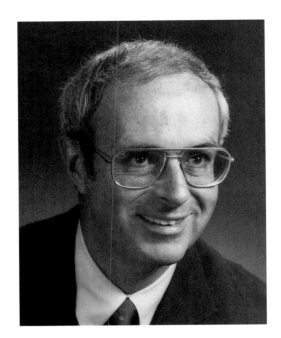

Russell Gibbons served as editor of the Association for the History of Chiropractic's Journal, Chiropractic History, *for over 15 years. The journal is indexed in the National Library of Medicine's* Bibliography of the History of Medicine.

Courtesy Russell Gibbons, Pittsburgh, Pennsylvania.

the demand. With this newly earned recognition and the resurgence in student populations came the opening of six new chiropractic colleges in the United States, one in Canada, one in Australia, one in France, one in South Africa, and two in Japan. In 1980, the Smithsonian Institution displayed its first exhibit on the history of the chiropractic profession. Also in 1980, the United States Olympic Sports Medicine Committee appointed chiropractors for the first time to their Alternative Methods subcommittee. Chiropractors were subsequently appointed to its athletes' health care team. Chiropractors with the United States Olympic Sports Medicine Committee have had frequent requests for chiropractic care from athletes of other nations during the games.

Chiropractic education took another step forward in 1980 when chiropractic students in the United States became eligible for the Health Education Assistance Loan (HEAL) program. Health Manpower legislation was signed into law authorizing the provision of guaranteed government loans of up to $50,000. Funding for chiropractic education, unlike most professional education, depends on tuition. Most chiropractic colleges' operating funds are more than 80% tuition-dependent. The average publicly supported medical school depends less on tuition monies since over 50% of their operating budgets are provided through tax dollars. Even private medical schools with large endowments to support their programs are not as tuition-dependent for their basic programs as chiropractic colleges are today. The federally guaranteed loans to chiropractic college students provided the colleges a more secure footing for financing their programs to meet the more demanding educational accreditation requirements of the Council on Chiropractic Education, as well as the increasing professional demands and standards of the chiropractic profession.

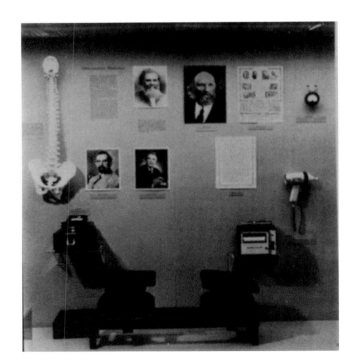

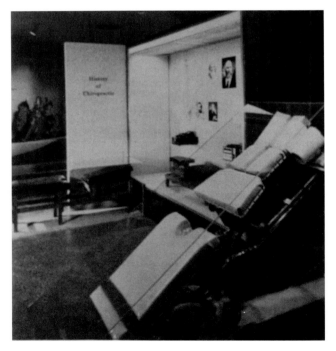

The first publicly sponsored exhibit on chiropractic at the Smithsonian's Museum of American History, Washington, D.C., opened in April 1980.
From Bulletin of the AHC June 1981.

CHIROPRACTIC RECOGNITION THROUGH FEDERAL LEGISLATION

As noted earlier, chiropractic was excluded from coverage benefits with the initial 1965 Medicare Act. Legislation that incorporated chiropractic for Medicare reimbursement was eventually signed into law in December 1972 and became effective July 1, 1973. Effective in July 1974, the Medicare Act also required that chiropractors planning to become a qualified Medicare provider must have graduated from a chiropractic college requiring 2 years of preprofessional education as of their enrollment in 1974. This served to both recognize chiropractic's positive health care benefits and to challenge chiropractic to reinforce a more unified and uniform educational program.

During 1974, chiropractic was included in two other federally supported health care programs. Chiropractic coverage was added to the Federal Employees Compensation Act (FECA) so that any federal employee injured on the job would be eligible for chiropractic manipulative services. Coverage was also added to the Federal Employee Health Benefits Plans (FEHB). In all, chiropractic coverage has been incorporated into nine federally supported health care plans.

A final piece of federal legislation signed into law by President Bush in 1992 was the authorization law for the commissioning of Doctors of Chiropractic into the armed services.

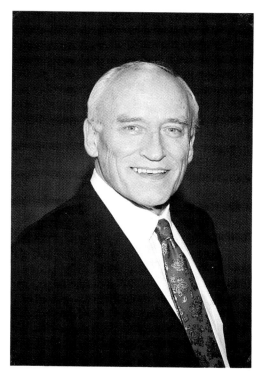

Jerome F. McAndrews, whose political career included serving as Executive Vice-President of the ICA, President of Palmer College of Chiropractic, and Vice-President of Professional Affairs of the ACA.

Courtesy American Chiropractic Association, Arlington, Virginia.

AMA ANTITRUST LAWSUIT

The most significant event for chiropractic, or series of events, over the past 20 years was the winning of the antitrust lawsuit filed against the American Medical Association (AMA) and a number of its related socie-

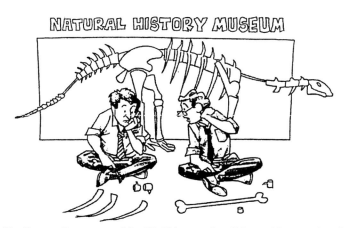

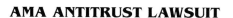

"Let's swallow our pride, Watkins, and call in a chiropractor."

A cartoon from Parade *magazine inferring that chiropractors are experts on the spine.*

Courtesy Bunny Hoest, Parade Publications, New York.

ties. The suit, Chester Wilk et al *v.* the AMA et al, was filed in 1976 and initially concluded in 1983, then retried, and concluded finally in January 1992. It is unfortunate that the story of this law suit and its effects have overshadowed the past 20 years of chiropractic history. However, the Wilk suit is indicative of the chiropractic profession's struggle to protect its rights and the rights of all patients to seek the health care of their choice.

In part, the Wilk case served to make chiropractic more commonly accepted by the general public and other health care professionals. As a result of the litigation, in 1980 the AMA changed its Code of Ethics to allow for some degree of interprofessional cooperation with chiropractors. The Chairman of the AMA's Board of Trustees, Lowell Steen, M.D., showed his support by stating, "It is hoped that the new American Medical Association provision will help to improve the public's perception of chiropractic and increase the utilization of its services with respect to the treatment of muscle, bone, joint and related conditions." Although bridges are slowly being built, the bitter rivalry between chiropractic and *political* medicine still exists.

The AMA's Official Chiropractic Position Before the Antitrust Lawsuit

In the early 1960s, the AMA watched the phenomenal growth of chiropractic while mired in its own members' concerns about the advent of Medicare and state sponsored health care programs. The AMA's public position regarding chiropractic was explicitly presented by Dr. Russell B. Roth, speaker of the AMA's House of Delegates, before the Ways and Means Committee of the United States House of Representatives during

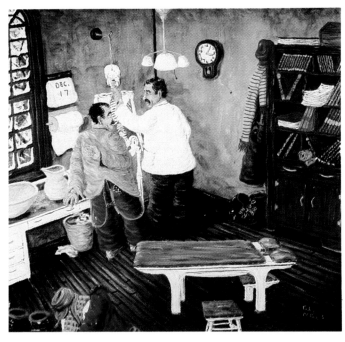

In the early 1980s, Gerald Nees, a quadriplegic artist who had been helped by chiropractic, painted a series of illustrations depicting chiropractic.

Courtesy Gerald Nees, Skokie, Ill.

220

the debate on Medicare laws. Congressman Barber B. Conable, Jr., of New York, questioned Dr. Roth:

I am a layman, and I am not knowledgeable about the various disputes between these two branches of the healing arts, but I am interested in whether or not there has been any revision of the relationship between the two groups as a result of the widespread licensing, most of which was directed at upgrading chiropractic as a healing art, and basing it on what at least from a medical viewpoint is a sounder basis than many people felt chiropractic had when it was unlicensed, when there was no public concern about the qualifications of those practicing chiropractic.

This is a complicated question, I realize sir, and it puts you in a delicate position to answer it, I am sure, but I, as a layman, would be interested in your response. I do feel that we here in Congress are in the middle of a comparatively irreconcilable contradiction in our public health programs.

Dr. Roth responds to Congressman Conable:

I would hope it is not an irreconcilable contradiction, Mr. Conable. I have no hesitation in suggesting that the American Medical Association, and I would say overwhelmingly, perhaps every one of its members, would subscribe to the remedy which we would propose. We indeed feel that your program should be consistent, and consistency should be achieved by eliminating payment for chiropractic from all of it.

I would only point out to you that there has been a magnificent eclectic track record for the medical profession in this country, and elsewhere in the world.

I think that none of you gentlemen would harbor in your minds for one moment the thoughts that if the magnificent departments of medicine and surgery of our Army and our Navy and our Veterans' Administration felt that chiropractic had one thing to offer to the well being of our wounded servicemen and our sick and disabled servicemen, they long ago would have ignored any other considerations except the welfare of their patients. Yet they have never accepted chiropractic services.

I think there was an excellent study made by the Department of Health, Education, and Welfare on independent practitioners under Medicare, which recommended a perfectly proper answer, which we of the American Medical Association would support 100 percent. May I read just one key paragraph from this: "Chiropractic theory and practice are not based upon the body of basic knowledge related to health, disease, and health care that has been widely accepted by the scientific community. Moreover, irrespective of its theory, the scope and quality of chiropractic education do not prepare the practitioner to make an adequate diagnosis and provide appropriate treatment. Therefore, it is recommended that chiropractic service not be covered in the medicare program."

I believe that we would wholeheartedly extend this to the point that it not be included in any other federally financed program. We believe this is an opportunity for two benefits: A savings of federal dollars and an improvement in the overall health care, since chiropractic is one of—I don't even want to use the word—disciplines that I have grouped under nonscientific substitutes for scientific medical care.

Mr. Conable then asks Dr Roth:

How do we reconcile this with the licensing of chiropractic by the States?

Dr. Roth: I come from the State of Pennsylvania, where this was long and bitterly fought over a number of years, and all I can say is that the guys with the white hats lost.

Mr. Conable: But apparently they have lost generally if chiropractic is licensed in most of the States. You understand our position here, don't you, sir?

Dr. Roth: I do.

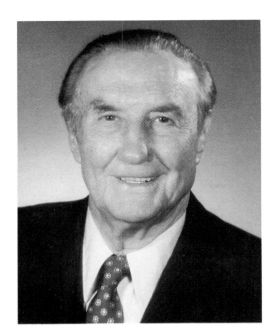

Senator Strom Thurmond of South Carolina, who introduced S.68, legislation to commission chiropractors as officers in the armed services.

Courtesy Senator Strom Thurmond, Washington, DC.

Mr. Conable: That we are in what could be described as a delicate position, as a group of laymen trying to evaluate the claims of not only the professions, but our constituents, many of whom are outraged by the fact that they cannot get chiropractic services, in which for one reason or another they believe.

Dr. Roth: They like their chiropractors.

Now, contrast that exchange in the 1960s with the testimony in 1992 of Senator Strom Thurmond of South Carolina. Before evidence was presented at the Wilk antitrust trial, it was not commonly known that this infamous HEW Report previously cited by Dr. Roth was "fixed" by the AMA and medical physician members of the Public Health Service. Senator Thurmond at the Committee On Armed Services of the United States House of Representatives, Subcommittee Hearings on Military Personnel and Compensation made this speech:

I appreciate the opportunity to appear today before the subcommittee to offer my strong support for H.R. 608, which would authorize the appointment of Doctors of Chiropractic as commissioned officers in the Armed Services.

It is good to see the sponsor of this bill, Representative Evans, and I commend him for introducing this legislation. I was pleased to introduce the companion legislation, S. 68, which now has 15 co-sponsors.

Presently, the members of our Armed Services who desire the care of a Doctor of Chiropractic are forced to pay for this care out of their own pockets, because the military does not recognize Doctors of Chiropractic as commissioned officers.

However, Doctors of Medicine, Doctors of Osteopathy, Dentists, Veterinarians, Optometrists, Pharmacists, Psychologists, Physical Therapists, Occupational Therapists, Dieticians, and Physicians Assistants may serve as commissioned officers.

This policy is not only unfair to our deserving men and women in uniform, but it is also outdated. The chiropractic profession is licensed in all 50 States and is an integral part of our Medicare, Medicaid and Federal Employees Health Care Systems.

Additionally, colleges of chiropractic are recognized by the Department of Education. Clearly, Doctors of Chiropractic are just as qualified in their area of expertise as any other profession accorded commissioned officer status. Their formal education includes a minimum of 2 years of

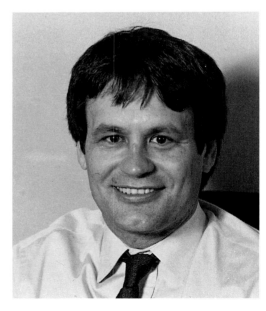

Congressman Lane Evans of Illinois, who sponsored H.R. 608, legislation to commission chiropractors as officers in the armed services.

Courtesy Congressman Lane Evans, Moline, Ill.

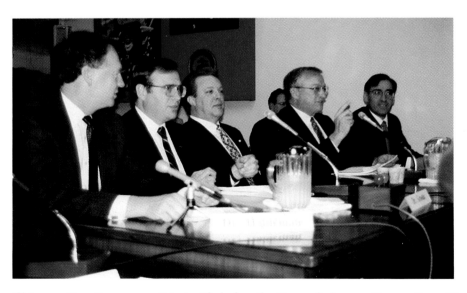

Chiropractic witnesses wait to testify before the House Subcommittee on the military commisions bill. Left to right, Scott Haldeman, Johm Grostic, John Hoffman, George McAndrews, and Jay Wipf.

From *ICA Review*, July/Aug 1992.

college work concentrated in the biological and basic sciences, and 4 years in a chiropractic college, which includes practice in a teaching clinic.

Denying our dedicated service members access to chiropractic care, which is otherwise widely available in our society, is an unfair policy.

The bill will put an end to that policy. It will ensure that members of our Armed Services have a full range of health care services available.

In October of 1992, President Bush signed into law the statute authorizing the commissioning of doctors of chiropractic as officers in the armed forces, a goal of the chiropractic profession, which took over 50 years to realize. The AMA tackled the problem of chiropractic as though it was the principal threat to the monopoly on health care delivery services enjoyed by its members. In 1963, the AMA set about to destroy, ("contain and eliminate") the competitive profession of chiropractic. The fundamental weapon was an ambitious nationwide boycott of every doctor of chiropractic.

Origins of Chiropractic's Boycott

With the subpoenaed documents from the Wilk suit, the boycott of chiropractic was given a primary impetus in Iowa in 1962. The Iowa Medical Society, a constituent society of the American Medical Association, through its General Counsel Robert B. Throckmorton, devised a plan in 1962 to contain chiropractic in Iowa. There were a relatively large number of chiropractors per capita in Iowa. Chiropractic had originated in Davenport, Iowa, and the Palmer School of Chiropractic was one of the profession's two most influential educational institutions. Thus M.D.'s had a relatively strong incentive to "contain and eliminate" chiropractors in Iowa because they were their health care market competitors.

The Iowa plan was published by Throckmorton in a speech to medical organization executives in November 1962. The AMA was a group in need of a "unity" campaign to counter the raging debate over national health insurance. Among the tenets of the Throckmorton plan were these points:

II. What Medicine Should Do about the Chiropractic Menace.
   F. Encourage chiropractic disunity.
   G. Undertake a positive program of containment. If this program is successfully pursued, it is entirely likely that chiropractic as a profession will 'wither on the vine' and the chiropractic menace will die a natural but somewhat undramatic death. This policy of 'containment' might well be pursued along the following lines:
   4. Encourage ethical complaints against doctors of chiropractic.
   5. Oppose chiropractic inroads in health insurance.
   6. Oppose chiropractic inroads in workmen's compensation.
   7. Oppose chiropractic inroads into labor unions.
   8. Oppose chiropractic inroads into hospitals.
   9. Contain chiropractic schools. Any successful policy of 'containment' of chiropractic, must necessarily be directed at the schools. To the extent that these financial problems continue to multiply, and to the extent that the schools are unsuccessful in their recruiting programs, the chiropractic menace of the future will be reduced and possibly eliminated.

Among the conclusions that Throckmorton presented were the following:

C. The 'mixers' (in chiropractic) may achieve their goal of emerging as 'medical men' if organized medicine remains apathetic to this problem.

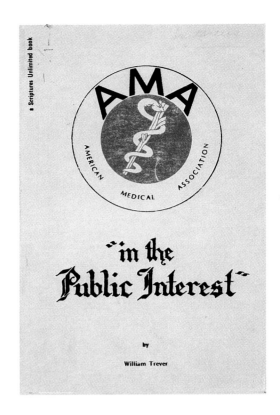

The cover from the book AMA: In the Public Interest, *which detailed the Committee on Quackery's campaign against chiropractic.*

From Trever W: *AMA: in the public interest*, 1972, Los Angeles, Scriptures Unlimited.

D. Any action undertaken by the medical profession should be directed toward:
   2. Containment of the chiropractic schools.
   3. The stifling of chiropractic schools.
E. Action taken by the medical profession should be . . . persistent . . .
   1. Behind the scenes whenever possible.
   3. Never give professional recognition to doctors of chiropractic.
F. A successful program of containment will result in the decline of chiropractic (PX-172, November 11, 1962).

The AMA Adopts the Iowa Plan to Contain and Eliminate Chiropractic

In 1963, Throckmorton was invited to become General Counsel of the AMA and to implement an AMA national "unity" program that would contain and eliminate chiropractic. On September 24, 1963 Robert Youngerman of the AMA reported to Throckmorton on the AMA's intention as follows: "It would seem from certain declarations of the House of Delegates and the Judicial Council, that the ultimate objective of the American Medical Association, theoretically, is the complete elimination of the chiropractic 'profession.' "

Soon thereafter, Throckmorton brought in Doyl Taylor to work on the program. Taylor had worked for the *Des Moines Register* for 35 years and his brother was the Executive Director of the Iowa Medical Society.

In October 1963, the AMA participated in the Second National Congress on Medical Quackery. However, the AMA was displeased with the results of the meeting. Due to the objections of the United States Food and Drug Administration and according to General Counsel Throckmorton, the AMA "was unable to put the spotlight on the primary target," chiropractic. The AMA was determined to form a Committee on Chiropractic. Acting through the AMA Board of Trustees on November 2-3, 1963, the Committee on Quackery was organized with its "major emphasis" to be "devoted to the chiropractic problem." The original Committee on Chiropractic was renamed the Committee on Quackery "to avoid lending dignity to the [chiropractic] profession."

By 1964, documents produced by the Committee made it clear that the AMA had formally implemented its plan. The Committee on Quackery had two goals: (1) "contain" chiropractic and then (2) "eliminate" it. Dr. Stevens, an orthopedic surgeon from Kentucky and a Committee on Quackery member from 1967 to 1974, testified under oath that the goal of the AMA was to "eliminate" and to "destroy" the entire chiropractic profession.

On January 4, 1971, the Committee on Quackery reported its mission to the American Medical Association Board of Trustees as follows:

> Since the American Medical Association Board of Trustees' decision, at its meeting on November 2-3, 1963, to establish a Committee on Quackery, your Committee has considered its prime mission to be, first, the containment of chiropractic, and, ultimately, the elimination of chiropractic.
>
> Your Committee believes it is well along with its first mission and is, at the same time, moving toward the ultimate goal. This, then, might be considered a progress report on developments in the past seven years.

Early in 1971 the AMA realized that chiropractors had far fewer malpractice actions filed against them than did medical doctors. Medical doctors were warned, "[The American Medical Association] urged that we stay clear of attempts to show civil malpractice situations. With the relative weight in numbers against the medical physicians, [The American Medical Association] felt we'd be playing with dynamite." (Blue Shield letter of February 3, 1971, PX-439.)

In its report to the American Medical Association Council on Long Range Planning and Development, April 9, 1971, the Committee on Quackery described its functions as follows:

> The American Medical Association's Committee on Quackery, since its formulation in 1964, has considered its prime mission to be, first, the containment of chiropractic, and, ultimately, the elimination of chiropractic as a recognized health-care provider . . . The Committee believes that the campaign against chiropractic is an effective unity mechanism for medicine at all levels and physicians at all levels must be made aware of this extremely beneficial side effect, particularly at this time.

Doyl Taylor's November 8, 1972 memorandum to the Executive Vice President of the AMA provided further insight into the Committee's goal: "When the American Medical Association Board of Trustees established the Committee on Quackery in 1964, it was made emphatically clear that the prime mission of the Committee on Quackery was and is to contain chiropractic and, hopefully eliminate it as a recognized health-care service to the people."

In 1972, the AMA and Doyl Taylor learned that the privacy of their documents, including those of the Committee on Quackery, had been compromised. Many appeared without permission in a book by William Trever entitled *In the Public Interest.* After learning of the public disclosure of its documents and the public outrage it generated, the AMA changed the phrasing of its "contain and eliminate" statements. For example, the Unity Plan, drafted by Taylor in 1974, added the underscored phrase "as a health hazard" as a postscript to the goal "eliminate." This postscript was tagged on in an attempt to "dress up" the actual plan by adding a philosophical twist to its goal, thereby tempering the anticompetitive emphasis of the earlier statements. It was hoped that this phrase would soften the finality of the phrase "eliminate" and make it appear that the AMA merely wished to "improve" the chiropractic profession not eliminate it. It was obvious the AMA authorities suspected that litigation would follow from the disclosure of the AMA documents.

While the phrasing may have changed, the real goals of the AMA and the other medical organizations in league with it did not. Taylor's trial testimony and the AMA's subsequent activities made this abundantly clear.

The courtroom testimony of Dr. Stevens, a Committee on Quackery and American Academy of Orthopedic Surgeons member, left no doubt that activities were intended to destroy the entire profession of chiropractic. As he admitted, he acted not in the interest of science but as an adversary to chiropractic. The AMA acted unfairly toward doctors of chiropractic, disseminated biased antichiropractic reports, and suppressed highly favorable medical reports about chiropractic, including a report by AMA Board member and orthopedic surgeon, Dr. Hendryson. This was done primarily in the economic interest of the medical profession.

Dr. James Sammons, Executive Vice President of the AMA and a member of the Board of Trustees of the AMA, reviewed and approved the goals, operations, and funding of the AMA's Committee on Quackery. The work of the Committee on Quackery was often covert. In fact, the Committee emphasized the desire to keep its activities from public view. In its efforts to "fix" the 1968 HEW Report and to keep its participation secret from Congress, the Committee on Quackery wrote to an influential medical physician who was a member of the Health Benefits Advisory Council that was helping to organize the HEW study: "We will be happy to supply these [antichiropractic documents] to anyone else in HEW or elsewhere in government who might have need for them in relation to the chiropractic study. I'm sure you agree that the American Medical Association's hand must not 'show' in this matter at this stage of the proposed chiropractic study." (Dated February 20, 1968.)

As explained by the Committee on Quackery to the American Medical Association Board of Trustees in 1971:

> The Committee has not previously submitted such a report because it believes that to make public some of its activities would have been and continues to be unwise. Thus, this report is intended only for the information of the Board of Trustees. The American Medical Association actively solicited the medical specialty societies and the M.D.-dominated groups, such as the American Cancer Society, the Arthritis Foundation, the National Council of Senior Citizens, Insurance Company Trade Associations, Blue Cross/Blue Shield, etc.,—some 600 groups in all, to adopt the American Medical Association position. "We have been working for several years now to have national voluntary health organizations, medical groups and others adopt statements of policy on chiropractic to back up the one adopted by the American Medical Association House of Delegates in 1966.

The AMA policy statement was the "necessary tool" by which it carried forward and expanded its antichiropractic boycott. The AMA had ghost writers write articles for certain nationally known columnists and financed certain authors to provide antichiropractic material. As a source of health care information, the AMA filled requests for information about chiropractic with hostile material while taking aggressive steps to make certain that materials supporting the profession were suppressed.

The Committee on Quackery sent letters to medical specialty societies, medical schools, medical specialty boards, and state and county associations reminding them that medical physicians should not voluntarily associate with Doctors of Chiropractic. The AMA stated that it was unethical to refer patients to, accept patients from, consult with, teach, or in any other way professionally associate with chiropractors.

But the AMA had overreached its bounds. Its membership was less than one half of the nation's M.D.s and even its own members frequently chose to ignore the ban. In an internal memo, the AMA noted: "One of the more surprising items brought to the attention of the Committee is reported to be professional cooperation and association between Doctors of Medicine and [chiropractors]."

This dilemma caused the AMA to turn to the Joint Commission on Accreditation of Hospitals, an organization over which the AMA exercises significant control. In 1971, the AMA had the Joint Commission incorporate into the accreditation standards of the nation's hospitals the sponsored ethics boycott of chiropractors. Thereafter any association with a chiropractor carried the possible sanction of the loss of hospital privileges, which would be a professional disaster for any M.D. After that strategic move, the chiropractic boycott blanketed the country. Few medical physicians had either the where-with-all or courage to challenge the stacked array of potential sanctions available to a medical society or hospital.

Throughout the 1960s and 1970s, chiropractors developed a combative mentality. Time after time, chiropractors sought legal redress and sued medical doctors and medical organizations for libel and slander. These cases were lost because "group" defamation is not wrong under the free speech and press provisions of the First Amendment. Chiropractors tried suing under the equal protection and discrimination provisions of the Constitution and the Civil Rights laws. Again, the cases were lost because the prerequisite race, creed, color, or sex could not be asserted as generally required to invoke those protections.

Finally, in October 1976, after 4 years of campaigning by Dr. Chester Wilk of Chicago to "do something—do anything" to stop the boycott, four doctors of chiropractic, including Dr. Wilk, Dr. Michael Pedigo of San Leandro, California, Dr. Pat Arthur of Colorado, Ohio, and Hawaii, and Dr. James Bryden of Sedalia, Missouri, filed an antitrust suit against the AMA and ten other medical associations to stop the boycott. They were to finally prove successful.

THE WILK SUIT AND MEDICAL ESTABLISHMENT ENLIGHTENMENT

The primary value of the Wilk et al v. AMA et al lawsuit was the exposure of the case and the tracking of the AMA's sophisticated use of propaganda and mean-spirited actions to suppress the rival chiropractic profession. Justice could only be served in a courtroom setting, where political power is neutralized and inequalities of size are taken out of the equation. Sworn testimony replaced manufactured propaganda and secret documents became part of the public record. The antitrust suit brought a better understanding of the actual value of chiropractic.

The Wilk suit may have had the value of causing M.D.s to question the "group-think" foundation of their own professional organization and to look more kindly and inquisitively on the "new kids on the block." The suit may also have caused some M.D.s to honestly ask themselves "What do chiropractors have to offer to the 17 million Americans who elect to seek health care from doctors of chiropractic each year?"

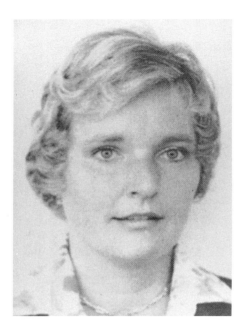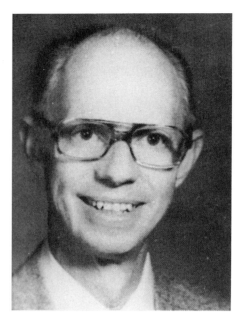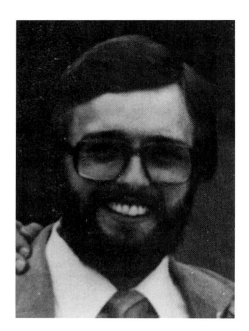

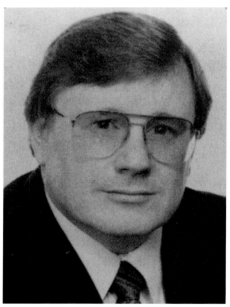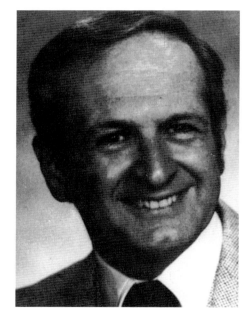

In October 1976, five chiropractors filed suit against the AMA and ten other health care associations to stop the boycott against chiropractic. Left to right (*top*), *Pat Arthur of Colorado, Ohio, and Hawaii; James Bryden of Sedalia, Missouri; Steven Lumsden of Washington; (bottom) Michael Pedigo of San Leandro, California; and Chester Wilk of Chicago.*

From *ACA Journal of Chiropractic,* November 1980.

The Fort Wayne *News-Sentinel,* on Friday, February 2, 1990, carried the following article:

> On a muggy morning in June 1989, Robert M. Centor, a prominent doctor of internal medicine from Richmond, Virginia, sat down at a congressional witness table and made a remarkable confession.
>
> When a patient comes to see him with a complaint, such as a sore throat or an aching back, Centor said he lacks the tools he needs to make a sound decision because medical science cannot tell him what kind of treatment works best for many common ailments.

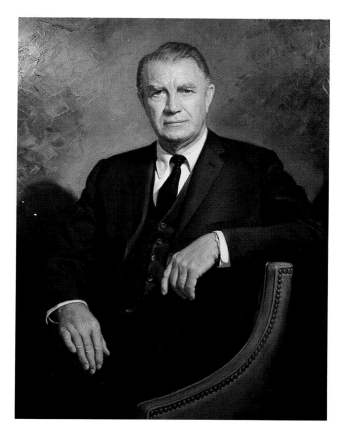

A 1966 oil portrait of David D. Palmer, 1906-1978.
Courtesy J. Anthony Wills, Houston, Tex.

"In order for me to make a good judgment, I need to have some data. And right now I don't have enough data to make that decision," said Centor, chairman of the division of general medicine and primary care at the Medical College of Virginia.

Centor's testimony—delivered on behalf of the 65,000 members of the American College of Physicians'—reflects a crisis of confidence that is just now being widely acknowledged in medicine.

With surprising candor, doctors are admitting that they are not sure what really helps their patients and what is useless or even harmful. Near the end of a century of extraordinary medical progress and generally improving health, doctors still do not always know what works. Meanwhile, doctors and surgeons continue to be plagued by doubts and disagreements about the accuracy of medical tests and diagnoses, about the value and safety of new machines and procedures, and about when, where, and how to cut, bore, and slice the human body.

"We don't know what we're doing in medicine," bluntly declared Dr. David Eddy, director of the Duke University Center for Health Policy Research, at a health-care conference in Atlanta. "The imperative for the 1990s is to fix that problem."

"The embarrassment of our ignorance about the efficacy of health-care practices is both hard for us to admit and hard for our clients to accept," Dr. Donald Berwick, vice president of the Harvard Community Health Plan, wrote in the *Journal of the American Public Health Association.*

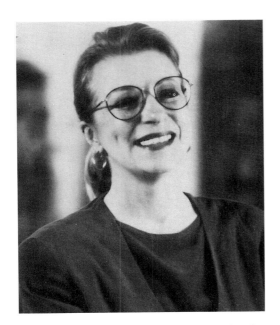

Judge Susan Getzendanner, circa 1990, who ruled that the AMA had been guilty of an illegal conspiracy against the chiropractic profession.

Courtesy Susan Getzendanner, Chicago, Illinois.

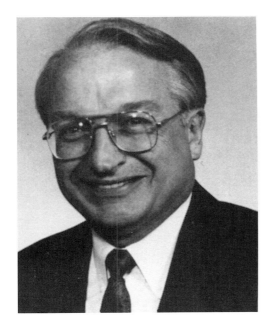

George McAndrews, the attorney representing the plaintiffs in Wilk v AMA.

Courtesy George McAndrews, Chicago, Illinois.

"It is difficult to face the disillusionment of the patients and the anger of the payers who ask: 'But how could this be? I thought you knew what you were doing.' "

Part of the evidence that much of modern medicine is still based on guesswork comes from the pioneering work of Dr. John Wennberg, a Professor of Community and Family Medicine at Dartmouth Medical School. For almost 20 years, Wennberg and his colleagues have been collecting evidence of inexplicable variations in treatment patterns between different cities, hospitals, and even different doctors, without any appreciable difference in outcome for the patient.

In view of the foregoing, there is a certain irony in US District Court Judge Susan Getzendanner's statement during the Wilk trial that the M.D.s delegated by the AMA with the task of destroying the profession of chiropractic "did not have minds open to chiropractic arguments or evidence." The Court of Appeals in affirming Judge Getzendanner found:

> But according to the court (and this is unchallenged), at the same time, there was evidence before the committee [on Quackery] that chiropractic was effective, indeed more effective than the medical profession, in treating certain kinds of problems, such as back injuries. The committee was also aware, the court found, that some medical physicians believed chiropractic could be effective and that chiropractors were better trained to deal with musculoskeletal problems than most medical physicians.

Clearly, well-intentioned medical physicians know that the medical model still leaves much to be desired. For instance, in 1967, medical educator John C. Wilson, Jr., M.D., chairman of the AMA's section on orthopedic surgery and later president of the American Academy of Orthopedic Surgeons stated that medical doctors and orthopedic surgeons were essentially ignorant of the causes or corrections of low back problems:

> When queried about the lower back a medical student soon to graduate from a far Western university revealed an enormous gap in his professional education. One instructor had given him a list of 125 causes of low back pain, from which the student had concluded that probably everyone with sciatica had a ruptured disc requiring surgery; another instructor had delivered a one-hour lecture on anterior interbody fusion. This young man, well informed concerning the cause and treatment of cardiac arrhythmias, electrolyte unbalance, and alterations in the DNA chain, displayed a disturbing ignorance of the cause and treatment of low back and sciatic pain—one of mankind's most common afflictions.
>
> The teaching in our medical schools of the etiology, natural history, and treatment of low back pain is inconsistent and less than minimal. The student may or may not have heard a lecture on the subject, he may have been instructed solely by a neurosurgeon, or the curriculum committee may have decided that clinical lectures are "out" and more basic sciences "in." The orthopedic surgeon, to his distress, often sees his hours in the curriculum pared to the barest minimum.
>
> A survey of orthopedic residents graduating from an approved program in a large urban area disclosed several alarming deficiencies in their training. Residents know very little about the natural history of degenerative disk disease in the lower part of the spine. The importance of the physician personally taking an accurate, detailed patient history had escaped them. They were too unsure of the technique of careful lumbar spine examination to include a search for early stages of neurologic deficit. They had too often been satisfied with interpretations of technically inferior x-rays, and their insufficient knowledge of diagnostic aids seldom permitted them to select the one most helpful in accurately establishing the level of a lesion. Residents knew least when to use a particular surgical procedure.
>
> At the postgraduate level, symposia and courses concerning the

cause and treatment of low back and sciatic pain are often ineffective because of prejudices and controversy.*

In a 1967 article from *JAMA*, "Low Back Pain and Sciatica," a doctor's incomplete information and understanding can lead to the following concerns:

1. Patients operated on after inadequate evaluations.
2. Reliance by physicians on poor quality x-ray films.
3. Surgery done only because of an abnormality in a myelogram without reference to plain films of the lower spine.
4. Exploratory surgery on the lower back done without sufficient clinical basis.
5. Extensive surgery done for solely subjective complaints.
6. Repeated attempts at spinal fusion—sometimes six or eight—by surgeons of limited experience.
7. Surgery authorized by industrial accident commissions comprised exclusively of laymen.
8. Extensive removal of posterior vertebral elements by neurosurgeons, making stabilization of the lower portion of the spine technically difficult if not impossible.

After the publication of Dr. Wilson's 1967 findings, the AMA adopted an informational concealment program, a program repeated many times over the years as it sought to destroy the credibility of any of chiropractic's known health care benefits.

The AMA wrote the following letter to Dr. Wilson:

Dear Doctor Wilson:

David B. Stevens, M.D., of Lexington, Kentucky, informed me of his recent conversation with you concerning the possibility of chiropractors quoting out of context items from your paper, "Low Back Pain and Sciatica," that appeared in *JAMA*, May 22, 1967.

With this in mind, you might consider writing a brief "Letter to the Editor" of *JAMA* to the effect that your article should in no way be construed as an endorsement of chiropractic, and perhaps point out why in your opinion chiropractic adjustments are contraindicated for low back pain and sciatica as well as being potentially harmful. Maybe you are aware of a case involving a chiropractor about which you have personal knowledge that resulted in harm to the patient, and which you might like to recount.

Dr. Wilson reacted as a thoughtful, open-minded scientist when he responded to the AMA's politically motivated request. He was not ready to condemn chiropractic:

I read your letter of September 6, 1967, very carefully and I regret that I am not able to comply with your request. The article which was written by me and which appeared in the American Medical Association on May 22, 1967, will, I believe, stand on its own merits. Should a chiropractor quote from my article without permission, I shall be pleased to take him to task. So far as I know, no such instance has as yet arisen, and I am not at this time desirous of engaging in an interchange with the chiropractor as to whether manipulative therapy is harmful or not.

In view of a number of recent studies regarding chiropractic's health care regimen for low back pain, it is traditional medical care that is being challenged today as the most appropriate approach for low back pain

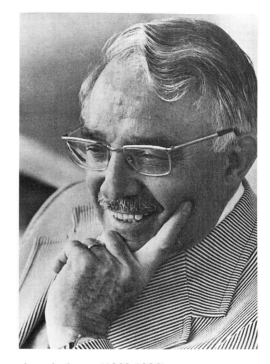

Joseph Janse (1909-1986).
Courtesy National College of Chiropractic, Lombard, Illinois.

During the AMA antitrust suit, the trial court also found that even the AMA's economic witness, Mr. Lynk, assumed that chiropractors outperformed medical physicians in the treatment of certain conditions and believed that was a reasonable assumption.

care. Chiropractic care is being scientifically established as the most suitable while the chiropractic profession is also validating scientifically its-value for a host of other health care problems.

As subsequent studies have shown, Dr. Wilson's caution was valid, as noted in the scientific conferences and reports published over the past 20 plus years. Not long before the Wilson exchange, in 1966, the AMA was informed by one of its trustees, a noted orthopedic surgeon and professor at the University of Colorado College of Medicine, Dr. Irvin Hendryson, that he had conducted a private, randomized test of chiropractic on Guadalcanal in World War II. His orderly was a chiropractor, and Dr. Hendryson praised the chiropractor's skills and the results obtained. Then, in the report cover letter to the AMA, Dr. Hendryson wrote specifically about chiropractic, back pain, manipulation, and pregnant women:

> As a final note in this regard, I must cite two cases which I think are of clinical significance. The first is that of an All-American football player who was "down on his back." This man was definitely not in the psychosomatic class nor was he neurotic. He was a commanding officer in an engineer battalion on Guadalcanal and about as tough a man as I have ever seen in my life. However, in reaching over to pick something out of his footlocker, his back "went out." Being the type of individual he was, he preferred to perform duty with the help of the medication given by his battalion medical officer but finally reached the place where he was completely incapacitated. Finally, he was sent to us and fell into the class of the next case for manipulation and after the routine million dollar roll, the osteopathic roll, the chiropractic punch and the osteopathic leg length maneuvers, this man was able to get off the table and say, "This is the best I've felt in days." I was impressed by this case and I still am. Granted, had he sought more competent medical attention early in the phase of his complaint, he may well have been ready to return to duty at the end of ten days. However, this was impressive.

> The second case, and one that I am not really at liberty to report objectively because it has to do with my own life, and yet I have heard from my friend in obstetrics and also in recent years in practice. However, it is commonly known that in the third trimester of pregnancy, unrelenting back pain is one of the prices that is paid for perpetuation of the race. I have learned from personal experience that general manipulations of backs in this particular condition has given these women a great deal of physical relief and has permitted them to go on to term and deliver without having to be bedfast during the latter term of this pregnancy.

> I would not for an instant indicate that it is manipulation alone that permits these women to go on and carry on normally for at the present time we are giving them manipulation to relieve them of their acute symptoms and also fitting them with support which is a well recognized medical practice. However, I must say that I am impressed by the many cases who are able to go on to term, to manage their households, to lead a comparatively comfortable third trimester without having to be hospitalized for traction, heat, support and all the rest of it.

> In spite of the fact that there are many more questions that I could raise as well as other analysts in this matter, I must say quite honestly that there are still aspects of the manipulative therapy itself which impress me and which I feel practicing clinicians should be using in the management of low back pain. Whether there is value in chiropractic or not, I am not prepared to say. However, I would also agree, as will you, that it has prospered through the years and it is a difficult thing to quarrel with success.

The Hendryson report was suppressed by the AMA because it was feared that it might be deemed by the public as favorable to chiropractic. It was brought to light only during the Wilk case. In the meantime, the public continued to be bombarded by the AMA with propaganda declaring that chiropractic was a menace to the population at large.

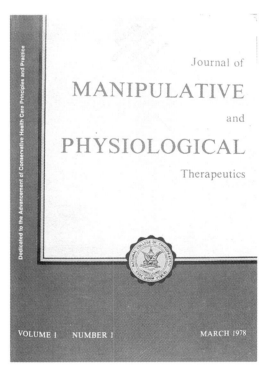

National College of Chiropractic's Journal of Manipulative and Physiological Therapeutics, begun in 1978, was the first chiropractic journal indexed in the Index Medicus.

From *Journal of Manipulative and Physiological Therapeutics,* March 1978.

Then, in 1972, the AMA learned of a study by Roland A. Martin, M.D., medical director of the Oregon Workmen's Compensation Board. The study suggested a two-to-one advantage of chiropractic care over medical care for comparable industrial injuries. Dr. Martin wrote:

Examining the forms of conservative therapy the majority received, it is interesting to note the results of those treated by chiropractic physicians.

A total of 29 claimants were treated by no other physician than a chiropractor. Of these workers, 82% resumed work after one week of time loss. Claims were closed without a disability award.

Their Examining claims treated by the M.D., in which the diagnosis seems comparable to the type of injury suffered by the workmen treated by the chiropractor, 41 percent of these workmen resumed work after one week of time loss.

Again, the AMA prevented the results of the study from being widely disseminated or used to the advantage of Doctors of Chiropractic or their patients. The AMA contacted Dr. Martin as they had Dr. Wilson. Dr. Martin then took steps to downplay his report:

I am writing you following contact with me by Mr. William J. Monaghan, Staff Associate of the American Medical Association. This pertains to some information published quoting portions of *A Study of Time Loss Back Claims* which I did more than one year ago.

I included this information in this report for two basic purposes only: one, I knew if I buried this tidbit in the body of the report, that if an M.D. read the report it would spark a comment to me and that if he did not make a comment, in all probability he did not read the report; secondly, I put it in hoping it might spark some interest by all of us to initiate a review of the treatment of back injuries with the thought in mind that perhaps there may be other and better methods found for the treatment of the patient with an injured back. As you are probably aware, the care and result of the care of workmen suffering back injuries is a continuing problem in workmen's compensation and those of us deeply involved in workmen's compensation affairs today are not necessarily satisfied with what we see happening to people once they have injured their backs.

If I can help you in any other matter, please contact me.

It is unfortunate that the discoverer of facts that could benefit millions of suffering people and possibly cut in half the societal and economic cost of the malady was importuned to apologize for his findings.

Another study of chiropractic's benefits was published in 1975 by C. Richard Wolf, M.D. Dr. Wolf published the results of his 1972 study of 629 workmen's compensation cases in California. The results almost tracked those from the Oregon study particularly the two-to-one ratio of chiropractic care over that of medical care of comparable industrial accidents:

Average lost time per employee: 32 days in the M.D. treated group, 15.6 days in the chiropractor treated group.

Employees reporting no lost time: 21% in the M.D. treated group, 47.9% in the chiropractor treated group.

Employees reporting lost time in excess of 60 days: 13.2% percent in the M.D. treated group, 6.7% in the chiropractor treated group.

Again no mention of this report appeared outside of chiropractic publications. The AMA, acting like a trade association, felt that it could not live with any facts that either called into question the education, background, or training of medical physicians or worse yet, any facts which may be seen to exalt the education, background, and training of Doctors of Chiropractic.

By 1979, a Royal Commission of Inquiry on Chiropractic in New Zealand, following an in-depth study, concluded:

34. The Commission has found it established beyond any reasonable degree of doubt that chiropractors have a more thorough training in

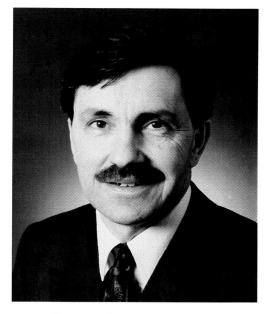

David Chapman-Smith, who represented chiropractors in the hearings of the 1979 Royal Commission of Inquiry on Chiropractic in New Zealand. The Commission concluded that chiropractors have a more thorough training in spinal mechanics and manual therapy than any other health professional.
Courtesy David Chapman-Smith, Toronto, Ont.

spinal mechanics and spinal manual therapy than any other health professional. It would therefore be astonishing to contemplate that a chiropractor, in those areas of expertise, should be subject to the directions of a medical practitioner who is largely ignorant of those matters simply because he has had no training in them.

79. Dr. Haldeman, in the course of his evidence, said that 12 months full-time training in spinal manipulative therapy following a medical degree would be appropriate.

The abstract of a government sponsored study, printed in the June 2, 1990 issue of the *British Medical Journal,* gives a good summary of the extensive, prospective study entitled "Low Back Pain of Mechanical Origin: Randomized Comparison of Chiropractic and Hospital Outpatient Treatment:"

Objective—To compare chiropractic and hospital outpatient treatment for managing low back pain of mechanical origin.

Design—Randomized controlled trial. Allocation to chiropractic or hospital management by minimisation to establish groups for analysis of results according to initial referral clinic, length of current episode, history, and severity of back pain. Patients were followed up for up to two years.

Setting—Chiropractic and hospital outpatient clinics in 11 centers.

Patients—741 Patients aged 18-65 who had no contraindications to manipulation and who had not been treated within the past month.

Interventions—Treatment at the discretion of the chiropractors, who used chiropractic manipulation in most patients, or of the hospital staff, who most commonly used Maitland mobilization or manipulation, or both.

Main outcome measures—Changes in the score on the Oswestry pain disability questionnaire and in the results of tests of straight leg raising and lumbar flexion.

Results—Chiropractor treatment was more effective than hospital outpatient management, mainly for patients with chronic or severe back pain. A benefit of about 7 percent points on the Oswestry scale was seen at two years. The benefit of chiropractic treatment became more evident throughout the follow up period. Secondary outcome measures also showed that chiropractic was more beneficial.

Conclusions—For patients with low back pain in whom manipulation is not contraindicated chiropractic almost certainly confers worthwhile, long term benefit in comparison with hospital outpatient management. The benefit is seen mainly in those with chronic or severe pain. Introducing chiropractic into NHS practice should be considered.

The rest of this complex study is what is so intriguing. Under "Economic Implications" the authors write:

The potential economic, resource, and policy implications of our results are extensive. The average cost of chiropractic investigation and treatment at 1989 prices was $273.90 per patient compared with $184.26 for hospital treatment. Some 300,000 patients are referred to hospital for back pain each year, "of whom about 72,000 would be expected to have no contraindications to manipulation." If all these patients were referred for chiropractic instead of hospital treatment the annual cost would be about $6,640,000. Our results suggest that there might be a reduction of some 290,000 days in sickness absence during two years, saving about $21,580,000 in output and $4,814,000 in social security payments. As it was not clear, however, that the improvement in those treated by chiropractic was related to the number of treatments, the cost of essential chiropractic treatment might be substantially less than $6,640,000. The possibility that patients treated in hospital would need more treatment during the second year than those treated by chiropractic also has to be borne in mind. There is, therefore, economic support for use of chiropractic in low back pain, though the obvious clinical improvement in pain and disability attributable to chiropractic treatment is in itself an adequate reason for considering the use of chiropractic.

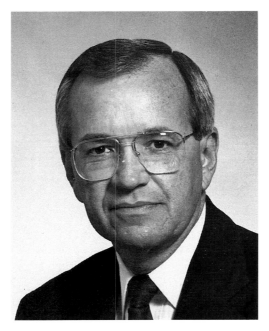

Michael Crawford, Chancellor, Palmer Chiropractic University, circa 1993.

Courtesy Palmer Chiropractic University, Davenport, Iowa.

Please note the fact that even though the "direct" payment to the chiropractor exceeds the direct payment for the hospital outpatient care, the researchers conclude that chiropractic care results in enormous cost savings to the system.

Dr. Tom Meade, the United Kingdom medical physician and researcher who directed the above study, was questioned about its implications:

> Well, how much better did you find chiropractic to be?
>
> We found it a lot better. I can illustrate it by saying that the improvement in the patients who were treated by chiropractors was between three quarters and twice as great as it was for the patients who had been treated in hospital. I can illustrate it in various other ways, for example, patients who had been treated by a chiropractor would not have very much pain, they would be able to lift weights, and they would not have very much pain, and they would be able to sit for as long as they wanted to. Whereas an average patient who had been treated in hospital would still have quite moderate and possibly severe pain, wouldn't be able to do much in the way of lifting weights, and would probably only be able to sit for twenty minutes or half an hour before having to get up and stretch and change position - - so it is quite a big difference.
>
> For how long did you follow these patients?
>
> We have followed patients now for up to three years since they came into the trial, which is two and a half years since they had their treatment, and one of the most unexpected findings was that the treatment difference "the benefit of chiropractic over hospital treatment" actually persists for the whole of that three year period. That was very unexpected but it looks as though the treatment that the chiropractors give does something that results in a very long term benefit.
>
> So, as far as low back pain treatment is concerned, Dr. Meade, you found really a clear cut advantage to chiropractic over hospital?
>
> Yes, this was not a marginal difference at all, it was a very big—a very important—difference.

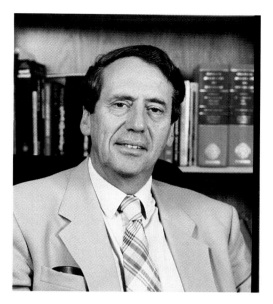

Tom Meade, a medical researcher, found chiropractic care to be more effective and less costly in his study of low back pain.
Courtesy Tom Meade, Harrow, Middlesex, England.

The AMA had been formally alerted to this phenomena by Dr. Hendryson in 1966. It is possible the AMA overall was ignorant of the millions of anecdotal reports by patients who had benefited from chiropractic care from 1895 through 1966. Yet, it appears the AMA chose to remain "ignorant" rather than question its own members' inappropriate education and training in the area of musculoskeletal maladies and related disorders.

Other chiropractic efficacy studies have followed. Most of them were favorable to the profession of chiropractic. It came as no surprise then, when in August 1993, the Manga Study, funded solely by the Ministry of Health of the Government of Ontario, was released. Its findings include:

> FINDINGS
>
> F1. On the evidence, particularly the most scientifically valid clinical studies, spinal manipulation applied by chiropractors is shown to be more effective than alternative treatments for LBP (low back pain). Many medical therapies are of questionable validity or are clearly inadequate.
>
> F2. There is no clinical or case-control study that demonstrates or even implies that chiropractic spinal manipulation is unsafe in the treatment of low-back pain. Some medical treatments are equally safe, but others are unsafe and generate iatrogenic complications for LBP patients. Our reading of the literature suggests that chiropractic manipulation is safer than medical management of low-back pain.
>
> F3. While it is prudent to call for even further clinical evidence of the effectiveness and efficacy of chiropractic management of LBP, what the literature revealed to us is the much greater need for clinical evidence of the validity of medical management of LBP. Indeed, several existing medical therapies of LBP are generally contraindicated on the basis of the existing clinical trials. There is also some evidence in the literature

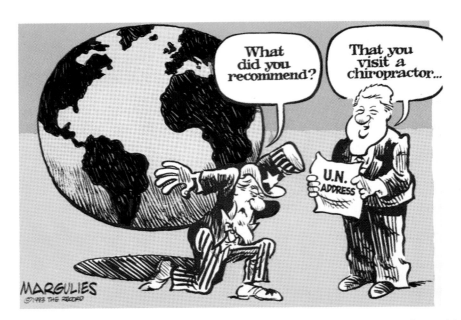

In this 1993 cartoon by Jimmy Margulies, President Clinton is prescribing chiropractic care for an overburdened "Uncle Sam."

From *The Record*, Hackensack, NJ.

to suggest that spinal manipulations are less safe and less effective when performed by non-chiropractic professionals.

F4. There is an overwhelming body of evidence indicating that chiropractic management of low-back pain is more cost-effective than medical management. We reviewed numerous studies that range from very persuasive to convincing in support of this conclusion. The lack of any convincing argument or evidence to the contrary must be noted and is significant to us in forming our conclusions and recommendations. The evidence includes studies showing lower chiropractic costs for the same diagnosis and episodic need for care.

F5. There would be highly significant cost savings if more management of LBP was transferred from physicians to chiropractors. Evidence from Canada and other countries suggests potential savings of many hundreds of millions annually. The literature clearly and consistently shows that the major savings from chiropractic management come from fewer and lower costs of auxiliary services, much fewer hospitalizations, and a highly significant reduction in chronic problems, as well as in levels and duration of disability. Workers' compensation studies report that injured workers with the same specific diagnosis of LBP returned to work much sooner when treated by chiropractors than by physicians. This leads to very significant reductions in direct and indirect costs.

F6. There is good empirical evidence that patients are very satisfied with chiropractic management of LBP and considerably less satisfied with physician management. Patient satisfaction is an important health outcome indicator and adds further weight to the clinical and health economic results favouring chiropractic management of LBP.

F7. Despite official medical disapproval and economic disincentive to patients (higher private out-of-pocket cost), the use of chiropractic has grown steadily over the years. Chiropractors are now accepted as a legitimate healing profession by the public and an increasing number of physicians.

F8. In our view, the constellation of the evidence of:

(a) the effectiveness and cost-effectiveness of chiropractic management of low-back pain.

(b) the economic efficiency of chiropractic care for low-back pain compared with medical care.

(c) the economic efficiency of chiropractic care for low-back pain compared with medical care.

(d) the safety of chiropractic care.

(e) the higher satisfaction levels expressed by patients of chiropractors, together offer an overwhelming case in favour of much greater use of chiropractic services in the management of low-back pain.

SCIENTIFIC CONFERENCES AND REPORTS

The past 20 years has seen the energetic development of chiropractic research and the beginning of what are now annual interdisciplinary scientific conferences. One of the first real breakthroughs for these scientific conferences was in 1975 when the National Institutes of Health and the Institute of Neurological Diseases and Stroke sponsored a Workshop on the State of the Art of Spinal Manipulative Therapy. The conference came about as result of a $2 million line-item in Congressional legislation directed toward "research on chiropractic and research performed by doctors of chiropractic." This conference was extremely successful precisely because it did not firmly establish the scientific basis of chiropractic adjustments. This conference *instead* laid the groundwork for further research on the understanding of manipulative therapy.

First Interdisciplinary Scientific Conference on the Spine

The first interdisciplinary scientific conference on the spine was held in 1978. No American M.D.s participated in this conference. However, M.D.s from Canada, Australia, and Western Europe presented papers.

From this, a number of governmental studies have been performed, primarily from the British Commonwealth. One of the first was a positive study relating to the education and practice of chiropractic. This study by the Royal Commission of Inquiry on Chiropractic in New Zealand, published in 1979, had a tremendous impact.

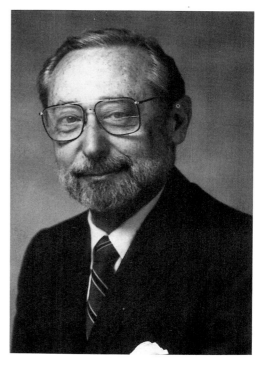

Murry Goldstein, Associate Director of the NINCDS, organized and chaired the 1975 landmark interdisciplinary conference on spinal manipulative therapy in Bethesda, Md.

Courtesy Murry Goldstein, Washington, DC.

Rand Study

Many of the studies done in the United States have dealt with the evaluation of worker's compensation claims in various states, including Oregon, Utah, California, and Iowa. During 1990, the American Chiropractic Association, the National Chiropractic Mutual Insurance Company, and the Consortium for Chiropractic Research working through the Foundation for Chiropractic Education and Research (FCER) funded the establishment of a multidisciplinary expert panel to be managed by the RAND Corporation. The deliberations of this panel led to the conclusion that spinal manipulation is an appropriate treatment for certain types of low back pain. A literature review showed that doctors of chiropractic provide 94% of spinal manipulations.

While the RAND report was conducted and compiled in the United States, another study was being carried out by the Ontario Ministry of Health. The Manga study, "A Study To Examine The Effectiveness and Cost Effectiveness of Chiropractic Management of Low-Back Pain" was released in August 1993.

Another recent panel report was completed in 1993. This panel was convened for the development and profession-wide dissemination of practice guidelines, which were published as *Guidelines for Chiropractic Quality Assurance and Practice Parameters* (1993). These were the first-ever guidelines for chiropractic practice in its 100-year history. They resulted from a 2-year-long effort by 35 participants, working in a consensus mode, who represented all significant elements of the profession in the United States and Canada. They have since been endorsed by the Federation of State Chiropractic Licensing Boards, the American Chiropractic Association, and others. The effort was initiated by the Congress of Chiropractic State Associations in 1992-1993. Periodic updating and refine-

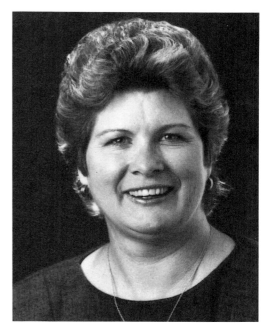

Jerilynn Kaibel, a Cleveland Chiropractic College graduate from San Bernadino, Calif, was the only chiropractor appointed to the Health Professional Review Group, a 47-member multidisciplinary health panel formed in 1993 to review the Clinton administration's health care reform package.

Courtesy Jerilynn Kaibel, San Bernadino, Calif.

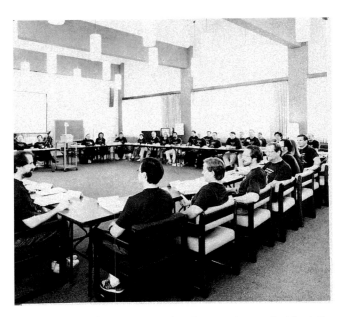

The process of consensus development was held at the Mercy Conference Center in Burlingame, California January 25-30, 1992. Private practitioners, representatives of chiropractic colleges, and representatives of national and state chiropractic associations developed the guidelines.

From *Journal of Chiropractic,* October 1992.

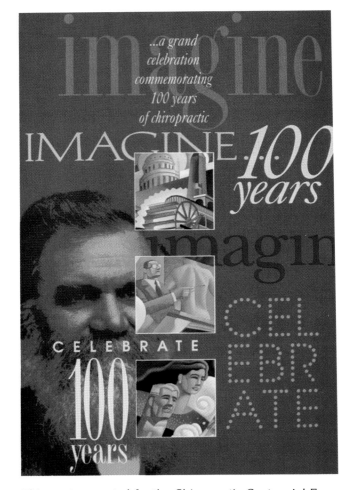

This poster, created for the Chiropractic Centennial Foundation in 1992, conveys the mood of celebration within the chiropractic profession as it approached its one-hundredth anniversary.

Courtesy Chiropractic Centennial Foundation, Davenport, Iowa.

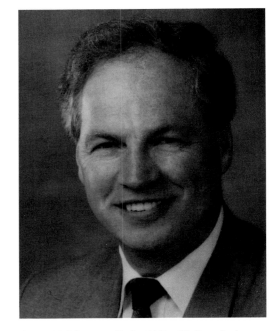

Scott Haldeman, D.C., M.D., Ph.D., chairman of the Commission for the Establishment of Guidelines for Chiropractic Quality Assurance and Practice Parameters. The process resulted in the first-ever guidelines for chiropractic practice developed by a cross-segment of the profession.

Courtesy Scott Haldeman, Santa Ana, Calif.

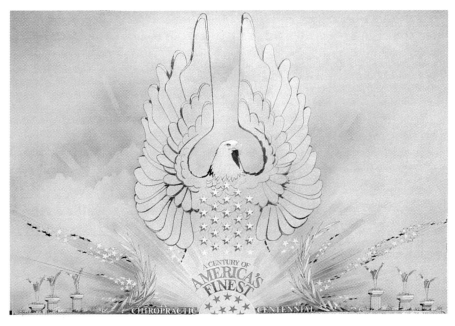

An artist's sketch of the Rose Parade float sponsored by the Chiropractic Centennial Foundation, to be built for the 1995 Rose Parade in Pasadena, Calif.

Courtesy Fiesta, Pasadena, Calif.

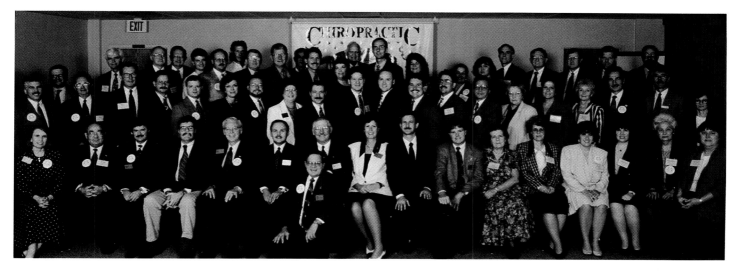

Chiropractic Centennial Foundation Constituency Meeting, September 18, 1993, Davenport, Iowa. Representatives of the Chiropractic Centennial Foundation's members, comprised of the ACA, ICA, Association for the History of Chiropractic, National Board of Chiropractic Examiners, World Federation of Chiropractic, Association of Chiropractic Colleges, 17 chiropractic colleges, 9 country associations, and 52 state associations met to plan the celebration of the 100th anniversary of chiropractic.

Courtesy Chiropractic Centennial Foundation, Davenport, Iowa.

ment in view of field experience and research is a part of the process of keeping the guidelines current.

RENAISSANCE: PERSEVERANCE

Through self-sacrifice, patient demand, and growing interprofessional acceptance, chiropractic's direction is toward scientifically validating its claim to effectiveness and efficiency in treating the host of ailments afflicting the human condition, particularly but not exclusively those that are believed to be responsive to the condition of the neuromusculoskeletal system.

Tens of thousands of chiropractors, long since gone, and tens of thousands of their successors have and are persevering. Their legacy is the improved well-being of countless patients—a quantum leap in the quality of life of those whom they serve. Progress demands challenge, change, personal growth, and making the education and skills of the members of the profession available to people around the globe.

The federal court's finding that the AMA's conduct was illegal did not say it all. The conduct was malicious and deeply detrimental to the health care of millions. It hurt the chiropractic profession, but more important, it hurt uninformed medical physicians and the patients of both professions.

Finally, if the renaissance of the past 30 years is to continue, progress will continue to demand perseverance. "See first that the design is wise and just; that ascertained, pursue it resolutely; do not for one repulse forego the purpose that you resolved to effect."—Shakespeare.

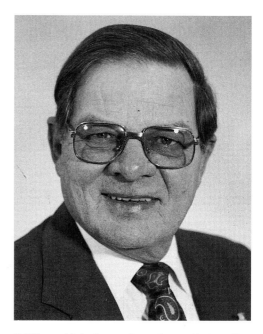

William Holmberg, President of the Chiropractic Centennial Foundation and Chairman of the Anti-trust Fund-raising Committee, which raised the funds for the legal expenses incurred in the lawsuit Wilk et al v. AMA et al.

Courtesy Chiropractic Centennial Foundation, Davenport, Iowa.

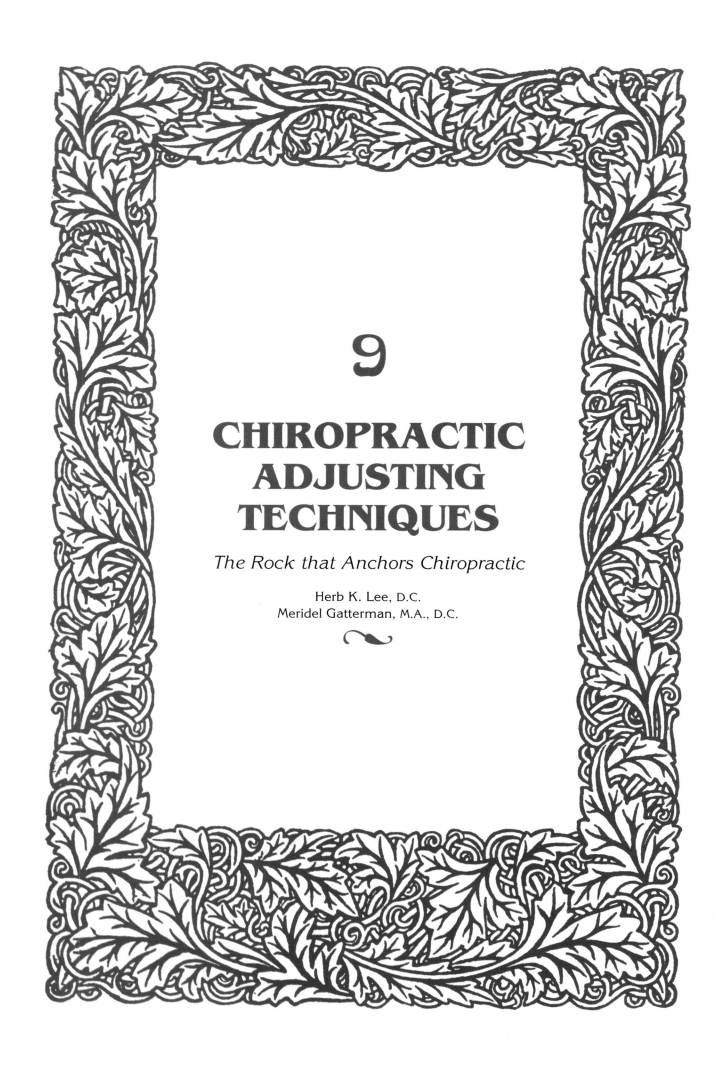

9

CHIROPRACTIC ADJUSTING TECHNIQUES

The Rock that Anchors Chiropractic

Herb K. Lee, D.C.
Meridel Gatterman, M.A., D.C.

The first application of chiropractic technique was performed by D.D. Palmer on September 18, 1895. From 1887 to that time, D.D. had been practicing as a magnetic healer in Davenport, Iowa. Palmer's approach to treating patients included direct contact at the site of complaint; there is speculation that this approach was a form of reflex technique. Harvey Lillard, the first chiropractic patient, was the janitor in the Ryan building where Palmer's practice was located. Lillard had told D.D. that one day as he bent over in a stooped position while working, he had felt something give way in his back and he became deaf almost immediately. According to Palmer, Lillard was so deaf for 17 years that he could not hear the racket of a wagon on the street or the ticking of a watch held close to his ear. The technique performed involved a "thrust," which D.D. described as: "I racked it into position by using the spinous process as a lever and soon the man could hear as before." Reflecting on this, Palmer became more emphatic after his second chiropractic case, stating:

> Shortly after this relief from deafness, I had a case of heart trouble which was not improving. I examined the spine and found a displaced vertebra pressing against the nerves which innervate the heart. I adjusted the vertebra and gave immediate relief.

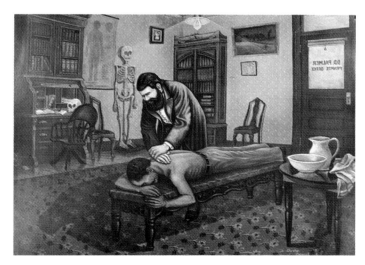

A watercolor rendition of the first Adjustment by C. & T. Paciorek, circa 1959.

Courtesy Chiropractic Chart Publications, Niagara Falls, New York.

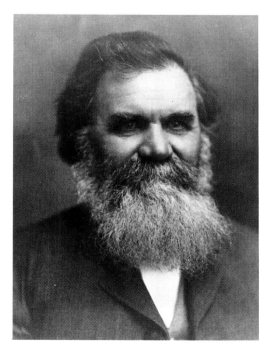

D.D. Palmer, the Founder of Chiropractic, 1909.

Courtesy Palmer College of Chiropractic Archives, Davenport, Iowa.

From these two cases Palmer reasoned that if two diseases, so dissimilar as deafness and heart trouble came from impingement, or pressure on nerves, perhaps other conditions were due to a similar cause? From this he began a systematic investigation for the cause of other diseases.

Palmer did not limit the application of chiropractic technique to the spine alone, having reduced the dislocated ankle of the daughter of the Reverend Samuel Weed. After the initial treatment she was able to walk home carrying her crutches. Weed, a scholar of the Greek language supplied Palmer with the terms *cheir* and *praktos* from which the term *chiropractic,* meaning done by hand, is derived. ∾

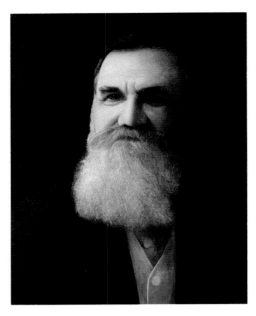

An oil portrait of Daniel David Palmer, artist and date unknown.

TEACHING CHIROPRACTIC TECHNIQUE

D.D. originally was quite secretive about his discovery, fearing others would steal it from him and become competitors. Heavy drapes covered the windows to prevent others from observing his palpations and hand treatments as D.D. called his early technique. Originally he may have been emulating the bonesetters who sought to keep their art a family secret to be passed on to the next generation. David D. Palmer, D.D.'s grandson relates a story told him by his father that:

> In D.D.'s treatment room there used to hang a long mirror which was used to see the patient's facial expressions during the adjustive thrust. The patient's face was always carefully kept turned away so he could not see the adjustment . . . If it was necessary for the patient to face the mirror, D.D. stood between the patient and the mirror.

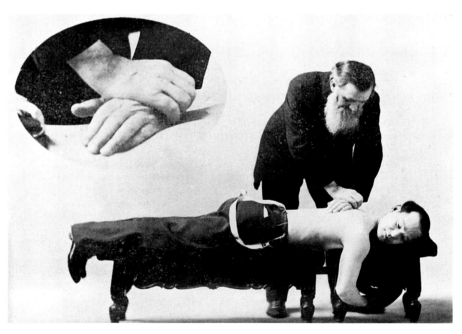

D.D. Palmer demonstrating the proper position and specific contact for correcting subluxation of lumbar vertebrae.

From Palmer DD, Palmer BJ: *The science of chiropractic: its principles and adjustments,* Davenport, Iowa, 1906, Palmer School of Chiropractic.

This became a bother after a time. One day, D.D. forgot his customary precaution. He noticed the patient carefully studying him. D.D. took the mirror from the wall and broke it into a thousand pieces. After that no mirror was allowed in the treatment room. In 1897 an incident occurred that D.D. recounted in *The Adjuster* causing him to change his mind: "Two years after the first adjustment was given I came near being killed at Clinton Junction, Ill. I then determined to teach the science and art to some one as fast as it was unfolded."

With that change of heart, D.D. opened the Palmer School and Infirmary of Chiropractic in 1897 and began teaching specific chiropractic adjusting with enrollment of the first student in 1898. D.D.'s reservations proved prophetic when many of the early graduates of this school immediately on completion of the program in a few weeks or months opened small schools elsewhere. Building on the Founder's theories and techniques, many of the early followers of D.D. became openly competitive. Notable among these are Solon Langworthy (a 1901 graduate), who with Oakley Smith (1899) and Minora Paxson (1899) opened the American School of Chiropractic at Cedar Rapids, Iowa. Authoring the first chiropractic textbook in 1906 called *Modernized Chiropractic,* Smith, Langworthy, and Paxson devoted close to 300 pages of the second volume to chiropractic technique. These authors promoted diagnosis of subluxations through movement analysis and hyperesthetic analysis in addition to Palmer's palpation for alignment. Langworthy refined chiropractic tables and developed and patented the Amplia-thrill, a traction table in 1904. Considerable specificity of contact and direction of thrust is described and illustrated in addition to the emphasis on traction. Adjustments were not confined to the spine with techniques for the extremities also precisely described.

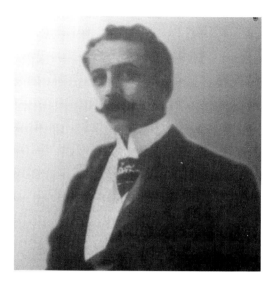

Solon Langworthy, a 1901 graduate of PSC, opened a competing school, The American School of Chiropractic, in nearby Cedar Rapids, Iowa in 1903.

Courtesy Palmer College of Chiropractic Archives, Davenport, Iowa.

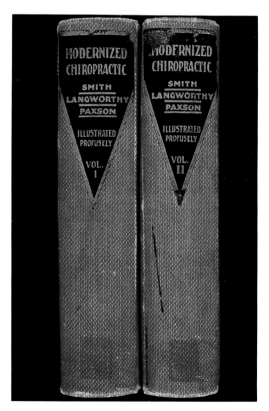

The first textbook of chiropractic, Modernized Chiropractic, published in 1906 by Solon Langworthy and two of his faculty, Oakley Smith and Minora Paxson.

Courtesy Palmer College of Chiropractic Archives, Davenport, Iowa.

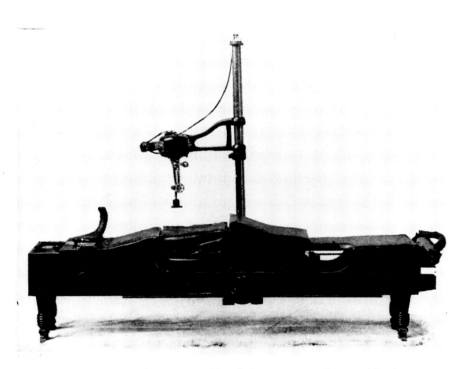

A traction adjusting table patented by Solon Langworthy in 1904, known as the Amplia-thrill.

From Smith O, Langworthy S, Paxson M: *Modernized chiropractic,* Cedar Rapids, Iowa, 1906, S.M. Langworthy.

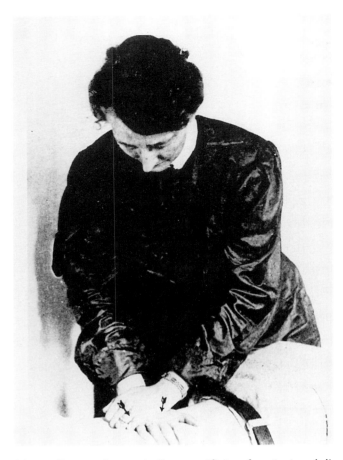

Minora Paxson demonstrating specificity of contact and direction of thrust for correction of lumbar subluxation.

From Smith O, Langworthy S, Paxson M: *Modernized chiropractic,* Cedar Rapids, Iowa, 1906, S.M. Langworthy.

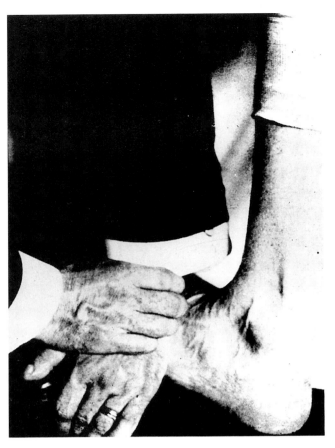

A contact for a cuboid adjustment.

From Smith O, Langworthy S, Paxson M: *Modernized chiropractic,* Cedar Rapids, Iowa, 1906, S.M. Langworthy.

Like pre-Flexner medical schools, numerous proprietary chiropractic institutions sprang up all over the country, many being short-lived. A number of early teachers of chiropractic technique entered into lively debate with D.D., including Willard Carver, Alva Gregory, Joy Loban, and A.P Davis.

Willard Carver: The Adjuster

Willard Carver, referred to as The Adjuster, was at variance with D.D. in his methods of instruction in the principles and practice of chiropractic and in his approach to chiropractic technique. Carver, an attorney and originally a patient of D.D's, graduated from the Parker College of Chiropractic located in Ottumwa, Iowa. Having offered free legal advice to D.D. in exchange for tuition, when turned down, Carver sought training from Parker. On graduation he opened a school of his own in Oklahoma City. Parker, who originally associated with Langworthy, later opened a school in his own name that closed 3 years later.

Carver applied chiropractic technique to all of the more than 300 joints of the human body. He stated that a subluxation is a "disrelationship or simple displacement that must be isolated, recognized, and pointed out by palpation." He theorized that the etiology of the subluxation was injury to the holding elements of the articulations. Philosophically he viewed chiropractic as "the science of relatology or the art of securing relations." Chiropractic technique therefore aimed to "relate distorted parts of the human organism with the only purpose of relating vertebrae to remove interference with the transmission of nerve stimulus."

Promoting the "Tracto-Thrust" system of chiropractic technique, Carver stressed traction followed by the thrust. He taught:

> The hand must be placed on the tissues in a gentle manner so as to prevent irritation, contraction and tension. It must be placed firmly to eliminate the possibility of slipping on the skin. The hand should not be allowed to slip on the skin: neither should the skin be permitted to slip on the muscles, or the bones to which they are attached.
>
> When the condition of the tissues, to be influenced by the thrust, has been determined and the direction of the thrust established, the hand should be placed over the area of contact and pressure applied slowly to test tissue resistance and the position of the application hand. When by test it is found that the application of the hand and the direction of the thrust are in a fixed and well determined line, pressure should be gently applied until all superficial resistance is removed, then a short quick, measured thrust is made, and stopped, before the tissues have had time to contract and become tense and resistant.

Also a proponent of correcting spinal distortions, Carver viewed the vertebral column as "the axis of the body around which the body of the vertebrae are so constructed as to form a base, around, over, and through which other structures may attach."

Studying the human body as a machine, Carver describes the spine as "a foundation for levers, pulleys, ropes and guys that sustain movement and hold other structures together in relative positions." In addition to procedures for adjusting spinal and peripheral joints, Carver developed techniques for treating muscles, fascia, ligaments, and visceral organs.

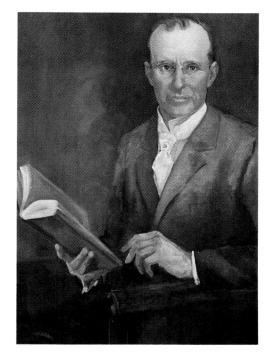

Willard Carver, an attorney turned chiropractor, promoted the "Tracto-Thrust" system of chiropractic, or traction followed by a thrust.
Courtesy Texas College of Chiropractic, Pasadena. Texas.

Alva Gregory

Alva Gregory, a medical doctor before studying chiropractic, formed a partnership with D.D. in 1907 and opened the Palmer - Gregory School of Chiropractic in Oklahoma City. In competition with Carver, the day Palmer was to lecture at the Carver school he joined forces with Gregory instead. Like many of D.D.'s ventures the Gregory association was short lived and after 3 months the affiliation ended.

In his 1919 book, *Spinal Treatment,* Gregory also emphasized adjustment under tension. He noted:

> In making an adjustment, observe the rule to always tighten the hand against the part to be adjusted, because if you slacken, or if you are not against the process before adjusting, you will usually fail to get the adjustment. After the quick application of force, get your hand away immediately, so as to permit a rebound movement.

Under the traction adjustment he described swaying, swinging, manual traction (auxiliary to the thrust), bimanual traction (traction with one hand while the other thrusts), vibrato traction, massage traction, and concussion stroke treatment. In addition to spondylotherapy Gregory promoted calisthenics. He developed a table that placed tension on the spinal column while the thrust was given. To D.D. such traction as "drawing or stretching the body by a machine . . . is orthopedic or osteopathic; it is not Chiropractic."

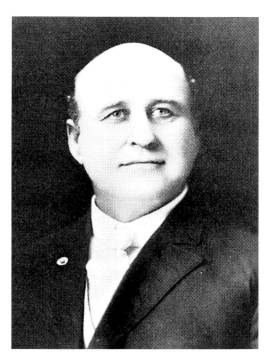

Alva Gregory, a medical doctor before studying chiropractic, operated for a short time with D.D. at the Palmer-Gregory School of Chiropractic. He emphasized adjustment under tension.
Courtesy Palmer College of Chiropractic Archives, Davenport, Iowa.

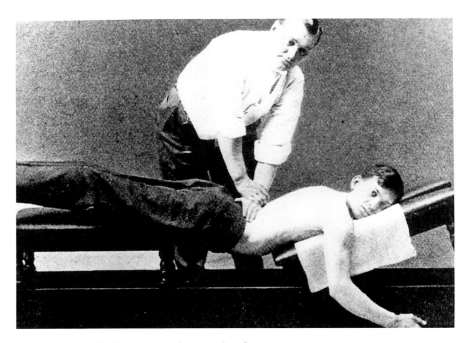

An old method of lumbar technique by Gregory.

From Gregory A: *Spinal treatment,* Oklahoma City, Oklahoma, 1912, Palmer-Gregory College.

Joy M. Loban

Joy Loban, an early lecturer in philosophy at the Palmer School of Chiropractic (PSC), left for private practice in 1909. Later he became President of the Universal Chiropractic College that opened in 1910 in Davenport following defection of 40 to 50 PSC students. After several years the school moved to Pittsburgh where it was operating in 1938. Loban emphasized a close-contact chiropractic technique that required taking out all of the slack before thrusting. He described the adjustment as "an instantaneous whip-like contraction" that is more of a "transmitted shock" than a thrust. This was recommended as a less painful form of chiropractic technique.

A.P. Davis

Blending ophthalmology, osteopathy, and neuropathy with chiropractic, A.P.Davis drew the wrath of D.D. who dismissed Davis as "talking thru his coat sleeve or beating the air." While sparring in print the two appeared to have remained friends, with Davis acknowledging Palmer's expertise. Davis attended four of D.D.'s lectures on specific adjusting and "I noted with satisfaction the elimination of superfluous adjustments used by many [other] chiropractors." Referring to Palmer's book, Davis stated:

> I hope to get great good and much new information out of your book. I have no words with which I can fully express my appreciation of your most wonderful science. I shall never be remiss in my efforts to advance the science of Chiropractic, and praise for its discovery.

Perhaps Davis was prophetic in noting the elimination of superfluous adjustments, since this course was followed to the extreme by D.D.'s son, B.J. Palmer.

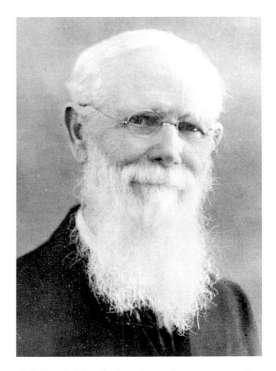

A.P. Davis blended opthamology, osteopathy, and neuropathy with chiropractic, drawing the ire of D.D.

Courtesy Palmer College of Chiropractic Archives, Davenport, Iowa.

B.J. Palmer: The Developer of Chiropractic

Since D.D. is known as the Founder of philosophy, art, and science of chiropractic, Bartlett Joshua (B.J.) Palmer is considered the Developer of chiropractic. Graduating from his father's school in 1902, B.J. later took over the Palmer Infirmary and Chiropractic School when the elder Palmer left for California. The relationship between father and son was frequently stormy. They entered into a partnership when D.D. returned in 1903, which was dissolved in 1906.

B.J.'s contributions to chiropractic technique are many and varied. Where early chiropractic technique relied on stiff arms with the elbows locked, B.J. developed the Palmer Recoil technique. The relaxation of the shoulders and arms of the chiropractor immediately before delivery of the adjustive force promoted greater relaxation by the patient and was much less painful.

In the early years, B.J. promoted full spine adjusting and with J.C. Wishart developed the Meric System. They worked out a system that divided the body into vertemeres listing the various forms of *dis-ease* caused by subluxations of the vertebra or vertebrae.

Around this time, 1910, x-ray became available at the PSC. In addition to this new diagnostic tool, spinal analysis included palpation of spinal "hot boxes," which preceded the development of the neurocalometer. Patented in 1925, the neurocalometer was used to detect temperature changes indicative of "tender nerve fibers." It was purported that the chiropractor may not have a uniformly accurate ability to detect "hot boxes" or "tender nerve fibres" through palpation and thus the neurocalometer was developed. Originally sold to individual chiropractors, it became the object of much controversy when it could only be leased through the Neurocalometer Department of the PSC.

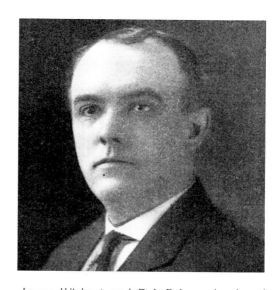

James Wishart and B.J. Palmer developed the Meric system for adjusting.

Courtesy Palmer College of Chiropractic Archives, Davenport, Iowa.

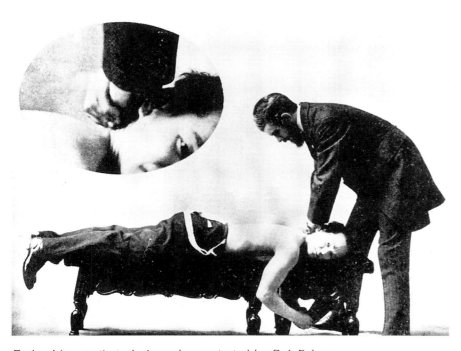

Early chiropractic technique demonstrated by B.J. Palmer.

From Palmer DD, Palmer BJ: *The science of chiropractic: its principles and adjustments,* Davenport, Iowa, 1906, Palmer School of Chiropractic.

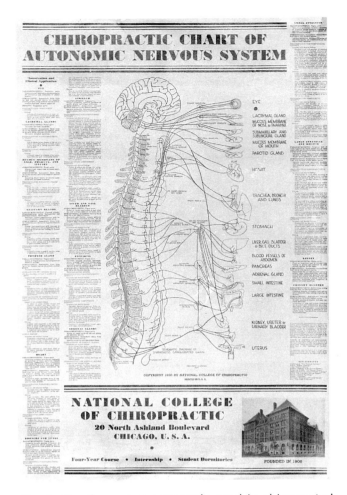

Charts like these were commonly used in chiropractor's offices.

Courtesy Palmer College of Chiropractic Archives, Davenport, Iowa.

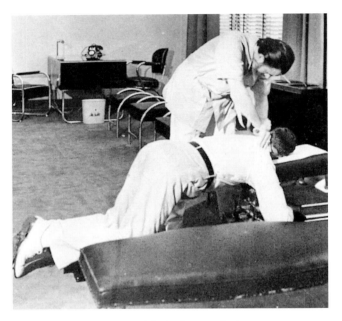

B.J. Palmer using the Hole-In-One technique.

Courtesy Palmer College of Chiropractic Archives, Davenport, Iowa.

As chiropractic technique evolved under the tutelage of B.J., the Palmer Toggle Recoil technique was developed whereby the pisiform contact was applied to the atlas and further refined to apply force directed externally to effect a torque or twisting movement in combination with both the recoil and toggle. As a last step in the evolution of chiropractic technique, B.J. developed the Hole-in-One (HIO), so that the external force was applied only in the superior cervical vertebrae at the atlas and axis. Palmer reasoned that the complete adjustment was not effected solely by the external force delivered by the chiropractor but was a combination of the external force and the "internal innate recoil force" within the patient. Thus the adjustment set the vertebra in motion and innately replaced it. The oscillation noted on cineradiography on delivery of a toggle recoil adjustment by B.J. exemplifies this innate tendency of the body to right itself.

THE EVOLUTION OF CHIROPRACTIC TECHNIQUES

As with most health care disciplines, chiropractic has developed a variety of approaches to the treatment of human dysfunction. Any approach at grouping chiropractic techniques is artificial to some extent but an attempt has been made to associate together for descriptive purposes the most common procedures used by the chiropractic profession. Some techniques fit the criteria of more than one category and have been arbitrarily discussed under one heading when it might as easily have been assigned elsewhere. While advocates of some techniques stressed unique methods of analysis and diagnosis, others became proponents of original methods of treatment or therapy.

TECHNIQUES DESIGNED TO RESTORE MOTION

Reference to normalizing segmental motion was made by Smith, Langworthy, and Paxson in the first textbook published on chiropractic (1906). In addition to palpation for misalignment and hyperesthesia they promoted diagnosis of subluxations through movement analysis. This rationale for the application of chiropractic technique was taught at both National College of Chiropractic and Western States Chiropractic College in the early 1920s, where a subluxation was defined as "the fixation of a joint in a position of motion, usually at the extremity of such motion. The concept of spinal fixation was popularized by Leikans and the Gillet brothers in Belgium. Henri Gillet was a prolific writer on spinal fixation, which he defined as "the element which in a subluxation holds the vertebra in its abnormal placement and hinders its normal movement."

The movement restriction component of the subluxation was emphasized in North America through the teaching of the vertebral subluxation complex paradigm by L.J. Faye. At the Canadian Memorial Chiropractic College and through the Motion Palpation Institute, which he founded, Faye emphasized the use of motion palpation to determine aberrant motion, with the goal of chiropractic technique to reverse kinesiopathology.

Motion palpation for the detection of manipulable subluxations is taught in chiropractic colleges today as part of the core curriculum with a multitude of chiropractic techniques used to restore normal motion.

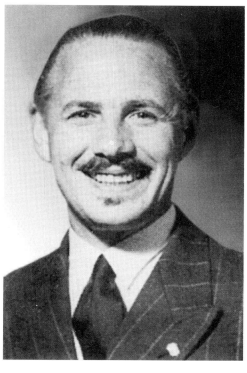

Henri Gillet, a Belgian chiropractor, popularized the concept of spinal fixation.
Courtesy Palmer College of Chiropractic Archives, Davenport, Iowa.

Low Force or Reflex Techniques

Less forceful forms of chiropractic technique, working through reflex mechanisms rather than thrust procedures, have been developed as another form of the chiropractic adjustment. Where the Palmers and their followers used the spinous and transverse processes of the vertebrae as levers to reduce subluxations, others relied on complex reflex mechanisms not totally understood but empirically effective in the treatment of spinal dysfunction.

Logan Basic Technique

Hugh Logan, a 1915 graduate of the Universal College established the Logan Basic Chiropractic College in 1935. With his son, Vinton, as dean, Logan developed and taught a nonthrusting technique. Logan Basic Technique contends that segmental subluxations are the result of body distortion. This may be caused by one or a combination of the following: deficient unilateral body support, delineated as unilateral sacral subluxation; leg length deficiency; or unilateral wedging of the fifth lumbar ver-

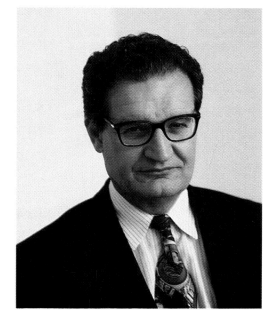

L. John Faye emphasized the use of motion palpation to determine aberrant motion.
Courtesy L. John Faye, Los Angeles, California.

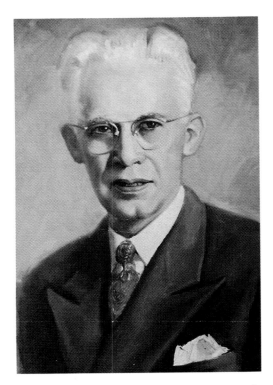

Hugh Logan developed a nonthrusting technique, which contends that segmental subluxations are the result of body distortion.

Courtesy Logan College of Chiropractic Archives, Chesterfield, Missouri.

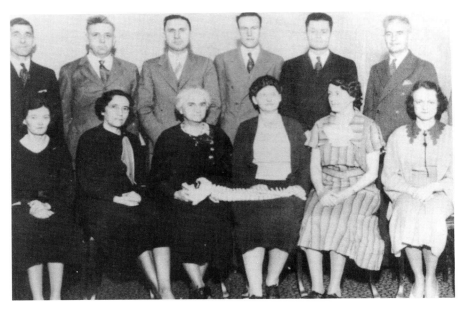

A Logan Basic Technique Group, circa 1940. Vinton Logan is standing third from the right. Sylva Ashworth is seated third from left.

Courtesy Russell Gibbons, Pittsburgh, Pennsylvania.

tebra. The diagnostic procedures used include positional analysis of the sacrum in the standing position, evaluation of leg length, and x-ray analysis. Correction uses manual pressure on the sacrotuberous ligament or apex of the sacrum for the purpose of leveling the sacrum and pelvis and straightening the spine. A useful technique where force is not appropriate, Logan Basic Technique continues to be used by many in the chiropractic profession.

Sacro-Occipital Technique

Influenced by both the study of chiropractic and osteopathy, Major B. DeJarnette began to research what was to become Sacro-Occipital Technique (SOT) in 1925. Spending the next 65 years studying and teaching this technique, DeJarnette promoted a unique method of diagnosis and reflex techniques in addition to manual force techniques. The basic diagnostic tests of SOT classify spinal distortion into one of three categories relative to the sacroiliac findings. The three categories require different systems of treatment with wedge-shaped blocks precisely angled under the pelvis in the prone or supine positions. Monitoring of corrective effects of body weight is performed by checking leg length discrepancies. To DeJarnette the sacrum and pelvis form a structural control base for the legs, spine, shoulders, and cranium; tests to determine which category applies to the patient are performed with the patient bearing full weight in the standing position and with the patient supine.

In addition to spinal distortion patterns, DeJarnette was a proponent of cranial and reflex techniques. Influenced by his early friendship with William Garner Sutherland while attending osteopathic college, DeJarnette further developed and taught cranial therapy and reflex techniques

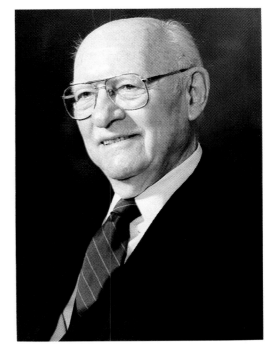

Major B. DeJarnette developed the Sacro-Occipital Technique and the Chiropractic Manipulative Reflex Technique ("bloodless surgery").

Courtesy Herbert K. Lee, Toronto, Ontario, Canada.

based on correlation of visceral and referred pain. The underlying principles of SOT state that the sacrum has a sagittal plane respiratory movement mechanism and is associated via the dura with the cranium. Based on this theory, manual methods of synchronizing cranial motion were developed to influence the circulation of cerebrospinal fluid that is thought to depend on normal inspiration and expiration and movement of the sacrum and cranial sutures. DeJarnette also felt that each vertebra is related to a visceral area, thus affecting all the internal organs. From this he developed the Chiropractic Manipulative Reflex Technique (CMRT) referred to as "bloodless surgery," whereby he delved into specific visceral manipulation.

DeJarnette was one of the last early pioneers in the profession. He died at the age of 93 in 1992, 3 years short of the one-hundredth anniversary of chiropractic. His influence on other chiropractors was not limited to practitioners alone, and he stimulated the development of other chiropractic techniques, most notably Applied Kinesiology.

Applied Kinesiology Technique

Applied Kinesiology Technique originated in 1964 when George G. Goodheart observed that postural distortion is often associated with muscles that fail to meet the demands of specific muscle tests. Apparent muscle dysfunction with both improved postural balance and outcomes of manual muscle tests respond to digital mobilization of palpable tender nodules in the origin and insertion of the involved muscles. A close clinical association was also observed between specific muscle dysfunction and related organ or gland dysfunction. Appropriately applied the Applied Kinesiology examination is used to enhance standard diagnostic procedures, not replace them. A variety of therapeutic approaches are used to treat the patient. In addition to manual force techniques Applied Kinesiologists employ various reflex and myofascial procedures, cranial technique, and meridian balancing.

Activator Methods

The Activator Method of chiropractic analysis and low-force spinal adjusting technique originated in 1965 through the collaborative efforts of Warren C. Lee and Arian W. Fuhr. Lee, a 1941 graduate of Northwestern College of Chiropractic, and Fuhr, a 1961 graduate of Logan Basic College of Chiropractic, integrated and further developed the works of Logan, Derefield, and Van Rumpt. Grounded in the concepts of the Logan Basic Technique, the structural unity of the skeletal system and the effects of gravity on the spinal column were further integrated. The leg length measurements of subluxation detection pioneered by the Derefields were then combined with the light toggle recoil thumb thrusts of the Directional Non-Force Technique developed by Richard Van Rumpt. A mechanical device originating from a combination of earlier adjusting devices and a dental impactor was developed to increase control of the speed, force, and direction of thrust and to reduce physical stress on the chiropractor. The activator device has undergone modifications and utilizes a hammer-anvil effect to produce a controlled force to osseous spinal structures.

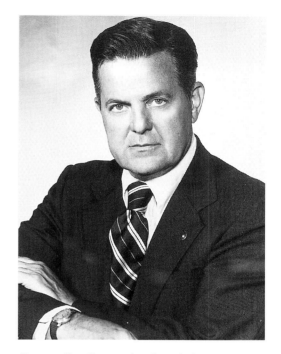

George Goodheart developed the technique of Applied Kinesiology in 1964.
Courtesy George Goodheart, Grosse Pointe Woods, Michigan.

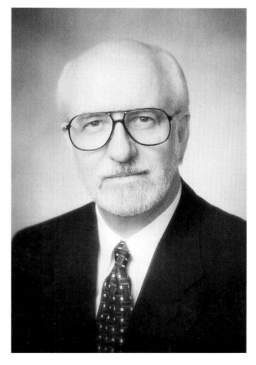

Arlan Fuhr (shown)*, along with Warren Lee, developed the Activator Method in 1965.*
Courtesy Arlan Fuhr, Phoenix, Arizona.

SPECIFIC CONTACT THRUST TECHNIQUES

Low amplitude, high velocity thrust procedures are probably the most widely recognized and commonly used of the chiropractic techniques. Characterized by joint gapping and the articular crack, cavitation, these techniques have become associated with chiropractic manipulation. The joint is typically tractioned to tension at which point a high velocity, low amplitude thrust is applied, with or without recoil. With recoil the thrust is immediately withdrawn.

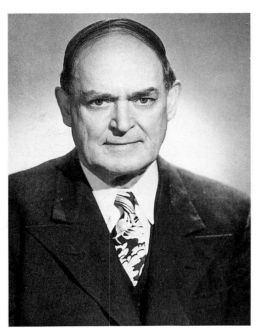

B.F. Wells, an osteopath and chiropractor, co-authored a book with Janse and Houser that describes more than 100 diversified procedures.

Courtesy National College of Chiropractic, Lombard, Illinois.

Diversified Technique

The origin of Diversified Technique cannot be traced to any one individual but rather the term *diversified* relates to the fact that the sources for these procedures are diverse. A few of the moves date back to the Palmers and are characterized by a specific contact and a high velocity, low amplitude thrust procedure. Some of the early methods are described by B.J. in his book *An Exposition of Old Moves.*

J.N. Firth also developed and refined a number of Diversified Techniques. Firth, H.E. Vedder, S.J. Burich, and A.G. Hendricks became known as the "Big Four" when they left the PSC in 1926 to form Lincoln Chiropractic College. They split with B.J. Palmer over the narrow "Hole-in-One" system regarding such limitations on learning as catastrophic and out of step with the teaching of D.D. Palmer.

Other procedures included under Diversified Technique can be traced to osteopaths and medical manipulators. John McMillan Mennell, M.D., is credited with developing a method of assessing specific articular movement that has been incorporated into Diversified Technique. Referred to as joint play, this procedure and static palpation, motion palpation, and joint challenge are now used to detect manipulable subluxations.

Wells, an osteopath and chiropractor, co-authored a book with Joseph Janse and Raymond Houser in 1937 that describes more than 100 Diversified procedures. Although not limited to a single school, Diversified Technique has had a strong association with National College of Chiropractic, which has taught Diversified Technique since its beginning. The *Manual of Spinal and Pelvic Technics,* written by Alfred States while at National College of Chiropractic, long formed the basis of Diversified Technique courses at many chiropractic colleges. Diversified Technique procedures have been described by Gittleman and Grice in 1980, Panzer in 1990, and by Gittleman and Fligg in 1992.

Diversified Technique is described by Bergmann, Peterson, and Lawrence as: "using the normal biomechanics of the spine and extremities to create motion at a vertebra or extremity joint." They conclude that its application becomes nearly universal, which may account for its widespread use within the chiropractic profession.

Gonstead Technique

Gonstead Technique uses engineering principles to analyze and correct dysfunction of the spine. Clarence Gonstead who had studied mechanical engineering before becoming a chiropractor, graduated from PSC in 1923. Similar to Logan's understanding of spinal distortion, Gonstead thought that any change in the level foundation offered to the spine by the pelvis and sacrum would result in spinal subluxations and com-

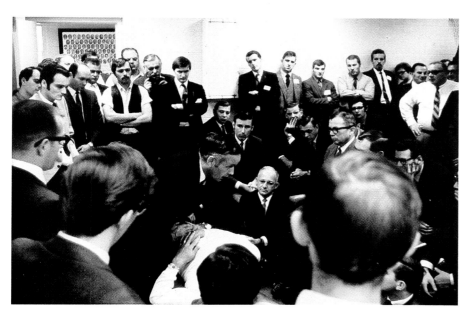

Alex Cox demonstrating the Gonstead technique.
Courtesy Herbert K. Lee, Toronto, Ontario, Canada.

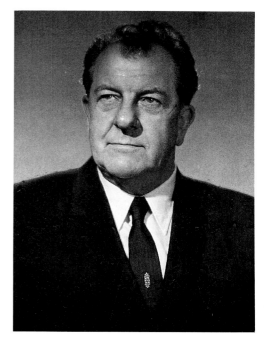

Clarence Gonstead, founder of the Gonstead Clinic and Gonstead Seminars, emphasized distingushing primary from secondary subluxations, preventing unnecessary overadjusting by treating only primary subluxations.
Courtesy W. Alex Cox, Mt Horeb, Wisconsin.

pensations. A compensation is thought to follow a primary subluxation elsewhere in the spine. This concept distinguishes primary from secondary subluxation preventing unnecessary over adjusting by treating only primary subluxations. According to Gonstead, both innominates are commonly involved in pelvic subluxations with the primary sacroiliac subluxation pulling the other in the opposite direction. The side of fifth lumbar body rotation is thought to be the side of the primary subluxation and the other side the compensation. Gonstead analysis depends on confirmation of subluxation findings on radiographs following the detection of temperature variations determined by a temperature differential instrument and motion palpation. The specifications of each corrective procedure include patient positioning, contact point, tractioning to tension, and direction of drive, before a thrust is applied. Innovative equipment was developed by Gonstead including the knee-chest table and cervical chair to improve Gonstead techniques. After Gonstead's death in 1978, his work was further promoted by Alex and Douglas Cox. A recent text by Plaugher ably describes Gonstead procedures.

UPPER CERVICAL TECHNIQUES

The forerunner of chiropractic Upper Cervical Techniques is B.J.'s "Hole-in-One." Common to Upper Cervical Techniques are systems for marking radiographs to determine the site and components of the subluxation. Discussed with this group are those chiropractic techniques that employ additional procedures along with upper cervical radiographic marking systems.

Palmer Upper Cervical Technique

Palmer Upper Cervical Technique is a method of measurement of atlas-axis misalignment as it relates to the foramen magnum. General considerations for this technique include angulation where a variation in angles from normal indicates misalignment, measurement from one point to another with deviation from normal indicating misalignment, and variation in size, shape, and location of corresponding descriptive parts. The "toggle" technique with a rapid recoil is applied to set the joint in motion, and correct alignment is thought to be achieved by the body's innate intelligence. The premise of misalignment concerns the relationship of a segment with the one above, the one below, or both. The thrust is varied in depth and speed with respect to patient requirements.

Grostic Procedure

The Grostic procedure had its origins in the Palmer Specific Upper Cervical technique. It was one of the techniques that developed as a result of the Palmer Standardized Chiropractic Council, which was formed to standardize chiropractic procedures and methods. Founded by Roy G. Labachotte under the direction of B.J. Palmer, this group provided a forum at which research and new ideas could be presented and exchanged. The Grostic Procedure was developed by John F. Grostic, also a member of this group, who presented his material as it was developed. In 1946 it was compiled in a "package" that was to become known as the Grostic Procedure.

The x-ray analysis is the core of the procedure, which has remained constant while the adjusting methods have been refined to improve the effectiveness of the procedure. Beginning with "Palmer Toggle," a much shorter and lighter thrust, which still resembles the "toggle," is employed to eliminate discomfort to the patient. The contact point, the pisiform, usually travels less than ¼-inch during the thrust, is thought to reduce the atlas misalignment more consistently and predictably.

In addition to radiographic analysis, the Grostic Procedure emphasizes methodology for x-ray machine alignment, patient evaluation, and calculation of the optimum vectors that can be used for reducing the subluxation either manually or by means of a mechanical adjusting instrument. Rotational misalignments between the atlas and the skull are measured on the vertex view by noting the angle formed by the intersection of the line drawn through the center of the transverse foramina of the atlas and a central skull line. Rotational misalignments between the atlas and the axis are observed and measured on the nasium view. John D. Grostic has further refined his father's work through computer-assisted x-ray analysis and x-ray safety through reduction of radiation hazards.

National Upper Cervical Chiropractic Association

The National Upper Cervical Chiropractic Association (NUCCA) was formed to promote techniques to reduce the detrimental effects of the atlas subluxation complex (ASC). NUCCA-approved techniques must fulfil specific criteria, including measurable evidence of the existence of vertebral misalignment, proof of the effects of the misalignments on the neurological component, a system or method of adjusting misalignments to or toward normal position, predetermined and controlled vectors, measurable and physical proof that the vertebral subluxation does in fact detrimentally influence the human organism, and measurable proof that reduction of the subluxation manifests itself as reduction in the physical distortions.

CHIROPRACTIC SOFT TISSUE TECHNIQUES

Chiropractic soft tissue techniques have been employed by chiropractors along with low force and osseous thrust procedures since the early decades of this century. Early proponents included Carver and Loban. Some techniques grouped elsewhere have a large component of soft tissue procedures included in their recommended approach to treating patients such as Applied Kinesiology Technique and SOT.

Although purists consider soft tissue procedures to be mixing and not within the scope of chiropractic practice, many practitioners today include soft tissue therapy as part of the management of patients. A number of chiropractors have developed specific soft tissue techniques that are unique to the chiropractic profession.

Spears Painless System

The Spears Painless System of chiropractic technique was developed by Leo and Dan Spears at their chiropractic hospital in Denver. Designed to reduce patient discomfort, the Spears Painless System involved soft tissue goading to hasten patient recovery. This technique was used to relieve a variety of conditions including sciatica, headaches, and acute arthritis.

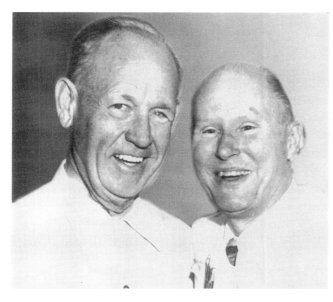

Dan and Leo Spears developed the Spears Painless System of chiropractic technique at their chiropractic hospital in Denver.

Courtesy William Rehm, Baltimore, Maryland.

Receptor Tonus Technique

Probably the most frequently used soft tissue technique used by chiropractors is the Receptor Tonus Technique that originated with Raymond L. Nimmo. Nimmo found noxious generative points in muscles that referred pain in characteristic patterns. Viewing these hypersensitive areas, the trigger points of Travell, as abnormal reflex arcs he developed a manual technique designed to reduce the irritable loci. He referred to the interrelationship of muscle tonus and the central nervous system as "reverberating circuits," whereby the stimulus was self-perpetuating until the cycle was broken. Nimmo's Receptor Tonus Technique utilizes manual pressure 5 to 7 seconds, which is strong enough to reproduce the patient's pain pattern but not so much to tense the affected muscle. This procedure referred to by Travell as ischemic compression offers a noninvasive chiropractic technique instead of the common medical practice of injection of the painful trigger points.

Soft Tissue Drainage Technique

Soft tissue procedures for the drainage of the lymphatic system, as well as the ears, nose, and throat, were developed and taught by Thomas Lake. This technique applies digital stimulation to improve respiration and drainage of congested areas.

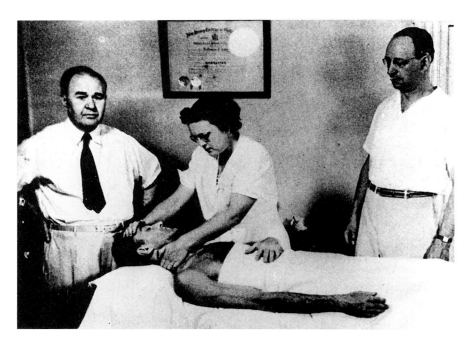

Cervical lymphatic drainage demonstrated by Thomas Lake (left) and an associate.

From Lake T: *Treatment by neuropathy and manipulative therapeutics,* 1946, [S.l.] Lake.

MECHANICALLY ASSISTED CHIROPRACTIC TECHNIQUES

After early development of tables designed to assist the chiropractor in delivering more effective adjustment a number of procedures have been developed utilizing specialized equipment.

Distraction Technique

Based on an early osteopathic table developed by McManus, James Cox has developed a method of manually controlled distraction applied to the intervertebral disc space and articular facets of the lumbar spine. Unlike traction that affects multilevels of the spine, distraction is applied to a specific level of the spine. In addition to tractioning the intervertebral disc, adjustments to the facet joints may also be applied. With the patient, prone ankle cuffs are applied and the caudal section of the table is distracted downward 1 to 2 inches while contact is made on the spinous process of a lumbar vertebral segment. This technique requires careful monitoring of the patient for pain and muscle spasm.

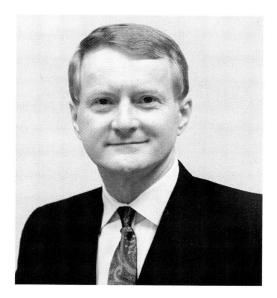

James Cox developed a method of manually controlled distraction applied to the intervertebral disc space and articular facets of the lumbar spine. A distraction table utilized by Cox's Distraction Technique.

Courtesy James Cox, Fort Wayne, Indiana.

Thompson Terminal Point Technique

Thompson Terminal Point Technique originated with J. Clay Thompson who developed a mechanical drop-section table. With drop pieces at the cranial, thoracic, abdominal, and pelvic sections, each section drops a short distance on the delivery of a chiropractic thrust followed by a sudden stop. Thompson has also produced a cervical head piece, which incorporates a torque mechanism that can be switched to clockwise or counter-clockwise. Thompson states that the free drop through space allows for the development of kinetic energy, which adds a unique dimension to the technique not seen in other procedures. The table extends the principle of the recoil technique for use at all spinal levels and allows the use of standard techniques assisted by a drop piece. The versatility of the table also helps to relieve stress on the doctor and can be set to adjust for differences in patient weight. The Thompson Terminal Point Technique relies on the Derefield leg check to determine subluxations in both the pelvic and cervical regions. Leg lengths are compared in both the prone and supine positions and with the legs straight or the knees bent. Cervical patterns are checked by comparing leg length with the head turned to either side.

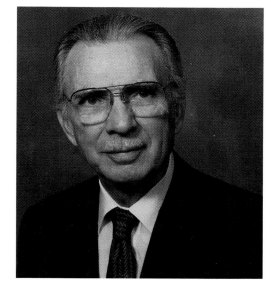

J. Clay Thompson, developer of the Thompson Terminal Point Technique.

Courtesy Portraits by Annette, Davenport, Iowa.

CHIROPRACTIC TECHNIQUE AT THE CENTENNIAL

Many exciting events have impacted on the chiropractic profession in the decade leading up to the centennial of the first application of chiropractic technique. Scientific validation of chiropractic techniques was promoted by publication of an algorithm that provides a model to study various chiropractic procedures. Stimulated by this model, Hansen convened a consensus conference held in Seattle in 1990 the outcome of which was two resolutions:

1. All chiropractic procedures should be submitted to a standardized scientific validation process. This process should include consensus methods and clinical research.
2. A steering committee should be established to facilitate the consensus process.

Since that time, annual consensus conferences have been held, cosponsored by the Consortium for Chiropractic Research and the California Chiropractic Association, each dealing with the validation of chiropractic procedures. Chiropractic procedures have been categorized by an algorithm recommended by the American Chiropractic Association's Council on Technique. With this algorithm a template for consensus development by the Consortium for Chiropractic Research is being developed.

Elaboration of these categories followed in 1993 with the publication of the Mercy Center Consensus Conference *Guidelines for Chiropractic Quality Assurance and Practice Parameters.* These guidelines offer ratings of levels of evidential support for various technique procedures.

Finally, terminology related to chiropractic technique has been developed through consensus methods and endorsed by the Consortium for Chiropractic Research and the Chiropractic Technique advisory council to the American Chiropractic Association. In keeping with the definitions outlined by the Rand Corporation report on *The Appropriateness of Spinal Manipulation for Low Back Pain,* it was agreed that manipulation would describe a manual procedure that involves a directed thrust to move a joint past the physiological range of motion, without exceeding the anatomical limit. The term *adjustment* is described as any chiropractic therapeutic procedure that utilizes controlled force, leverage, direction, amplitude, and velocity, which is directed at specific joints or anatomical regions. It was further agreed that chiropractors often use such procedures to influence joint and neurophysiological functions.

Chiropractic technique has taken many roads in the past 100 years. Many variations of technique procedures have been developed giving the chiropractor multiple vehicles by which to restore function and enhance the body's natural healing mechanisms. The table on pp. 260-261 lists many but not all chiropractic techniques and developers.

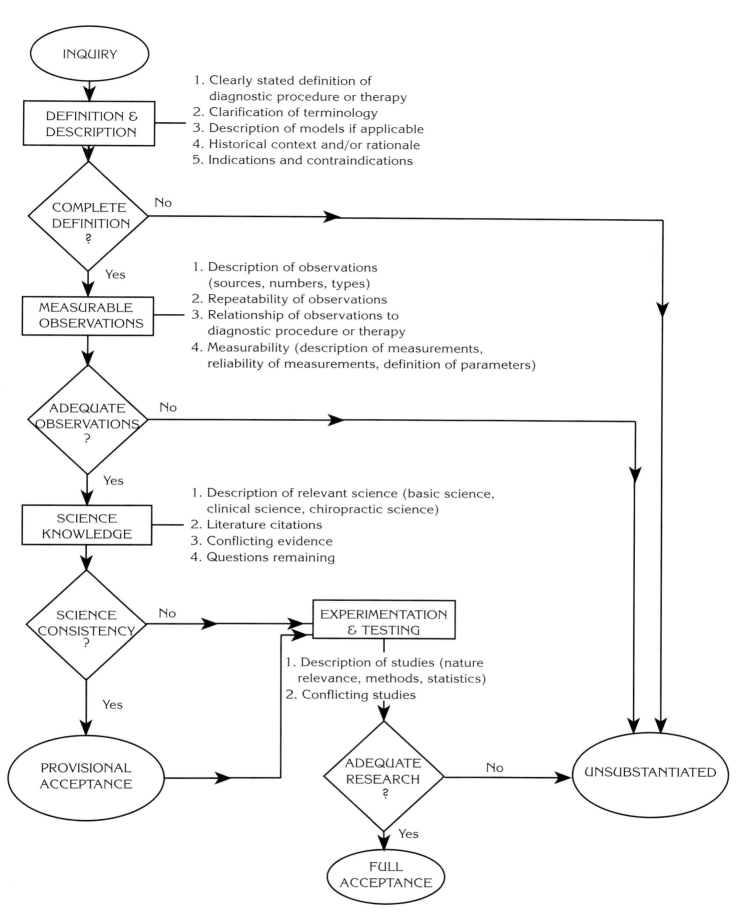

A model for the evaluation of chiropractic methods.
From *Chiropractic Technique,* February 1992.

NAMED CHIROPRACTIC TECHNIQUES ∽

Technique	Developer
Access Seminars	Weigant, Bloomenthal
Activator Technique	Arlan Fuhr, Warren Le
Alternative Chiropractic Adjustments	Robert Wiehe
Applied Chiropractic Distortion Analysis	William J. Kotheimer
Applied Spinal Biomechanical Engineering	Aragona
Applied Kinesiology	George Goodheart, Walters, Schmitt, John Thie
Aquarian Age Healing	John Hurley
Arnholz Muscle Adjusting	Walter W. Arnholtz
Atlas Orthogonality Technique	Roy Sweat
Atlas Specific	A.A. Wernsing
Bandy Seminars	Bandy
Bio Kinesiology	Barton
BioEnergetic Synchronization Technique-BEST	M.T. Morter
Bioenergetics	Richard Broeringmeyer
Biomagnetic Technique	Hermen Stoffels, Borham, Richard Broeringmeyer
Blair Upper Cervical Technique	Blair
Bloodless Surgery	Lorenz, Ralph M. Failor, Major B. DeJarnette
Body Integration	Espy
Buxton Technical Course of Painless Chiropractic	A.G.A. Buxton
Chiroenergetics	Edwin H. Kimmel
Chiro Plus Kinesiology	Dowty
Chirometry	Quigly
Chiropractic Concept	Clarence Prill
Chiropractic Spinal Biophysics	Donald Harrison
Chiropractic Manipulative Reflex Technique-CMRT	Major B. DeJarnette
Chiropractic Neuro-Biochemical Analysis	—
CHOK-E System	—
Clinical Kinesiology	Alan G. Beardall
Collins Method of Painless Adjusting	Frederick W. Collins
Concept Therapy	Thurman Fleet, Dill
Cranial Technique	Major B. DeJarnette, Denton Goodheart
Craniopathy	Nephi P. Cottam
Diversified Technique	Homer Beatty, Joseph Bonyun, Carver, Crawford, Frank P. DeGiacomo, Frank, Grecco, Logan LeBeau, Metzinger, Otto C. Reinert, Alfred States, Richard D. Stonebrink, Stierwalt
Directional Non-Force Technique-DNFT	Richard Van Rumpt, Johns
Distraction Technique	James Cox, Markey, Leander, Tom Hill
Endo-Nasal Technique	Walter Gibbons, Thomas Lake, Richard Broeringmeyer
Extremity Technique	Burns, Grecco, Christenson, Gertler, Hearon, Malley, Schawn
Focalizer Spinal Recoil Stimulus Reflex Effector Technique	Phillip George
Freeman Chiropractic Procedure	Freeman
Fundamental Chiropractic	Ray Ashton
Global Energetic Matrix	Babinet
Gonstead Technique	Clarence Gonstead
Herring Cervical Technique	Herring
Holographic Diagnosis and Treatment	Franks, Gleason
Howard System	Frank Howard
Keck Method of Analysis	W. Frederick Keck
King Tetrahedron Concept	Wallace King
Lemond Brain Stem Technique	Lemond
Logan Basic Technique	Hugh B. Logan, William Coggins

Technique	Developer
Master Energy Dynamics	Bartlett
Mawhinney Scoliosis Technique	R.B. Mawhinney
McTimody Technique	McTimody
Mears Technique	—
Meric Technique System	C.S. Cleveland, B.J. Palmer, J.M. Loban, A.L. Forster, J.S. Riley
Micromanipulation	Young
Motion Palpation	Henri Gillet, John L. Faye
Muscle Palpation	Spano
Muscle Response Testing	Lepore, Fishman, Grinims
MusculoSkeletal Synchronization and Stabilization Technique	Krippenbrock
Nerve Signal Interference	Craton
Network Chiropractic	Epstein
Neuro Emotional Technique	Walker
Neuro Organizational Technique	Ferrari
NeuroLymphatic Reflex Technique	Chapman
NeuroVascular Reflex Technique	Bennett
Olesky 21st Century Technique	I.H. Olesky
Ortman Technique	Ortman
Pettibon Spinal Biomechanics Technique	Burl Pettibon
Pierce-Stillwagon Technique	Walter Pierce, Glenn Stillwagon
Posture Imbalance Patterns	Sinclaire
Perianal Postural Reflex Technique	R. Watkins
Polarity Technique	
Pure Chiropractic Technique	G.M. Morreim
Reaver's 5th Cervical Key	Reaver, Walter Pierce
Receptor Tonus Technique	Raymond Nimmo
Riddler Reflex Technique	Riddler
Sacro-Occipital Technique	Major B. DeJarnette
Soft Tissue Orthopedics	Rees
Somatosynthesis	Ford
Spears Painless System	Leo Spears
Specific Majors	Harry Nemiroff
Spinal Stress (Stressology)	Lowell E. Ward
Spinal Touch Technique	W. Lamar Rosquist
Spondylotherapy	Arthur Forester, Joe Riley
Thompson Terminal Point Technique	J. Clay Thompson, Stucky, Mitchell
Tiezen Technique	Tiezen
Toftness Technique	I.N. Toftness
Upper Cervical Technique-HIO, Toggle	B.J. Palmer, DUFF, John F. Grostic, Michael Kale, Life College, NUCCA
Top Notch Visceral Techniques	Portelli, Marcellino
Tortipelvis/Torticolis	Fred Barge
Touch for Health	John Thie
Total Body Modification	Frank
Truscott Technique	Leon Truscott
Ungerank Specific Low Force Chiropractic Technique	Ungerank
Variable Force Technique	Leighton
Von Fox Combination Technique	Von Fox
Zindler Reflex Technique	Zindler

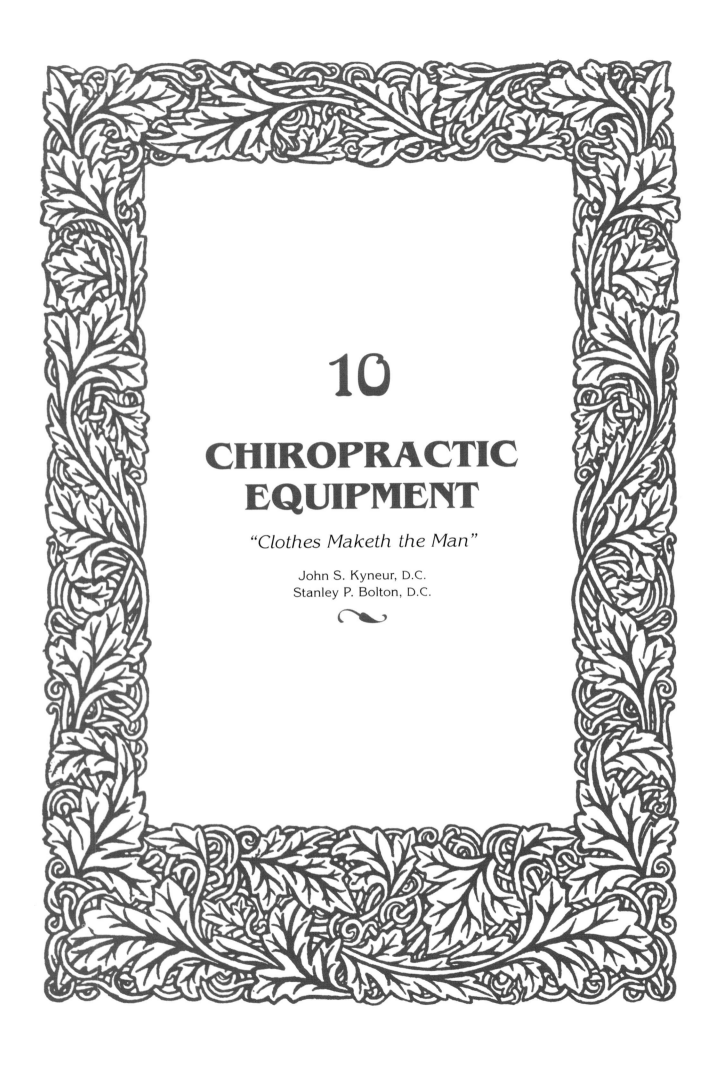

10

CHIROPRACTIC EQUIPMENT

"Clothes Maketh the Man"

John S. Kyneur, D.C.
Stanley P. Bolton, D.C.

What distinguishes the world's newest evolving health profession? To the academic it might be the curriculum leading to the qualification "Doctor of Chiropractic." To the lawyer it might be enabling legislation regulating the chiropractic profession in 79 jurisdictions around the world. To the scientist it might be the gathering evidence of the efficacy of chiropractic principles and practice. To the journalist it might be the drama of health regained by natural noninvasive chiropractic care.

But to the average person, the patient, it is the visible features that distinguish the chiropractor from other health professionals—from the physician, the dentist, the optometrist, and physiotherapist. These visible features are the things in the professional office that are germane to chiropractic methods and treatment of patients—the equipment.

Equipment helps the chiropractor identify a spinal subluxation (spinal vertebrae misalignments with neurological insult in classical terms) that can cause and/or relate to health problems of wide ramification. Spinal subluxations are at the core of the chiropractic discipline. Some equipment helps the chiropractor focus on specific spinal adjustment needs while other equipment monitors changes made and progress achieved in the course of chiropractic care. Still other types of chiropractic equipment assist in the adjustment process. Combined with clinical signs and symptoms, knowledge, and experience, the use of chiropractic equipment aids the chiropractor in making a professional judgment of when to adjust, how to adjust, where to adjust, and when not to adjust.

The history of the development of chiropractic equipment underlines the story of the development of the unique role of the chiropractor in the community of health disciplines. ᘐ

POSTURAL ANALYSIS

The first chiropractic adjustment was made by D.D. Palmer on Harvey Lillard in Davenport, Iowa, in 1895. It restored Lillard's hearing. Before the adjustment, Palmer had questioned Lillard and observed and palpated his spine. Superficial as this might seem by today's standards, Palmer had conducted a history-taking and an examination. In examination he had used his fingers in palpation to identify "the bump" in Lillard's spine. Palpatory skills are an important part of chiropractic practice. These palpatory and observation skills were supplemented by the development of plumblines in spinal analysis.

Use of the single or double plumbline and grid was a main form of spinal analysis in the early half of the twentieth century. In a review of the history and development of spinal analysis, Triano cites the Fipps grid system in 1906 as having an important bearing on the development of future spinal and postural analysis.

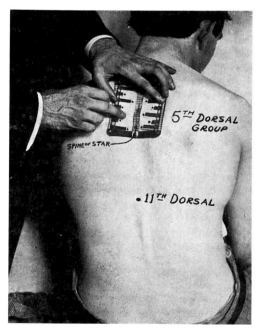

Smith's Spinal Locometer was used as early as 1906 to help the chiropractor locate positions on the spine when palpating.

From Smith O, Langworthy S, Paxson M: *Modernized chiropractic,* Cedar Rapids, Iowa, 1906, Laurence Press.

263

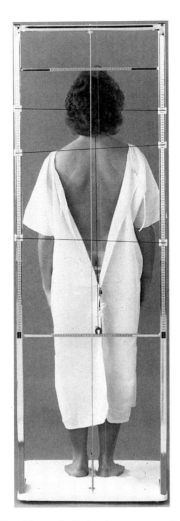

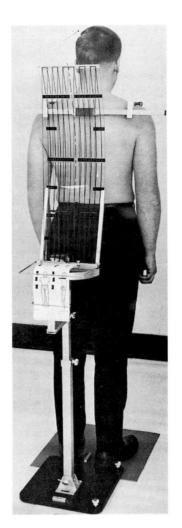

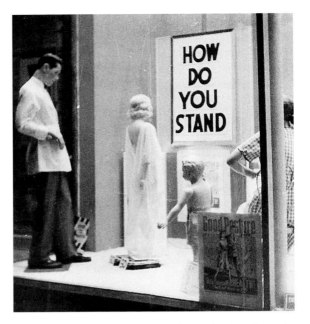

An early chiropractor's storefront display featuring the benefits of postural analysis.

Courtesy Palmer College of Chiropractic Archives, Davenport, Iowa.

The Master's Spinalyzer, manufactured by the Lloyd Table Company, is an example of a postural analysis device used today.

Courtesy Lloyd Table Company, Lisbon, Iowa.

The Gravity Stress Analyzer (GSA) is an automatic recording plumbline posturometer.

Courtesy Larry Allen, Sun City, Arizona.

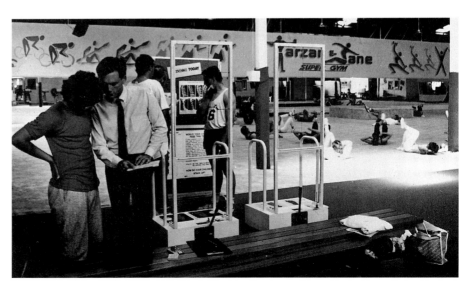

A Spinal Analysis Machine (SAM) being used for posture screening.

Courtesy John Kyneur, New Lambton, New South Wales.

Fipps' equipment, called the *scoliometer,* consisted of a scaled grid-lined celluloid sheet, a plumbline, a footplate for repeatable examination evaluations, and moveable cords stretched between the upright supports that could also allow for shoulder and pelvic level comparisons.

Several similar systems to Fipps' scoliometer have been developed in recent decades. These units include the Johnston Posturometer, developed at Canadian Memorial Chiropractic College (CMCC); the Master's Spinalyser; the Distortion Analyser; James Parker's PARD; and William Lange's Spinal Analysis Machine (SAM). In both the Posturometer and the Distortion Analyser, systems of calibration were developed to enable more objective comparisons.

Another postural analysis method developed within the chiropractic profession used body weight scales, both bilateral and four quadrant scales. Bilateral scales date from the 1930s in a procedure recorded by New York chiropractor, Roy Ashton. Development of four-quadrant weight scales stems from the work of Swiss chiropractor Fred Illi and was developed by Joseph Janse and Adrian Grice at National College of Chiropractic, Chicago.

The four quadrant weight scales gave information about both side-to-side and front-to-back body weight distribution. The latter suggests links between sway-back spinal posture and excessive body weight carried on the heels bilaterally. CMCC's Lyman Johnston and David Drum called this the positive gravity line syndrome. Illi's original work, however, was to determine the need for heel lifts in patients with true unilateral short-leg lengths.

Using modern technology, photographic contour scans, including moire contourography, emerged. Moire contourography, or moire topography, was introduced by Tennessee chiropractor Ronald Free in 1973. It is a contour analysis of the patient's back that topographically maps elevations in both static and moving positions. As a noninvasive method, using a light source to produce light and dark bands, circles and shapes emerge that when photographed enable a permanent record to be made. Moire contourography became popular in the 1970s, but because of extreme sensitivity to changes of either body position or muscle tension it became difficult to standardize for effective comparisons. Despite concerted research efforts to standardize methodology by Eilbert and Spector at the New York Chiropractic College, it is difficult to find a chiropractor using contour scans today.

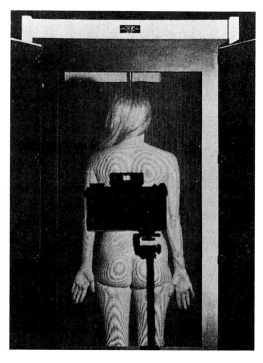

Moire topography produces a topographic elevation of the patient's back in both static and moving positions.

From *The Digest of Chiropractic Economics,* January/February 1975.

CHIROPRACTIC ADJUSTING TABLES

Highly specialized chiropractic adjusting tables developed from the simple, hard flat bench used by D.D. Palmer in 1895. The unpadded, leather-covered oak and pine 'nosebreaker' bench on which patients lay face down for spinal adjustment, soon gave way to the flat bench with a 45-degree sloping headpiece. This was supplemented by pads and pillows under the upper chest and hips, both to secure more comfort for the patient and, principally, better positioning for the adjustment.

Chiropractic historian August Dye records that as adjustment techniques developed in type and range, the one-piece table was superseded in 1904-1905 by a two-piece adjusting table. The headpiece had an upward slant that supported the upper edge of the sternum, while the lower

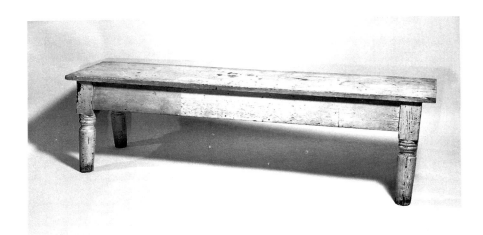

The table on which D.D.'s first chiropractic patient rested, called "the nose-breaker," because it had no nose hole or padding to accommodate the patient's face.

Courtesy Palmer College of Chiropractic Archives, Davenport, Iowa.

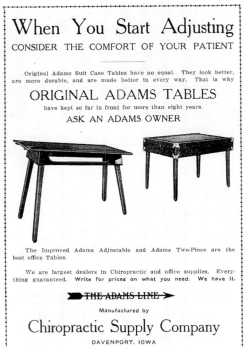
The Adams "suitcase" adjusting table was widely used by early chiropractors to adjust patients who were unable to leave their homes.

Courtesy Palmer College of Chiropractic Archives, Davenport, Iowa.

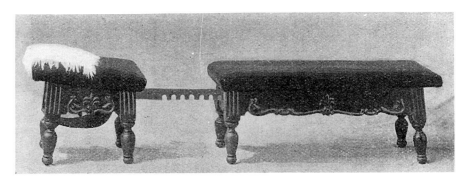

The padded two-piece adjusting table soon evolved to accommodate patients of varying sizes.

From *The Chiropractor*, April 1905.

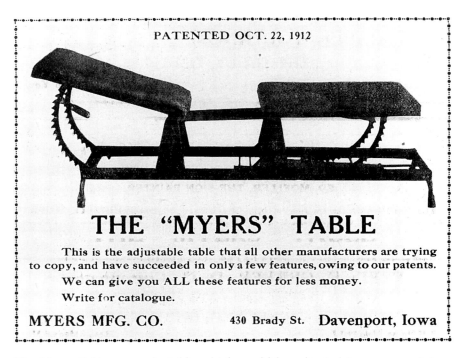

The Myers Table, an early table which could be adjusted to accommodate patients of varying sizes, circa 1914.

From *The Chiropractor*, March 1914.

piece was a shorter replica of the flat table that supported the remainder of the body from the hips down. Both sections were slightly padded with a cut-out for the male genitals.

From 1905 to 1916 a dominant manufacturer of chiropractic adjusting tables was Adams, a carpenter of Davenport, Iowa, whose production at the time was almost exclusively occupied by supplying the chiropractic profession with adjusting tables.

Limitations of the two-piece adjusting table with a freely suspended abdomen and frequent need to move the two sections to accommodate to shorter and taller people led to further variations. A return to a single bench-type adjusting table with a central fixed split abdominal support and two moveable end sections guided by floor rails emerged. A split headpiece enabling the patient's head to be directed straight downward was also incorporated.

According to Wells, Willard Carver used a side posture table in 1908 in early development of cervical adjustments. Wells noted that the Palmer recoil adjustment began development then, although it was not until 1935 that the Palmer "Hole-in-One" combining spinography, instrumentation, and toggle recoil adjustment along with knee and side posture tables was presented to the profession.

Hy-Lo Tables

In 1911 the first mechanically moveable adjusting table, the early Hy-Lo table with metal components, was invented by Bert Clayton. Although cumbersome and difficult to operate, using compressed air for smooth movement variations, it led to a rapid development of this adjusting table concept. It enabled the whole spine to be adjusted freely and was ideal for the majors and minors system of spinal adjustment and the later developing Meric system of adjustment. The development of the Hy-Lo adjusting table was a benchmark in the evolution of chiropractic adjusting tables.

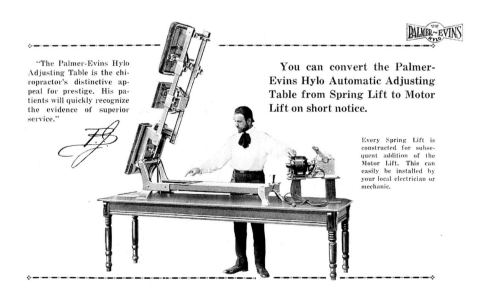

"The Palmer-Evins Hylo Adjusting Table is the chiropractor's distinctive appeal for prestige. His patients will quickly recognize the evidence of superior service."

You can convert the Palmer-Evins Hylo Automatic Adjusting Table from Spring Lift to Motor Lift on short notice.

Every Spring Lift is constructed for subsequent addition of the Motor Lift. This can easily be installed by your local electrician or mechanic.

B.J. Palmer demonstrating an early Hy-Lo adjusting table marketed by the PSC.
Courtesy Palmer College of Chiropractic Archives, Davenport, Iowa.

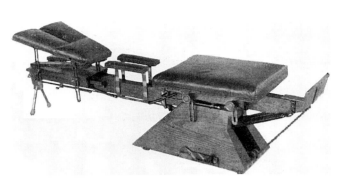

The Naysmith adjusting table, another early version of a Hy-Lo.
From *The Chiropractor*, May 1914.

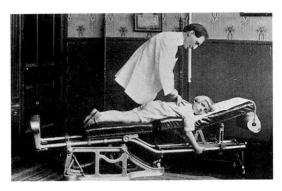

An early Hy-Lo table in use in a chiropractor's office.
Courtesy Palmer College of Chiropractic Archives, Davenport, Iowa.

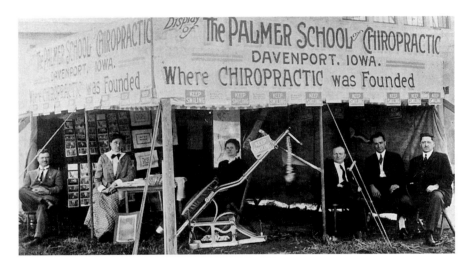

Another early Hy-Lo table featured in a PSC equipment display.
Courtesy Palmer College of Chiropractic Archives, Davenport, Iowa.

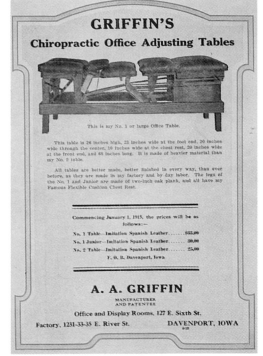

A Griffin spring-loaded adjusting table, circa 1915.
From *The Chiropractor*, January, 1916.

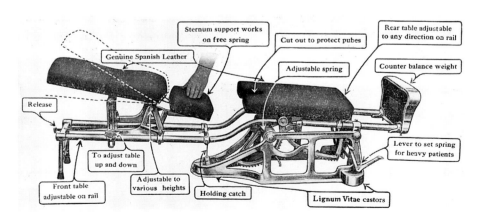

The Styles Hy-Lo adjusting table, developed about 1923, relied on springs for its lift and changed in the early 1930s to an electric motor as the source of its power.
Courtesy Palmer College of Chiropractic Archives, Davenport, Iowa.

Many mechanical variations were developed in the evolution of the Hy-Lo adjusting table. Ease of operation, better patient access, and accommodation to developing sophistication and specificity of spinal adjustment techniques were the criteria demanded by the profession.

Early spring-loaded Hy-Lo tables contained some thirty springs of the type used in closing screen doors. The Griffin Company of Davenport, Iowa, patented these spring-loaded Hy-Los in 1913. These numerous lighter springs gave way to fewer, more specifically directed heavier springs for balance and counter-balance in mechanical operation refinement of spring-loaded tables.

Changing from compressed air for movement of the components of the Clayton Hy-Lo to springs, Dossa Evins, in conjunction with Styles, developed the Styles Hy-Lo adjusting table about 1923. In the early 1930s the electric motor was used as its source of power.

The modern sophisticated Zenith Hy-Lo adjusting table with split- and variable-angle headpiece; shaped dorsal spring and firm support sections; and ankle supports and footplate, which takes the patient comfortably from the standing position to the prone position for adjustment and return by use of a foot control, is now found in most chiropractors' professional offices.

The development and evolution of chiropractic tables parallels development and evolution of adjusting techniques. Thus evolving adjusting techniques of different types led to the development of other well known types of adjusting tables also found in the chiropractors' professional rooms. These included the knee-chest table, a product of the mid-1920s and the side-posture table for specific upper cervical adjusting further developed from the 1930s. The Thompson drop headpiece for side posture tables of 1955 was a further refinement. In the 1960s and 1970s the Cox flexion/distraction tables, the Pettibon bench-instruments, and the Sweat instrument table all contained variations directed to several spinal adjusting techniques and methods.

In 1987, there were some 20 table companies servicing the chiropractic profession. Some were small, some were large, and a few had a wide range of different table models available; others were limited to special technique methods.

The Zenith Hy-Lo adjusting table is manufactured by the Williams Manufacturing Company of Moline, Illinois, the oldest of the current chi-

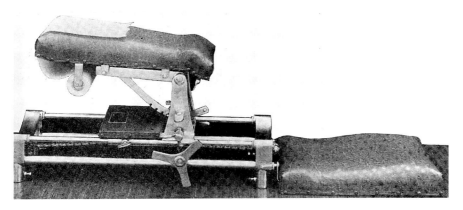

The knee-chest table is an example of a table developed for a particular technique, specifically the upper cervical techniques.
Courtesy Palmer College of Chiropractic Archives, Davenport, Iowa.

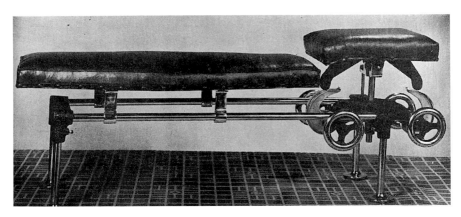

The side-posture table is another example of a table designed for use with a specific technique. This table is sized for a child.
Courtesy Palmer College of Chiropractic Archives, Davenport, Iowa.

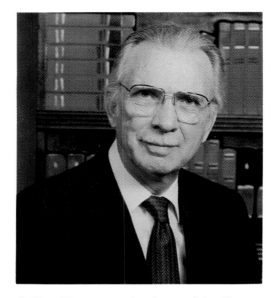

J. Clay Thompson, developer of the Thompson drop headpiece.
Courtesy Portraits by Annette, Davenport, Iowa.

ropractic adjusting table manufacturers. Founded by a chiropractor, G. Williams in 1916, the H910 product line has evolved through the spring-assisted, the electric worm-driven, and the electric hydraulic Hy-Lo table models of today.

In addition to the Hy-Lo, Williams Manufacturing also produces side-posture tables, flat benches, tables with drops, and now produces a Zenith-Cox flexion and distraction table. Although not the only manufacturer of adjusting tables specifically designed by and for the chiropractic profession, Williams Manufacturing is probably the most widely known.

Drop sections in adjusting tables were further refinements of the Thompson drop headpiece developed in the early 1950s by chiropractor J. Clay Thompson. The drop pieces were developed mainly at Clearview Sanitarium, a chiropractic mental institution in Davenport. Devised to make adjustments less fatiguing to the chiropractor and less painful to the patient, particularly toggle recoil type adjustments, the mechanism was patented by Dr. Thompson in 1956. It originally involved a manual mechanical cocking device and magnetic catch to hold the piece in cocked position ready for the toggle thrust. In thrust the headpiece and patient's head move in the direction of the thrust to bottom out during the toggle recoil mechanism. Later, both pneumatic and hydraulic cocking mechanisms were developed. Although originally designed for the cervical vertebrae region, the drop piece can also be built into other sections of adjusting tables such as the thoracic and lumbar vertebrae areas.

Re-Lax-O products was started in 1944 by chiropractors L.T. and Bernie Widmoyer and family. Re-Lax-O initially made accessories for existing adjusting table models developing pads that notably incorporated the "Dorsal Roll." These innovations led to development of a standard stationary table with all of the pads' features. The Company claims to have displayed the first electric hydraulic Hy-Lo table.

The Lloyd Table Company, founded by chiropractor Lloyd S. Steffensmeier in the late 1950s, was typical of the kind of development in table production over the years. As a student at PSC, he saw the need for a lighter, more stable portable adjusting table. House calls by the chiropractor for acute and nonambulatory patients made the need for portable adjusting tables, combining strength and light-weight construction. But unlike others who when they entered a busy practice they left the field of

ZENITH-THOMPSON PNEUMATIC

Chiropractic Table

*The Standard
Of
Excellence
In
Chiropractic
Equipment*

AIR POWER

A touch of your toe on these special switches and your pneumatically cocking recoil sections are in position and set to go. Air power does all your work - except to deliver the thrust.

ELECTRIC POWER

An advertisement for the Thompson Pneumatic Table, developed in the 1950s by J. Clay Thompson.

Courtesy Williams Manufacturing, Elgin, Illinois.

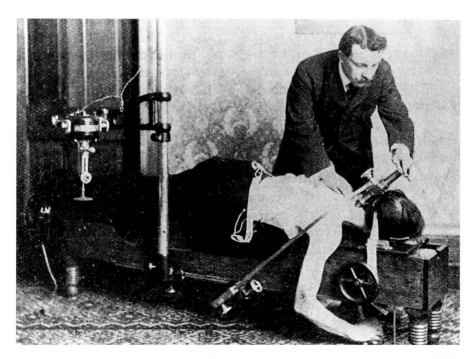

Solon Langworthy demonstrating the use of an early traction table, circa 1906.

From Smith O, Langworthy S, Paxson M: *Modernized chiropractic,* Cedar Rapids, Iowa, 1906, Laurence Press.

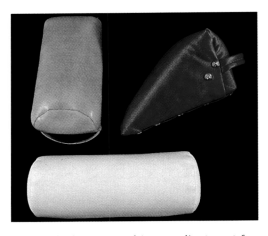

These blocks are used in an adjustment featuring the Sacro-Occipital Technique (SOT).
Courtesy Photographer, Palmer College of Chiropractic, Davenport, Iowa.

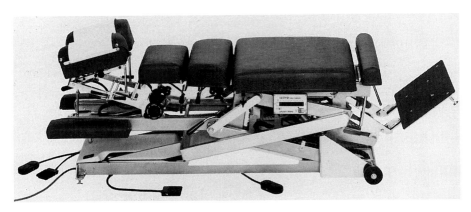

The 900HS is an example of a modern adjusting table.
Courtesy Lloyd Table Company, Lisbon, Iowa.

table design, Steffensmeier developed his own table and manufacturing company to satisfy not only his own needs but specialized needs within the profession. In 1963 he redesigned a knee-chest table and later produced pelvic blocks, block boards, sternal rolls, anterior dorsal blocks, all relevant to Dr. Major De Jarnette's Sacro-Occipital Technique (SOT). He also manufactured an adjusting bench and side-posture table.

Traction Tables

While the chiropractic profession was developing its own adjusting tables centered around developing techniques for correction of spinal subluxation, the parallel profession of osteopathy, with its emphasis on the whole body's blood supply, was developing its own tables. Osteopaths combined the examination function with functions of general manipulation, massage, and lymphatic drainage treatment. The osteopathic concepts of axial traction and intersegmental traction influenced the development of chiropractic adjusting tables.

As a form of treatment, traction methods date from the time of Hippocrates, about 400 BC. Traction has been described as involving binding of the patient's head, pelvis, knees and/or ankles, and stretching, somewhat in the same way as the rack of medieval times. The former was used

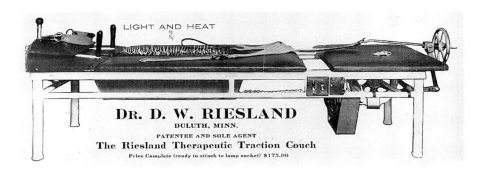

An example of an early traction table that also provided massage, produced by D.W. Riesland during the 1910s.
Courtesy Palmer College of Chiropractic Archives, Davenport, Iowa.

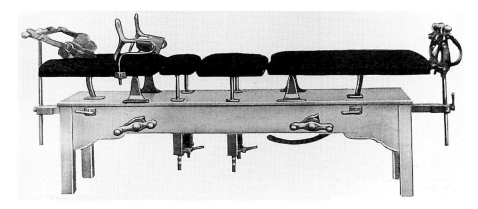

The Cropp "All-in-One" traction table was marketed to both chiropractors and osteopaths.

Courtesy Palmer College of Chiropractic Archives, Davenport, Iowa.

sometimes employing a stout beam along the back of the prone patient in traction for therapeutic purposes while the rack was used with the body supine, as an instrument of torture.

Wells also reports that in the early 1900s, Swofford developed the first gravity inversion table for spinal traction, and in 1913 the Pandiculater Company began production of an axial traction table followed by the Cropp 'All-in-One' table designed to provide best traction with best positioning. It was marketed both to medical and nonmedical drugless practitioners to administer "the very important science of tension therapy in the treatment of disease, the correction of deformities, injuries, etc."

Wells describes production of intersegmental traction tables by the Spinalator Company developed by osteopath O.N. Donahoe in 1937. While essentially used for traction techniques, it developed limited use for specific areas of the spine as distinct from general traction of the whole spine.

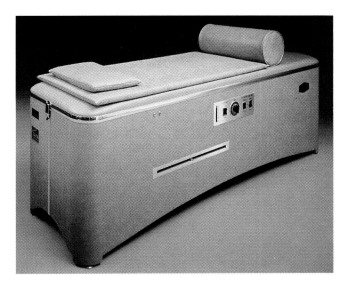

The Spinalator intersegmental traction table, developed by osteopath O.N. Donahoe, has a stationary top with moveable rollers.

From *The Journal of Chiropractic,* March 1984.

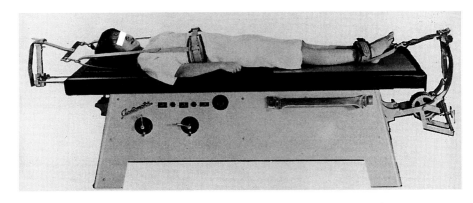

The Anatomotor traction table features a moveable table top with stationary intersegmental rollers.

From *The Digest of Chiropractic Economics,* September/October 1974.

In application, intersegmental traction could be achieved in two ways. A stationary table top with moveable intersegmental rollers might be used or, alternatively, a moveable table top with stationary intersegmental rollers could be used. The Spinalator table uses the former while the Anatomotor table uses the later.

Cox-McManus Table

But probably the most significant impact of osteopathic tables on the chiropractic profession was when James Cox, a chiropractor, developed in the 1960s the Cox-McManus table for the lumbar distraction work developed by Cox.

As early as 1909, an osteopath named McManus patented his table, which combined flexion, extension and rotation in addition to axial traction. Use of the universal joint in this table provided multidirectional movement to spinal segments and sacroiliac joints in addition to its primary traction function. It was this mechanical principle that Cox borrowed to develop a table suited to his lumbar distraction techniques later used by the chiropractic profession.

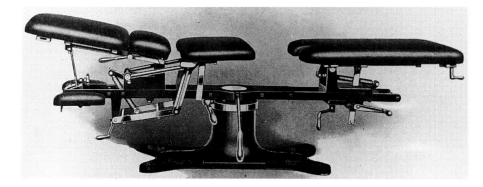

The McManus table was patented in 1909 by an osteopath and featured flexion, extension, and rotation in addition to axial traction.

Courtesy Palmer College of Chiropractic Archives, Davenport, Iowa.

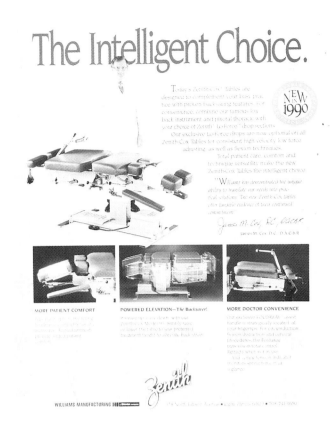

James Cox adapted some features from the McManus table to develop this table suited to his lumbar distraction technique.

Courtesy Williams Manufacturing, Elgin, Illinois.

ADJUSTING INSTRUMENTS

Adjustment techniques have traditionally been delivered to the patient by the chiropractor's manual dexterity skills of "by hand only," about which many textbooks have been written. However, some investigations have been made into the use of mechanical devices to deliver adjustments. One such device is the Activator Adjusting Instrument (AAI) developed by Drs. Warren C. Lee and Arlan W. Fuhr of Redwood Falls, Minnesota in the late 1960s.

Warren Lee graduated from Northwestern College of Chiropractic in 1941. He then completed a 1-year residency at the Logan Basic College of Chiropractic in St. Louis and studied the works of Toftness and Radionics. Arlan Fuhr, a former patient of Lee, enrolled at Logan in the autumn of 1958 and later became associated with Dr. Lee in practice. Radionics was dropped from their practice when warned that officials of the United States Food and Drug Administration were confiscating the machines.

Radionics was replaced by the preadjustment and postadjustment analysis of Richard Van Rumpt, D.C. which utilized leg-length checking and double thumb-lock adjusting procedures. In a busy practice, Lee and Fuhr found the repetitive use of Van Rumpt's thumb toggle tiring. Arlan Fuhr relates the story of waking in the morning with sore elbows that he placed in hot water to loosen up and then in ice water after his days work to reduce discomfort from adjusting.

In 1967 a Redwood Falls dentist, Dr. Steve Inglis, gave Lee and Fuhr a small dental impactor designed to force amalgam into tooth cavities.

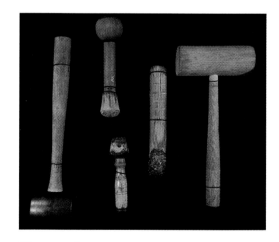

These mallets and chisels were framed and displayed by B.J. Palmer as "unscientific tools used by pseudo-chiropractors" who used them to attempt to drive protruding spines into line.

Courtesy Palmer College of Chiropractic Archives, Davenport, Iowa.

275

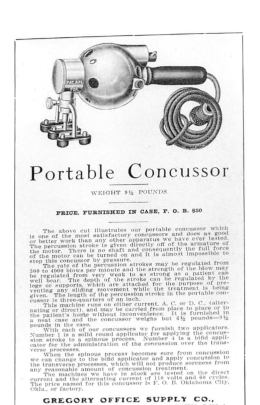

Portable Concussor

WEIGHT 9½ POUNDS

PRICE, FURNISHED IN CASE, F. O. B. $50

The above cut illustrates our portable concussor which is one of the most satisfactory concussors and does as good or better work than any other apparatus we have ever tested. The percussion stroke is given directly off of the armature of the motor. There is no shaft and consequently the full force of the motor can be turned on and it is almost impossible to stop this concussor by pressure.

The rate of the percussion strokes may be regulated from 300 to 4000 blows per minute and the strength of the blow may be regulated from very weak to as strong as a patient can well bear. The depth of the stroke can be regulated by the legs or supports, which are attached for the purpose of preventing any sliding movement while the treatment is being given. The length of the percussion stroke in the portable concussor is three-quarters of an inch.

This machine runs on either current, A. C. or D. C., (alternating or direct), and may be carried from place to place or to the patient's home without inconvenience. It is furnished in a neat case and the concussor weighs but 6½ pounds—9½ pounds in the case.

With each of our concussors we furnish two applicators. Number 1 is a solid round applicator for applying the concussion stroke to a spinous process. Number 4 is a bifid applicator for the administration of the concussion over the transverse processes.

When the spinous process becomes sore from concussion we can change to the bifid applicator and apply concussion to the transverse processes, which will not produce soreness from any reasonable amount of concussion treatment.

The machines we have in stock are tested on the direct current and the alternating current of 110 volts and 60 cycles. The price named for this concussor is F. O. B. Oklahoma City, Okla., or factory.

GREGORY OFFICE SUPPLY CO.,
Box 3   OKLAHOMA CITY, OKLA.

This portable concussor, marketed by Alva Gregory around 1910, was used for massage and may have been used for adjusting.

Courtesy Palmer College of Chiropractic Archives, Davenport, Iowa.

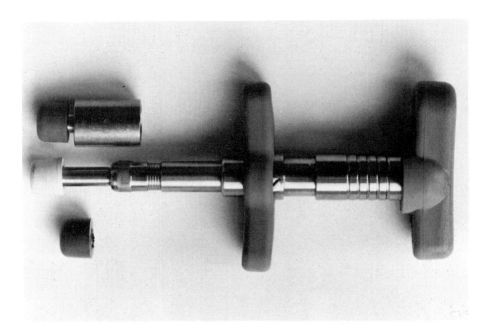

The activator instrument is reported to be used by over 21,000 chiropractors worldwide.

Courtesy Arlan Fuhr, Phoenix, Arizona.

Unsuccessful as an adjusting device, a surgical impact mallet designed for splitting impacted wisdom teeth was later successfully used. The original AAI was manufactured by Union Broach of New Jersey. Since 1976, Lee and Fuhr activator instruments have been manufactured by a Swiss-American firm. The name *Activator* was chosen because it was taught at Logan College of Chiropractic that an adjustment "activated" the bone. The AAI has been well-received by chiropractors. Australian chiropractor and Activator technique instructor, Dr. Dennis Richards, reports that over 21,000 chiropractors and chiropractic students have attended Activator Methods seminars and courses. He estimates that over 30,000 instruments are being used by chiropractors around the world.

In the early 1980s, Dr. Phillip George and other faculty members of Palmer College developed a light, disc-shaped force applicator known as the *"focalizer."*

More recently a computerized force-applying instrument, the Precision Spinal Adjustor, was developed. Conceived by Dr. Thomas Allegrezza, a Boise, Idaho chiropractor, it was developed in 1986 by Joseph Evans, a Ph.D. in civil engineering, and Rex Moore, a co-worker in industrial design. The Precision Spinal Adjustor has an internal microprocessor that monitors the energy level and changes this level when needed, selects the proper adjusting head, and activates the head when the proper patient contact is achieved. Three prototypes have been produced including tabletop, wall-mounted, and rolling stand models.

Upper Cervical Adjusting Instruments

Whereas hand-held mallets and computerized devices are essentially for use on the full spine, a more specialized series of instruments and

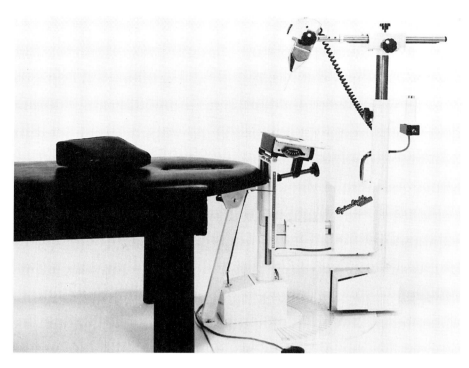

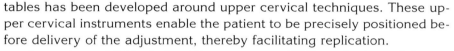

The Spinalight specific adjusting instrument designed by Dr. Roy Sweat.
Courtesy John Kyneur, New Lambton, New South Wales.

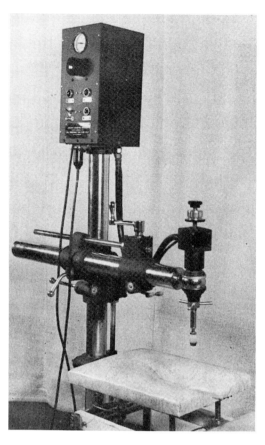

Arden Zimmerman's early mechanical adjusting instrument designed in 1941.

From Zimmerman A: The research and development of the specific adjusting machine, *The Digest of Chiropractic Economics*, May/June 1964.

tables has been developed around upper cervical techniques. These upper cervical instruments enable the patient to be precisely positioned before delivery of the adjustment, thereby facilitating replication.

As early as 1941, Arden Zimmerman, a PSC graduate and former Stanford engineer, discussed the possibility of developing a machine to adjust upper cervical vertebrae with two Stanford engineers who were former classmates and patients of Zimmerman. Encouraging Zimmerman to pursue the idea, these engineers did an investigative time, speed, and motion study of Zimmerman performing a manual adjustment. The resulting 27-page report was titled "Analysis of specific adjustments." In May 1948, the compressed-air driven instrument was completed. After preliminary tests the first upper cervical instrument adjustment was performed on June 6, 1948.

Zimmerman's instrument had been developed as a mechanical duplication of the toggle recoil manual adjustment. Along similar lines, Burl Pettibon developed his adjusting instruments in the 1960s to produce a repeatable force imitative of the triceps pull adjustment first used by A.L. Wernsing, D.C., in the 1940s and further developed by Drs. John Grostic and Ralph Gregory.

Similar instruments with additional features have been developed by chiropractors Roy Sweat and Don Harrison. Dr. Sweat produced a solenoid stylus instrument manufactured by the Spinalight Corporation. Dr. Harrison's instrument features an electric solenoid head, which is unique in that the table part of the machine has five small cushioned parts that can be raised and lowered to allow the stressing of patients into a myriad variety of configurations. The first model was produced in November 1983.

RADIOGRAPHY

History is replete with coincidences; for example, chiropractic was discovered in the United States in 1895, the same year x-ray was discovered in Germany. Without the early introduction of the use of x-ray into chiropractic practice the development of chiropractic as a unique discipline centered around spinal studies and treatment would probably never have developed as fully as it has. The use of x-ray by chiropractors in the development of chiropractic from 1910 on not only supplemented palpation and external examination of the spine but led to more detailed and scientific pictorial examination of segmental units of the spine and its adjacent structures. The use of x-ray, although its introduction was controversial, signalled a major step forward in the development of modern chiropractic.

X-ray equipment specially designed for the chiropractic profession emerged, and auxiliary devices used in alignment, safety, and quality control of the films produced were developed within and for the chiropractic profession.

A variety of special head clamps by W. Blair, Burl Pettibon, and J. Clay Thompson emerged in cervical spinography in conjunction with specific adjustment techniques. S.W. Bolton designed a direct x-ray beam pointer. The Felix-Bauer aluminum filters and gonad shields combined reduced radiation with improved film clarity and definition. Cervical spine analysis instruments, such as the Protractoscope and Grostic templates were developed to interpret x-ray photographs. Special moveable chairs for reproducible posture constants in x-ray positioning were designed. These and other developments were all devised by chiropractors as aids in producing spinal x-rays for the chiropractor's special needs. These x-ray films became known as spinographs.

Three-dimensional or stereoscopic x-ray films were also used by chiropractors in an attempt to improve on the normal two-dimensional films taken. Following the initial work by Dr. Fred Illi of Geneva, Switzerland,

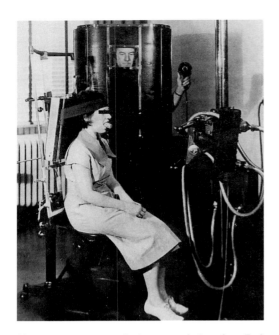

X-ray equipment being used in the B.J. Palmer Clinic, circa 1940.
Courtesy Palmer College of Chiropractic Archives, Davenport, Iowa.

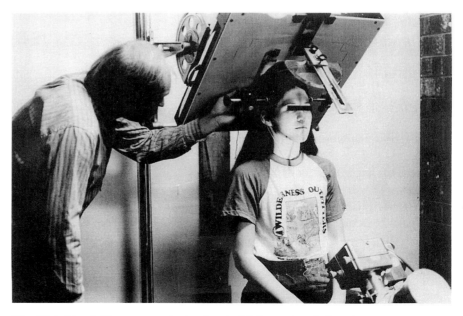

The Blair Head Clamp was devised to hold the patient's head in the proper position for taking x-ray photographs.
Courtesy John Kyneur, New Lambton, New South Wales.

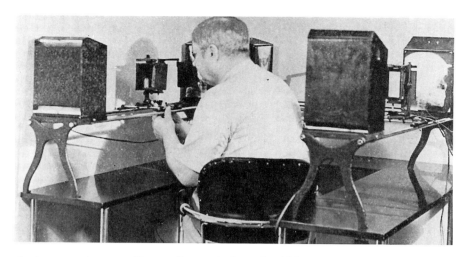

A stereoscopic x-ray film reading unit from the 1930s.
Courtesy Palmer College of Chiropractic Archives, Davenport, Iowa.

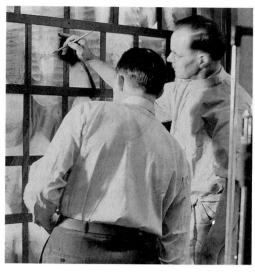

Chiropractors reading x-rays, which became an important adjunct for chiropractic spinal analysis and was incorporated as the major analysis tool for several chiropractic adjusting techniques.
Courtesy Palmer College of Chiropractic Archives, Davenport, Iowa.

Lincoln Chiropractic College and Kodak produced x-ray movies of spinal dynamics in cineroentgenology during 1940. A specifically designed and produced x-ray unit called the *Chiroprax* further attests to the special needs of the chiropractor in the field of x-ray examination recognized by commercial manufacturers. All these innovations in the development of chiropractic x-ray equipment and design are linked directly to specialized chiropractic x-ray analysis and spinography.

The use of x-ray is a standard procedure in chiropractic spinal analysis. Its primary role in chiropractic practice is to identify specific biomechanical components of the classical chiropractic subluxation.

Because of potential abnormalities, anomalies, or pathologies, an x-ray may either indicate which particular technique to use from the types available to the chiropractor; a need to modify adjustive techniques; or contraindication to spinal adjustment at given levels or even to any spinal adjustment.

THERMOELECTRICAL INSTRUMENTATION ANALYSIS EQUIPMENT

Of equal importance and complementary to the use of x-ray in chiropractic practice was the development of instruments designed to aid in determining the existence of spinal subluxation and changes following spinal adjustment. Chiropractic instrumentation, combined with spinography, supplemented by a case history, neurological testing and orthopedic examination are essential elements in clinical identification of the chiropractic subluxation.

Palpatory and nerve tracing skills were extensively used in early chiropractic practice and then were developed into electrical devices such as the Neurocalometer, the Visual Nerve Tracer, and the Ellis Microdynameter. The following three types of electrical devices categorize chiropractic instrumentation:

1. Bioelectrical
2. Photoelectrical
3. Thermoelectrical

Bioelectrical Instrumentation

Bioelectrical instruments measure skin resistance to the passage of a small electrical current of galvanic skin response. The best known example was the Ellis Microdynameter (MDM), which was a popular instrument of the 1940s and 1950s. Bioelectrical instruments have all but disappeared from contemporary chiropractic practice following the U.S. Department of Health, Education and Welfare's Food and Drug Administration (FDA) attack in the 1950s on its advertised use as a danger to patients' health. The Microdynameter was the main bioelectrical instrument utilized by chiropractors during the period 1931 until its dramatic ending in the early 1960s. This instrument was invented by Francis Cutler-Ellis in 1923, and distribution commenced in 1931. It was widely accepted by chiropractors as an additional aid in chiropractic instrumentation in the search for vertebral subluxations and became the main bioelectrical instrument utilized by chiropractors for some 30 years. It came to a sudden end when in 1961 Robert Ellis, president of Ellis Research Laboratories was enjoined by Federal Judge William J. Campbell to cease interstate transport of his product. The Judge claimed the equipment was wrongly branded and could not do what the makers claimed.

Despite this, similar bioelectrical devices have been used in research by the osteopathic and medical professions.

Photoelectrical Instrumentation

Photoelectrical instruments, not in common use in chiropractic today, include the Analyte and the Visual Nerve Tracer (VNT), or the "Photoelectrical visual nerve tracing instrument," which were developed by Adelman and Weiant. These instruments consist of a matched pair of photoelectrical cells that evaluate the reflection of light from engorged vascular beds under the skin. Kimmel and Triano recognize these instruments as forerunners to modern day thermography, variations of which (such as liquid crystal and telethermography) may be found in some chiropractors' offices.

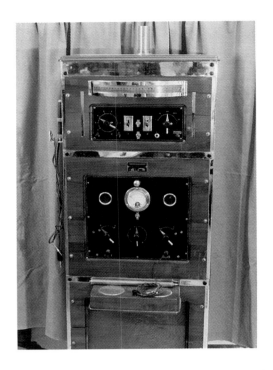

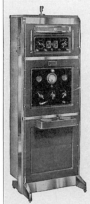

The Ellis Microdynameter of the 1930s measured galvanic skin response. This instrument was used during the 1940s and 1950s until the Food & Drug Administration removed it from the market.

Courtesy Logan College of Chiropractic Archives, Chesterfield, Missouri.

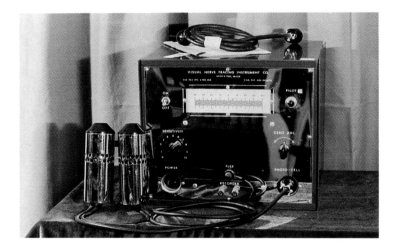

The Visual Nerve Tracing Instrument, a photoelectrical instrument, is a precursor to modern day thermography.

Courtesy Logan College of Chiropractic Archives, Chesterfield, Missouri.

Thermoelectrical Instrumentation

Thermoelectrical instruments, using a thermocouple principle, initiated instrumentation in chiropractic clinical practice. Thermoelectrical instruments measure paraspinal skin temperature and are thought to monitor the heat of spinal nerves via their sympathetic components. Thermoelectrical instruments are the most widely used of chiropractic instruments today.

Historically the development of thermoelectrical instruments stems from the early chiropractor identifying "hot spots" along the spine as potential trouble spots and sites of subluxations.

Quigley describes how B.J. Palmer taught that warmer spots along the spine signalled a subluxation. He referred to these areas as "hot boxes" from a common rail-road car problem in which the lack of lubrication in the wheelbox allowed friction to develop an extremely hot box and often a fire. The chiropractor was trained to seek out these hot areas with the more sensitive back of his hand as a preliminary to spinal adjustment in the early days at the Palmer School of Chiropractic.

DOSSA EVINS AND THE NEUROCALOMETER

Dossa Evins is reported by August Dye to have worked on this spinal heat concept as a facet of the chiropractic spinal subluxation complex from 1920 to 1922. Born in Blodget, Missouri, on February 13, 1896, Evins studied engineering at the University of Arkansas and served during World War I in the radio department of the U.S. Secret Service. He contracted tuberculosis and spent several years in a sanitorium. His search for health led him to Dr. R.S. Marlow of San Antonio, Texas, a chiropractor from whom he greatly benefitted. During treatment he noted that his chiropractor used the back of his hand on patients' backs, in a sort of exploratory fashion, and was told that chiropractors looked for "hot spots" as an indication of "nerve pressure." In 1920 he enrolled at PSC and, after graduation in 1922, practiced in Kansas City, Missouri, where he took up in earnest the development of an instrument to detect "hot spots."

Evins introduced and applied the thermocouple principle to spinal analysis. The thermocouple principle, as a method of measuring heat differentials, was discovered by T.J. Seebeck of Germany in 1829.

Seebeck found that an electrical current will flow in a circuit consisting of two dissimilar metallic conductors with two junctions of these wires a distance apart, a *thermocouple,* when one junction is at a higher or lower temperature than the other. The electromotive force (EMF) producing this current is known as the Seebeck Thermal EMF. The instrument invented by Evins was made up of a number of thermocouples in two probes, termed *thermopiles,* which were connected to a galvanometer set in a hand-held instrument case. It is used to compare paraspinal heat by straddling the spine and aids more accurately than palpation in pinpointing "hot spots." It was called a Neurocalometer (NCM). B.J. Palmer realized the potential of the NCM and worked to have the instrument patented in time for the 1924 Lyceum.

At the August 1924 Lyceum, B.J. introduced the NCM. Lyceums and Homecomings were regularly held at PSC and drew chiropractors from all over the world.

The name, *neuro-calo-meter* (nerve-heat-meter), was a composite designation devised by B.J. to describe the instrument's purpose. But the main objections to the NCM were the cost and B.J.'s insistence that it be used by chiropractors. The NCM was not to be sold, B.J. explained, but

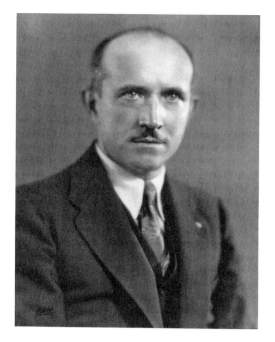

Dossa Evins, an engineer who graduated from the PSC in 1922, invented the Neurocalometer.

Courtesy Palmer College of Chiropractic Archives, Davenport, Iowa.

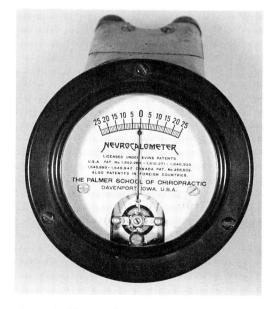

An early Neurocalometer, which B.J. Palmer introduced to the profession at the PSC's August 1924 Lyceum.

Logan College of Chiropractic Archives, Chesterfield, Missouri.

The Scientific Health Service

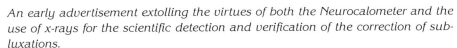

IT HAS long been a problem in the Chiropractic profession to develop a workable means by which to arrive at some immediate demonstrable proof of the effects of interference with spinal nerve transmission; demonstrable proof that such interference was removed by proper adjustment of the causative subluxation, by showing the disappearance of its associated phenomena with the subsequent elimination of attending symptoms.

The discovery, by the German physicist Roentgen, of the X ray, made it possible to prove the vertebral subluxation. With the use of the X ray, the chiropractor produces a picture of the spine, called a Spinograph, and thus scientifically determines the exact position of the vertebral subluxation.

Then came the invention of the Neurocalometer. The Neurocalometer is a scientific instrument designed to detect very minute tempera-

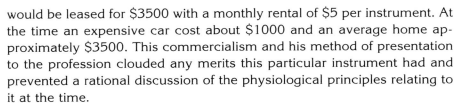

ture differences along the spine. It locates accurately the point of spinal nerve interference. The detector used is a very delicate thermopile which makes a comparative heat reading that is registered through the medium of a galvanometer. With the use of the Neurocalometer, the chiropractor is able to determine the point of nerve pressure in the spine, and, after a Chiropractic adjustment has been given for the purpose of releasing such pressure, further use of the instrument provides accurate knowledge as to whether the nerve pressure has been released, and in what degree.

Chiropractic is no longer the practice of theoretical principles. These have now been established as scientifically demonstrable facts, by the use of scientific equipment. Chiropractors who use the Neurocalometer and the X ray in their practice are equipped to deliver modern, scientific Chiropractic health service to their patients.

An early advertisement extolling the virtues of both the Neurocalometer and the use of x-rays for the scientific detection and verification of the correction of subluxations.

Courtesy Palmer College of Chiropractic Archives, Davenport, Iowa.

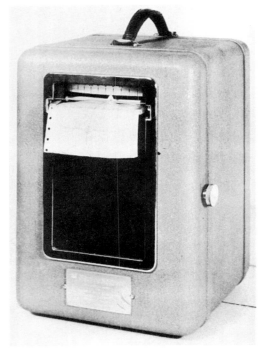

The Neurocalograph, introduced in 1939, produced a graph-recording of NCM readings and eliminated the human element of error in NCM work.

Courtesy Palmer College of Chiropractic Archives, Davenport, Iowa.

would be leased for $3500 with a monthly rental of $5 per instrument. At the time an expensive car cost about $1000 and an average home approximately $3500. This commercialism and his method of presentation to the profession clouded any merits this particular instrument had and prevented a rational discussion of the physiological principles relating to it at the time.

Initially rejected by a large section of the profession, the NCM did survive and came to be used by a significant number of practitioners. Many in the profession regard the NCM's importance in the "scientific" practice of chiropractic as similar to the importance of the use of x-ray to chiropractic practice. The introduction of x-ray by B.J. in 1910 had caused a PSC walkout of faculty and students. Similarly, the introduction of the NCM, equally controversial, was the commencement of the use of chiropractic analysis instrumentation in chiropractic practice and caused another wave of faculty and student walkouts at PSC.

Graph-recording of NCM readings by mechanical means was a logical development of visual and handwritten NCM readings. By 1939 the Neurocalograph (NCGH), developed by the PSC consultant engineer Otto Schiernbeck, appeared as a sophisticated self-recording NCM. Its introduction eliminated the human element of error in recording neurocalometer work and allowed more accurate comparisons.

OTHER THERMOELECTRICAL ANALYSIS INSTRUMENTS

Other heat-reading instruments, similar to the NCM, were later manufactured by independent companies and appeared on the market. Among the better-known instruments were the Nervoscope (NS) and the Neuropyrometer (NPM).

The Nervoscope, manufactured by Electronic Development Laboratories, New York, was developed in the 1940s. Its graphing companion is the Analgraph (AG). In addition, a table-top galvanometer, the Analascope (AS), was manufactured. The AS allowed the patient to see the

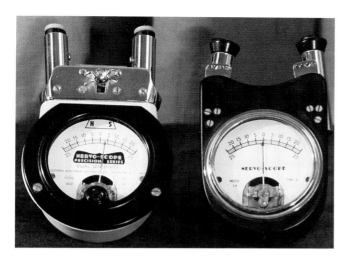

The NervoScope was introduced during the 1940s as an alternative to the Neurocalometer.

Courtesy Logan College of Chiropractic Archives, Chesterfield, Missouri.

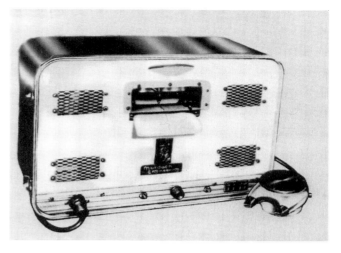

A ThermoScribe graphing instrument produced by Murdoch Engineering during the 1950s.

From *The ICA International Review of Chiropractic,* May/June 1991.

reading as it was being made. The AS may be described as a high-gain, vacuum-tube, voltage-controlled amplifier.

Murdoch Engineering of California produced the Neuropyrometer (NPM). The NPM later became known as the Thermeter (TM) with the Thermoscribe (TS) as its graphing partner.

All of these heat-reading instruments are still marketed today. All are available for individual sale except the NCM, which until the mid-1980s, was available for lease only. All make use of the thermocouple principle and measure comparative heat by conduction from skin-contact probes straddling the spine.

With these spine-straddling comparative heat-readers it was realized that there was no way to know if an area was bilaterally hot or bilaterally cold. Further, contact-fixed probes could be improved by reaching closer to the transverse processes of the spine and hence the neurological bed, particularly in the upper cervical spine.

Thus heat-reading instruments were devised to fill this gap. In the 1950s the Chirometer and the Vasotonometer (VTM), the latter leading to the Synchrotherme, emerged. The development of the VTM emerged from the study of vasomotor control and thermoregulation taken up by Dr. A.R. Petersen of Davenport, Iowa in 1951, to fulfill the need for bilateral temperature comparisons. It led to development of the Synchrotherme (ST).

Considerable work on development and interpretation of the Synchrotherme was done by Petersen, Himes, Watkins, Haldeman, Grice, Gitelman, and Bailey at the Canadian Memorial Chiropractic College, Toronto, in the 1960s and 1970s. But despite thousands of hours spent in development and research of this instrument, the Synchrotherme is no longer available to the profession.

In the 1960s, Vernon Pierce of Dravosberg, Pennsylvania developed the Dermathermograph (DTG). This instrument, using different technology, is an infrared, heat-sensitive instrument that measures skin surface temperature by radiation without direct skin contact.

Interest in paraspinal heat readings waned in the 1970s, but in the 1980s the correlation between thermal anomalies and vertebral subluxa-

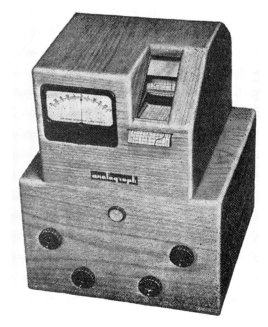

The Analagraph used the same principles as the NervoScope with the added benefit of recording the results onto graph paper.

From *The Journal of the National Chiropractic Association,* April 1954.

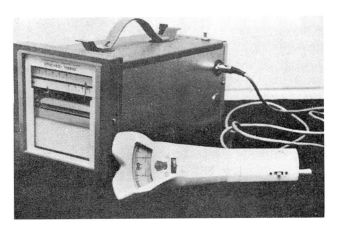

The Synchrotherme, a bilateral temperature reading instrument that was developed and tested at Canadian Memorial Chiropractic College in Toronto during the 1970s.
From *The Journal of the Canadian Chiropractic Association*, 14(1), 1970.

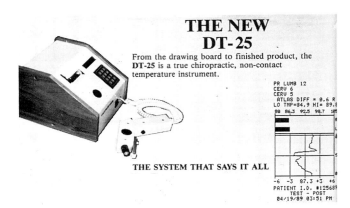

The Derma-thermograph, another temperature measuring diagnosis device developed by Vernon Pierce. This device is an infrared heat-sensitive instrument that measures skin surface temperatures.
From *The Digest of Chiropractic Economics*, May/June 1989.

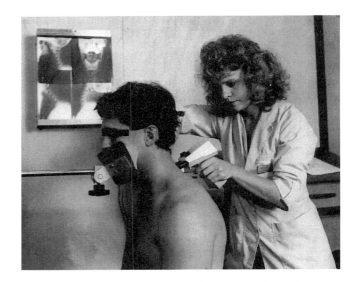

A student reading temperature differences along the spine with an Accolade III instrument.
Courtesy John Kyneur, New Lambton, New South Wales.

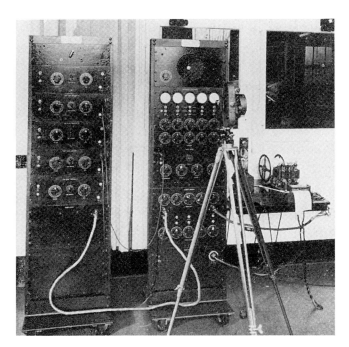

The Electroencephaloneuromentimpograph was designed and developed at the B.J. Palmer Chiropractic Research Clinic in the 1930s. The machine was used to measure nerve impulses from the brain and is considered a precursor to the EEG.
Courtesy Palmer College of Chiropractic Archives, Davenport, Iowa.

tions was studied. The writings of Hart, Crowder, Kale, Duff, Gelardi, Rush, Plaugher, Stillwagon, and others continue to develop interest in this field.

The electroencephaloneuromentimpograph, or timpograph, was a special instrument developed to play a particular role in the B.J. Palmer Chiropractic Clinic at Davenport, Iowa, from 1935 to 1961. A precursor to the electroencephalogram (EEG), it was used to measure and calibrate nerve impulse flow between brain and body in clinical assessment of the subluxation complex and sought to validate the specific upper cervical (or Hole-In-One) adjustment regimen. It was essentially a clinical research instrument.

OTHER EQUIPMENT USED BY CHIROPRACTORS

Standard diagnostic equipment found in chiropractic rooms may include the stethoscope, sphygmomanometer, and opthalmascope, which supplemented by laboratory tests help to assess the patient's physiological status. The Cameron Heartometer introduced in the 1960s is a discgraph mechanical ink-recording device combining a record of pulse rate and standard systolic and diastolic blood vascular pressures.

In addition to the equipment used in adjusting the patient—the tables, the posture analyzers, and the adjusting instruments—many chiropractors use charts, models, and other patient education tools to help the patient understand what the chiropractor's adjustment is doing. The Fleet Spinal demonstrator is one example of such equipment. Based on x-ray findings, the chiropractor can position the model so that it is a replica of the patient's spine, visually showing the patient what the chiropractor is doing.

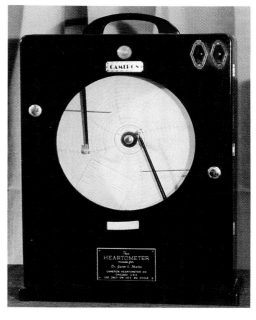

The Cameron Heartometer from the 1960s was a device that recorded the pulse rate and systolic/diastolic blood pressures.
Courtesy Logan College of Chiropractic Archives, Chesterfield, Missouri.

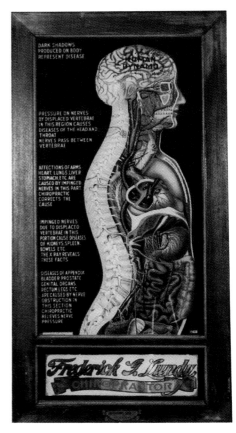

Patient education tools like this colorful spine mounted in a light box were designed to demonstrate what the chiropractor would do.
Courtesy Logan College of Chiropractic Archives, Chesterfield, Missouri.

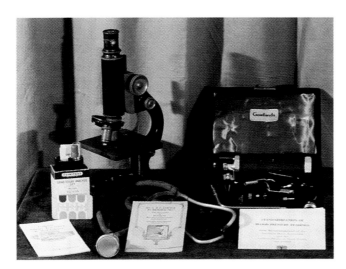

Some early diagnostic instruments found in a chiropractor's office would include a stethoscope, a sphygmomanometer, an opthalmascope, and a microscope.
Courtesy Logan College of Chiropractic Archives, Chesterfield, Missouri.

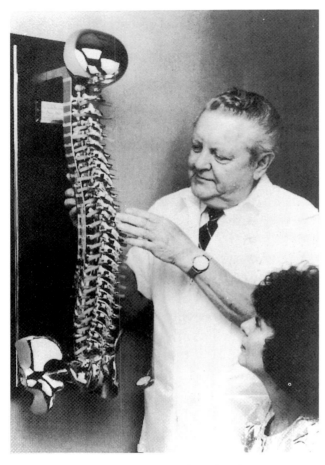

Fleet's Spinal Demonstrator enables the chiropractor to re-produce the patient's spinal distortion, helping the patient understand the spinal condition.

From *The ICA International Review of Chiropractic,* November/December 1991.

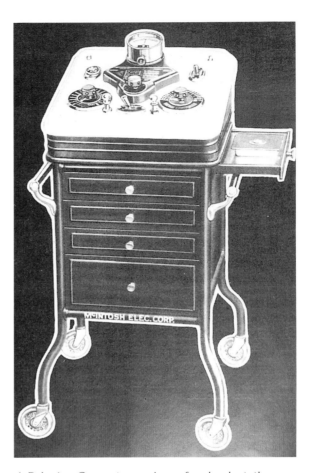

A Polysine Generator, a piece of early electotherapy equip-ment used by some chiropractors.

Courtesy Logan College of Chiropractic, Chesterfield, Missouri.

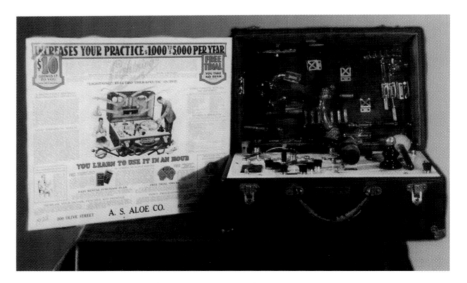

Electrotherapy, such as this "Lightning" Electro-Therapy Kit, was used by some chiropractors. Although this particular model may have had therapeutic value, it was marketed for its profitability and ease of use.

Courtesy Logan College of Chiropractic Archives, Chesterfield, Missouri.

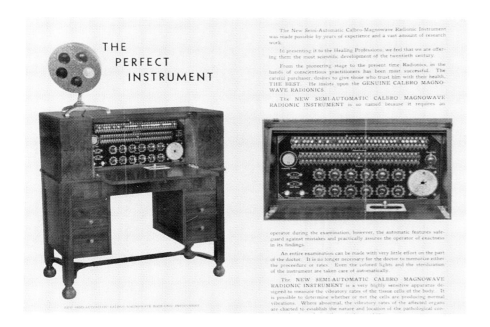

An advertisement for a Calbro Magno-Wave Radionics Instrument, which was used by a few chiropractors during the 1940s and 1950s.
Courtesy Palmer College of Chiropractic Archives, Davenport, Iowa.

As early as the days of Solon Langworthy, many chiropractors used ancillary methods to treat their patients, in addition to the chiropractic adjustment. Such methods may employ heat, electrotherapy, hydrotherapy, acupuncture, acupressure, vitamin therapy, as well as rehabilitation equipment. The disagreement over whether ancillary procedures are in the purview of the chiropractor has formed the basis of the debate between the "straights" and the "mixers."

Like dentistry and optometry, special equipment devised and developed within and for the chiropractic profession focuses on the unique role of the chiropractor within the community of health services available to the public.

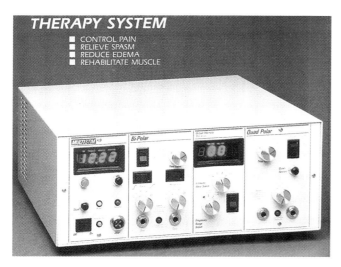

An example of contemporary electronic devices used today by some chiropractors to control pain and rehabilitate muscle.
Courtesy Palmer College of Chiropractic Archives, Davenport, Iowa.

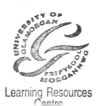

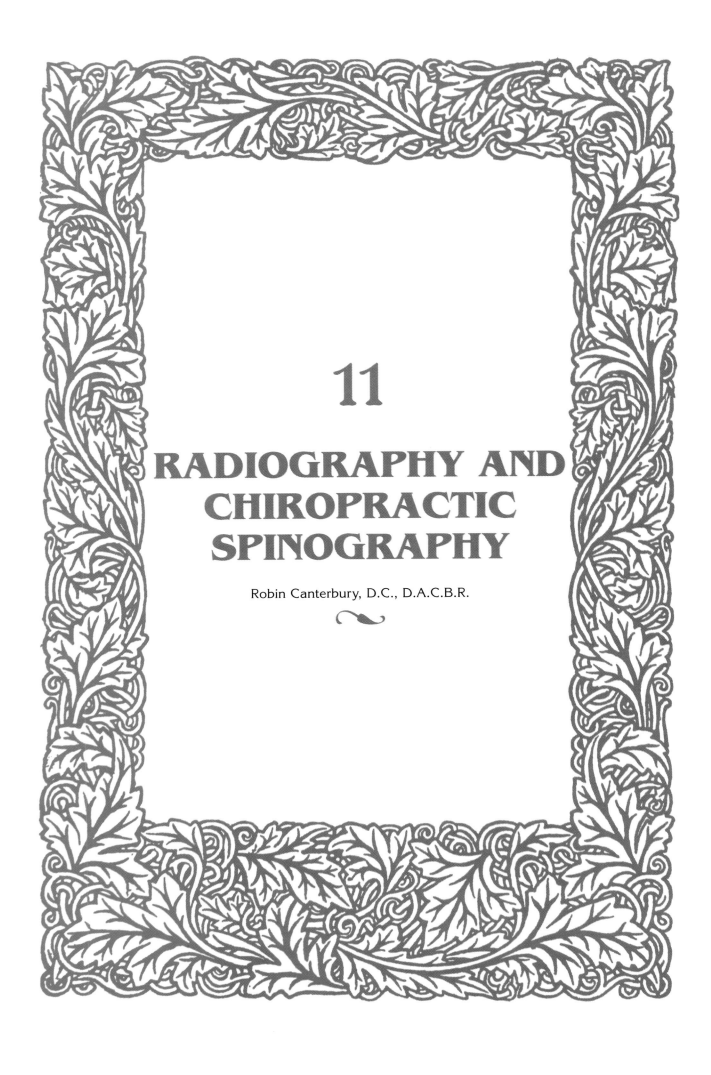

11

RADIOGRAPHY AND CHIROPRACTIC SPINOGRAPHY

Robin Canterbury, D.C., D.A.C.B.R.

The year 1895 was momentous in the advancement of the health care sciences. It was the year in which the discoveries of chiropractic, during September, and x-ray, during November, were made, both more or less by accident, and both ideas having been done before but without organized reasons behind them. The news of the discovery of x-rays spread quickly and was met with a great deal of public interest, as well as catching the attention of physicists, electrical scientists, photographers, and a few physicians. Chiropractic, on the other hand, was not widely heralded, the news was disseminated slowly, and the theory was not understood by the established medical community.

It was not until 15 years later, although some historians say 13, that x-ray found its way into the relatively new healing art of chiropractic. Its utilization in chiropractic was probably delayed because of the poor images of the deeper bony structures, specifically the spine, which were produced by the still infantile x-ray equipment, as well as because of the reported burns and soft tissue damage suffered by early workers and the occasional patient. Organized medicine did not take to the roentgen ray with zeal either. As Eisenberg said, "Physicians were not readily adopting the new science even though the public was clamoring for its use." When x-ray was introduced to the chiropractic profession in 1910 by B.J. Palmer, president of the Palmer School of Chiropractic in Davenport, Iowa, it was not widely accepted; in fact, its use even met with rebellion.

To explore adequately both the impact that the inclusion of x-ray had on chiropractic and the developments that occurred with radiology within the profession and outside of it, one must start at the beginning with

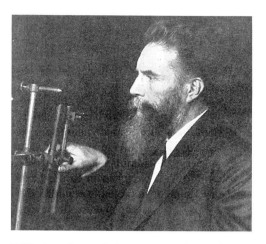

Wilhelm Conrad Roentgen, the acknowledged discoverer of the x-ray.
Courtesy Burndy Library, Norwalk, Connecticut.

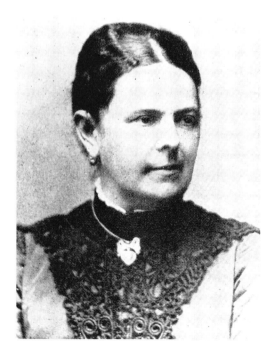

Anna Bertha Roentgen, Wilhelm Roentgen's wife and the first human subject (other than himself) of his x-ray discovery. Sources say she was horrified at the sight of the bones in hand.
From Glasser O: *W.C. Roentgen,* Springfield, Ill, 1933, Charles C Thomas.

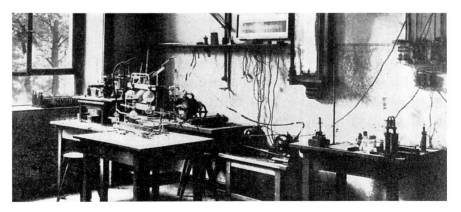

Roentgen's laboratory in Wurtzburg, Germany, which looks today much the way it did in the 1890s.
From Kaye GWC: *Roentgenology: its early history,* 1928, Hoeber.

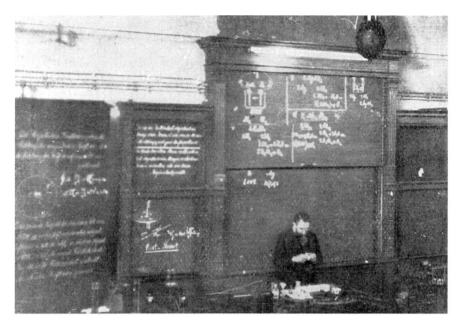

Wilhelm C. Roentgen in a physics class in Wurtzburg, Germany.
From Glasser O: *W.C. Roentgen,* Springfield, Ill, 1933, Charles C Thomas.

Roentgen. Though this history is dealt with here in only an abbreviated fashion, a more detailed investigation of the progression of x-ray can be found in *Radiology: An Illustrated History* by Ronald L. Eisenberg, M.D., and *The Trail of the Invisible Light* by E.R.N. Grigg, M.D.

On a Friday in November 1895, professor Wilhelm Conrad Roentgen, a physicist and director of the Physical Institute of the University of Wurzburg, Germany, discovered a new light which he called *x-ray.* The discovery was accidental, occurring when he attempted to duplicate an experiment by the physicist Philipp Lenard using cathode rays and fluorescence.

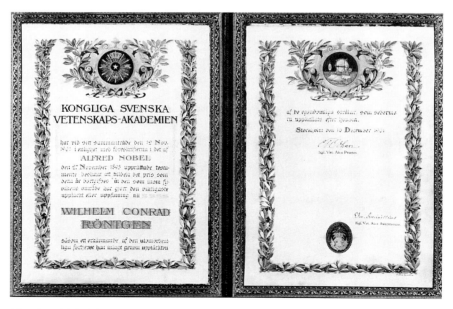

The first Nobel Prize in Physics was awarded in 1901 to Wilhelm Conrad Roentgen for the discovery of x-rays, a decision that upset Lenard until his death.
From Eisenberg R: *Radiology: an illustrated history,* St. Louis, 1991, Mosby.

Roentgen spent the next 7 weeks isolated in his laboratory until he was sure of what he had discovered. In December he submitted his first written communication on the subject and in January 1896 made his first oral presentation and public demonstration of his discovery. ◠

EARLY MEDICAL EDUCATION AND USE

The emergence of x-ray caught the attention of physicists, photographers, and a few electrical manufacturers, but it was not until some physicians found that they could see inner structures, particularly bones and metallic foreign bodies, that they could see the clinical potential. The few farsighted and mechanically minded doctors who were attracted to it eventually influenced others, and with much experimenting, new discoveries and improvements produced better image quality and safer production.

The medical doctors who were excited about x-ray did not have many colleagues who shared their enthusiasm, but whenever a few of the innovators would get together, they shared experiences and plates. This informal sharing was the first method of training for radiologists. As articles appeared and texts were written on the subject, they read them. Originally most early books were technical in nature. In 1910, Ernest Codman wrote his first book on pediatrics. Other authors from 1912 to 1921 produced books dedicated to specialty areas, such as the alimentary canal, diseases of the kidney, diagnosis of diseases of the head, and in 1921, injuries and diseases of bones and joints. Groups of interested doctors got together, formed societies, and held conventions where they could learn from one another.

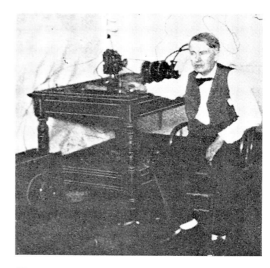

Photograph of Thomas Edison x-raying his own brain as a publicity stunt.
From Eisenberg R: Radiology: an illustrated history , St. Louis, 1991, Mosby.

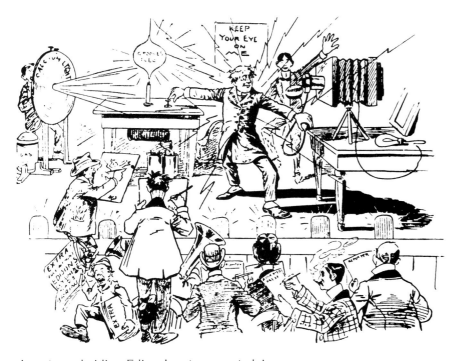

A cartoon deriding Edison's extravagant claims.
From Grigg ERN: Trail of the invisible light, Springfield, Ill, 1965, Charles C. Thomas.

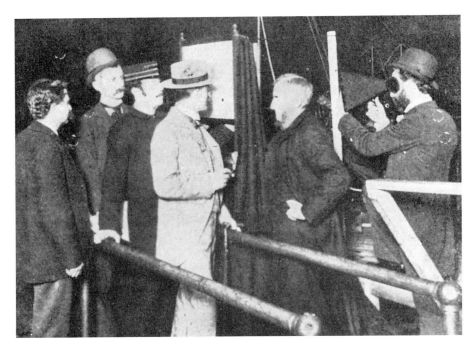

Thomas Edison's x-ray exhibit at the 1896 New York Electrical Exposition. He hoped to sell his "vitascope" to the general public.

From Elsenberg R: *Radiology: an illustrated history,* St. Louis, 1991, Mosby.

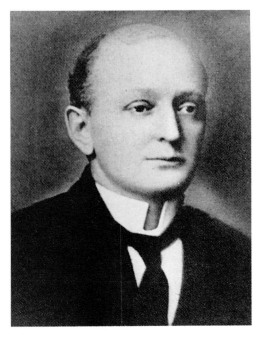

Clarence Dally, Edison's friend and worker, was the first known x-ray radiation fatality in 1904 and the reason Edison stopped working with x-ray.

From Brown P: *American martyrs to science through the Roentgen ray,* Springfield, Ill, 1925, Charles C Thomas.

There was no formal education in the early days of which they could avail themselves. Newer doctors coming out of college, who were interested in radiology, could seek out and learn from those who already had experience. Even by 1930, few American universities had postgraduate programs that would lead to a diploma in radiology, and many of the early courses lacked fundamental education in technology and physics. They tended to be geared to the physician who wanted to learn about an area of special interest in a course that would last only a few weeks.

Undergraduate education was also very slow in developing. A 1930 survey by Preston Hickey found that only 53 medical schools taught a course in radiology. One medical school taught x-ray before 1900. Fifteen additional colleges took up the subject by 1910 and 37 more by 1928. Hickey's survey showed that 36% of the institutions taught x-ray in connection with anatomy in the first year, 46% taught 10 hours in connection with anatomy and physiology in the second year, and about 80% gave instruction in the third year averaging 30 hours. An additional 25 hours was offered in 98% of the schools that stressed the clinical application of radiology. Even today there are few hours of x-ray education in medical schools, with most doctors relying on the specialists in radiology for interpretation and recommendations for further studies.

In 1933 James T. Case wrote about the state of x-ray in medicine. "The vicious tendency on the part of incompetent or dishonest laymen, and even unscrupulous physicians, to commercialize radiology is a natural danger of too rapid expansion of the specialty of radiology and a consequent faulty and insufficient training of physicians entering it." It was obvious that the science had to be regulated and have standards set.

One-and two-year fellowships began to appear at some teaching centers, but they lacked uniformity. By 1934 the American Board of Radiology (ABR) was formed and held its first examination. There were three

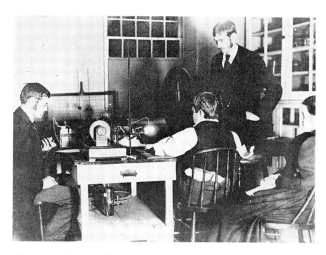

The first "clinical" x-ray plate was produced in the physics laboratory of Dartmouth College in 1896.

From Grigg ERN: *The trail of the invisible light,* Springfield, Ill, 1965, Charles C Thomas.

categories of candidates: "outstanding radiologists" with years of experience, most of whom were certified without testing; doctors with less experience; and new graduates from established radiology programs. The grading scale for the first few years of the ABR, however, was imaginary. It used the letters of the word *x-ray: x* for scores of 100% to 90%, *r* for 80% to 89%, *a* for 79% to 70%, and *y* for below 70%, or failure.

Use of x-ray was a low priority for hospitals and, therefore, slow to develop in that setting as well. America's oldest hospital, Pennsylvania Hospital, purchased its first x-ray unit in 1897, but roentgenograms were not recorded as having been taken that year. By 1902, it is reported that "the x-ray machine was rarely used and then only out of curiosity, not for patient care. Even a decade later, in 1912, roentgenographic examination was still quite an unusual event for hospitalized patients." More ambitious, however, was the Children's Hospital in Boston, which started radiography in 1899 with Ernest Codman as its first "skiagrapher." By 1901 he had produced some 300 glass plate roentgenograms, which was quite a feat since the hospital was not yet furnished with electricity, lighting still being supplied by gas. It is reported that he received the needed current by running a wire from a nearby opera house. When the opera was in progress, then he could proceed with the x-rays.

CHIROPRACTIC'S EARLY USE

The first use of x-ray in chiropractic occurred in early 1910. B.J. Palmer, president of the Palmer School of Chiropractic (PSC) in Davenport, Iowa, purchased his first x-ray unit from the Scheidel-Western X-ray Coil Company of Chicago, and installed it in a bedroom on the second floor of a building that the school owned at 828 Brady Street. The actual year of procurement of the first x-ray unit has been in doubt and speculations range from the year 1908 to 1910. This confusion in the date of purchase of Palmer's initial x-ray machine arises from his conflicting

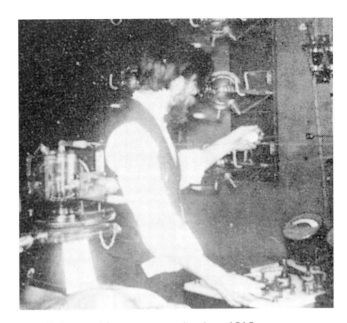

B.J. Palmer with an x-ray unit, circa 1910.
Courtesy Chance-Peters Chiropractic Collection, Wagga Wagga, New South Wales, Australia.

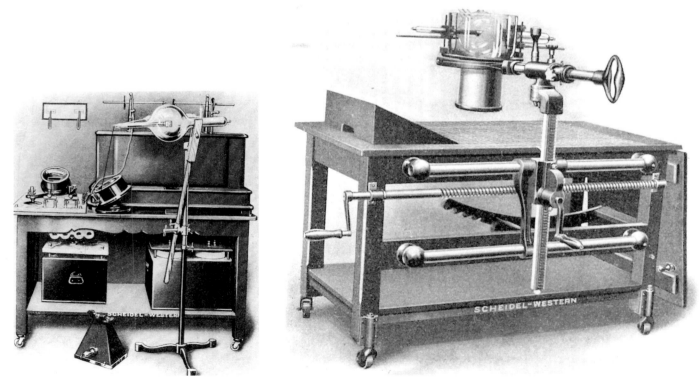

The Schiedel-Western x-ray units purchased by the Palmer School of Chiropractic in 1910.
From *Annual Announcement*, Davenport, Iowa, 1910, Palmer School of Chiropractic.

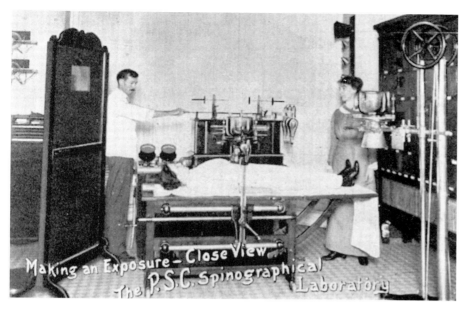

James McGinnis using the Scheidel-Western equipment at the PSC, circa 1912.
From *Glimpses of the PSC*, Davenport, Iowa, 1913, Palmer School of Chiropractic.

statements. In September 1910, however, Palmer stated before the Universal Chiropractors Association (UCA) convention that he had "worked with the machine for ten months," and an advertisement in March 1910 stated "only installed two months ago." These early utterances seem to have validity. Although x-ray machines were already in use in Iowa, this was apparently the first in Davenport.

Apparently Palmer was captivated by the relatively new penetrating device and its potential for chiropractic, since he had attended the annual electrical shows in nearby Chicago for 5 years and had communicated with x-ray companies about suitable units for exposures of the spine. When he decided to order the Scheidel-Western, he claimed that "he found a unit that would penetrate the spine and he ordered it." Since spinal films had been performed by Monell as early as 1902, Palmer may have been talking about a unit that could penetrate and produce a detailed and clearer image, which ongoing developments in the x-ray eventually brought out. No doubt with his concentrated work with the spine, he contributed to the development of better techniques and procedures.

X-RAY AND SPINOGRAPHY

B.J. Palmer coined the term *spinography* in February 1910 for his work in radiographing the spine. The term was an obvious extension of radiography, coined with the Latin root, *spine,* and the Greek root *graphy,* which means "to write."

The 1910 school announcement does not reflect the term *spinography* but instead reflects the common usage of the day, *spinal photography department* and *spinal skiagraphs,* a common term of the day for the radiographic print. By February, the spinal photographic department became the spinographic department, and spinographs, instead of skia-

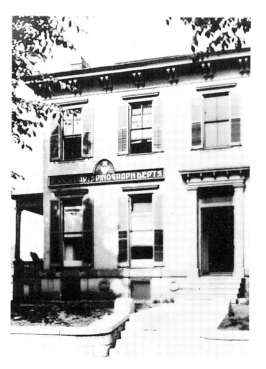

The second building to house the x-ray department at the PSC.

From *The Wivern*, Davenport, Iowa, 1960, Palmer School of Chiropractic.

295

graphs, were taken of the spine. Of course, the spinographic department x-rayed other body parts, but these were simply called skiagraphs or roentgenographs.

With the introduction of the x-ray into the Palmer School came dissention among Palmer's faculty, students, and alumni. Many of the faculty rebelled against the idea, with many members of these groups feeling that the science of chiropractic did not need this addition. After all, their skills with palpation of the spine had been very well developed, and their patients had experienced beneficial results. They did not know why chiropractic needed x-ray in 1910 when it had not in 1895. B.J. Palmer reminisced about the events in 1930, stating,

> My early faculty called me crazy and advised the students to pay little attention to my ravings. I suggested introducing it as an additional subject for instruction into the school. The faculty refused and the student body rebelled even to petitions against it. We were told that if we enforced its introduction they would secede to another school where they were not asked to study a useless subject.

Several of the PSC faculty told Palmer, "if you do [introduce x-ray, presuming in any form] we will quit the PSC." Palmer said that when he introduced it, many students and faculty, some say around 45 people, immediately walked out and went down to the foot of Brady Hill and started a new school. This school established at the foot of Brady Hill in the month of April was the Universal Chiropractic College, not to be confused with the Universal Chiropractic Association, and the head of it was Joy Loban, Palmer's former director of the Chiropractic Analysis Department. Loban was not among those that had walked out, however, but had left for school on February 15 and had entered into private practice with Palmer's praises. Whether or not Universal College came about over the x-ray issue is in dispute. The material printed by the college does not mention x-ray pro or con but does reflect a dissatisfaction with Palmer's leadership of his school.

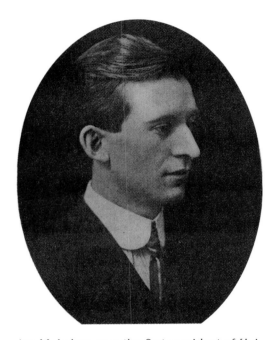

Joy M. Loban was the first president of Universal College in 1910. His split with Palmer probably was not over Palmer's use of x-ray.
From *Universal College of Chiropractic Catalog,* Davenport, Iowa, 1911.

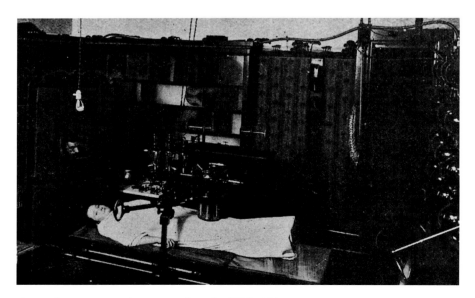

An early x-ray unit being used at the PSC, 1911.
From *Annual Anouncement,* Davenport, Iowa, 1911, Palmer School of Chiropractic.

Loban left the Universal Chiropractic College in Davenport to become dean of the Pittsburgh Chiropractic College in 1916, 2 years before the merger of the two schools. He later became president of the Universal Chiropractic College of Pittsburgh, the product of the merger. Loban was supportive when Universal instituted x-ray and when the first upright x-ray of the pelvis and lower spine was performed for the determination of the effects of gravity, or weight-bearing changes, by Leo Steinbach, dean of the college, and Edwin Garbisch, director of the school's x-ray department.

What of D.D. Palmer, founder of chiropractic, during this period, and what did he think of x-ray? The only written statements found by him mention that x-ray burns are a health problem and that "x-ray causes spinal caries."

Theories developed by the historians of the profession range from the opinion that the elder Palmer was against x-ray because it would detract from the doctor's emphasis on the nervous system and place it on the spinal vertebra, to the feeling that he was ambivalent about the whole thing and by these later years may not have given x-ray much thought because of failing mental health. Of interest is the fact that D.D. Palmer had returned to Davenport at different times to speak at Loban's Universal College and must have been aware of the situation, if not before certainly by the time of his last visit in 1913.

As B.J. Palmer put it, "The principal chiropractic use was the analysis of vertebral subluxations, nothing more, nothing less." Palmer further claimed that "the advent of the x-ray into chiropractic was to prove that vertebral subluxations did actually exist and could, by use of the x-ray, be made visible to the eye." B.J. also contended, "Whereas once medical books said that a vertebral subluxation was impossible without a fracture or dislocation now almost every book acknowledges them as of common occurrence, in fact, some books go so far as to state that almost everyone has them."

Palmer, however, did become interested in x-rays for revealing pathological conditions. As he stated, "Having established this phase of our work, the x-ray would have gone into the discard, but there was a more valuable use for it. Spinography does more than to read subluxations—it proves the existence, location and degree of exostosis, ankylosis, abnormal shapes and forms; all of which may prevent the early correction to normal position of the subluxation." Palmer's interest in "pathological plates", combined with the claim that palpation was often in error, sealed the fate of x-ray inclusion in the chiropractic profession forever.

One wonders when this transformation occurred, but it apparently did not take long, since in Palmer's address before the September 1910 UCA convention he even talked about and demonstrated spinal abnormalities as well as plates of the extremities and the sternum.

On the occasion of Palmer's address before the association, Palmer shared the platform with Mr. A.G. Magnuson of the Scheidel-Western X-ray Coil Company of Chicago, who was there to answer technical and equipment questions, not to mention getting names and addresses of those doctors interested in obtaining x-ray equipment. On October 16th, a local Davenport newspaper, the *Davenport Democrat and Leader,* reported that, "Any person having any fracture, dislocation of suffering with all of the conditions that are usually radiographed by radiographers can have it done at PSC." Obviously Palmer had no intention of treating these conditions but offered to take the radiographs and give the patient prints to take to their medical doctor. The students of the school were told that

If it isn't an

Eastman
It isn't a

Kodak
———

If it isn't branded

The P. S. C.
It isn't a

Spinograph
———

Eastman invented Kodak
The P. S. C. coined Spinograph

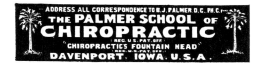

A 1910 advertisement by the PSC for their Spinographs, comparing Kodak and Eastman to Spinograph and PSC.
From *The Chiropractor,* June 1910.

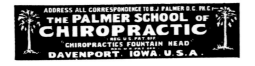
A 1910 advertisement for a Spinography Lecture at the Universal Chiropractors Association Convention.

From *The Chiropractor,* June 1910.

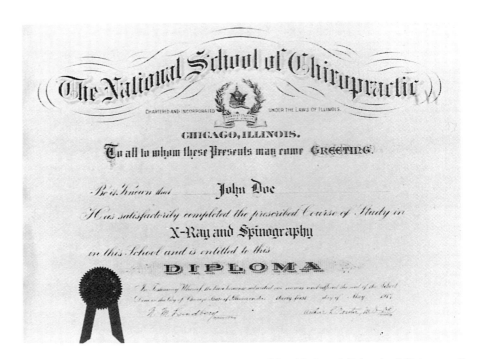

The X-ray and Spinography diploma issued by National School of Chiropractic in 1918.

From *Catalog,* National School of Chiropractic, 1918.

"many conditions revealed, such as dislocations and fractures, are not for the chiropractor but for the surgeon."

B.J. Palmer's first lecture on x-ray occurred in April 1910 at the lecture hall of the school before patients, lay people, and doctors. It is said that he demonstrated "abnormalities of vertebra, hands, feet, arms, etc." and expounded on the "evils of the corset," which not only "jam[med] and deform[ed] the liver of females but deformed ribs downward."

Spinography caught on in chiropractic circles, and the other chiropractic colleges used it as they established their x-ray departments, including National School of Chiropractic of Chicago, Pacific College of Portland, Cleveland Chiropractic College of Kansas City, Los Angeles College of Chiropractic, and Missouri Chiropractic College of St. Louis, to name a few. Universal Chiropractic College, initially in Davenport and later Pittsburgh, seemed to avoid Palmer's term but, nevertheless, taught x-ray by 1921.

By the late 1920s to early 1930s all the college curriculums included x-ray, and as new schools started, an x-ray–spinographic department was included. The addition of the term *spinograph* to the rapidly expanding field of radiography, and the host of other new terms for various procedures, also contributed to confusion. Even E.R.N. Grigg, M.D., author of *The Trail of the Invisible Light,* did not grasp the idea, feeling that some might think that "spinography was x-raying after the patient has eaten spinach." To B.J. Palmer's delight, and probably to the sarcastic Grigg's annoyance, spinography found its way into dictionaries such as the *Unabridged Merriam-Webster* and *Gould's Medical Dictionary.*

Through the years, spinography has come to mean the comparison of spinal segments for alignment. Usually measurements of symmetrical parts of a vertebra are made comparing the right and left side to a midpoint of the segment. Comparison with the segments above and below is then considered to ascertain if a vertebra is displaced or misaligned.

A PSC reading service announcement.
Courtesy Palmer College of Chiropractic Archives, Davenport, Iowa.

One of the major criticisms of measurement methods used in spinography is that the right and left parts of the segment being measured are not truly symmetrical. Of course those using spinography effectively know this, and Palmer, after studying untold specimens from his enormous osteological collection, and his faculty knew it well and stated as such many times. The small asymmetries, inherent in the basically symmetrical human spine, would be considered by the person interpreting the radiograph, as would be distortions from imperfect patient positioning, which was minimized in Palmer's clinics as much as possible.

P.S.C. Film Reading Service

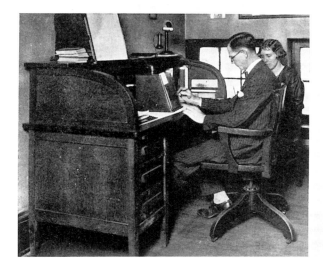

An advertisement for the PSC film reading service picturing E.A. Thompson, 1924.
From *The Chiropractor*, November 1924.

Even though Palmer felt in the early years that spinal radiographs proved the existence of subluxation, his belief was not shared by all in the profession. In fact, by 1924, with the introduction of the neurocalometer, Palmer had agreed with others that the x-ray could show spinal misalignments but that these might or might not be significant from the standpoint of neural aberrations. It was at this point that Palmer advocated means other than the x-ray to determine what segment(s) to adjust. He wrote, "Reading the spinograph is not a mathematical problem because the descriptive parts are not symmetrical. Therefore, the seeming problem is only an estimate."

Spinography's popularity in the lexicon has all but died out. Today most doctors of chiropractic refer to spinal radiographs or x-rays and the interpretation includes biomechanical evaluation and evaluation for abnormalities such as pathologies.

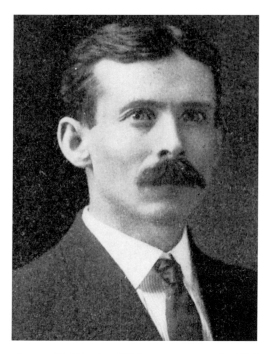

James McGinnis, 1912, was an early PSC photographer and Spinographer.

From *Annual Announcement,* 1910, Davenport, Iowa, Palmer School of Chiropractic.

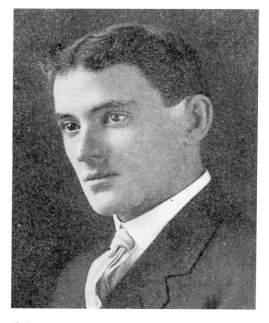

C.R. McAdams, D.C., Director of the PSC Spinographic Department in 1911.

Courtesy Palmer College of Chiropractic Archives, Davenport, Iowa.

EARLY CHIROPRACTIC EDUCATION

The inclusion of x-ray meant that chiropractic faced the same challenge as the medical profession in developing methods of education for those already practicing as well as for those earning their degrees in the educational institutions. For the established chiropractor, the x-ray companies would teach them how to work the equipment in a few days, but classes on the interpretation of the radiograph would have to be taught by chiropractors who had already mastered the art.

B.J. Palmer announced he was in charge of the Spinographic Department in February 1910. James McGinnis was the first person at the Palmer School other than Palmer to take and probably teach x-ray. In this first year all students and faculty doctors who wished to have x-rays performed on their patients were to request them through Joy Loban for approval. By 1911, C. R. McAdams was put in charge of the spinography department, and in 1912, James McGinnis was given the title of school photographer and spinographer; in those days it was common for photographers to become involved with x-rays. McGinnis had worked with Palmer and his x-ray unit since 1910, while he was completing the chiropractic program. Later in 1912, McGinnis, having graduated, left to open a practice. By 1914 Dr. E.A. Thompson took over the helm and stayed in that position until 1925 when he resigned and moved to Baltimore, Maryland, to open a private practice and x-ray reading service for field doctors. An historical sidenote is that McGinnis turned up in California at the Golden State Chiropractic College as a director from 1921 to 1922. In the 1940s he headed up the Advanced Manipulative Chiropractic Association, which dealt with soft tissue manipulative techniques.

The earliest mention of classes for undergraduate students at the Palmer School is found in the 1911 school announcement. A class in x-ray was not included in the regular curriculum but offered as an extended course, which also included other subjects. This first x-ray course was optional because of the experimental state of development, but even then many of the faculty did not want it taught at all. This opposition forced Palmer to take x-ray out of the extended course and develop an extracurricular x-ray class in 1916. By 1922 x-ray and spinography became part of the required curriculum for all those studying to be doctors of chiropractic at PSC.

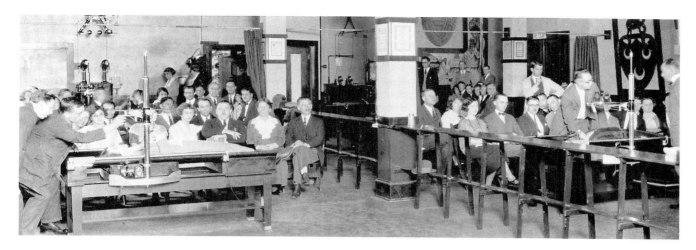

An early spinography class at the PSC.
Courtesy Palmer College of Chiropractic Archives, Davenport, Iowa.

Under Palmer's direction as head of the school, the emphasis in radiographic interpretation was primarily focused on the biomechanical findings with the use of spinography. There were a few examples of spinal pathologies depicted in the pages of Thompson's text, *Chiropractic Spinography,* and he wrote, "Always be very careful when reading plates that you do not fail to observe any abnormal conditions other than just the subluxation." In 1931 Thompson, then of Baltimore wrote,

> During my last few years as a teacher (at PSC), I incorporated the subject of abnormalities (and) I felt it right that the chiropractor not only be taught during his training the diseases and conditions in which he could naturally expect satisfactory results but also some of the conditions where good judgement and discretion would be advisable for accepting such cases.

B.J. Palmer stated, "A chiropractor must be able to recognize abnormal conditions of the spine."

During P.A. Remier's long tenure as chairman of the Radiographic Department at PSC from 1938 to 1966, he advocated the need for chiropractors to x-ray the site of a patient's complaint, not just the spine, and to interpret all radiographs for abnormalities such as pathologies. He taught in his classes and illustrated in his texts patient positioning and machine settings for the entire skeleton, as well as the chest, gastrointestinal tract, teeth, and sinuses. Remier's attitude was also reflected by B.J., as witnessed by those close to them. Some of the PSC graduates, however, apparently ignored their advice and professed to others that the x-ray should only be used by chiropractors for the determination of subluxations or misalignments of spinal segments. Just how this attitude developed is thus far unknown.

The first organized course by PSC for the practicing doctor was held May 1916 at the Palmer School. This "spinographic and x-ray class" ran for a month on campus and had four doctors graduate: H.N. Leland from Pennsylvania, W.B. Buck from New York, M.M. Markwell from Texas, and Alfred H. Post from New Jersey. The next class was offered to doctors as well as students of the school, since Palmer announced on May 1st that the "spinographic and x-ray work had been divorced from PSC courses" because of faculty objections to x-ray. There were 57 enrolled, among whom were two leaders of the emerging specialty, Warren Sausser and S.E. Julander, as well as Carl S. Cleveland, Sr., and Ruth Ashworth, who

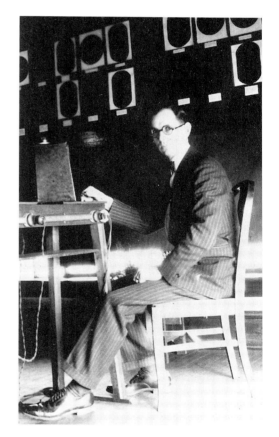

Ernest A. Thompson, the author of the first book on chiropractic use of x-ray and head of the PSC Spinography Department from 1914-1925.

Courtesy Palmer College of Chiropractic Archives, Davenport, Iowa.

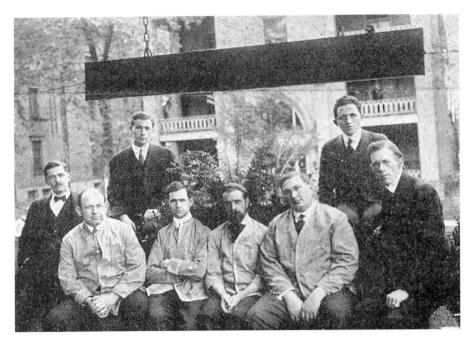

The first PSC spinography and x-ray class.
From *The Fountain Head News,* June 1916.

later went on to found the Central Chiropractic College to be renamed Cleveland Chiropractic College of Kansas City, Missouri.

As the other colleges included x-ray, they too offered special and postgraduate courses for the doctors.The National College of Chiropractic in Chicago was using and teaching x-ray by 1917, and perhaps even before that, under the direction of Nels Moody Lundberg, as the college's roentgenologist who came from the West Suburban Hospital and Cook County General Hospital where he served for 3½ years. In 1919 or 1920, the department and postgraduate x-ray classes were under the direction of C. Bernhard Herrmann, who held a medical and chiropractic degree.Of interest is that National College had access to Cook County Hospital from 1908 to 1924, where they were allowed to observe in the laboratories. National's own x-ray department taught spinography for the detection of suspected subluxations, as well as x-ray pathology of all body systems, including lung, heart, gastrointestinal tract, gallbladder, sinuses, teeth, kidney, uterus, and fetus. These courses were part of the core curriculum requirements before one could obtain a D.C. degree. By 1924 the Dean of the college, William Schulze, cited that the profession had "adopted the x-ray."

Los Angeles College of Chiropractic also required x-ray in 1917, as part of the curriculum under the direction of Clement Joynt. By 1922 Manley Gamage was the college's roentgenologist and John Koer served as an instructor in the department.

In 1919, the Pacific Chiropractic College of Portland, Oregon, wrote, "Spinography is a very essential thing for every chiropractor to know." Under the watchful direction of Nellie Byrd, x-ray and fluoroscopic work was taught. The Eclectic College of Los Angeles also taught x-ray in 1919, with W.J. Daly in charge and later Frank Pyott.

The Eclectic College of Chicago had x-ray by 1920, headed by H.H. Snyder, a D.O. as well as D.C. The college also shared privileges at Cook County Hospital with the National College. The Missouri Chiropractic Col-

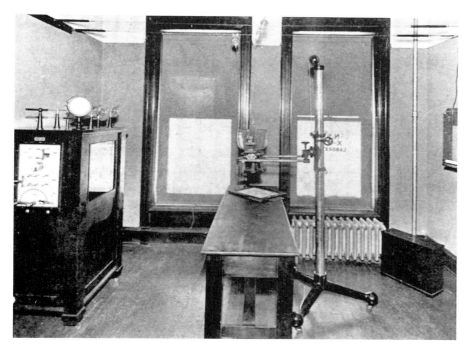

An early radiology laboratory at National College of Chiropractic, circa 1917.
Courtesy National College of Chiropractic, Lombard, Illinois.

lege in St. Louis was incorporated in 1920 with a mission to "teach the philosophy, science and art of chiropractic and chiropractic spinography," as stated in the articles of incorporation. The Mecca College of Newark, New Jersey, added their x-ray department in this year as well, under Arthur Herdling as roentgenologist.

In 1921 the Universal College offered x-ray in the undergraduate as well as postgraduate programs "for those who desire to fit themselves for this specialistic work." While this description may lead one to believe that x-ray was an optional course, like Palmer's at the time, indications are that x-ray was taught in the sophomore, junior, and senior terms. X-ray diagnosis was included in the senior year with "plate reading," which according to Universal College "is considered a fundamental of chiropractic knowledge." Even more ironic than having Pacific College, a descendant from the elder Palmer's school in Oregon, mandating x-ray education for all students, is that one year before PSC, Universal College printed that x-ray courses "are included without extra tuition fee to all matriculants of the three year and postgraduate courses." That year also found the Evans School of Washington, D.C., with x-ray requirements for all students. Their catalog stated that "it is the popular belief that within a short time, every REAL chiropractor will own an A-1 x-ray apparatus."

The other chiropractic institutions that taught x-ray by 1923 included Golden State College, with Edwin Fortin teaching spinography as well as obstetrics and serving as dean and treasurer of the school until 1925, when he became President but still remained in x-ray. Fortin had his own "pathological and x-ray laboratory" in 1921 and advertised as an "expert spinographer." The Central College of Kansas City, Missouri, later to become the Cleveland Chiropractic College, also taught x-ray in 1923. Texas Chiropractic College began x-ray sometime in the 1920s, with D.A. Gregory head of the department.

As the other colleges in existence continued to institute their radiology departments, and newer schools opened with departments already

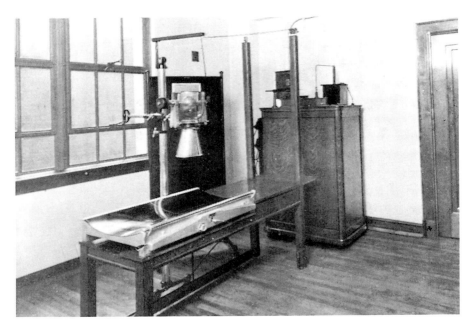

An early x-ray laboratory at Lincoln College of Chiropractic.
From *The Lincoln Post*, volume 1, 1926.

intact, there was one prominent institution that was not willing to take this progressive step until somewhat later. In 1922 Willard Carver, president of the Carver College, described x-ray as a means

> by which shadows of bones, cartilages, and dense tissue may be dimly distinguished, but these tests only dim shadows, and do not in any sense reveal the structures, and of course, are of no value in the observation of adverse functional processes.

By the 1950s, however, he had instituted x-ray, with Paul Parr, Richard Shipman, and Goldia Young in his department of roentgenology.

X-ray opened up a whole new world of study, and many graduates of the special courses and early college classes wanted advanced education in radiology. They knew of and used the methods of evaluating patient's spines biomechanically, and they knew of the smattering of disease processes of bone and soft tissue, but they were not satisfied and

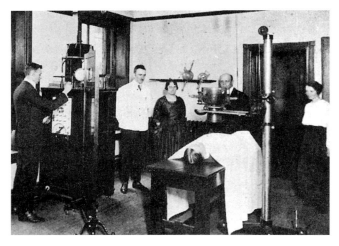

An early National College x-ray laboratory, 1920.
Courtesy National College of Chiropractic, Lombard, Illinois.

desired to learn more. The doctors also desired to meet with others who used x-ray to discuss mutual problems and interesting cases and to show their interesting films. They also wanted to explore more of the diverse appearances of disease processes on films. Having already read and studied medical texts of the day, they felt that dissemination of the information attained would be beneficial to the profession and that it could also be included in the undergraduate work to prepare the doctor of chiropractic for the disease processes that would have a direct bearing on the patient's health and well-being.

This desire, no doubt, brought about a change in emphasis among some of the schools' undergraduate programs from the biomechanical evaluation to the pathological processes seen on the radiographs. Some of the colleges that advocated the pathological aspects as paramount over the biomechanical aspects in undergraduate training were National of Chicago, Los Angeles College, Lincoln of Indiana and, later, Northwestern College in Minnesota. The colleges that maintained the biomechanical emphasis over the pathological included Palmer, Cleveland of Kansas City, and Logan of St. Louis.

ADVANCED POSTGRADUATE EDUCATION

The early years found many of the radiographers and spinographers involved in establishing x-ray laboratories serving the chiropractors who desired radiographs of their patients but did not have the equipment. These laboratories were particularly numerous along the East Coast and in California. Another arena for education was brought on by World War I. During the height of the war, 1916, few people knew how to run the still primitive x-ray units. Those chiropractors and students who had early classes in radiology at Palmer School, like Warren Sausser, could be channeled into the noncombatant roll of radiography in the medical corps. This provided a unique opportunity for them to take the government's radiography course, which not only gave them federal recognition and licensure as a radiographer but also the important educational experience of working with some of the leading medical radiologists of the time. With World War II, the same chance occurred for virtually all of the recent chiropractic graduates young enough to serve, since they were all required to take x-ray in chiropractic college. It is this era that found Earl Rich working with a medical orthopedic specialist named Ferguson, of lumbar spine fame with his measurements, angles, and lines, an experience which had a very definite influence on him. Of course many doctors of chiropractic were not only involved in the military during war time, but also when the country was at peace. Some of these individuals who also participated in military service were John Teranel, J.O. Epringham, L.A. Nash, Ronald Watkins, Joseph Howe, and James Winterstein. Their experiences provide but a few examples of a situation in which a seeming interruption in one's career turned into a golden opportunity.

Advancement in the postgraduate arena took two forms. First, articles dedicated to roentgenology were added to existing chiropractic journals and papers, becoming regular features in the national organization's periodicals and the state radiological journals. The biomechanical aspects were far from ignored in these early articles; in fact, many articles appeared on the subject with various new developments and procedures being promoted. Second, the lecture circuit, including both state and national association conventions, welcomed the news of x-ray and spinography.

Lectures to the graduate doctors on roentgenology and spinography were very popular in the early days and occurred at many state and national meetings as well as college homecoming seminars. In 1922 the Palmer Lyceum dedicated one entire day for radiographic lectures, which included L.W. Heath, Jr., of the school on spinographic technology; C.W. Parsons, from Los Angeles, on adjusting from the spinograph entirely; A.W. Schwietert, of South Dakota, on the Universal Spinographic Society; and Leo Wunsch, of Denver, on radiological laboratories. Most of the colleges provided radiology faculty for meetings and lectures off and on campus, and also provided extension faculty to promote x-ray interests at various locations.

Classes at the postgraduate level took two forms. The first was for the general practitioner who wanted to keep current on developments and study areas they either did not get in school or had forgotten because of rarity and not encountering them in their years of practice. The second arena of postgraduate education was for those delving into study for preparation to become a specialist and, in the late 1950s, to lead toward eligibility for certification by the board in radiology.

The educators who were school based did much to promote radiology from both the biomechanical and pathological standpoint, including from the 1940s to the 1960s such notables as Earl Rich and Tom Goodrich from Lincoln College; Fred Baier, Lester Rehburger, and Ralph Powell from Missouri College; Roland Kissinger, Joseph Janse, Leonard Richie, and Joe Howe from National; John Teranel from The Standard School of New York; E.O. Epringham, Duane Smith, C.B. Eacrett, and Amedeo Vampa of Los Angeles College; Robert Ridler and Robert Whitnig from

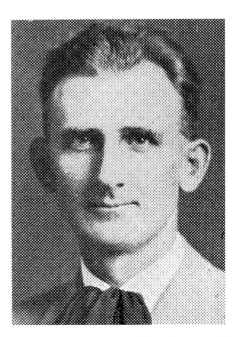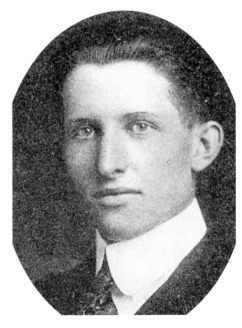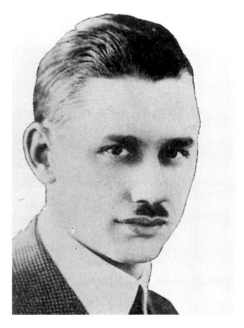

Organizers and officers of the 1923 Spinographic Society. Left to right, *A.W. Sweitert, President, Warren Sausser, Vice-President; Waldo Poehner, Secretary-Treasurer.*

Courtesy Palmer College of Chiropractic Archives, Davenport, Iowa.

Northwestern; Appa Anderson from Western States; and Ronald Watkins from the Canadian College.

Some practicing specialists got into the act, as did some of those institutions' employees who had left the college and were invited to be extension faculty of the schools. Those who maintained their private practice but taught part-time for colleges included Waldo Pohner of Illinois, Leo Wunsch of Denver, Earl Swallen of Ohio, Donald Hariman of North Dakota, Michael Giammarino of Pennsylvania, Douglas Ray of Texas, and Russell Erhardt of Wisconsin. They, like the school men, taught both to the general practitioner and to doctors in courses preparing for board examinations. Most outstanding of these in the arena of a private practitioner teaching upgrading and refresher classes was Russell Erhardt, who at the request of many of his fellow practitioners in Milwaukee, started lecturing locally without college involvement. As his program spread, he became a member of the extension faculty at many of the chiropractic colleges and holds the distinction of having lectured, in his extraordinary style, to more doctors than anyone else in the profession, instilling the desire in untold numbers of them to seek specialization and certification. As a result of his dedication to upgrading chiropractic in this aspect of practice and his generosity to the teaching institutions, both Palmer College and Parker College named their radiology departments after him.

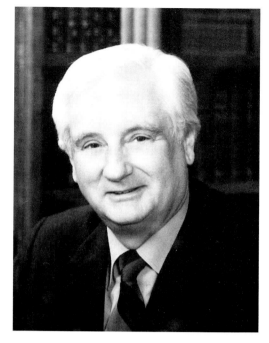

Russell Erhardt, D.C., D.A.C.B.R., is a world-renowned lecturer on radiology in chiropractic.

Courtesy Russell Erhardt, Dunwoody, Georgia.

CHIROPRACTIC ORGANIZATIONS DEDICATED TO X-RAY

The Spinographic Society, the first organization to be formed in chiropractic dedicated to the specialty of radiology, was founded at the Palmer School's annual Lyceum in 1923, under the auspices of the UCA. This came about due to the efforts of the three doctors who were elected the first officers. These officers were A.W. Sweitert, president; Warren Sausser, vice president; and Waldo Poehner, secretary-treasurer. The board of director members were B.J. Palmer, S. Julander, F. Suebold, W. Danforth, and D. Johnson. After the development of the neurocalometer, pressure was applied to this society to merge with the newly formed neurocalometer society in 1924. In the same year a merger occurred, and the new organization was named the Neurocalometer and Spinographic Society. The officers were C.W. Johnson, president; William Brownell, vice president; and Waldo Poehner, secretary-treasurer. The board of directors consisted of A.W. Schweitert, Frank O. Logic, William Casper, and J. Ralph John. In *The Chiropractor* articles appeared from members of the group concerning the continued use of spinography and the addition of the neurocalometer in practice. The president of the society, C.W. Johnson, talked about a research project correlating findings from both devices, and in November 1924 Leo Wunsch wrote an article, "Observations and Deductions in the Spinographic Laboratory," using illustrations from Thompson's book and discussing the research on tuberculosis at the Johnson's office in Denver. Waldo Poehner also wrote articles for the society published in the same journal heralding the development of the neurocalometer and its use with x-ray. Friction developed quickly between the two groups, and it became very evident that the spinographic specialty was losing its identity with this merger, which frustrated spinographic members.

In October 1924, B.J. Palmer called for the society to disband. In an

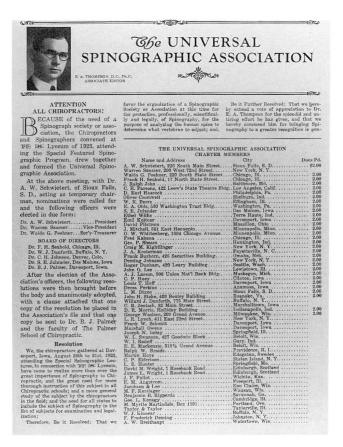

The Universal Spinographic Association Charter Membership listing from 1923.

From *The Chiropractor*, November 1923.

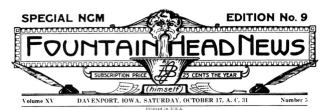

An open letter announcement in 1925 by B.J. Palmer calling for the dissolving of the Neurocalometer and Spinographic Society.

From *The Fountain Head News*, October 17, 1925.

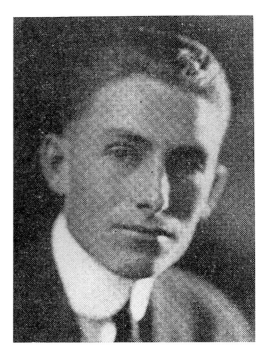

C.W. Johnson, D.C., President of the 1924 Neurocalometer and Spinographic Society.

From *The Chiropractor*, November 1924.

article in *The Fountain Head News* he criticized the officers of the society and stated that "the honorable president never was in step, except as it was a spinographic society." There was no active national organization in existence at this point, and the profession did without one for about 8 years, probably because these years were taken up with the furor created by Palmer's control of marketing arrangements for the neurocalometer. As a result, Palmer left the UCA to form the Chiropractic Health Bureau the forerunner of the International Chiropractors Association (ICA). Additionally, four of his most trusted and admired faculty left the school to form Lincoln Chiropractic College in Indianapolis, Indiana, which would figure prominently in the growth of radiology in the profession. Even E.A. Thompson moved out of Davenport and opened a spinographic laboratory in Baltimore, Maryland, while serving as a director for Lincoln. In 1932 at the meeting of the National Chiropractic Association (NCA), formed by a merger of the UCA and the old American Chiropractic Association (ACA) in 1930 in Detroit, Michigan, the Board of Counselors of Chiropractic Spinographers and X-ray Operators was formed, with Warren Sausser as president, A.W. Schwietert as vice president, O.A. Ohlson as secretary, and E.A. Thompson as chairman of research. By 1936 the name had changed to the National Council on Chiropractic Roentgenology (NCCR). The NCCR lasted until the NCA merged with members of the International Chiropractors' Association to form the American Chiropractic Association (ACA) in 1963. The NCCR had changed its name to the Council on Roentgenology of the American Chiropractic Association.

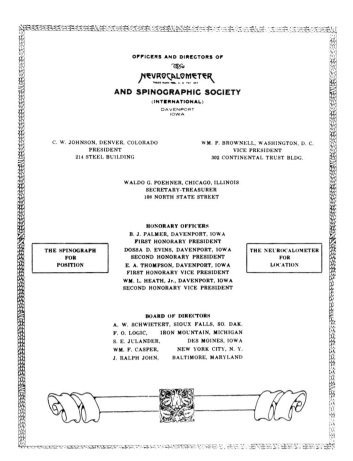
The 1924 merger announcement of the Spinographic and Neurocalometer Societies. The merger lasted 1 year.
From *The Chiropractor*, November 1924.

Officers listed in the first *ACA Journal of Chiropractic* were J.J. McCarthy, president pro tem; J. Clay Thompson, spinography section; Rhea D. Caster, diagnostic section; and Earl Rich, cineroentgenology section. In 1986 the Council underwent another title change with the inclusion of a group of doctors representing thermology, and became the Council of Diagnostic Imaging. These councils and specialty groups have always been open to any doctor of chiropractic who is a member of the parent organization and holds an interest in imaging.

An ad for E.A. Thompson's film reading service in Baltimore after leaving PSC.
From *NCA Journal* 1(2):1931.

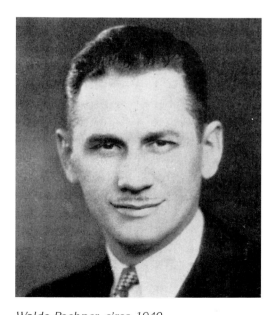

Waldo Poehner, circa 1940.
Courtesy Palmer College of Chiropractic Archives, Davenport, Iowa.

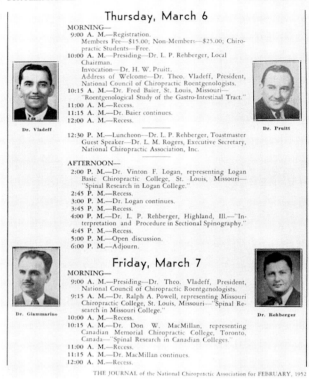

Spinograph *and* X-Ray

Dr. Warren L. Sausser, 200 W. 72d St., New York City, is President of the Board of Counselors of Chiropractic Spinographers and X-Ray Technicians. Dr. E. A. Thompson, 516 N. Charles St., Baltimore, Maryland, is Chairman of Research. This department solicits your X-Ray problems.

THIS X-RAY ANALYSIS IS STANDARD. Approved by the National Board of Spinographers.

I. SUBLUXATION is a condition in which the articulating surfaces of one vertebra have lost their normal relationship with the articulating surfaces of one or both of the adjacent vertebrae.

II. RELATIVE POSITION is a consideration of the spinal column in its entirety, in which the position of each vertebra is listed as regards the position of the spinous process with its body, also body tipping, not necessarily a subluxation.

III. BENT SPINOUS PROCESSES, or Long Prongs, are recorded right (R), or left, (L), according to the direction in which they are bent or elongated, from the junction of the laminae.

IV. CURVATURES. Any deviation of the spinal column, laterally, posteriorly, or anteriorly, from the normal.

V. ROTATIONS refer to a condition wherein the bodies of the vertebrae are rotated upon their axis in comparison with their spinous processes. In listing a rotation the body is the consideration, not the spinous process.

KEY TO SYMBOLS USED IN SPINOGRAPHIC ANALYSIS

X=Probable points of impingement.
)=Indicates transitional area.
-|-|-|-| =Thin disc.
=Compression of disc on right or left.
> =Apex or break as marked.
=Points to area of ankylosis.
=Points to exostotic areas.
L:=Spinous to left of median line, or left subluxation.
R=Spinous to right of median line, or right subluxation.
S=Superior subluxation.
I=Inferior subluxation.
RI=Combination as right and superior.
LI=Combination as left and inferior.
TIR=Body tipped inferior on right; no laterality.
TIL=Body tipped inferior on left.
TRANSITION=Opposite rotation of two adjacent vertebrae.

Anterior Views Reveal:...........
Lateral Views Reveal:...........

X-RAY ANALYSIS OR SPINOGRAPHIC READING OF

NAME............ PLATE NO...........
REFERRED BY
DOCTOR............
DATE............

THE CHIROPRACTIC JOURNAL

An x-ray analysis form developed by the Board of Counselors of Chiropractic Spinographers and X-Ray Technicians in 1934.
From The NCA Journal, *April 1934.*

Official X-ray Symposium Program
National Council of Roentgenologists
MARCH 6th, 7th and 8th, 1952
STATLER HOTEL   ST. LOUIS, MO.

Thursday, March 6

MORNING—
9:00 A. M.—Registration.
Members Fee—$15.00; Non-Members—$25.00; Chiropractic Students—Free.
10:00 A. M.—Presiding—Dr. L. P. Rehberger, Local Chairman.
Invocation—Dr. H. W. Pruitt.
Address of Welcome—Dr. Theo. Vladeff, President, National Council of Chiropractic Roentgenologists.
10:15 A. M.—Dr. Fred Baier, St. Louis, Missouri—"Roentgenological Study of the Gastro-Intestinal Tract."
11:00 A. M.—Recess.
11:15 A. M.—Dr. Baier continues.
12:00 A. M.—Recess.

Dr. Vladeff   Dr. Pruitt

12:30 P. M.—Luncheon—Dr. L. P. Rehberger, Toastmaster Guest Speaker—Dr. L. M. Rogers, Executive Secretary, National Chiropractic Association, Inc.

AFTERNOON—
2:00 P. M.—Dr. Vinton F. Logan, representing Logan Basic Chiropractic College, St. Louis, Missouri—"Spinal Research in Logan College."
2:45 P. M.—Recess.
3:00 P. M.—Dr. Logan continues.
3:45 P. M.—Recess.
4:00 P. M.—Dr. L. P. Rehberger, Highland, Ill.—"Interpretation and Procedure in Sectional Spinography."
4:45 P. M.—Recess.
5:00 P. M.—Open discussion.
6:00 P. M.—Adjourn.

Friday, March 7

MORNING—
9:00 A. M.—Presiding—Dr. Theo. Vladeff, President, National Council of Chiropractic Roentgenologists.
9:15 A. M.—Dr. Ralph A. Powell, representing Missouri Chiropractic College, St. Louis, Missouri—"Spinal Research in Missouri College."
10:00 A. M.—Recess.
10:15 A. M.—Dr. Don W. MacMillan, representing Canadian Memorial Chiropractic College, Toronto, Canada—"Spinal Research in Canadian Colleges."
11:00 A. M.—Recess.
11:15 A. M.—Dr. MacMillan continues.
12:00 A. M.—Recess.

Dr. Giammarino   Dr. Rehberger

THE JOURNAL of the National Chiropractic Association for FEBRUARY, 1952

A page from the Symposium Program for the 1952 National Council of Roentgenologists.
From *Journal of the NCA,* May 1952.

The first annual symposium of the National Council of Chiropractic Roentgenologists (NCCR) was held in Chicago on June 7, 1946. The 1947 symposium held in February drew larger numbers, even exceeding the Council's expectations. The presentations included speakers of the caliber of Leo Wunsch on x-ray interpretation of the gallbaldder, stomach, and colon; Fred Baier on bone pathology, sinuses, and skull; and John Teranel on chest and genito urinary conditions. M. R. Lewis of Chicago gave a podiological x-ray presentation (the first of many medical doctors to address the chiropractic radiology groups).

In November 1964, the first "workshop" was conducted by the chiropractic doctors certified in radiology at Lincoln College in Indianapolis, with 19 of the then 36 D.A.C.B.R.s present. This group continued to meet annually, separate from the Council, and in 1968, the certified body of radiologists formed the American Chiropractic College of Radiologists, principally due to the efforts of Douglas Ray of San Antonio. The annual meeting of the Diplomates became a function of the college and has attracted many of the outstanding medical radiologists of today as lecturers.

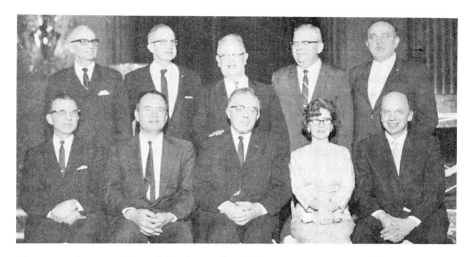

The annual symposium of the Council on Chiropractic Roentgenology of the ACA, held in Cincinnati in 1964. Back row, left to right, J.M. Howard, V.D. Good, A.J. Fitzgerald, O.M. Krogh, E.L. Kropf. Front row: J.C. Thompson, R.D. Caster, J. Janse, M. Caster, E.A. Eliopulos.

From the *ACA Journal of Chiropractic,* June 1964.

In the mid-to-late 1960s, many involved in radiology in the chiropractic profession participated in courses sponsored by the Bureau of Radiological Health of the Health, Education, and Welfare Department in Rockville, Maryland, with Gerald Levine serving as liaison for the chiropractic profession.

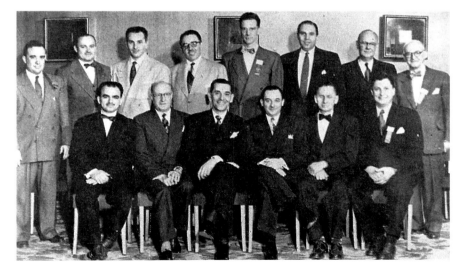

Speakers and officers of the National Council of Chiropractic Roentgenologists at the 1957 St. Louis convention. Front row, left to right, Michael Giammarino; Leo Wunsch; Theodore Vladeff, President; Hillary Pruit, Secretary; Waldo Poehner; Lester Rehberger. Back Row, left to right, Ralph Powell; Earl Rich; Roland Kissinger; Joseph Janse; D.W. MacMillan; Carl Cleveland, Jr.; L.M. Rogers; James Long Lovz.

Courtesy Michael Giammarino, Coatesville, Pennsylvania.

CERTIFICATION OF THE RADIOLOGIST IN CHIROPRACTIC

Michael Giammarino, one of the first board members, reminisced about the history of radiology certification in chiropractic at a lecture in California in 1986:

> For several years during the 1950s, the certification of chiropractors in x-ray was the topic of discussion at symposia and other meetings. Great interest was shown by the NCCR officers and members, as well as officials of the NCA.
>
> At the 1957 spring symposium held in Cleveland several of us including Drs. Poehner, Wunsch, Baier, and NCCR officers met to discuss plans for a certification program. On September 14 to 15, 1957, a committee composed of Edward Kropf, president of the Council, Waldo Poehner, Fred Baier, Leonard Van Dusen, secretary, Joseph Janse, representing the Council on Education, and I, as chairman, met at the Morrison Hotel in Chicago to formulate plans for a certification program.
>
> After this meeting, and much letter writing, rules and requirements for candidates qualifying for the board examination were proposed and sent to the Council on Education of the NCA for their approval. Drs. Poehner, Wunsch, and Baier were recommended as Board members by the NCCR officers.

The board members and data pertaining to the examination were approved by the National Council on Education in a letter dated January 20, 1958, as submitted. The NCA also recommended that two additional members be added to the board: Duane M. Smith of Huntington, California, and Michael A. Giammarino of Coatesville, Pennsylvania, were proposed by the council officers and approved by the National Council on Education.

The board members were accredited by virtue of their years of experience, including their attendance at roentgenology lectures, symposia, and state and national meetings, as lecturers and authors of x-ray articles.

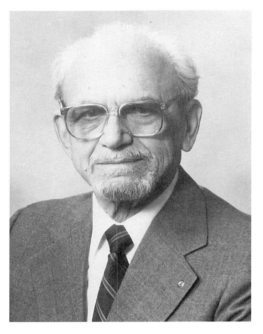

Michael Giammarino, D.C., DACBR, original board member of NCCR.
Courtesy Michael Giammarino, Coatesville, Pennsylvania.

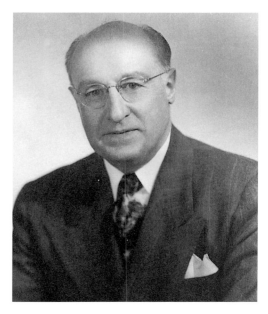

Leo Wunsch, D.C., DACBR, original board member of NCCR.
Courtesy Leo Wunsch, Jr., Sun City, Arizona.

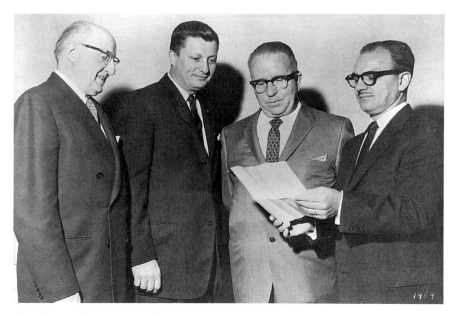

Leo Wunsch, Lester Rehberger, Duane Smith, Michael Giammarino, NCCR-certified roentgenologists board, 1959.
Courtesy Michael Giammarino, Coatesville, Pennsylvania.

The original name of this board as it appeared in the 1958 *NCA Journal* was Certification Board of the National Council of Chiropractic Roentgenologists; however, the official title shortly became National Board of Chiropractic Roentgenologists," then with the change from NCA to ACA, The American Board of Chiropractic Roentgenologists, and then Roentgenologists was changed to Roentgenology. To better reflect the fact that roentgenology is, in fact, roentgenology, whether it be medical, osteopathic, or chiropractic the name became American Chiropractic Board of Roentgenology. As a result of the more popular and widespread use of the term *radiology,* it was voted to change the title to the American Chiropractic Board of Radiology. The doctors certified by this group are termed *Diplomates of the American Chiropractic Board of Radiology* and are designated with *DACBR* after their names.

CERTIFICATION REQUIREMENTS

By March 1958 eligibility to apply for the examination by the newly formed Board of Chiropractic Roentgenology required the completion of 200 organized lecture hours plus the maintenance of an active practice in chiropractic with practical use of x-ray for 5 years. Since there were no formal complete courses at the time, private tutorials were allowed. Chiropractors also studied the same books used by medical radiologists. Lincoln College instituted the first college-based course, started by Earl Rich in 1965. Shortly afterward National College, Los Angeles, Western States, and Northwestern Colleges also started 200-hour courses leading to board eligibility.

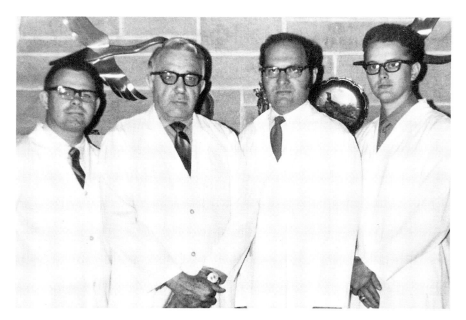

First National College Resident Program Participants, 1968. Donald Tompkins, Senior Resident; Joseph Janse, DACBR, College President; Leonard Richie, DACBR, Radiology Department Chairman; James Winterstein, Junior Resident.
Courtesy James Winterstein, Lombard, Illinois.

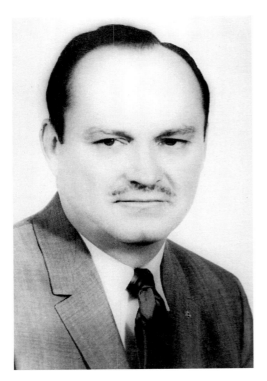

Earl Rich, a Lincoln College President, was active in the ACA's Council on Roentgenology and author of the landmark text, Atlas of Clinical Roentgonology.

Courtesy Mary Rhoades, Davenport, Iowa.

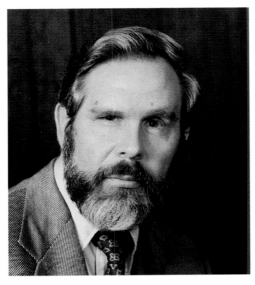

Joseph W. Howe, circa 1990, a chiropractic educator who developed a radiology residency program at National College and later at Los Angeles College.

Courtesy Joseph Howe, Sylmar, California.

By 1966 the requirements had grown to 250 hours, and in 1967 Douglas Ray, Joseph Howe and Thomas Goodrich organized a 300-hour course in addition to the 5-year hands-on experience and the needed outside study of incalculable hours. Early teachers in this extended syllabus included Thomas Goodrich, Douglas Ray, Earl Swallen, Donald Hariman, Joseph Howe, Michael Giammarino, and Leonard Richie. After the 300-hour course was mandated, Logan College and Texas College also offered the classes. By 1966 all postgraduate training leading towards eligibility for certification was sponsored by the educational institutions, mainly as a result of the untiring efforts of Earl Rich and others. This was also the year that the first extension course was offered at a location other than a college campus through the postgraduate divisions. The college heads met in 1969 at the Associates' Diagnostic and Research Center in Tallmadge, Ohio, to further standardize the syllabus for the postgraduate courses.

In 1955 Earl Rich had actually received approval from the National Council on Education for an on campus residency program that started in the undergraduate senior term of chiropractic college. This course produced Thomas Goodrich, who also completed the 250-hour extension course, which was still a requirement of the board. Rich had also produced two landmark books that served as a syllabus for the postgraduate course and were used in the undergraduate curriculum: the *Atlas of Clinical Roentgenology* and the *Manual of Radiographic and Diagnostic Roentgenology.* Upon Rich's death, the residency was continued by Goodrich's trainee, Jerald Balduf, until 1968, at which time he left the college.

In 1966 Northwestern College instituted a similar program under the direction of Robert Ridler, with Robert Whiting its first resident. Phillip Rungston was the first successful resident from a full-time course at the Los Angeles College under the direction of Nilson Santos, who started the program. Also in that year, these residencie's carried the requirements of the board for the extension of class hours.In 1967, National College, under the direction of Leonard Richie, submitted the first modern day residency syllabus, which was approved by the board as the first full residency without the additional extension hours. This was for 2000 hours of total postgraduate work presented in 2 calendar years. He trained James Winterstein and Donald Tompkins as his first residents.

In 1969 Joseph Howe, who was cofounder of the Associates Diagnostic and Research Center in Tallmadge, Ohio, was approved for a radiology residency through National College. His first residents were Michael Buehler and John Danz. After this facility closed, Howe filled a vacancy as Department Chairman at National College, succeeding James Winterstein, and trained Terry Yochum, Ray Conely, Larry Pyzic, and Donald Taylor in the next National class. He moved to California and headed up the radiology department at Los Angeles College of Chiropractic, accepting more residents than any other college. So great were his teaching abilities that one of his National residents, Sharon Jaeger, followed him to Los Angeles to complete her program under his tutelage. Howe went on to maintain the longest running radiology residency in chiropractic, producing half of all the radiology specialists.

The postgraduate radiology residencies first required 2 full years of full-time study, but soon grew to 3 full calendar years. Now radiology residency programs are in place in almost all of the accredited chiropractic institutions, and the graduates of these programs make up the majority of the candidates to the examining board.

EXAMINATIONS OF SPECIALISTS

The first examinations were held by the newly formed National Board of Chiropractic Roentgenologists, consisting entirely of Michael Giammarino, Leo Wunsch, and Duane Smith, in Omaha, Nebraska, March 1958; Waldo Poehner and Fred Baier had both passed away within 1 month of the testing. The 15 doctors that sat for the examinations were Lester Rehberger, Edward Peterson, Carl Anderson, H. Gustarson, Joseph Janse, H.T. Virgin, O.E. Bude, Richard Lange, D.E. McCarty, W.O. Womer, Earl Rich, Ronald Watkins, Neil Conley, T.L. Lilyhorn, and E.S. Barker. Of these, Joseph Janse, Lester Rehberger, and Earl Rich were certified, a pass rate that was to become typical of these grueling examinations. The designation of diplomate of the American Board of Chiropractic Roentgenologists was suggested a year later by James J. McCarthy, a new board member.

In response to a request from a group of doctors who had completed a concentrated course at National College, in addition to the regular postgraduate studies, the Board held a second examination in May 1958, and among those who were successful in the group were Ronald Watkins; Leonard Richie, a partner of Waldo Poehner in a radiology office and faculty member of National College from 1953 to 1956 and 1963 to 1973 as department head; and Roland Kissinger, who headed the department at National from the late 1940s until his death in 1961.

In Canada chiropractors formed the Canadian Council on Chiropractic Roentgenology in 1952, with D.W. MacMillan as president, C.A. Greenshields as vice president, W.C. Sundy as secretary, and H.D. Whatmough as treasurer. Since its formation, the council has maintained a liaison with its American cousins, with doctors such as Rudy Muller filling this position. There has always been cooperative intercouncil symposia attendance, with a large Canadian contingency always present at the annual American meetings. In 1972 six of the certified roentgenologists in Canada, Eric Shrubb, Ronald Collett, Gerald Kremer, Robert Thurlow, John Macrae, and Laurent Boisvert, formed the Chiropractic Council of Radiologists (of Canada) with the help of American specialist Donald Hariman. Many of the United States specialists have gained honorary membership in the Canadian group for their active participation in Canadian-sponsored classes. Such individuals include Donald Hariman, Roy Ottinger, Edward Maurer, Joseph Howe, Robert Whiting, and Thomas Goodrich. The Canadian group maintains a correspondent agreement with the American Chiropractic Board of Radiology.

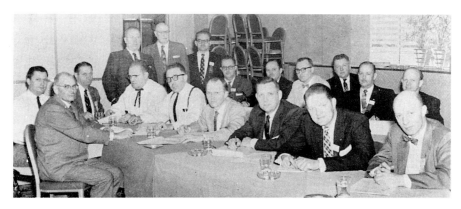

First class to be examined by the National Council of Chiropractic Roentgenologists. The examination were held in March 1958 in Omaha, Nebraska.

From *The Journal of the National Chiropractic Association,* May 1958.

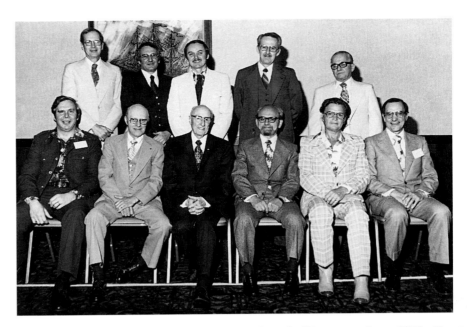

Past members of the American Chiropractic Board of Roentgenology, 1970s. Front row, *Joseph Howe, J.J. McCarthy, Leo Wunsch, Michael Giammarino, Douglas Ray, John Muilenburg.* Back row, *Earl Swallen, John Bestgen, Thomas Goodrich, Donald Hariman, Brian Davis.*
Courtesy Robin Canterbury, Davenport, Iowa.

Predating the formation of the NCCR's examining board was a certifying group in California working in cooperation with doctors of osteopathy who specialized in radiology. Graduates of this course, who were granted reciprocity by the American Chiropractic Board of Radiology, included J.O. Epringham, C.B. Eacrett, Duane Smith, and C.B. Moran. The Los Angeles College started teaching this certifying course in radiology in 1948 with Epringham; Eacrett, who had previous x-ray experience; G.T. O'Sullivan; Clyde Hall; Thor Halsteen; F. Hatfield; and R.J. Huff.

The International Chiropractors' Association set out to develop councils in areas of specialty in the early 1980s, including a Council on Skeletal Roentgenology. This council, to date, has not met with a great deal of acceptance for several reasons. Many felt that it was a duplication of an already established and accepted radiology specialty in the profession. In addition, the practice of studying only skeletal abnormalities was limited in scope, since a patient's system cannot be isolated and diseases often cross over to other body areas. The organization also proposed only 100 hours before eligibility was obtained. It should be stated, however, that this early group does have individuals who are very well versed in osseous pathologies. Another factor that may have lessened acceptance of the Council on Skeletal Roentgenology was that in the 1980s the American Board of Chiropractic Radiology became an autonomous body, removing requirements that would mandate membership in the ACA.

DEVELOPMENTS IN DEVICES AND PROCEDURES

Early x-ray equipment was cumbersome, noisy, and frightening for the patient. It probably made many patients think that they were next to a lighting bolt! The tubes had to be replaced often, and the doctor had to

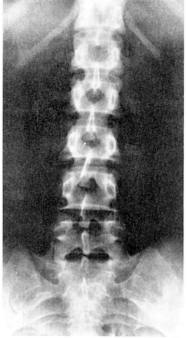
Advertisements for early x-ray units from the Engeln Electric Company, Cleveland, Ohio.

Courtesy Palmer College of Chiropractic Archives, Davenport, Iowa.

know spark gap settings and varied electrical dangers. Images taken by these machines left a lot to be desired, but eventually they became clearer and safer to produce because of improvements in both the x-ray equipment and the receptor products, intensifying screens, and film. The actual time of exposure to x-ray by the patient went from minutes to seconds and then to fractions of seconds. Improvements in the equipment not only brought about what the doctor wanted but also what the patient wanted, more comfort.

As more chiropractors used x-ray, they would discuss their displeasure with the standard types of x-ray units and express a desire to have modifications that would make their work more efficient and accurate. The early organizations contacted x-ray companies to develop machines for chiropractic use. It was not long before some of the x-ray companies made the desired changes and began to target the chiropractic market. Gearing the machine to the private office, with limited space, and the chiropractic specifications, particularly with the popularization of weight-bearing studies that had its beginning in the 1920s, some of the companies actively solicited and advertised for chiropractic use.

Going from the glass plate to celluloid film was a change partly necessitated by World War I and the difficulty in obtaining the Belgian glass, which was preferred for manufacture of the plates, but film would have eventually replaced glass anyway. The film had great advantages with its light weight: a 14 inch × 17 inch film weighs 1.5 ounces, but a glass plate

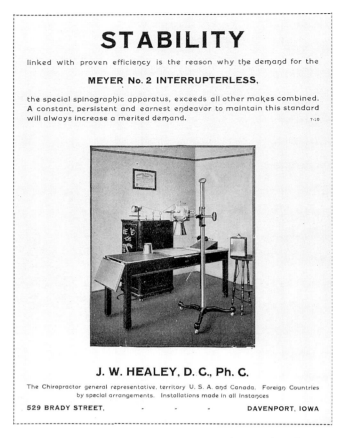
The Meyer No.2 Interrupterless, manufactured in Davenport, Iowa by J.W. Healey, 1920.
From *The Chiropractor*, July 1920.

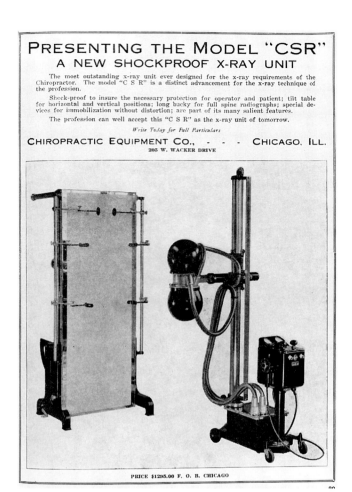
An advertisement for an x-ray unit from the Chiropractic Equipment Company of Chicago, Illinois, 1935.
From *The NCA Journal*, May 1935.

of the same size weighs 2 pounds. Easier storage and shorter exposure times also gave film the advantage.

The size of the photographic receptors, either plate or film, also changed. In 1910 McAdams, at Palmer, was reportedly using up to 12 inch × 20 inch plates, but mostly the standard size of 5 inch × 7 inch and 8 inch × 10 inch were cheaper and easier to handle. For the doctor of chiropractic who wanted to see the entire spine, there was an obvious dilemma. It took a lot of time and effort to expose the entire spine accurately, but this was done and taught by Thompson with three 8 inch × 10 inch films and one 5 inch × 7 inch film for the open mouth. Another 8 inch × 10 inch film could be added if the sacrum and coccyx was an area that the doctor wanted to see. Many began to use the sacrum-coccyx film routinely.

As P.A. Reimer reminisced in his 1938 book, *Modern X-ray Practice and Chiropractic Spinography,* five 8 inch × 10 inch films were used for the entire spinal column, which allowed adequate overlapping for easier comparison and included the base of the occiput, sacroiliac joints, and coccyx. This technique discarded the 5 inch × 7 inch upper cervical projection, replacing it with the bigger 8 inch × 10 inch. Then came the 14 inch × 17 inch film used in a procedure placing a 1/16 inch sheet of lead over half of the cassette, vertically splitting off the film for half of the spine,

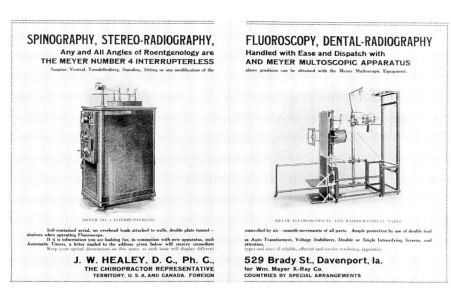

Ads of Spinography and Dental Radiography machines produced by the Healey Company of Davenport, Iowa, circa 1922.

Courtesy Palmer College of Chiropractic Archives, Davenport, Iowa.

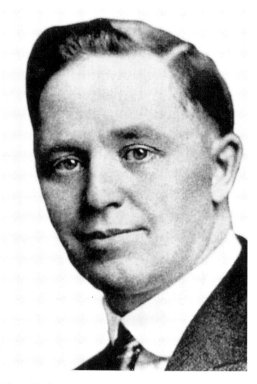

Ray Richardson introduced filming the entire spinal column on a single film in 1930.

From *The Recoil,* February 1925, Davenport, Iowa, Palmer School of Chiropractic.

then moving the lead over to the side of the cassette that was exposed, and x-raying the other half of the spine on the unexposed half of film. This process would in effect create two side by side 7 inch × 17 inch images of the entire column. Nevertheless, this procedure was abandoned, probably because of the time it took to perform it, its inconvenience, and the resulting distortion.

The major solution to fragmented spinal column images came about in 1930 when Ray Richardson of the Palmer School introduced a process for filming the entire spinal column on a single film which measured 8 inch × 36 inch. The technique, which took 5 years to develop, used an 8

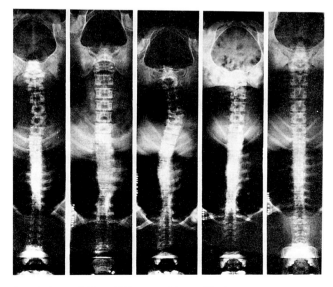

Depiction of 8′ × 36′—one film with two exposures, produced by Ray Richardson in 1930.

From *The Chiropractor,* April 1931.

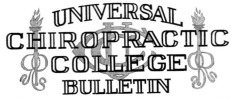

UNIVERSAL
CHIROPRACTIC
COLLEGE
BULLETIN

VOL. 14, No. 5   PITTSBURGH, PA., AUGUST, 1924   Edited by JOY M. LOBAN

The Erect Spinograph

Remarkable Advancement in Spinal Radiography
Achieved in Universal College Laboratory

A TREMENDOUS scientific achievement, overshadowing any Chiropractic discovery or invention of the past decade, and destined to save thousands of lives, reduce the cost of X-Ray equipment by doing away with the table, and furnishing the most convincing and absolute proof of the truth of Chiropractic that could be devised or imagined, is the contribution of Universal College for 1924.

It is the Erect Spinograph.

For years, Chiropractors have dimly realized that Spinal Radiography was imperfect. Skilled palpaters compared X-Ray pictures of the spine with their findings and were bewildered and puzzled by the results in a certain percentage of cases. The X-Ray sometimes confirmed palpation and inspection but sometimes flatly contradicted these methods and seemed to give the lie to Chiropractic. Cases of undoubted abnormality showed a straight spine and only minor defects in the plate. It was not only discouraging but often humiliating in cases where the X-Ray had been brought in as final proof, to the patient, that the Chiropractor's analysis was correct. When the plate denied the analysis, the Chiropractor was in a distinctly uncomfortable position.

Some Chiropractors met this situation by concluding that palpation and observation were inaccurate methods, despite the fact that they had been safe reliances for many years. They said, "The X-Ray cannot lie. I must be wrong." Losing faith in their palpation, they presently lost skill in it. Others, unwilling to doubt their own senses, developed a distaste for the X-Ray, which here and there flared out in open opposition to its use. Physicians, making spinal pictures, were able to declare that these pictures refuted the Chiropractic theory and it was hard to convince them otherwise.

Dr. Erwin H. Garbisch, U. C. C. Roentgenologist, and Dr. L. J. Steinbach, Dean of U. C. C. Faculty, were unwilling to adopt either attitude and approached the subject with detached scientific mind, determined to get at the truth. We will not here set down all the details of the laborious years of research by which, through trial and error, they gradually reached the correct conclusion. Nor shall we describe all the steps of the painstaking process by which they investigated and proved their conclusion. It is enough to say that they found the answer to the riddle and that the riddle exists no longer. The answer can be indicated in one word—stresses!

When a patient lies prone in the ordinary position for an X-Ray picture, he relaxes and relieves his spine of all the stresses to which it is normally subjected. It no longer supports

Announcement from Universal College of upright filming of the spine in 1924.

From *Universal Chiropractic College Bulletin*, August 1924.

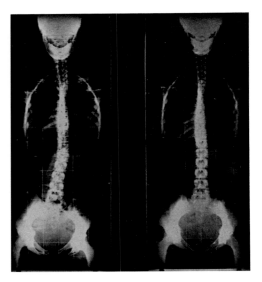

14" X 36' full spine films illustrating before and after chiropractic care.

From *Logan Basic College of Chiropractic Catalog*, 1950.

inch × 36 inch film cassette with double intensifying screens and a 36 inch bucky diaphragm for the radiographic table. If a bucky was not available in that size, the procedure could be done without a bucky. The upper 4 inches of the cassette was covered with lead, and the third cervical through the coccyx was exposed. The portion of the film that was then exposed was covered with lead, and the upper part was then exposed after the tube was centered over the open mouth, thus eliminating distortion of the upper cervical region. The tube distance initially used was 44 inches, but then 53 inches was instituted. Eastman double contrast film and Eastman screens were developed for this procedure.

The 8 inch × 36 inch film was received with enthusiasm by many. Some, however, did not spot film the upper cervical region. This failure led to distortion resembling fusion of the upper cervical spine, which Reimer later talked about. He suggested that the 8 inch × 36 inch film could be used with a moving jaw technique that would blur the mandible and make the entire cervical spine visible with one film and one exposure. He later abandoned this idea, thinking that the motion of the jaw caused some muscles to contract, resulting in head motion, which blurred the image. Another reason for his discarding the procedure was that in the late 1930s the Palmer School was working with stereoscopic x-ray procedures and the blurred mandible made it difficult to visually fuse the films.

Since upright filming was introduced into the profession in 1924, it was natural that many doctors used Richardson's idea but stood the patient up instead of laying him down. Standing patients were harder to center, and the film's 8 inch width left very little room for carelessness. If there was a marked scoliosis, the chiropractor would miss it. It became apparent, particularly to those who advocated upright filming for evaluation of the pelvis and hips, that the 8 inch × 36 inch film was not wide enough. The film reader could see the sacroiliac joints but not the appearance of the entire pelvis and hip joints and the effect gravity had on them.

It fell to Warren Sausser, a New York chiropractor who took Palmer's early spinography course and served in the army as an x-ray technician during World War I, to do something about it. Sausser had met Hugh B. Logan, founder of the Logan Basic Technique and a Universal College of Chiropractic graduate at one of the latter's postgraduate courses in November 1932. He became interested in Logan's technique, which required examination of the spine in the weight-bearing posture. The two men discussed their desire to see the entire spine and pelvis of a patient altogether as it would naturally appear under the stress of gravity, and in response Warren Sausser developed a procedure for what would popularly become known as the full-torso, or more recently full-spine, film.

The desire for one film and one exposure of the entire spinal column and pelvis was a challenge. Sausser made arrangements for equipment from the Standard X-ray Company of Chicago; Eastman Kodak supplied the film measuring 14 inch × 36 inch, as well as 14 inch × 36 inch screens and developing frames; and the Alberene Stone Company made the soapstone developing tank. The Improved Mailing Case Company made indestructible 4 inch × 14 inch mailing tubes, and the John C. Schwend Company made viewing boxes.

A 42 inch bucky was mounted on a counter-balanced frame, a level platform was built, and an aluminum filter was used to produce a uniform density on the film. Sausser used a 54 inch tube distance, and the technique setting for the anterior-posterior film for an "average 150 pound patient was 5 inch spark gap, 30 ma 22 seconds." A lateral film was also made, which he said was "fairly successful."

In July 1933, Sausser, then president of the Board of Counselors of Chiropractic Spinographers and X-ray Operators, wrote of his procedure in an article titled "New Spinographic Technique" in the *Journal of the National Chiropractic Association:*

> The advantages of this work on a single film are numerous," among the most important being a more accurate interpretation as to subluxation, rotations, curvatures, additional vertebrae, less vertebrae. Abnormal relationship of the entire osseous structure from the pelvis to the occiput. Exact length of the spine can be recorded.

Arthur W. Fuchs, son of the famous roentgen pioneer Wolfram Conrad Fuchs and author of the widely read and popular text, *Principles of Radiographic Exposure and Processing,* produced a 14 inch × 36 inch film 3 years later, which was reported in the December 1936 Kodak journal, *Radiography and Clinical Photography.* In his article, "Radiography of the Spine—a New Method," Fuchs wrote about the advantage of visualizing the entire spine with one exposure instead of using sectional films, and he also advocated the erect posture for spine filming as "desirable." He used a 54 inch tube distance and filtration, as did Sausser, and produced an anterior-posterior as well as a lateral film. This "new" procedure was reported by the Kodak journal as a first; however, upon being notified of Sausser's accomplishment 3 years earlier, an acknowledgement was printed in their August 1937 journal crediting him with the technique.

The full-spine film was a boon to the Logan technique, and Hugh Logan is credited with the popularizing of its use in chiropractic circles. Later Clarence Gonstead promoted the full-spine x-ray among his followers, and other chiropractors developed adjustive procedures, which utilized the 14 inch × 36 inch film. Gonstead added a twist in the procedure, however. In an effort to balance the varied densities of the body, he used split intensifying screens for a better spinal image. This technique worked to a degree in improving film quality but at the expense of patient exposure. His clinic did add filtration of the beam at a later date. Another Gonstead variation was to take the lateral film with two different exposures, which cut down on distortion but negated viewing the entire spine together normally, since invariably, a patient would move between the two projections, leaving an offset of the spine on the 14 inch × 36 inch film.

Sausser did not stop there. His next project was the development of a full-body x-ray, again using Kodak products in both the anterior-posterior and lateral positions. While this was an impressive site, it lacked practicality. Many thought Sausser had originated the practice, but it had already been done in 1896, and Sausser wrote in his article that Dr. Robert Janker of Germany displayed his in 1934. Fuchs also accomplished full-body x-rays, but his efforts were not practical either. Ray Richardson developed an extraordinary film measuring 18 inches × 40 inches which included both hips and shoulders, when the full spine was x-rayed, and allowed taking a lateral cervical projection and a lateral lumbosacral at the top by the head. His procedure was to center the patient on a tilting table in the upright position standing on a foot plate, which he developed, and then to lower the table and take the film in the recumbent position. He felt, then, that the pelvis would be positioned as it was in the standing posture, and he would get a better quality image since recumbency would level the abdomen and stabilize the patient. Earl Rich, who did not like the full-spine film because of image quality problems, remarked that he would accept Richardson's procedure when a full-spine was necessary.

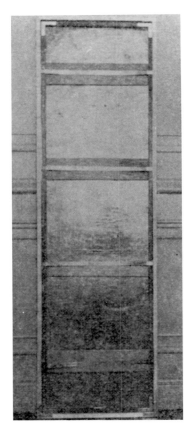
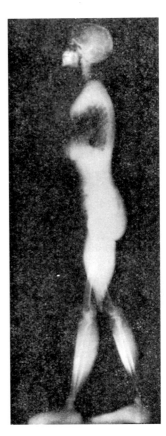

A lateral full body radiograph produced by Warren Sausser in 1935. The 20′ X 72′ cassette weighed 54 pounds.
From *The Chiropractic Journal*, February 1935.

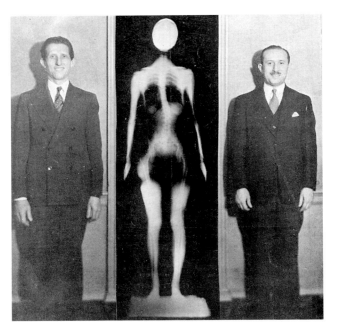

Warren Sausser (left) and Sol Goldschmidt (*right*) with a full-body x-ray using Kodak film, 1934.
From *The Chiropractic Journal*, February 1935.

The full-spine film became, and has remained, very popular, not just with chiropractors, but also with the medical orthopedists who use it for scoliosis evaluation. The main criticism of the full-spine film has been the difficulty in assuring good image quality, because of all the variables of bodies. Even though filtration is used, there are still limitations. The full-spine film came to be so popularly identified with chiropractic use that the syndicated game show *To Tell the Truth* once had three contestants on stage with their full-spine films in front of them claiming to be "Miss Perfect Posture." Of course only one was.

Development of better filtration occurred over the years. Most notably, Felix Bauer of Australia came up with a variable filtration system circa 1967 that is still the vanguard of today. His devices, though developed for sectional spinal films, have probably produced the best films around. He is also responsible for developing several filming innovations to improve film quality with reduction of patient exposure to x-ray. Bauer almost single-handedly saved Australia's and New Zealand's chiropractors from losing the right to x-ray patients.

Dr. John Noland of New Zealand, another innovator, followed Bauer's lead and developed his own variable filtration system, adding devices for the full-spine film, and today has one of the most popular filter systems. Back at the Palmer School of Chiropractic, J. Clay Thompson, an innovator and inventor of many widely used chiropractic devices, made an intriguing filtration system for improving the x-ray image that used lead and aluminum. His x-ray timing apparatus used a shutter system that de-

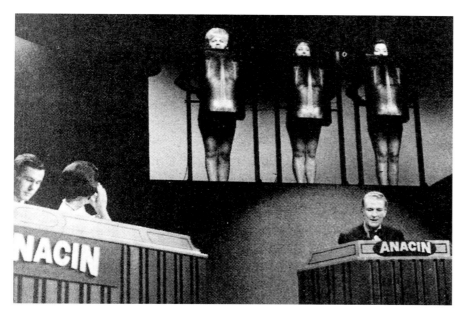

Full spine x-rays on "To Tell the Truth" with Bud Colyer, host, and panelists Kitty Carlisle and Johnny Carson.

From *The Digest of Chiropractic Economics,* January/February 1962.

scended in front of the tube during the exposure to lessen the exposure of the cervical and upper thoracic spine. Even though Thompson successfully applied for a patent in 1960, he was so busy inventing and developing other pieces of chiropractic equipment, as well as practicing chiropractic and teaching at the school, that he never got around to manufacturing the system.

Another system of filtration to emerge was the Sportelli-Winterstein aluminum wedge. Louis Sportelli of Pennsylvania worked closely with one

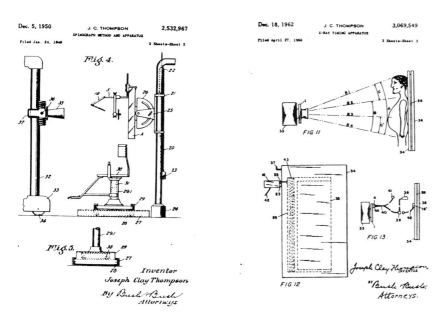

Pictures of full spine filter device and cervical positioning apparatus designed by J. Clay Thompson as submitted to the U.S. Patent Office in 1949 and 1960.

Courtesy J. Clay Thompson, Bettendorf, Iowa.

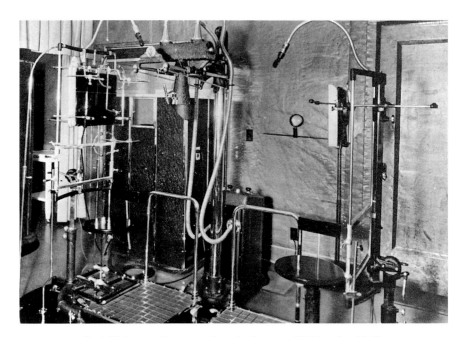

Stabilizing and measuring devices at PSC in the 1940s.
From *The PSC Announcement,* Palmer School of Chiropractic, circa 1940.

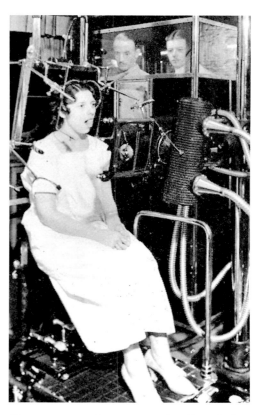

The x-ray equipment in the B.J. Palmer Clinic, circa 1945. Note the head clamp to assure proper positioning for the cervical films.
From *The B.J. Palmer Chiropractic Clinic,* Palmer School of Chiropractic, 1947.

of his postgraduate radiology instructors, James Winterstein, to develop an aluminum filter that tapered for gradual diminution of the x-ray beam before it reached the patient or film. Further developments made by Sportelli made the wedged-shaped aluminum filter variable.

Another area that chiropractors were interested in was patient stabilization and alignment to minimize technical factors that could mislead the doctor in his interpretation of the spinal radiograph. J. Clay Thompson developed head clamps to assure that the patient did not move but was centered to the film when positioned for cervical films. Medical doctors were already using head clamps for the skull and some cervical spine films, but these functioned differently, with the sides operating independently. Fuchs also used head clamps for his full-spine anterior-posterior and lateral x-rays, and a centering device that the doctor could use to make sure the head was centered, thus assuring some degree of accuracy. Pads that could be moved in on both sides of the patient's body to stabilize and center were also made for full-spine films, and a measuring and calculating system was used to be able to take films at different times on a patient and assure the exact same positioning. B.J. Palmer called this work "posture constant." It was used for researching the change that occurred after care. Wes Culwell of Texas also developed a body clamping system to assure proper patient positioning, resulting in improved accuracy.

With the Palmer School's specialization in the upper cervical spine, head clamping was essential, as was positioning the patient on a stool or chair for cervical films. This practice led to the development of a chair that was movable in all directions, so the doctor could move any patient, no matter how twisted, into a true anterior-posterior position, as well as other positions like lateral and oblique. A tilting bucky was developed so the film could be moved for different views of the upper cervical spine while keeping the patient immovable. In 1950 J. Clay Thompson patented his head clamps, movable chair, and tilting bucky under the name of *spinograph methods and apparatus.* Since then similar chairs and head clamps have been made with minor modifications.

Theodore Vladeff of Detroit, Michigan, also desired specificity of the entire spine and pelvis. He developed a centering device, a turntable for full spine upright films, and a chair. These became popular and were endorsed by Joseph Janse, Warren Sausser, Waldo Poehner, D.W. Poupard, and Arthur Hendricks of the Lincoln College, who made up a committee from the NCCR. Vladeff also produced precision sitting and standing spinographic procedures in 1943, developed the Vladeff fixation theory, and developed several devices, including his own brand of head clamps.

Other devices that came on the scene included the orthoprotractor by A.A. Wersing for analyzing upper cervical films. He also developed the Vernier Table for x-ray placement and the atlas slide rule for calculating errors in placement for upper cervical spine analysis. In 1946 Sanford Ulrich, a member of the New York Chiropractic Research Foundation, developed a full-spine lateral positioning apparatus to accomplish accurate repositioning for lateral follow-up films. In 1947 a distortion corrector was developed by S.H. Nihswander to measure object film distance and correct for film distortion. In 1948 Jack S. Pry invented the Pry rule to correct off-centering for full-spine films, using the Logan basic system. In the 1950s Travis Utterbach developed a frame to make sure that the x-ray equipment, especially tube, would not be jarred from its centered position, keeping it in alignment so that this technical factor could be eliminated when the doctor interpreted the films. He also invented self-centering head clamps, used in the upper cervical technique to help assure accurate patient positioning. Compression bands had been used for a number of years, tightening around the abdomen from one side. Many felt that this caused some rotation of the standing patient and distorted the spine. Felix Baurer addressed this problem by developing a band that could tighten on both sides simultaneously, thus stabilizing the upright patient while compressing the abdomen. Marshal Dickhotz also contributed many devices for the upper cervical techniques.

Resolution of Appreciation

DECEMBER 3, 1944

ACTING UPON THE INVITATION OF A GROUP OF SCIENTIFICALLY-MINDED CHIROPRACTORS OF THE STATE OF MICHIGAN, WE, THE UNDERSIGNED, WERE PRIVILEGED TO EXAMINE AND STUDY THOROUGHLY THE EQUIPMENT, METHOD AND PROCEDURE EMPLOYED BY DR. THEODORE VLADEFF OF THE CHIROPRACTIC X-RAY AND RESEARCH LABORATORIES OF DETROIT, MICHIGAN, FOR THE PURPOSE OF ARRIVING AT A MORE EXACTING AND SPECIFIC X-RAY PROCEDURE TO BE USED IN DETERMINING THE NATURE, TYPE AND LOCATION OF SPINAL AND PELVIC DISTORTIONS, ESPECIALLY THE MAJOR VERTEBRAL SUBLUXATIONS.

WE HAVE FOUND THE EQUIPMENT, INCLUDING A TURNTABLE AND CENTERING DEVICE, USED IN THE ACCOMPLISHMENT OF THIS AIM, BOTH ORIGINAL AND EXACTING, ALLOWING A MARKED IMPROVEMENT IN THE SCIENCE OF CHIROPRACTIC RADIOGRAPHY.

HIS METHOD OF SPINOGRAPHIC INTERPRETATION IS DISTINCTLY UNIQUE, AND IS SUGGESTIVE OF REVOLUTIONARY POSSIBILITIES THAT CERTAINLY MERIT CONTINUED RESEARCH AND INVESTIGATION.

THEREFORE, CONSCIOUS OF THE FACT THAT A SOUND, STANDARD TECHNIC OF TAKING SPINAL X-RAYS FOR PRECISION WORK IS NECESSARY AND SHOULD BE UNIVERSALLY INSISTED UPON, WE, THE UNDERSIGNED, WHOLEHEARTEDLY ENDORSE THE MECHANICAL FEATURES AS ADVANCED BY DR. VLADEFF AND WOULD SINCERELY SUGGEST THAT HE CONTINUE HIS INVESTIGATIONS ON X-RAY INTERPRETATION UNTIL WARRANTED CONCLUSIONS MAY BE DRAWN.

WE CALL ON ALL PROGRESSIVE GROUPS AND LIBERAL-MINDED AGENCIES WITHIN THE PROFESSION TO ENCOURAGE AND SUPPORT THE CONTINUANCE OF THIS WORK.

(Signed) WARREN SAUSSER, D. C.
(Signed) W. G. POEHNER, D. C.
(Signed) ARTHUR HENDRICKS, D. C.
(Signed) JOSEPH JANSE, D. C.
(Signed) D. W. POUPARD, D. C.

Resolution by members of the Council of Roentgenologists of the NCA concerning Theodore Vladeff's x-ray laboratory.

From *The National Chiropractic Journal,* January 1945.

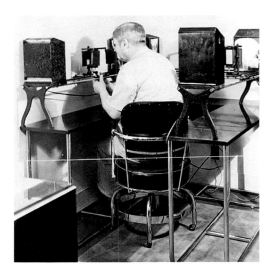

Dr. R.W. Stephenson reading stereoscopic x-rays in the B.J. Palmer Clinic, circa 1935.

From *The B.J. Palmer Chiropractic Clinic,* Palmer School of Chiropractic, 1935.

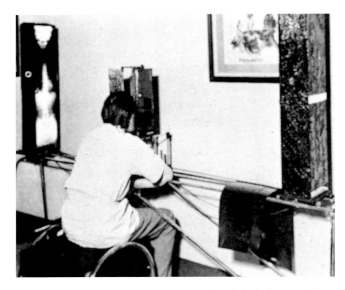

B.J. Palmer viewing stereoscopic 8' X 36' full spine films for 3-D image.

From *The B.J. Palmer Chiropractic Clinic,* Palmer School of Chiropractic, 1947.

In the 1930s, B.J. Palmer was seeking the best possible way of seeing the upper cervical spine and came across stereoscopic radiographs, which gave a 3-D image. While this technique had been done first in 1896, it was still very popular and remained so for some time. Arthur Fuchs advocated it for the traumatized cervical spine. This work required a tube shift and two films for each position as well as double the viewboxes and mirrors for viewing. The images were great, but the procedure died out, probably because of difficulty in finding machines that were easy to manipulate and the excessive amount of time involved with the taking and viewing of the films. The B.J. Palmer Clinic at first used it often, then later "primarily for difficult cases." Stereoscopic radiographs vanished from Palmer College after the death of B.J. Palmer in 1961 and the closing of the B.J. Palmer Clinic. Even though the school's public clinic was almost exclusively using upper cervical techniques, the B.J. Palmer Clinic was not as limited. Palmer devised a stereo viewing apparatus that could handle the 8 inch × 36 inch full-spine studies. Even Fuchs, in his article on full-spine films, wrote that "supplementary stereoradiographs are valuable also when the entire spine radiographs yield evidence of local disease or injury".

Cineradiography, x-ray images in motion, was first performed in 1898 by Roux on film, although an x-ray pioneer McIntier came up with the idea by putting pictures together in 1897. Felding, in 1956, performed cine cervical spine studies. Cineradiographic studies were first performed in the chiropractic profession in 1957 by Fred Illi of Geneva, Switzerland. A great investigator, Illi obtained a Phillip's cine unit from the company in the Netherlands for his Institute for the Study of Statics and Dynamics of the Human Body in Geneva. He had previously developed a method of taking upright full-spine films at 4 meters with synchronized exposures from numerous tubes. He was the first chiropractor to perform orthogonal radiography as well. In 1939, 1940, and 1942, Illi studied at the National College with Joseph Janse in dissection work, primarily on the sacroiliac joint, and discovered a previously unknown ligament, which is today termed *Illi's ligament.* His numerous studies have earned him the

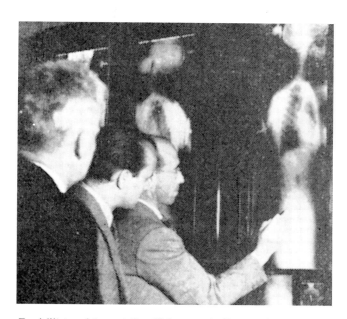

Fred Illi teaching at the Chiropractic Research Institute in Geneva, Switzerland.

From the *NCA Journal*, January 1946.

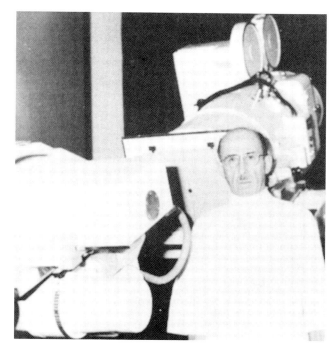

Fred Illi of Geneva with Phillips cineradiography unit.

Courtesy Claude Illi, Geneva Switzerland.

reputation of being the premiere expert on lumbar spine and sacroiliac motion.

Lincoln College, with Earl Rich heading up the radiology department and later becoming president, started cineradiographic work for the evaluation of spinal motion in the United States. In 1961 to 1962 Rich received an offer to install the appropriate equipment from the Picker or-

N.C.A. TO PURCHASE

CINEROENTGENOLOGY

Moving Pictures X-Rays Will Aid Research

Lincoln Chiropractic College soon will receive $32,000 worth of new X-ray equipment as a result of action taken here by the Executive Board of the National Chiropractic Association.

The cineroentgenology equipment will be installed at the college as a project of the Foundation for Accredited Chiropractic Education.

Dr. Earl Rich, designated chairman of this Foundation project by the NCA board, will work under the general direction of the NCA director of research.

Staff members from other NCA accredited Chiropractic Colleges will be invited to participate in the project's research as the need arises. Copies of all X-rays made in the project will be sent to each

of the other NCA accredited colleges as soon as the films are available.

Funds to carry out the project will be made available from the Research Fund of Foundation for Accredited Chiropractic Education.

The NCA Executive Board approved the $32,000 purchase agreement with Picker X-ray Co., at its meeting held in connection with the 66th Anniversary Convention of the NCA here June 11-16.

Picker is designing the special cineroentgenology equipment and will deliver it to Lincoln College upon completion.

The equipment will be labeled as the property of the Foundation for Accredited Chiropractic Education.

A National Chiropractic Association announcement for support of cineroentgenologic equipment for Lincoln Chiropractic College.

From The Digest of Chiropractic Economics, July-August 1961.

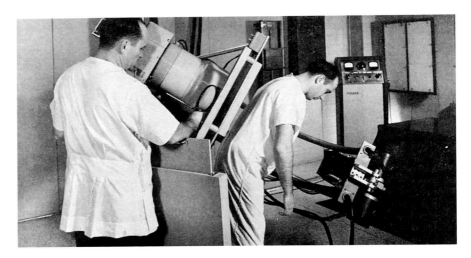

Dr. Earl Rich of Lincoln Chiropractic College, with cineroentgenographic equipment of the early 1960s.

From *The Journal of the NCA*, February 1963.

ganization, which would donate half of the cost plus a donation of $30,000 from the NCA. With this funding, Rich started to work with the able assistance of Thomas Goodrich, who took over the studies after Rich's death in 1967. Rich had made the unit available to all of the radiologists in chiropractic, and of the ones that worked with it, Ronald Watkins and Joseph Howe were the most prolific. Howe continued the work after Goodrich left Lincoln College, and also continued to study spinal motion at the Talmidge, Ohio, Center in 1974, and at National College when he assumed the position of radiology department head there. The Northwestern College also obtained a cine unit a few years later.

Shortly after this progress in cineradiography, videofluoroscopy be-

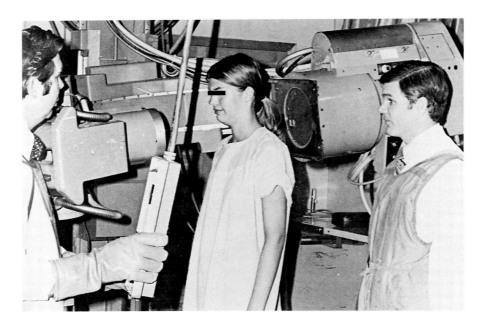

Joseph Howe, D.C., D.A.C.B.R., with patient and Senior Resident Terry Yochum, circa 1973.

From the *Journal of Clinical Chiropractic*, November/December 1973.

came popular. James Mertz and John Danz obtained a unit and started studies at their facility in St. Louis, Missouri. Other schools used fluoroscopy but not necessarily with videotaping to the extent that Mertz and Danz did. Fluoroscopy's use among radiologists was limited, but others in the field of chiropractic who were not certified in radiology began to take it up somewhat later. Kevin Robinson, James Noia, and Eugene Bell, who purchased Mertz's unit in St. Louis, and a few medical doctors who saw the advantages of spinal motion studies and did not mind bucking the medical establishment by associating with chiropractors professionally, began to study and teach their findings on the postgraduate level. Walter Pierce also started videofluoroscopic work at a slightly later date but in a different way than most others were viewing it. Instead of looking for areas of hypermobility from ligamentous tearing and instability, he looked for fixations of spinal joints as one of the criteria to decide what vertebral levels in the cervical region should be adjusted.

Conventional tomography has also been performed by some of the radiology specialists in chiropractic for enhancement of suspected lesions. In addition, magnetic resonance imaging (MRI) has been delved into by many. Some chiropractors have opened or been involved in the establishment of MRI centers and have taken fellowships offered by medical radiologists, as well as having taught classes for medical personnel. The examining board for the radiologists in chiropractic includes both MRI and computed tomography to some degree.

UPRIGHT RADIOGRAPHY AND ITS CONTROVERSY

In the early years, 1910 to 1924, spinography was performed in the recumbent supine position. Although Monell did write of upright spinal films in 1902, there is no evidence they were done for evaluation of the stresses of gravity on the body, but rather more for convenience of the operator, and this type of equipment did not last long. In 1924, though, the Universal College, under the presidency of Joy Loban, announced the accomplishment of the first standing x-ray of the lumbar spine and pelvis for the visualization of the effects of gravity on the spine and pelvis. This feat was accomplished by Leo Steinbach, dean of the college, and Edwin Garbisch, college roentgenologist, after several years of technique variations and equipment modifications.

The proponents of this change felt that the biomechanical variations of the spine and pelvis that could be seen in the recumbent films would be exaggerated by the pull of gravity on the patient's body in the standing posture, thus exaggerating any spinal segmental displacements and making them more visible. The standing radiograph should also more closely correlate to the findings of the doctor's palpation, which was most often performed in the seated position. The standing x-ray answered the nagging complaint of many chiropractors who had palpated curvatures only to lay the patient down for x-ray and not find the curve they had told the patient was there. It was also felt that with the standing position, the foundation of the spine—the pelvis, sacrum, and hips—would demonstrate unleveling that might also be the cause of curvatures, or even subluxation. This later reasoning particularly underlay the first upright film of the pelvis. Steinbach wrote numerous papers comparing x-rays in the upright and recumbent positions, and many articles in the journals of the

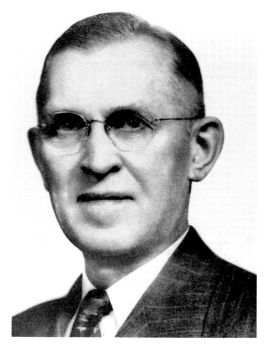

Leo J. Steinbach of Universal College of Chiropractic, circa 1946.

From *The National Chiropractic Journal,* January 1946.

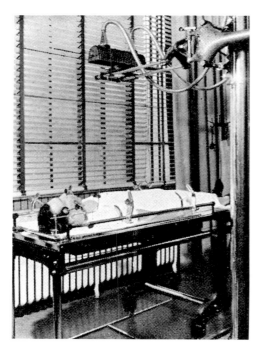

Recumbent spinal filming at PSC with device to assure duplicated position.

From *The B.J. Palmer Chiropractic Clinic*, Palmer School of Chiropractic, 1947.

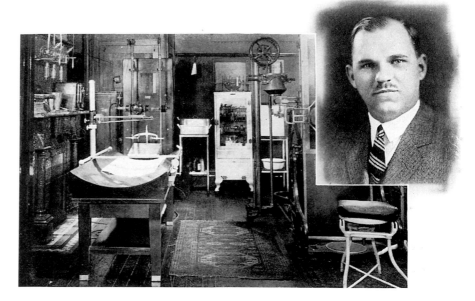

Edwin H. Garbisch and his x-ray laboratory at Universal College of Chiropractic where he and Steinbach developed upright filming of the spinal column.

From *Universal Chiropractic College Catalog*, 1919-1920.

day announced this logical advancement in patient evaluation. Steinbach concluded that the standing position was far superior to the recumbent position for demonstrating biomechanical, abnormal spinal, and pelvic alignments.

Ray Richardson had stated in 1924 after Universal's "upright" announcement that "from the experiments that we have made, we find that spinographs taken with the patient in the dorsal position are more accurate, the patient being relaxed and more free from any movement than in the erect posture." This would indicate that he had previously worked with

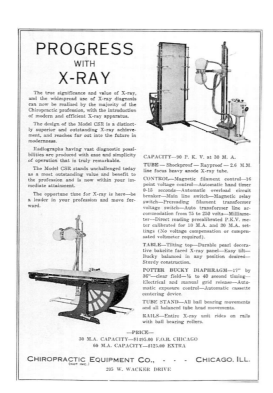
An ad for equipment from the Chiropractic Equipment Co., Chicago, Illinois, 1937.

From *The NCA Journal*, June 1937.

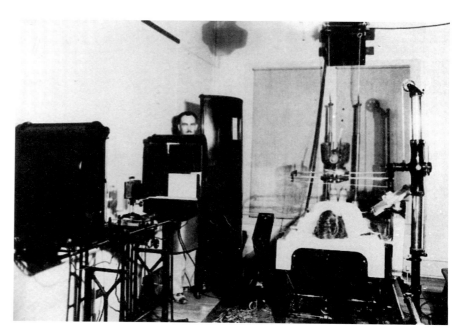

An early x-ray laboratory at Texas Chiropractic College.

From *What Chiropractic Is Doing*, 1937.

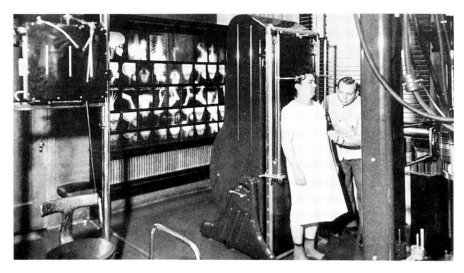

Upright spinal filming during the late 1940s at the B.J. Palmer Clinic.
From the *PSC Announcement,* Palmer School of Chiropractic, 1950.

upright filming only to abandon it. The Palmer School accepted this work in the late 1930s, after Ray Richardson, who was an advocate of the recumbent posture, left. Remier stated in 1938 that "for the lumbar and thoracic spine, the standing position was superior while for the cervical spine, the seated position was better."

D.W. Poupard of the Universal College was one of the strongest advocates of upright work in the 1930s, as were Warren Sausser and the Logans. With the popularization of the full-spine film in the mid-1930s, standing posture became exceedingly popular, and it predominates in the profession today even to the point that some assume when one talks of spinography that a weight-bearing film has been taken.

In 1934 Poupard in the *Journal of the NCA* wrote a background of the historical developments with upright filming. He explained that the "horizontal type of machine was the only one then in use. Later, a vertical machine was constructed from specifications furnished by chiropractors, but it was first offered to the medical profession at a convention in the city of Wheeling, West Virginia. Strangely, however, this first model was purchased by a member of our profession and was installed by Dr. E.H. Garbisch, who did much research work. Hundreds of films were

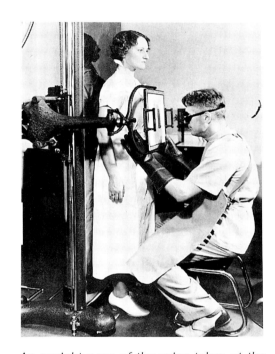

An upright x-ray of the spine taken at the B.J. Palmer Clinic in 1947.
From *The B.J. Palmer Chiropractic Clinic,* Palmer School of Chiropractic, 1947.

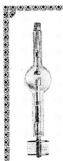

"Spinographically Speaking"

By

Dr. E. A. Thompson, Baltimore, Md.

EDITOR'S NOTE: This department will be glad to consider any of your X-ray problems. We consider ourselves very fortunate in obtaining so able an authority as Dr. E. A. Thompson to edit this page. Dr. Thompson is the pioneer spinographer. For many years head of this department in The Palmer School of Chiropractic and since specializing in X-ray work and film reading, he has undoubtedly had more intensive X-ray training and experience than any other person in the chiropractic profession.

In addition to writing Chiropractic Spinography, *E.A. Thompson also edited a column on radiology, "Spinographically Speaking."*
Courtesy Palmer College of Chiropractic Archives, Davenport, Iowa.

taken and countless comparisons between films taken in both the horizontal and the vertical positions. He further stated that "the addition of x-ray for the study of the spine had been a step forward of no little importance." The major consideration in those days appears to have been directed to the discovery of two things: subluxations and structural pathology. The horizontal technique served this purpose quite well in the early days of development. However, the Horizontal technique, or the picturization of the spinal column in the recumbent position, did not and could not show the maximum strain on nor the forced degree of displacement of the vertebral column."

Nevertheless, some still advocated recumbent filming. Dr. Carl Cleveland of the Kansas City Cleveland College had equipment modification done from the standard upright devices to perform experiments in the 1950s. His work consisted of three full-spine films in the anterior-posterior position: the first with the patient standing, the second with the patient in the recumbent position with greater tube distance than before, and the third with the patient suspended from a bar by their knees in an inverted position. He found that curvatures changed but that he could correlate on all three studies the same radiographic misalignment that was in a state of fixation. He concluded that the recumbent posture was superior for film quality and reduced curvatures and the effects of gravity that were compensatory, thus leading to more confusion on the film. His next experiment, also performed with three full-spine films, but all standing, x-rayed the patient in their worn down shoes, a new pair of shoes, and barefooted. He noted a lot of differences, at times, in pelvic and sacral tilt, but could still find the fixated misalignment, thus concluding that the pelvic shift did not significantly alter the intersegmental dysfunction.

Cleveland was not alone. In the early 1970s Joseph Howe made the following observations: "Recumbency allows distribution of abdominal structures and will give far better visualization of all structures than will upright films except in very thin patients. Another matter worth considering is that while the weight-bearing relationships are seen in upright radiographs, so are antalgic and compensatory mechanisms. These may hide the true problems. Recumbency shows non-stressed vertebral relationships and a disrelationship seen recumbent is probably more significant than one seen upright. Often the only way to assess the importance of an apparent intervertebral disrelationship is to see it both upright and recumbent." He cites Robert Ridler and Leo Wunsch as being in agreement, as is Russell Erhardt, who has stated that once he gets a doctor to take recumbent lumbar films, he has not seen one go back to the upright work.

CHIROPRACTIC RADIOLOGICAL PUBLICATIONS

Early articles on x-ray became regular features, "Spinographically Speaking" in the UCA publication, edited by E.A. Thompson, and "Visualizing Chiropractic" by L.A. Nash in the earlier ACA periodical. Articles continued in the later NCA Journal of Chiropractic, today's ACA, and occasionally the ICA journal. Several state associations and school-supported magazines such as the Chirogram, also ran x-ray related information. In 1937 The National Spinographic Society in New York produced the journal The Spinographer, with William P. Schmeelk, editor.

The first textbook written by a chiropractor specializing in roentgenology was *Chiropractic Spinography* by Ernest A. Thompson in 1918. This Palmer School publication covered physics of the early equipment; technology, including machine settings for spine and extremities; techniques for soft tissue contrast media studies of the esophagus, stomach, and colon; and a few spinal osseous pathologies and procedures for spinal measurements. It became the standard text in virtually all the colleges of the day with an x-ray department and was revised in 1919, 1921, and 1923. The Palmer School also published P.A. Remier's *Modern X-ray Practice and Chiropractic Spinography* in 1938, 1947, and 1957. Palmer had his own printery on campus, which produced *The Chiropractor* and *The Fountain Head News* and some of the books used as texts by the school until B.J.'s death in 1961. Remier's texts covered the technology of all systems, except those studied by invasive procedures, and gave the techniques and machine settings for each, as well as an in-depth dissertation on different systems of spinography, including the upper cervical Palmer advocated at this period. The books did not contain pathological films, but these were covered in class by the instructor, mainly Remier.

In addition to Rich's *Atlas,* a 1947 publication, *X-ray Technic and Spinal Interpretation,* by A.G. Hendricks, one of the founders of Lincoln College and a leader in early x-ray, and Earl Rich, was a popular text. Other popular texts included the following: H.E. Turley's *X-ray in Chiropractic,* published by Texas College in 1947; Lester Cheal's *Manual of Precision Spinography* in 1950; Fred Illi's outstanding text, *The Vertebral Column Life-Line of the Body* in 1950; John Teranel's *Chiropractic Orthopedics and Roentgenology,* another leading book of its day in 1953; James Winterstein's *Chiropractic Spinographology* in 1970; John Macrae's *Roentgenometrics used in Chiropractic* in 1974; the very prolific Roy W. Hildebrandt's *Synopsis of Chiropractic Roentgenographic Technology* in 1974, and his first of three editions of *Chiropractic Spinography* in 1977; Russell Erhardt's *Chiropractic Reference of Clinical Radiographic Studies*

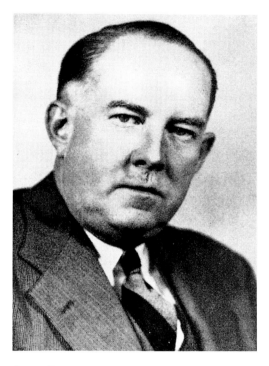

Percy Remier, long-time department chair at the PSC and author of Modern X-Ray Practice and Chiropractic Spinography.

From Remier P: *Modern x-ray practice and chiropractic spinography,* 1938, Palmer School of Chiropractic, Davenport, Iowa.

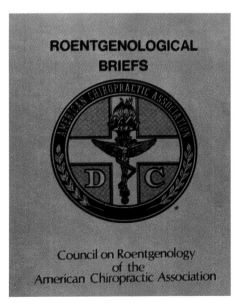

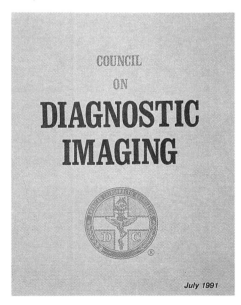

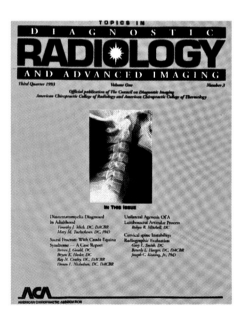

A trio of publications sponsored by the American Chiropractic Association.

From *Council on Roentgenology: roentgenological briefs,* Grand Forks, North Dakota, 1982, The American Chiropractic Association; *Council on diagnostic imaging,* Arlington, Virginia, 1991, The American Chiropractic Association; and *Topics in diagnostic radiology and advanced imaging,* Arlington, Virginia, 1993, The American Chiropractic Association.

in 1983, a standard for the practicing field doctor; and Peter Kogan et al.'s *A Synopsis of Clinical Roentgenology* in 1986.

Until fairly recently the many books written by doctors of chiropractic on the subject of radiology were all privately published, but in recent years major publishers have started handling and even seeking out these works. The first such book was published by Williams and Wilkins in 1983 and titled *Practical Applied Roentgentology* by Edward Maurer and geared to the undergraduate student preparing for examining boards.

In 1985 the same publishing house also printed a revision of Roy Hildebrandt's *Chiropractic Spinography.* Other books by major publishers include *Atlas of Radiographic Positioning: Normal Anatomy and Developmental Variance* by Sharon Jaeger, published by Appleton and Lange, and *Case Studies in Chiropractic Radiology* also by Sharon Jaeger with Debra Pate, published by Aspen. The most widely used text today is *Essentials in Skeletal Radiology* authored by Terry Yochum and Lindsey Rowe, Yochum's first resident from his Australian days as department head at the Preston Institute's International College of Chiropractic, with Gary Guebert, Joseph Howe, Margaret Seron, Bryan Hartley, and David Thomas as contributors. This work has become the standard today and is required in all of the accredited chiropractic institutions, as well as being found in many medical school libraries and private collections of medical radiologists. Yochum bridged the gap between medical and chiropractic radiologists and has joined the teaching staff of The School of Medicine of the University of Colorado and received the "Outstanding Clinical Radiologist Award Teacher of the Year."

RADIOLOGICAL REGULATIONS

X-ray in the early years was basically unregulated, but as the dangers became apparent, restrictions from both the scientific community and the state legislatures began to appear. It was not until the 1930s that the medical association's specialists began to control radiology in their own realm and even tried to restrict its use only to the medical profession. One of the early fears on the part of some M.D.s about chiropractic use was raised by the practice of a practitioner named Andrew P. Davis, M.D., D.O., and D.C.—one of the first graduates of D.D. Palmer's school in Davenport, Iowa. In his practice and the school he established, Davray in 1902 in Michigan, Davis used x-ray as a therapeutic device. Some thought that this practice would become a part of chiropractic, which is probably one reason one finds early chiropractic school catalogs stating that x-ray is not used for therapy, as well as why many state laws governing chiropractic specifically prohibit x-ray therapy. Davis also operated under his medical degree, thus making his therapeutic use legal.

The fact that x-ray therapy was not used in chiropractic did not deter the medical associations from fighting tooth and nail to ban any use of x-ray in chiropractic. An example of the extent of their opposition occurred in New York City where an army trained x-ray technologist and graduate of Palmer's x-ray course and school, Warren Sausser, opened an x-ray laboratory that catered to chiropractors. Around 1924, he was arrested for operating an x-ray laboratory without a permit, and other chiropractors operating similar labs in the city were told to close them. The case was tried before the Board of Health which refused to grant a permit after a 6-month delay. The UCA entered to support Sausser, and the decision was appealed to the Superior Court, which upheld the decision of the Board of Health. The UCA then appealed to the Appellate Division of the Supreme Court, which upheld the decision of the Superior Court. The UCA then made application to the Appellate Division for a writ of error to the Court of Appeals, which was denied. Sausser, growing weary of litigation, refused to have anything more to do with the case after the Supreme Court decision. The UCA persevered and appealed to the Court of Appeals, for a writ of error, which was finally granted. So successful was the case that not only Sausser was allowed to x-ray people, with his army radiological technology degree, but the other chiropractors in New York with x-ray training could also operate x-ray laboratories.

Restrictions got so tight, however, that in some places chiropractors who were well trained to use the equipment, even more so than the medical doctor, lost or were in danger of losing their right to use x-ray. State by state, chiropractors had to get involved in convincing senators, representatives, and governors either to keep x-ray as a method of examination in the chiropractic laws that had already been enacted or to include it in any proposed laws governing the profession. There have been many legal battles concerning x-ray in chiropractic from state to state and nationally. Even though the country was moving state by state to license chiropractic and award it the same status as the medical profession, New York continued in its opposition. In 1963 the Court of Appeals, by a five to two vote affirmed a regulation of the Public Health Council prohibiting chiropractors from using x-ray for diagnosis. In the dissenting opinion, New York Chief Justice Charles Desmond stated, "New York is the only state that had ever enacted a law making it impossible for chiropractors to take or even use x-ray pictures." He went on to state, "Taking and reading of x-ray photographs is a customary and legal activity of chiropractors and does not constitute the practice of medicine. I am convinced that (this) regulation violates the Constitutional rights of chiropractors to follow their chosen calling free from unreasonable governmental influence."

With the eventual passing of a chiropractic law by the New York legislature, and with its signing by Governor Nelson Rockefeller in 1963, came one of the most bizarre twists in chiropractic legislation in the country's history. Having formed a commission of medical and osteopathic association representatives, Rockefeller supported their recommendation to limit chiropractors' use of x-ray to "persons over 18 years of age" and at "a level above the top of the first lumbar vertebra." The chiropractors in the state were split over whether to support the legislation. Based on the idea that a restrictive law was better than no law at all, chiropractors accepted it, and Governor Rockefeller signed the act on April 30, 1963, making New York the forty-seventh state to license doctors of chiropractic. David Redding, an upstate practitioner, later won a legal battle removing the restrictions, which finally allowed chiropractors to x-ray the low back and extremities and patients under the age of 18.

California was another state that saw a legislative battle for chiropractic radiology. The first state radiation control act passed in 1968 with Governor Ronald Reagan's signature, and a copy was sent to the United States Department of Health, Education, and Welfare as model legislation that other states could base their laws on. Before its passage, however, many battles were fought, with the California Medical Association trying to keep chiropractors out and the California Chiropractic Association attempting to assure chiropractic inclusion. Robert Jackson, who was chairman of the legislative department of the chiropractic association, met Senator Walter Stiern, who introduced the first radiation control bill in 1965. Stiern had agreed to put chiropractic into his legislation, but because of the demands of the American Medical Association, the bill was withdrawn. Another attempt was made in 1967. When the final vote came, the bill could not be passed without the chiropractic inclusion. In the 1968 session, Senator Stiern asked Robert Jackson to write in the chiropractic section, which was the final draft that received the governor's signature.

For many years the state of Washington had a restrictive law that limited the doctor of chiropractic to x-raying and treating only the spine. If a patient came into the chiropractor's office with a complaint in the arm or leg, the chiropractor, even though there was clinical justification, could not legally x-ray that part of the patient. Some states still cling to this restrictive standard, although legally, in most places, a primary health care provider is responsible for examining the area of the patient's body that is the complaint.

All primary health care providers have two-tiered systems of control: one set of standards for the private practitioner and another for the radiologist. There are still a fair number of medical and osteopathic doctors who perform in-office procedures but the majority use the services of the specialists. In chiropractic, the majority of doctors own their own x-ray equipment and either have a radiologic technologist, general or limited, perform the procedures or do it themselves. The reason for this practice, no doubt, goes back to refusal on the part of many medical radiologists to accept referrals from a chiropractor and the refusal to have x-ray procedures performed for a doctor of chiropractic; consequently, it fell to the chiropractor to do it.

The regulatory agency for the chiropractic practitioner is the state, which has a board of examiners that tests a graduate on all standard subjects, including x-ray. The graduate or senior student is also required to take a national board, usually before the state board, which examines basic and clinical sciences, including x-ray procedures and interpretation.

PARAPROFESSIONAL RADIOLOGICAL TECHNOLOGISTS

It became apparent that chiropractors were in need of assistance in spending the needed time and care for producing quality radiographs of patients. To free up this time that could be spent for treating patients, P.A. Remier devised and started an x-ray course to train technologists in the later part of the 1930s or early 1940s and continued until the early 1960s. This was a program specializing in x-ray, as well as performing instrumentation (neurocalometer), which lasted 4 months. It trained students in all radiographic procedures of the skeletal system as well as in noninvasive contrast media techniques such as that for the gastrointestinal tract, which was performed most often without the aid of fluoroscopy. Upon completion, and passing examinations, the individuals were granted a certificate titling them as "chiropractic technologists."

In addition to functioning as clinical radiographers in private offices, graduate chiropractic technologists were able to work in chiropractic colleges teaching x-ray positioning. One such individual was Wilma Schroeder, who functioned in this capacity at Palmer College from the day of her graduation in the mid-1940s to 1982. In her earlier years, before 1961, she was involved in performing many of the radiographic procedures on patients in the Clearview Sanitarium as well as in the B.J. Palmer Chiropractic Clinic. In this capacity she reminisced over the many contrast media procedures, including barium enemas, that were ordered by many of the doctors on staff, including Lyle Sherman, whose name now graces one of the chiropractic institutions known for its conservative philosophy.

In 1967 the Remier course had ended. However, Palmer College received a federal grant under the Manpower Development Training Act to be used in the establishment of a chiropractic assistant's course under the direction of Roy Hildebrandt. As other chiropractic assistant courses sprung up throughout the various chiropractic colleges, the emphasis was placed on other office procedures, including clerical activities. Eventually, many of the courses began to institute radiological technology, but with quite diverse standards.

For years the American Registry of Radiologic Technology (ARRT) would not renew the Radiologic Technologist (RT) status for those medically trained technologists who worked for a chiropractor. Nor would they renew membership in the organization if the ARRT member became a chiropractor. In 1976 a member of the ARRT, Stephanie Bohnsack-Canterbury, the first full-time radiological technologist at Palmer College, asked to have the credentials of DACBR-certified radiologists in chiropractic accepted for annual renewal. After review of the credentials this request was eventually approved. She then with the urging and support of her department head, Leon Coehlo, D.C., asked that the doctor of chiropractic degree be accepted just as the M.D. and D.O. degree had been. After consideration of the curriculum containing the hours of education devoted to radiology, this request was granted as well.

Today, the American Chiropractic Registry of Radiologic Technologists (ACRRT) has filled the need for the limited radiological assistant for chiropractic offices. This organization is largely a result of the efforts of Edward Maurer of Michigan, who instituted and developed the commission on education of the ACRRT, a board made up of diplomates of the American Chiropractic Board of Radiology and of members from the ARRT, the medically sanctioned organization of radiographers. The ACRRT was established in 1982 and probably is the only paraprofessional group in chiropractic to have state as well as professional recognition. It was initially organized in response to a federal dictate that standardization of education and credentialing be undertaken for those non-physician users of ionizing radiation, and it serves the need for standardization of education in all chiropractic assistance programs using x-ray. The guidelines call for a minimum of 300 hours of education experience provided through an accredited chiropractic college; to date, 28 states accept the ACRRT status in lieu of state examinations. Currently 10 states have no existing regulation for non-physician generated radiography, and 12 have preexisting boards that have not been challenged for reciprocity.

With the myriad of chiropractic techniques for treating the patient, and with many of these techniques having variations in x-ray work, a patient will find a wide variety of x-ray procedures in the chiropractic office. Radiographs may be taken with the patient standing, sitting, or lying on a table. There may or may not be stabilizing devices used, and, of course, different measuring devices for the films may also be used. The patient should know, however, that the doctor of chiropractic has been trained in safe and effective radiographic procedures in the accredited colleges, with many more hours of education in x-ray protection, technology, and interpretation than the medical doctor. The radiographic education in colleges today includes somewhere between 400 to 500 classroom hours. The radiologists in chiropractic often will be called upon to render expert opinions on many cases, and in a growing number of offices, radiographic studies are evaluated to get the most information possible from the film.

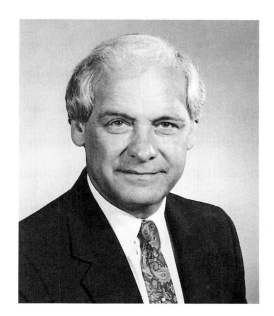

Edward Maurer, author of Practical Applied Roentgenology, *1983, was largely responsible for the organization of the American Chiropractic Registry of Radiologic Technologists.*

Courtesy Edward Maurer, Kalamazoo, Michigan.

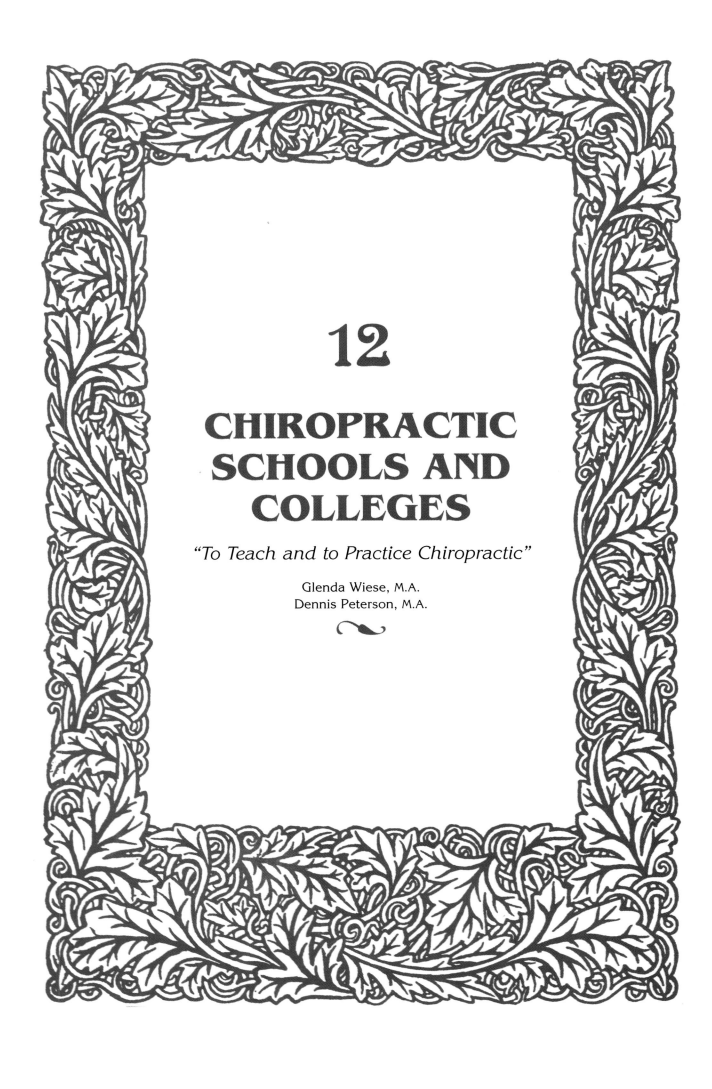

12

CHIROPRACTIC SCHOOLS AND COLLEGES

"To Teach and to Practice Chiropractic"

Glenda Wiese, M.A.
Dennis Peterson, M.A.

Daniel David Palmer's early life has been outlined and described in many books and articles. It is generally thought he was a man who, not unlike many men and women of the late nineteenth century, was a gifted and profoundly driven individualist. As he had done throughout his life, D.D., who was perpetually curious, studied continously. He read the leading medical books, newspapers, and periodicals of his day, and he traveled throughout the whole of the Upper Mississippi River Valley.

It is from this industriousness that the story behind D.D.'s leap from magnetic healing to a new art, chiropractic, is woven. From 1885 on, when D.D. began his magnetic healing practice, he prospered at helping "sick people get well." Accompanying his magnetic healing practice, D.D. also established an infirmary and boarding house, which eventually occupied the entire fourth floor of the downtown Davenport Ryan Building.

The story is well known within the profession about how D.D. came to perform the first chiropractic adjustment on September 18, 1895, on Harvey Lillard. Following his success, D.D. continued to develop chiropractic in his magnetic healing office, using his new found healing art on his magnetic healing patients when he thought appropriate. He was reluctant to openly share his new discovery with others. Though he shared his thoughts with a few close friends, he kept his notes and discovery to himself. It was not until a near escape from death in a railway accident near Clinton, Iowa, in 1897, that D.D. decided to teach chiropractic even though he had not finished formulating his theory.

As was still the customary mode of professional training at the end of the nineteenth century, D.D. at first wanted only two students at a time to "read" with him and learn chiropractic. LeRoy Baker of Fulton, Illinois, was his first student in his offices in the Ryan Building on Davenport's riverfront, and in fact, treated D.D. for the injuries suffered in the railway accident. However, Baker never completed the course.

In 1897 D.D. reorganized his infirmary and was legally incorporated as the Palmer School and Cure. In January 1898, William A. Seeley became the first full-fledged student. Later, A.P. Davis, an M.D. and an osteopath, enrolled. The tuition was $500, and the course of instruction was limited to 3 weeks of training. By 1902, D.D. had renamed his school as the Palmer Infirmary and Chiropractic Institute and had graduated 15 students as Doctors of Chiropractic. Among those early graduates was D.D.'s son, Bartlett Joshua, or B.J., as he preferred to be known.

Late in 1902, D.D. received an urgent messsage from the family of Tom Storey, an early graduate. D.D. went to California, found Storey, and stayed to start a school in Santa Barbara. Oakley Smith and Minora Paxson, two early graduates, then traveled out to California and were the faculty of the Santa Barbara School of Chiropractic. B.J. had stayed behind

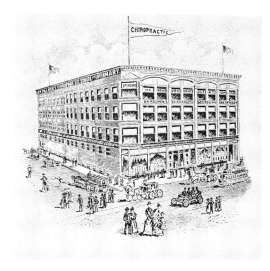

This rendering of the Ryan Building was commissioned by the Palmers. Notice the chiropractic flag, undoubtedly the artist's addition.

Courtesy Palmer College of Chiropractic Archives, Davenport, Ia.

in Davenport to manage the infirmary. When D.D. returned to Davenport in late 1903, he and B.J. established an equal partnership, which would continue until May 1906.

In 1905 the Palmer School moved from the downtown riverfront Ryan Building location to atop residential Brady Street Hill, 828 Brady Street. B.J. and his bride, the former Mabel Heath of nearby Milan, Illinois, lived in the building, which served as both a classroom and boarding house. D.D. and his wife lived nearby on Perry Street, then called Pershing Avenue.

In October 1905, D.D. was indicted for practicing medicine without a license by the Scott County District Attorney's Office, to which he pled not guilty. While D.D. had been working as a magnetic healer, he had irregularly published a newspaper-sized promotional piece called *The Magnetic*. After his work with Harvey Lillard, he changed the name of this journal, which contained numerous testimonials, to *The Chiropractic,* and eventually, in 1904, began publishing a testimonial journal called *The Chiropractor.*

The prosecution used the statements professing to cure in *The Chiropractor* as evidence that Palmer was guilty of practicing medicine without a license. In March 1906 D.D. was tried and found guilty of practicing medicine without a license. Palmer refused to pay the $350 fine and was sentenced to 105 days in the Scott County jail.

On April 21, 1906, after 23 days in jail, the 60-year-old D.D. relented and paid his $350 fine. Then on April 30, 1906, B.J. and D.D. signed an agreement whereby B.J. purchased D.D.'s half of the school for $2196.79. ⌒

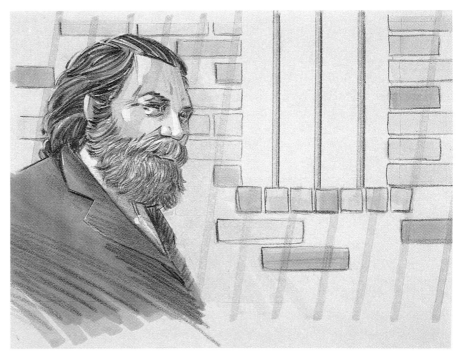

D.D. was jailed in 1906 for practicing medicine without a license.
Courtesy Palmer College of Chiropractic Archives, Davenport, Iowa.

SCHOOL PROLIFERATION

Chiropractic education during the years 1906 to 1924 saw an explosion in the number of chiropractic schools and their student populations. As had been the healing arts custom, when a student graduated from the Palmer Infirmary, D.D. issued a diploma declaring that the holder was competent to both "Practice and Teach Chiropractic." As a result, the founder's school in Davenport soon was to have numerous rivals.

The number of schools increased from 17 in 1906 to 64 in 1924. Although figures are not available for total student enrollment, the enrollment at the PSC increased from eight in 1906 to almost 3000 in 1924. The standard course increased from 3 months to 18 months during this same period, and an effort was made by the International Association of Chiropractic Schools and Colleges to discuss standardization, curriculum, and other educational policies.

One of the earliest rival schools was the American School of Chiropractic in Cedar Rapids, Iowa. It was founded in 1903 by Solon Langworthy, a 1901 graduate of D.D.'s school. Two other early Palmer graduates, Oakley Smith and Minora Paxson, joined him as faculty in 1903, soon after their return from California and D.D. Palmer's Santa Barbara School.

About the time D.D. was leaving Davenport, Willard Carver was graduating from the Parker School of Chiropractic in Ottumwa, Iowa, the hometown of D.D. Palmer's magnetic cure mentor Paul Castor. Carver, who had been the family attorney for D.D., joined forces with another Parker graduate to form the Carver-Denny Chiropractic College and Sanitarium in Oklahoma City. He went on to create three other chiropractic schools. Carver published a journal, the *Chiropractic Record,* and authored several textbooks.

When D.D. left Davenport in May 1906, he went to Oklahoma City, where he soon established a partnership with Alva Gregory, a recent Carver graduate. The partnership lasted less than a year. D.D. was soon conducting his own separate institution in Oklahoma City, the D.D. Palmer School of Chiropractic. Sometime in 1908 D.D. went to Portland and

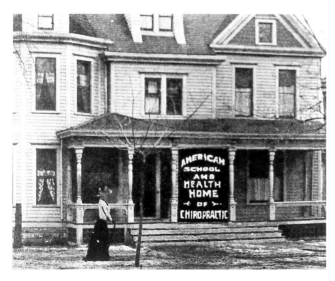

Solon Langworthy's American School of Chiropractic in Cedar Rapids, Iowa, circa 1903 was the first serious competitor to the Palmer School.

Courtesy Palmer College of Chiropractic Archives, Davenport, Iowa.

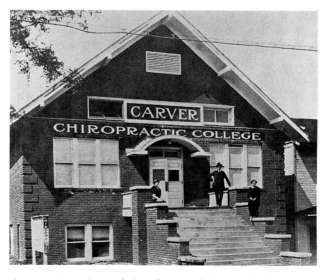

An exterior view of the Carver College of Chiropractic, Oklahoma City, Oklahoma, circa 1921.

Courtesy Palmer College of Chiropractic Archives, Davenport, Iowa.

started another chiropractic school with one of his former students. D.D.'s association with the school in Portland did not last long, and he began traveling along the West Coast working on compiling his notes, correspondence, and criticisms into his 1910 textbook, *The Chiropractor's Adjustor.*

In 1906 John Howard, a student at the Palmer School of Chiropractic, or the "Fountainhead" as B.J. proclaimed, along with a number of other Palmer faculty and students, started the National School of Chiropractic in the same Ryan Building at 2nd and Brady in downtown Davenport that had housed D.D.'s offices for some 15 years. The National School moved to a downtown Chicago location in 1908, becoming well established in the Chicago area and even developing an informal clinical arrangement with Cook County Hospital that was to last for several years.

During the decade following his father's death, B.J. Palmer was the undisputed leader of the profession. From its humble beginnings at 828 Brady Street, where B.J. and Mabel cooked and cleaned for boarding students as well as taught, the Palmer campus expanded rapidly. The D.D. Palmer Memorial Classroom Building was built in 1916; the Administration Building and the B.J. Palmer Classroom Building soon followed in 1920 and 1921, respectively. The school population had grown from 400 in 1911 to a peak of 3000 in 1923. B.J. was a leader in the use of Roentgen's x-ray in chiropractic, introducing an x-ray lab at the PSC in 1910.

B.J.'s initial osteological collection was purchased from D.D., and then he expanded it. The osteological collection was praised by an Ameri-

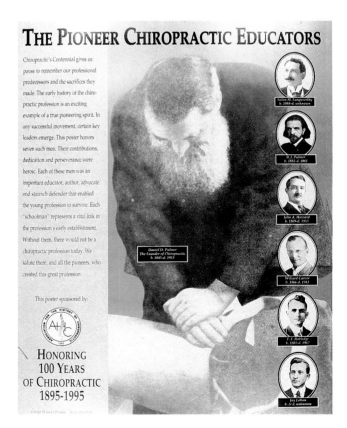

A poster honoring the pioneer chiropractic educators.

Courtesy *Association for the History of Chiropractic,* Davenport, Iowa.

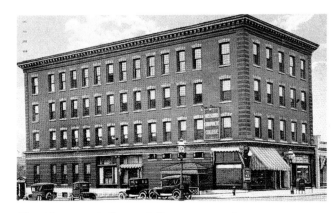

The Missouri College of Chiropractic, St. Louis, Missouri, circa 1922.

Courtesy Palmer College of Chiropractic Archives, Davenport, Iowa.

can Medical Association inspection team as being "the best collection of human spines in existence." The Universal Chiropractors Association (UCA), led by B.J., with the guidance of attorney Tom Morris, was defending chiropractors all across the country against charges of practicing medicine without a license, and B.J. was one of its most flamboyant witnesses. His printing presses produced millions of chiropractic pamphlets and tracts every year, and his radio station, WOC, was selling the message of chiropractic to the whole country.

In 1910 Joy Loban, a faculty member at the Palmer School of Chiropractic, started Universal Chiropractic College at 608 Brady Street, just three blocks down Brady Street Hill from the Palmer School. The Universal College stayed in Davenport for 8 years, moving in 1918 to Pittsburgh.

In 1922 Carl S. Cleveland, Sr., a PSC graduate, founded the Central Chiropractic College in Kansas City, Missouri. Two years later he changed the name to the Cleveland Chiropractic College. In 1951, he acquired the Ratledge Chiropractic College of Los Angeles and renamed it Cleveland Chiropractic College—Los Angeles.

In 1926 four PSC faculty resigned and started a school in Indianapolis, Indiana—the Lincoln Chiropractic College. Lincoln Chiropractic College was prominent in the movement toward the 4-year curriculum. It inherited the charter of Universal Chiropractic College in 1944. Lincoln itself was eventually absorbed by National College of Chiropractic in 1969.

A decline in the number of schools followed the economic depression. The number of chiropractic schools dropped from 82 in 1925 to 69 in 1927 to 59 in 1932. Enrollment fell from over 3000 in 1925 to 1400 in 1932.

THE REFORM AND EXPANSION OF CHIROPRACTIC EDUCATION

The Council on Medical Education and Hospitals of the American Medical Association issued a very critical report of the chiropractic educational system in 1927. The medical educational community had been struggling successfully to improve its own standards and was highly critical of the lack of standards in chiropractic. In 1910 the Council on Medical Education had issued the *Flexner Report,* which was critical of medical education at that time. The *Flexner Report* became an invaluable aid in the fight to raise the educational level in America's medical schools.

During the 1930s a similar effort was made by the National Chiropractic Association (NCA) to raise the educational standards of the profession. In 1935 the Committee on Educational Standards was created. In 1947 the Council on Chiropractic Education (CCE) was created. During the period 1941 to 1960, the committee, under the leadership of John Nugent, worked to strengthen chiropractic education. Many of the weaker institutions were closed, and by 1960, the number of chiropractic schools had decreased to 22.

With the influx of the baby boomer generation, the 1960s saw the beginnings of important advances in profession-wide standards. The National Board of Chiropractic Examiners was formed in 1962, and the first exams were held in 1965. The CCE was incorporated as an autonomous organization separate from the American Chiropractic Association in 1971 and was officially recognized by the United States Office of Education in 1974.

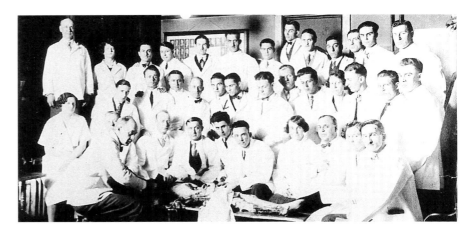

Dissection Lab at the Missouri College of Chiropractic, St. Louis, Missouri, circa 1920.
Courtesy Logan College of Chiropractic Archives, Chesterfield, Missouri.

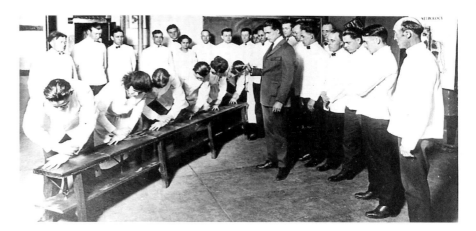

A technique class at Central States Chiropractic College, Indianapolis, Indiana, circa 1925.
Courtesy Palmer College of Chiropractic Archives, Daventport, Iowa.

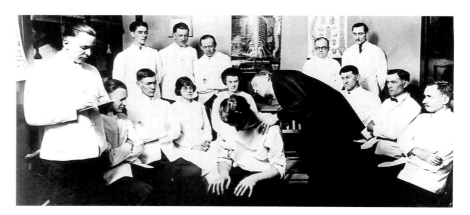

A technique class at Bebout Chiropractic College in Indianapolis, Indiana, circa 1940.
Courtesy Russell Gibbons, Pittsburgh, Pennsylvania.

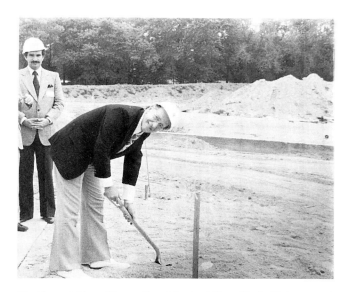

Dr. Ernest Napolitano, President of New York Chiropractic College, breaking ground at the Old Brookville, Long Island campus in the 1970s.
Courtesy New York Chiropractic College, Seneca Falls, New York.

Partially as a result of the profession's increasing educational standards, and partially because of the maturation of the first of the baby boomers, the early 1970s saw increasing enrollments in all the chiropractic colleges. By 1975 there were 5000 students, by 1978 enrollment stood at 8570, and today there are over 9880 students.

During the 1970s physical expansion on almost every campus was taking place. Palmer College built the Alumni Auditorium and the David D. Palmer Library Building. National College moved from its inner-city site to its suburban Lombard location and built a student center, on-campus housing, and a 48-bed patient and research center. The Columbia Institute acquired a new campus adjacent to the New York Institute of Technology and gained affiliation with the State University of New York system. Texas Chiropractic College acquired a new location in Pasadena and built several buildings. Logan College moved to a spacious suburban campus, as did Northwestern and Western States. Los Angeles College built a new classroom building. Canadian Memorial Chiropractic College added a new building and a satellite clinic.

CHIROPRACTIC COLLEGES OF TODAY

With the continuation and strengthening of several of chiropractic's long-standing college programs, the 1970s also saw the birth of several new colleges. Life Chiropractic College started classes during 1975 in Marietta, Georgia. Pacific States College of Chiropractic began classes in 1978, then became Life Chiropractic College—West in San Lorenzo, California. Northern California College of Chiropractic also began in 1978 and then during 1980 became Palmer College of Chiropractic—West in San Jose, California. Pasadena College of Chiropractic began classes in 1977, then rechartered to become Southern California College of Chiropractic.

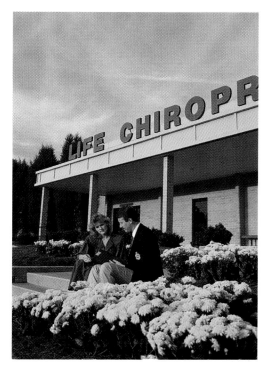

An exterior view of one of the first buildings on the Life Chiropractic College Campus, which was founded in 1975.
Courtesy Life of Chiropractic College, Marietta, Georgia.

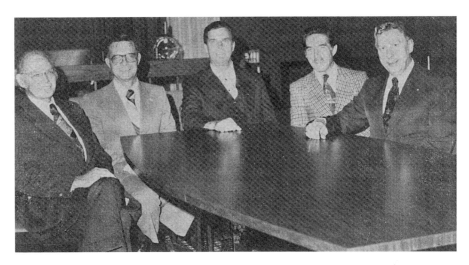

In a 1-year span, circa 1977, new people took the helm at five chiropractic colleges. They were (left to right) *Dr. H. W. Quigley, Los Angeles College of Chiropractic; J. B. Barfoot, Texas Chiropractic College; Galen Price, Palmer College of Chiropractic; Donald Sutherland, Canadian Memorial Chiropractic College; and R. H. Timmons, Western States Chiropractic College.*

Sherman College of Straight Chiropractic was chartered in 1977 in Spartanburg, South Carolina. ADIO Institute of Straight Chiropractic was charted in 1977, and later became Pennsylvania School of Straight Chiropractic.

During the 1980s, Parker College of Chiropractic in Irvine, Texas, was the only new North American college founded. Now in the 1990s two North American chiropractic colleges are beginning classes. In 1991, the University of Bridgeport, Bridgeport Connecticut, enrolled its first students in its School of Chiropractic. Then, after over a decade of study and consideration, a second Canadian college opened its program at the Universite du Quebec á Trois Riviers.

Worldwide, several chiropractic colleges are currently teaching students to become Doctors of Chiropractic. The Anglo-European College of Chiropractic in Bournemouth, England was established in 1965. The

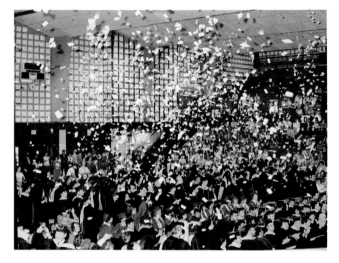

Student clinic cards are tossed into the air as these students are pronounced "Doctors of Chiropractic" at a Palmer College graduation ceremony, circa 1990.
Courtesy Palmer College of Chiropractic, Davenport, Iowa.

Institute of Chiropractic in Paris, France, began classes in 1983. The Philip Institute of Technology—School of Chiropractic and Osteopathy in Bundoora, Victoria, Australia began classes in 1981. The Macquarie University—Centre for Chiropractic and Osteopathy in Summerhill, New South Wales, Australia, absorbed the Sydney College of Chiropractic in 1989.

There are also new programs being planned and established worldwide. Although Japan has yet to legislate a national jurisdiction and accreditation act primarily because of its strong natural healing arts heritage and traditions, two schools have been established. The Chukyo School of Chiropractic in Nagoya, Japan, and the Japan Chiropractic College in Tokyo. At the Odense University, Odense, Denmark, a prechiropractic curriculum has been established for Scandinavian students. The implementation of a chiropractic clincial curriculum for the Scandinavian countries is being planned. At the Technikon Natal in Durban, South Africa, a chiropractic clinical curriculum is being implemented beginning in 1994.

With its centennial approaching, all the struggles and hardships many of the colleges have had to endure over the past 90 years seem to have put the surviving educational institutions on as strong a footing as they ever have been. With the merger of several programs and the establishment of 10 others since the 1970s, chiropractic education and research is entering a new era of intraprofessional cooperation that is bound to enhance its promising future.

Outlined below are brief descriptions of these programs that will be preparing for the profession's second century of dedication to health care service and "helping sick people get well."

Cleveland Chiropractic College—Kansas City

Cleveland Chiropractic College—Kansas City was founded in 1922 as Central Chiropractic College in Kansas City, Missouri, by Dr. C.S. Cleveland, Sr., Dr. Ruth Rose Ashworth Cleveland, and Dr. Perl B. Griffen. On December 23, 1922, the college was chartered as the first non-profit college of chiropractic. The college began classes with three students in a residence located at 436 Prospect in the northeast section of Kansas City. In 1924 the college was renamed Cleveland Chiropractic College.

The 27-month curriculum consisted of 3 academic years of 9 months each, and was one of the first to include x-ray and human dissection, considered advanced offerings for the time. Early college promotional materials, circa 1923, announced the college offering a D.C. degree, a Ph.C., and a Master of Spinography certificate for x-ray coursework. The faculty and subject areas in 1923 included the following: C.S. Cleveland, Sr., D.C., symptomatology, orthopedy and chiropractic analysis; Perl B. Griffen, D.C., physiology, histology, and technique; Ruth R. Cleveland, D.C., anatomy, gynecology, palpation, and nerve tracing; and R.C. Jackson, D.C., x-ray and spinography.

Tuition costs in 1923 were $360 for the day course, $450 for the evening course, and $50 for spinography (the study of spinal x-rays). A husband and wife could complete coursework for $100 in addition to the single tuition rate. Required textbooks, written by such chiropractic educators as Palmer, Vedder, Firth, Craven and Burick, cost a total of $40 to $60.

The early years at Cleveland Chiropractic College—Kansas City were

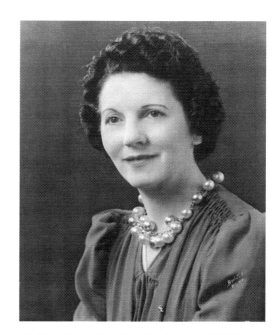

Ruth Ashworth Cleveland, circa 1923, and her husband Carl started the Cleveland Chiropractic College.

Courtesy Cleveland Chiropractic College—Kansas City, Missouri.

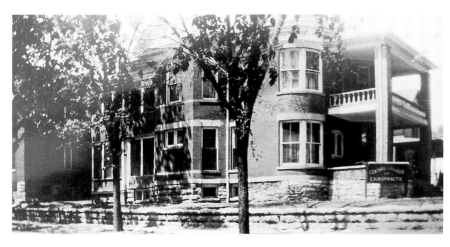

Central College of Chiropractic was renamed Cleveland Chiropractic College in 1924.
Courtesy Cleveland Chiropractic College—Kansas City, Missouri.

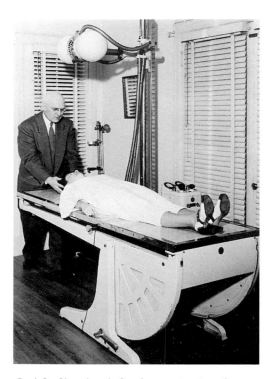

Carl S. Cleveland, Sr. demonstrating the use of an x-ray machine.
Courtesy Cleveland Chiropractic College—Kansas City, Missouri.

marked by the struggle for recognition and licensure of the chiropractic profession. At that time, chiropractors were arrested and jailed based on laws in the state of Missouri that interpreted the practice of chiropractic as the practice of medicine without a license.

Dr. C.S. Cleveland, Sr., a 1917 graduate of Palmer, was a chiropractic philosopher, educator, and political activist who created public awareness and political advocacy by bringing attention to the plight of jailed chiropractors. Dr. Cleveland, Sr., raised monies for the jail fund to provide food for the families of such chiropractors during their time of incarceration, provided a portable adjusting table in the chiropractor's jail cell so patients could continue to receive care, and hired a brass band to play outside the jail to bring attention to the persecution of doctors of chiropractic. Through his mobilization of patients and chiropractors statewide, Dr. Cleveland, Sr., lobbied aggressively for the Chiropractic Practice Act, which was signed by Missouri Governor Sam A. Baker on March 14, 1927.

Cleveland Chiropractic College—Kansas City survived the depression, and as the need grew to expand the college, a new site was established at 37th and Troost in 1929. During the almost 50-year span that the college was located there, several nearby buildings were purchased and renovated to create a multibuilding campus.

Cleveland Chiropractic College—Kansas City grew steadily until World War II, when the majority of its students were drafted. Instructors were laid off as enrollment dropped. At one point Dr. Cleveland, Jr., was teaching every class, day and night, and treating approximately 18 patients a day in the clinic.

Following the war, the advent of the G.I. Bill bolstered enrollment. In the 1940s the curriculum was expanded from the 27-month program to an optional 36-month program, and in 1946 Cleveland Chiropractic College—Kansas City presented its first 36-month diploma. By 1951 the 36-month course was standard.

By the early 1970s the need for additional space was evident, and the Board of Trustees approved the purchase of property at 6401 Rockhill Road, the present location of the campus. The college has since purchased additional buildings and land to expand these facilities.

Today's student population at Cleveland Chiropractic College—Kansas City ensures a healthy mix of ideas and cultural points of view. Cur-

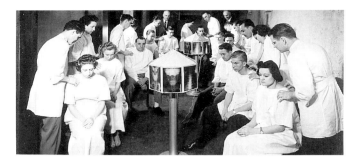 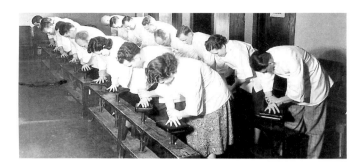

A palpation class (left) and adjusting class (right) at Cleveland Chiropractic College in the mid-1940s.

Courtesy Cleveland Chiropractic College, Kansas City, Missouri.

rent students range in age from 20 to 60, and many are career changers. Approximately 30% are women, and many are from foreign countries.

Cleveland Chiropractic College—Kansas City offers a residency program in Chiropractic Radiology to qualified graduates or to persons nearing completion of degree programs at other accredited chiropractic colleges. The radiology program requires a minimum of 36 months full-time residency.

Students benefit from the college's affiliation with the neighboring University of Missouri-Kansas City. A state-of-the-art recreation center is open to all Cleveland students, as are a variety of intramural and individual sports. Other services include child care and counseling.

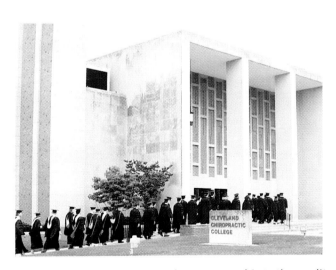

Faculty and graduating students proceed into the auditorium for commencement on the Rockhill Road campus of Cleveland Chiropractic College—Kansas City, circa 1991.

Courtesy Cleveland Chiropractic College—Kansas City, Missouri.

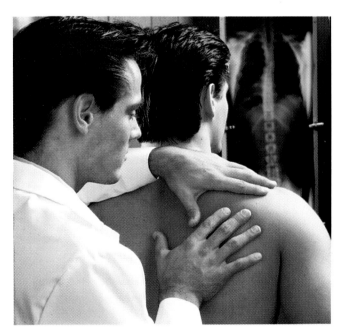

The correlation between motion palpation and x-ray analysis is a key component of chiropractic education at Cleveland Chiropractic College—Kansas City.

Courtesy Cleveland Chiropractic College—Kansas City, Missouri.

Cleveland Chiropractic College—Los Angeles

Cleveland Chiropractic College—Los Angeles was founded by Dr. Tullius de Florence Ratledge, 1881 to 1967, and traces its origins to the Ratledge system of chiropractic schools, first established in Guthrie, Oklahoma, in 1908, with colleges located in Arkansas City, Kansas, and in the Kansas state capital of Topeka. The fourth in the system of schools, later to become Cleveland Chiropractic College—Los Angeles, was opened in September 1911 in Los Angeles.

Dr. Ratledge, a 1908 graduate of the Carver/Denny College of Chiropractic in Oklahoma and an early pioneer and political activist, first introduced a chiropractic bill in the California legislature in 1912. Dr. Ratledge's visible and open advocacy of chiropractic in the unlicensed state caught the attention of medical authorities. "I was soon visited by representatives of official medicine in California and told to remove my signs and cease the 'practice of medicine' or face arrest," Dr. Ratledge recalled in 1953. In 1914 Dr. Ratledge was arrested, convicted, and sentenced to serve 90 days in Los Angeles County Jail for "practicing medicine without a license." Dr. Ratledge's incarceration was proudly worn as a badge of courage throughout the rest of his career, and he encouraged other D.C.'s not to pay fines but to serve their jail terms in order to generate public sympathy for the cause of chiropractic licensure in the state of California.

Dr. Ratledge repeatedly introduced bills in the legislature each year until 1922. Despite significant medical opposition, the voters of California approved the chiropractic bill on Nov. 7, 1922. The first Board of Chiropractic Examiners was appointed in early 1923, and the first chiropractic licenses were issued. Throughout its first 4 decades of operation, the Los Angeles branch of the Ratledge system offered a 24-month course of study in those basic and clinical subjects that Dr. Ratledge considered essential to chiropractic practice. The location of the Los Angeles school changed a number of times during its first 40 years, including once to the 2415 Southwestern Avenue facility, former residence of prize-fighter Jack Dempsey.

Dr. Ratledge offered to sell his for-profit school to his close friend and colleague, Dr. C.S. Cleveland, Sr., for the sum of $40,000. Dr. Cleveland, Sr., assumed leadership of the one-building school and its 17 students in 1950. Dr. Cleveland, Sr., extended the curriculum to a 4000-hour, 36-month program, added an x-ray machine and diagnostic equipment, and

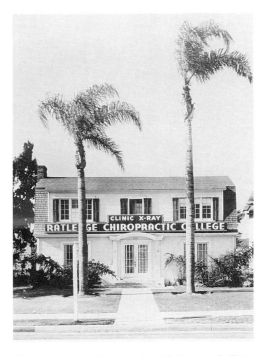

The campus of Ratledge College of Chiropractic, circa 1950.

Courtesy Cleveland Chiropractic College—Los Angeles, California.

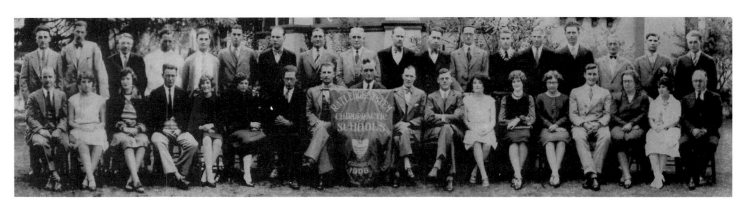

An early class of the Ratledge College of Chiropractic.

Courtesy Cleveland Chiropractic College—Los Angeles, California.

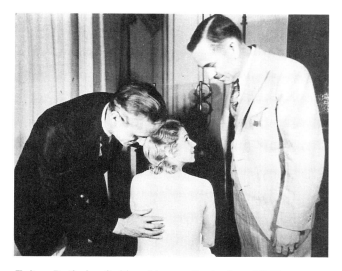

Tulius Ratledge (left) *with a patient, circa 1950.*
Courtesy Cleveland Chiropractic College—Los Angeles, California.

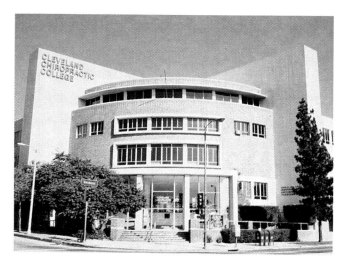

An exterior view of the Cleveland - Los Angeles campus, circa 1990.
Courtesy Cleveland Chiropractic College—Los Angeles, California.

expanded the curriculum to include symptomatology and diagnostic coursework. The college was rechartered as Cleveland Chiropractic College of Los Angeles and later obtained non-profit status. The facility was relocated to its present site at 590 North Vermont in 1976, at the prominent intersection of Vermont Avenue and the Hollywood Freeway in central Los Angeles.

The present student body at Cleveland Chiropractic College—Los Angeles strongly reflects the multiculturalism of Southern California, representing Armenia, Australia, Brazil, Cambodia, Canada, China, Colombia, Cuba, Denmark, Ecuador, Egypt, Mexico, Morocco, Nicaragua, Peru, Philippines, Russia, South Korea, Sweden, Switzerland, Taiwan, Turkey, Vietnam, and the former Yugoslavia. The student body includes both the young (early twenties) and the mature (late fifties), and 36% are women.

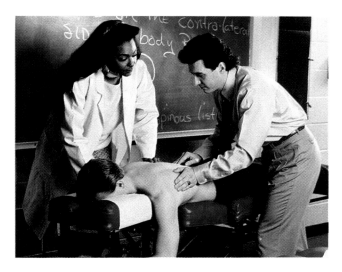

A strong emphasis is placed on personalized instruction in chiropractic technique at Cleveland Chiropractic College—Los Angeles.
Courtesy Cleveland Chiropractic College—Los Angeles, California.

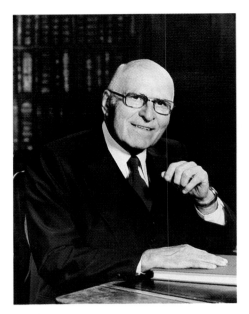 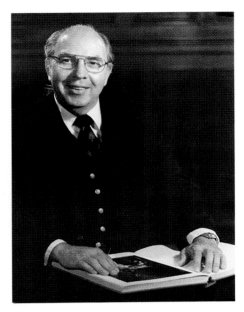 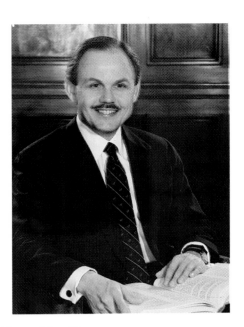

Three generations of the Cleveland family have served as President of the Cleveland Colleges. Left to right, *Carl Cleveland, Sr., Carl Cleveland, Jr., and Carl Cleveland III.*
Courtesy Cleveland Chiropractic College—Los Angeles, California.

The role of the doctor of chiropractic as an integral member of the health care system is evolving. Today's Cleveland students learn the skills necessary to consult with other providers in an interdisciplinary role. Through an affiliation agreement with Coast Plaza Doctors' Hospital, clinic interns learn hospital protocols by rotating through various departments.

Three generations of the Cleveland family have now served as president of Cleveland College: Dr. C.S. Cleveland, Sr., was president of Cleveland Chiropractic College—Kansas City from 1922 to 1967 and president of Cleveland Chiropractic College—Los Angeles from 1950 to 1982. The retirement of Dr. Cleveland, Sr., in 1982 completed his 60-year tenure as a chiropractic college president. Dr. Carl S. Cleveland, Jr., was president of Cleveland Chiropractic College—Kansas City (1967 to 1981) and Cleveland Chiropractic College—Los Angeles (1982 to 1992). He now serves as chancellor of the multicampus system. Dr. Carl S. Cleveland, III, became president of Cleveland Chiropractic College—Kansas City in 1982 and now serves as president of the multicampus system.

Life College

Life Chiropractic College, later renamed *Life College* to reflect the broader scope of its mission, was founded in 1974 by Drs. Sid and Nell Williams. With 600 staff and faculty members to serve its 3600 students, the college is the largest of its kind in the world and is located in Marietta, Georgia, a northern suburb of Atlanta. The campus has 15 buildings located on 125 acres, including a 5.5-mile running trail. With access to two city parks and additional acreage, Life College has nearly 200 acres to accommodate its public and student needs.

Accredited by the Council on Chiropractic Education (an agency recognized by the U.S. Department of Education) and the Southern Association of Colleges and Schools, Life College continues to place an em-

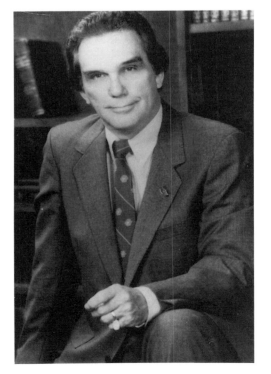

Dr. Sid Williams, President and founder of Life Chiropractic College.
Courtesy Life Chiropractic College, Marietta, Georgia.

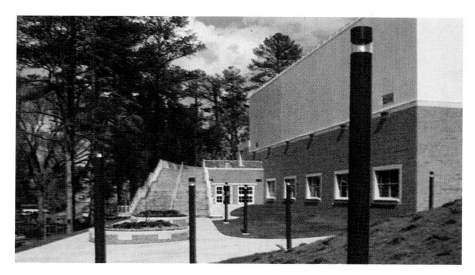

The Sports Health Sciences Center on the Life campus, circa 1992.
Courtesy Life Chiropractic College, Marietta, Georgia.

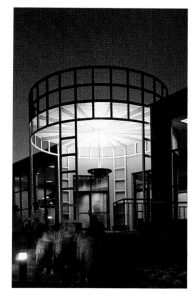

An exterior view at night of the Nell Williams Learning Resource Center, named after Dr. Nell Williams, wife and co-founder of Life College.
Courtesy Life Chiropractic College, Marietta, Georgia.

phasis on the philosophy of the science of chiropractic, which includes the biological, clinical, and academic sciences; special diagnostic skills; and various techniques for spinal subluxation correction. Supplemental to a firm foundation in traditional basic academic and clinical training, Life College places a heavy emphasis on "hands-on" training with patients. In addition to its clinic on campus, major out-patient clinics for student practicums are located in downtown Atlanta and northern Marietta.

In addition to its doctor of chiropractic degree, Life College also offers a master's degree in sports health science, with plans for other degrees in such specialities as diagnostic imaging, neurology, and orthopedics. The undergraduate program offers a degree in nutrition for chiropractic sciences; dietetics, leading to a dietician's certificate; a chiropractic technicians program, leading to a certificate; and a B.B.A. in business administration (with minors in management for coaches and trainers) as well as regular and accelerated preprofessional studies programs to qualify students for entry into chiropractic, medical, dental, and other health-related fields of study. A graduate program offering a Ph.D. in health sciences research now being developed will increase campus research and help to qualify Life College's application for university status within the near future.

A well-rounded school with a host of student activities, Life College has already gained a national and international reputation in sports with its basketball, team which was the runner-up in the NAIA championship playoff; a world-class rugby team; and excellent cross-country track team; and beginning with the 1994 season, a NAIA soccer team.

Life Chiropractic College—West

In 1976, Drs. George Anderson and George Wentland had a vision of establishing a chiropractic college with a sound foundation in chiropractic philosophy. They wanted to provide that education in their home region of northern California, where there were no chiropractic schools at the time.

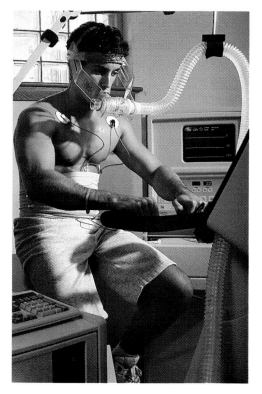

A student in the exercise physiology lab of the Life campus.
Courtesy Life Chiropractic College, Marietta, Georgia.

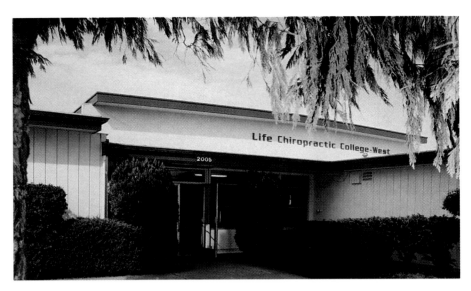

An exterior view of Life Chiropractic College— West, founded in 1976 as Pacific States Chiropractic College and reorganized as Life Chiropractic College—West in 1981.

Courtesy Life Chiropractic College—West, San Lorenzo, California.

The two men opened the doors to their vision two years later in a former elementary school building in San Lorenzo, California, under the name of Pacific States Chiropractic College, today's Life Chiropractic College—West.

During 1976 and 1977, Pacific States began the process of developing an educational institution and preparing the college to receive its first class of students. In April 1978 the charter class of Pacific States began its training, which included then, as it does today, full-spine and upper cervical adjusting methods.

In January 1980 the growing institution moved to a larger facility, another public school building in the same town. But despite the expansion, times were tough for the fledgling college. The effects of a rapidly changing economic situation, combined with other institutional setbacks,

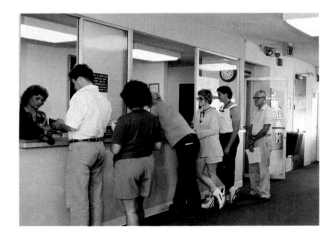

An interior view of the Hayward Public Clinic of Life Chiropractic College West, circa 1990, where interns obtain clinical experience.

Courtesy Life Chiropractic College—West, San Lorenzo, California.

caused the Board of Regents of Pacific States to consider entering a relationship with an established institution in the profession.

In March 1981 through the efforts of Dr. Sid E. Williams, president and founder of Life College, and Drs. Anderson and Wentland, an agreement was reached between Life College (then Life Chiropractic College) in Marietta, Georgia, and Pacific States Chiropractic College.

The college was renamed Life Chiropractic College— West, and shortly thereafter, Dr. Gerard W. Clum was appointed president.

The college has been profoundly influenced by the objectives, dedication, commitment, and enthusiasm that have been the hallmarks of Dr. Williams and the entire Life community, while maintaining the vision of Drs. Anderson and Wentland.

Life—West was granted Recognized Candidate (RCA) status by the Commission on Accreditation (COA) of the Council on Chiropractic Education in February 1983 and became accredited July 24, 1987.

The college continues to grow in the same location today with a current enrollment of 600 full-time students.

Logan College of Chiropractic

Logan College of Chiropractic was founded in 1935 by Hugh B. Logan, D.C., at St. Louis, Missouri. The college was originally named Logan Basic College of Chiropractic, referring to the specific system of body mechanics and adjusting developed by Dr. Logan, which gives particular attention to the sacrum and pelvis and the base of the spine. The Logan basic system of body mechanics was founded upon the principle that the human structure represented an integrated unit. The college was renamed Logan College of Chiropractic in 1964 after a merger with Missouri College of Chiropractice.

Logan College has had a history marked by innovations within the chiropractic profession. It was the first chiropractic college to institute a D.C. degree program consisting of 4 academic years. Throughout its his-

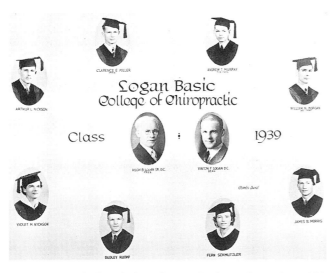

Logan Basic College's first class, which graduated in 1939.
Courtesy Logan College of Chiropractic Archives, Chesterfield, Missouri.

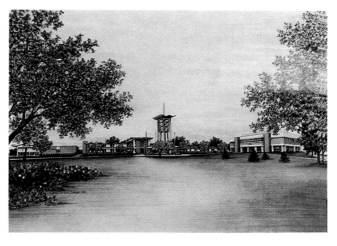

A watercolor sketch of the Logan College Campus, featuring its distinctive campanile.
Courtesy Logan College of Chiropractic Archives, Chesterfield, Missouri.

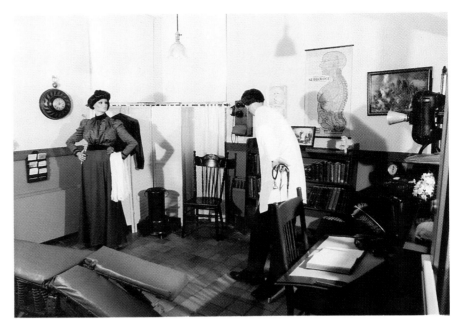

A museum display of an early chiropractor's office, located on the campus of Logan College.

Courtesy Logan College of Chiropractic Archives, Chesterfield, Missouri.

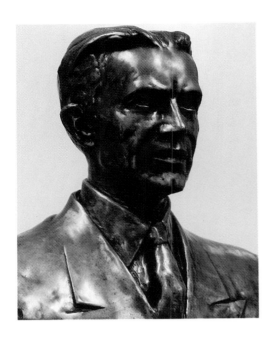

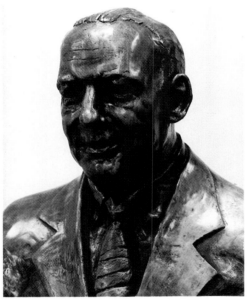

Hugh Logan (top) *was the founder and first president of Logan College. Vinton Logan* (bottom), *his son, was second president of Logan College.*

Courtesy Logan College of Chiropractic Archives, Chesterfield, Missouri.

tory, Logan College has been a strong supporter of standardization of chiropractic education and has played an integral part in the CCE, the accrediting agency for chiropractic colleges.

In 1973 Logan College moved to its current campus, located at Chesterfield, Missouri. This campus is a 103-acre wooded area situated in a growing suburban area of St. Louis. The Chesterfield campus had a considerable expansion of the clinic facilities with the construction of the Dale C. Montgomery Health Center in 1982.

The year 1985 marked the golden anniversary of the founding of the college, as well as a commitment to expansion by constructing the Science, Research, and Ergonomics Center, which was dedicated in 1988. The addition of this building expanded and modernized the research and basic science laboratories and represents a commitment to teaching and research in the area of ergonomics, as it relates to chiropractic.

Chiropractic is uniquely qualified to expand the body of knowledge pertaining to the design of the workplace as it relates to human biomechanics and work habits. The establishment of the ergonomics program at Logan has enabled the college to implement consulting and ergonomic training activities for the prevention of workplace injuries and to work with companies and government agencies in Missouri and elsewhere.

In addition to its on-campus health center, the college also operates satellite health centers located throughout the St. Louis community. Two of the health centers are affiliated with local Salvation Army Facilities and provide health care services to the homeless and other low-income individuals.

It has been the history and goal of Logan College to provide innovative and contemporary education to the chiropractic profession, preparing men and women to fulfill this necessary and unique health care need to society. The celebration of the one-hundredth anniversary of the founding of the chiropractic profession, and the sixtieth anniversary of the founding of Logan College of Chiropractic is an exciting opportunity to continue the tradition of educational and health care excellence.

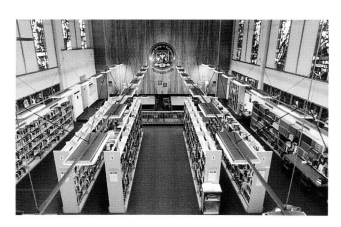

The library at Logan College, which reflects the buildings original use as a chapel.

Courtesy Logan College of Chiropractic Archives, Chesterfield, Missouri.

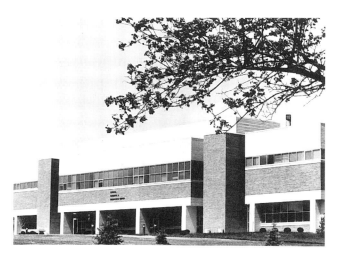

Exterior view of the Science, Ergonomics, and Research center, circa 1990.

Courtesy Logan College of Chiropractic, Chesterfield, Missouri.

Los Angeles College of Chiropractic

A horseless carriage—one of the few—"sped" down mud and brick roads. A pioneer fervor dominated the thinking of progressive leaders. Los Angeles, "The City of Angels," was a bustling city of 319,000 citizens. Movies were in their infancy . . . still silent.

Into this milieu, Dr. Charles Cale and his wife Linnie, committed themselves to educate others and disseminate the knowledge of a little known, yet ancient, healing art—chiropractic. Dr. Cale sought to formalize the training of chiropractic physicians.

By 1911, when modern chiropractic was 16 years into its history, Dr. Cale applied for and received a charter for the Los Angeles College of Chiropractic (LACC). The Cales began the first classes in their home—a course of study 9 months long which included anatomy, chiropractic principles, and technique.

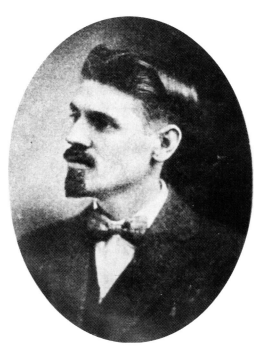

Dr. Charles Wood, president of Eclectic College of Chiropractic, one of the colleges absorbed by the Los Angeles College of Chiropractic.

Courtesy Los Angeles College of Chiropractic, Whittier, California.

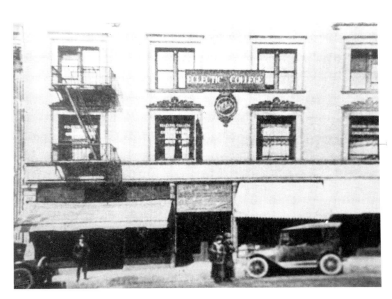

An exterior view of the Eclectic College of Chiropractic, circa 1920.

Courtesy Palmer College of Chiropractic Archives, Davenport, Iowa.

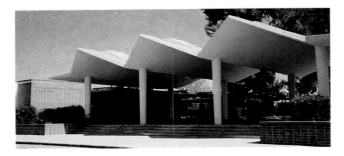

An exterior view of Los Angeles College of Chiropractic's Glendale campus, circa 1975.

Courtesy Los Angeles College of Chiropractic, Whittier, California.

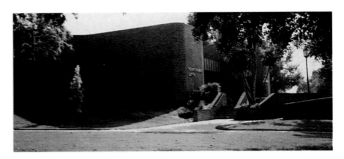

An exterior view of Los Angeles College of Chiropractics Performing Arts Building, 1993.

Courtesy Los Angeles College of Chiropractic, Whittier, California.

Eleven years later, 1922, the college had moved to progressively larger and more modern facilities. The curriculum was now 18 months of study. During this period, the college had absorbed the Eclectic College of Chiropractic, a progressive yet fledgling school with a 5-year history.

The Chiropractic Initiative Act of 1922 provided the mechanism for the college to continue upgrading its offerings and improving its facilities.

The succeeding 28 years were marked with continued curricular improvements and material expansion. In those years, LACC acquired many institutions: Golden State College of Chiropractic; Dr. Cale's second school, the Cale Chiropractic College; the College of Chiropractic Physicians and Surgeons; Southern California College of Chiropractic; Continental Chiropractic College; and the California College of Natural Healing Arts.

Voluntarily over the years, the course of study had extended to 32 months. In the late 1940s a non-profit corporation was organized. The California Chiropractic Educational Foundation (CCEF) acquired several colleges, including the Los Angeles College of Chiropractic. As a holding company, the CCEF created a new chiropractic college, which retained the name of Los Angeles College of Chiropractic.

By 1950 the course of study had expanded to 4 years. The school moved to Glendale that year, consolidating its basic science subjects and chiropractic sciences into one comprehensive curriculum taught in one modern facility.

For over 20 years, Dr. George Haynes provided able leadership for the college. He promoted educational standards for chiropractic education, urged progressive methods of instruction, and expanded the Glendale campus for academic growth.

The Board of Regents, directors of the college, boldly moved the institution in a new direction in the late 1970s. Determined to improve and develop a progressive chiropractic college, they sought professional educational administrators to assure academic planning, facility usage, and economic independence. In 3 short years, the board had succeeded in creating a responsive and responsible institution.

To guarantee continued growth in a high-technology society, to educate health care professionals for the nation's millions, and to provide outstanding leadership for the 1980s, Dr. E. Maylon Drake was appointed President February 1, 1980. His contributions to LACC are measured by improved morale, sound management procedures, and the development of teamwork.

In 1980 the governing Board of Regents expanded the size and composition of its membership, adding four positions, which have been filled by visionary lay professional persons of great experience.

The LACC realized a dream-come-true when it purchased a new 38½ acre campus in November 1981 in Whittier, California. The new site affords the college ample opportunities to increase enrollment, strengthen its academic offerings, and develop new programs for health care professionals and consumers.

National College of Chiropractic

The college was established in 1906 in Davenport, Iowa, as the National School of Chiropractic, a part of the pattern of a growing profession with the need for increased avenues of education. In 1908 the school settled at 1732 West Congress Street, Chicago, across the street from Presbyterian Hospital, where it was incorporated under the laws of the state of Illinois.

In 1920 the student enrollment had increased to such an extent that larger quarters were required. A 5-story stone and brick building was purchased at 20 North Ashland Boulevard. The name was then legally changed to the National College of Chiropractic. To fulfill a need for more extensive clinical experience in all phases of chiropractic practice, Chicago General Health Services was established in 1927 in connection with the college.

In 1941 National College became a non-profit educational and research institution in accord with the corporate laws of Illinois and the requirements of the United States Department of the Treasury governing tax-exempt institutions.

From 1936 to 1965, the professional training program at National College was 4½ academic years. In 1965, the program was expanded to 5 academic years. In 1968 the 2-year professional requirement for admission became effective. Additional qualitative requirements for admission have been adopted from time to time. In 1995 the preprofessional requirement will increase to a minimum of 75 credit hours. In 1997, 90 credit hours will be required, and in 1999 the baccalaureate will be required.

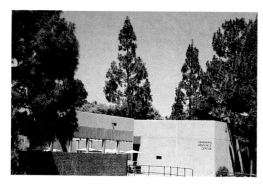

An exterior view of the Learning Resource Center on the Los Angeles College of Chiropractic's Whittier campus, circa 1990.

Courtesy of Los Angeles College of Chiropractic, Whittier, California.

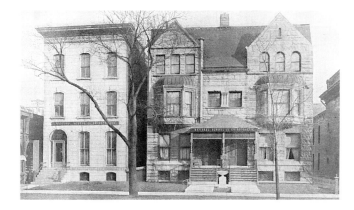

The campus on 20 South Ashland Boulevard, home of the National School of Chiropractic from 1920-1963.

Courtesy National College of Chiropractic, Lombard, Illinois.

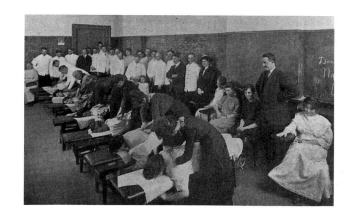

John Howard lecturing before a class at the National School of Chiropractic, circa 1910.

Courtesy Palmer college of Chiropractic Archives, Davenport, Iowa.

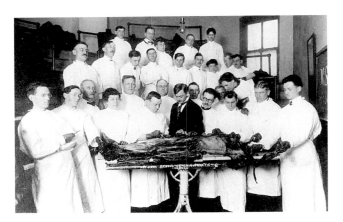

An early dissection class at the National School, circa 1908.

Courtesy National College of Chiropractic, Lombard, Illinois.

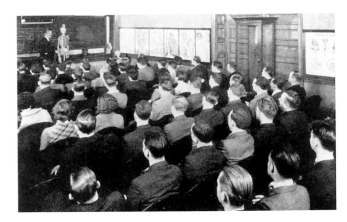

A lecture class at National College of Chiropractic, circa 1930.

Courtesy National College of Chiropractic, Lombard, Illinois.

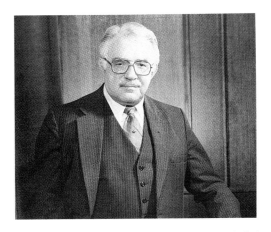

Dr. Joseph Janse, president of National College of Chiropractic from 1945-1983.

Courtesy National College of Chiropractic, Lombard, Illinois.

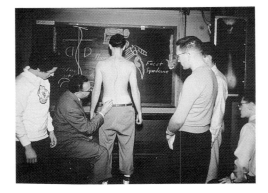

Joe Janse in the classroom at National College, circa 1960.

Courtesy National College of Chiropractic, Lombard, Illinois.

The Office of the Superintendent of Public Instruction of the state of Illinois granted official status to National College as a degree-granting institution in 1966 for both the Bachelor of Science and the Doctor of Chiropractic degrees. The Doctor of Chiropractic program was approved by registration with the State Education Department of the State of New York in 1972. In 1974 the College was recognized as a candidate for accreditation by the North Central Association of Colleges and Secondary Schools and was accredited by North Central in 1981.

The National College of Chiropractic has long been a leader in chiropractic education. It has been at the forefront of introducing laboratory procedures into the teaching of the basic sciences; teaching the clinical approach to diagnosis; incorporating other therapeutic measures into a chiropractic spinal adjustive procedure; researching the scientific basis for the practice of chiropractic; introducing a minimum of a 2-year preprofessional program admission requirement; and seeking accreditation and approval of the college and its programs by state, regional, and federal accrediting bodies and agencies.

In 1963 the college moved to Lombard, Illinois, where its facilities occupy approximately 30 acres. By 1979 this Lombard campus provided science-based chiropractic curriculum and clinical experience of the highest standards for 1000 students from all over the world. It now has six teaching clinics for its interns: the Student Clinic, National College Chiropractic Clinic—Aurora, National College Chiropractic Clinic—Chicago, National Chiropractic Center at Lombard, and two Salvation Army clinics.

National College of Chiropractic's educational and professional leadership led to a number of far-reaching contributions to the health science community, including publishing a referenced, internationally indexed, chiropractic scientific journal, the *Journal of Manipulative and Physiological Therapeutics;* constructing and operating a Spinal Ergonomics and Joint Research Laboratory; constructing and operating a 56,000 square foot National College Chiropractic Center on campus for chiropractic health care and research; developing the Practice Consultants Clinical Research Center; developing a Training and Assessment Center; and installing and operating a magnetic resonance imaging system for patient care and research.

360

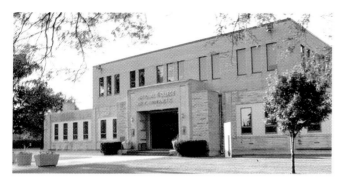

An exterior view of Janse Hall, National College of chiropractic's "Old Main," the first building constructed on the Lombard campus in 1963.
Courtesy National College of Chiropractic, Lombard, Illinois.

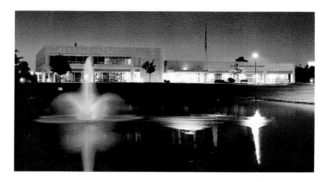

A night-time view of the National College of Chiropractic's campus.
Courtesy National College of Chiropractic, Lombard, Illinois.

In addition to the preparation of ethical, competent doctors for the general practice of chiropractic, the college offers continuing education to practicing chiropractic physicians, conducts clinical research, and functions as an upper division, postsecondary institution offering programs and conducting research in the biological sciences. National College believes that its purpose is best achieved through competent instruction, sound scholarship, and adequate clinical experience.

New York Chiropractic College

Founded in 1919 by Dr. Frank E. Dean, New York Chiropractic College (NYCC) has emerged as one of the profession's most prestigious educational institutions. Formerly known as Columbia Institute of Chiropractic, NYCC is the oldest Chiropractic College in the Northeast. In 1954, the College merged with the Columbia College of Chiropractic of Baltimore, Maryland. A decade later, a second merger took place with the Atlantic States Chiropractic Institute of Brooklyn, New York.

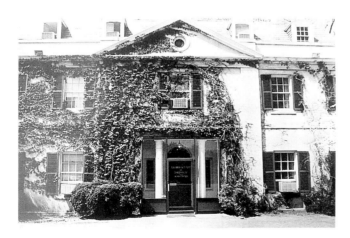

This building housed the Columbia College of Chiropractic, New York. Columbia later merged with Columbia College in Baltimore and Atlantic States Chiropractic Institute of Brooklyn to become New York Chiropractic College.
Courtesy New York Chiropractic College, Seneca Falls, New York.

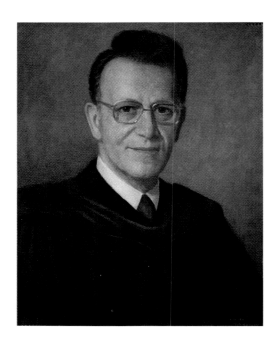

Dr. Earnest Napolitano, president of C
bia Institute of Chiropractic and later
York Chiropractic College from 1959 un
death in 1985.

Courtesy of New York Chiropractic College, Seneca Falls,
New York.

In 1959 the Board of Trustees appointed Dr. Ernest G. Napolitano as president. Under his leadership, the college became one of the leading chiropractic institutions in the United States. An extensive renovation plan was completed in 1961, and in the 1970s, with increasing demands for chiropractors and increasing enrollments, relocation plans were developed to help the college expand. The Old Brookville campus was purchased and clinics opened in Greenvale and Levittown, Long Island.

In 1976 the college was granted status as a recognized candidate for accreditation by the CCE. The next year, a provisional charter was granted by the regents of the University of the State of New York. At that time, the college acquired its new corporate name: New York Chiropractic College. In 1979 the CCE granted NYCC accredited status, and the regents of the State of New York awarded the college an absolute charter.

In 1980 the 50-acre Old Brookville campus opened its doors, and two years later the Anatomical Research Center was completed.

The Commission on Higher Education of the Middle States Association of Colleges and Schools granted accreditation status to NYCC in 1985; that same year, the untimely death of Dr. Napolitano ended an era in the institution's history. Alumnus and former vice president Dr. Neil Stern was appointed acting president; in 1987, Dr. Keith Asplin was named president, and served for a 2-year period.

In response to the continued growth of the college, further expansion was considered. In May 1989 the Board of Trustees approved the acquisition of the former Eisenhower College in Seneca Falls, New York, putting plans in motion to relocate to a new campus. In October 1989 Dr. Kenneth W. Padgett was elected president; his extensive experience in the chiropractic profession and his familiarity with upstate New York prepared him well for the challenges during what became known as the college's "Tradition in Transition" period.

In January 1991 the college opened the Syracuse Health Center in Syracuse, New York, to serve the needs of patients in the Syracuse area and offer another internship option to students.

The college moved its main campus to Seneca Falls, New York, and in September 1991 classes began at the new campus, the former Eisenhower College campus on the northern tip of Cayuga Lake. Nestled in the heart of the Finger Lakes region in upstate New York, the college is

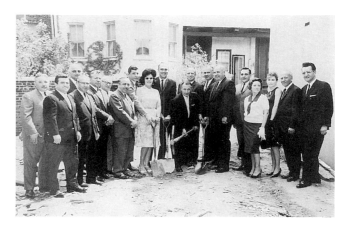

Ground breaking for renovation of the original building of Columbia Institute of Chiropractic, circa 1960. President Ernest Napolitano is at the far right.

Courtesy New York Chiropractic College, Seneca Falls, New York.

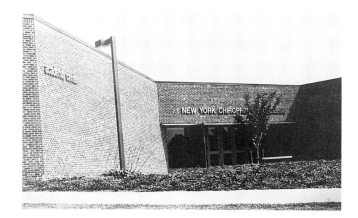

An exterior view of the academic center on the Long Island campus of New York Chiropractic College, circa 1980.

Courtesy New York Chiropractic College, Seneca Falls, New York.

at the epicenter of a triangular area including the cities of Syracuse, Rochester, and Ithaca, an area known for its excellent universities, wineries, and recreational opportunities.

The new campus rests on 286 acres and includes an on-campus student health center within the Academic Building; an athletic center which includes a 25-meter swimming pool, a gymnasium, and tennis, basketball, and racquetball courts; a library, whose lower level houses an anatomy center; residence halls for married couples, families, and single students; and an administration building.

On campus, students work with state-of-the-art technology and brand new equipment in their classrooms, technique labs, x-ray facilities, and anatomy lab. Off campus, students complete their education through internships at one of the campus health centers, located in Levittown (Long Island), Syracuse, or Buffalo, New York.

Chartered by the regents of the University of the State of New York, and accredited by the CCE and the Middle States Association of Colleges and Schools, NYCC offers a doctor of chiropractic degree program over 10 trimesters, which includes 40 months of intensive, full-time study, and over 5000 hours of clinical internship at the college's outpatient centers. The challenging rigors and rewards of the NYCC program, along with the college's association with other educational institutions and civic organizations, have brought the college international recognition and an overall reputation for excellence.

In October 1991 the Ernest G. Napolitano Postgraduate Center was named. Constructed in 1991 to 1992, it adjoins the Levittown Health Center, providing a home for the college's extensive postgraduate programs. The 5000 square foot annex opened February 1, 1992.

As the college continued to grow, plans were put in motion in 1993 to establish a third outpatient center in Buffalo, New York, as well as to renovate more classroom and residential living space on the campus.

Northwestern College of Chiropractic

Northwestern College of Chiropractic (NWCC) was founded June 2, 1941, in response to the need in the midwestern states for an educational institution offering a liberal course in chiropractic sciences, built upon a comprehensive background of basic sciences. Immediately after the college was established on Nicollet Avenue in Minneapolis, World War II began and enrollment plunged. A postwar influx of veterans raised the total enrollment to 280 by 1949. NWCC prospered as a school because of the rigorous academic goals it established, and because of the excellent quality of the students and faculty it attracted. In this period the college became a member of the CCE.

During June 1949, in order to best advance the interests of the chiropractic profession in Minnesota, it was reorganized under a non-profit corporate structure. The new organization obtained as governing members on its Board of Trustees representatives from the Minnesota Chiropractic Association, the Minnesota Chiropractic Foundation, and the public. Dr. John Wolfe remained as president. The college moved to a campus on Park Avenue in Minneapolis, purchased with funds given in response to a capital drive by the alumni association.

After 1950 declining veteran enrollment led to retrenchment until the Korean War G.I. Bill boosted enrollments again to 160 in the period from 1955 to 1958. Once again, though, enrollments declined. In 1964 a re-

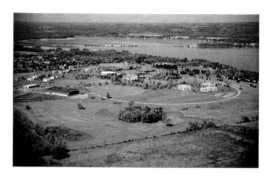

An aerial view of the Seneca Falls campus of New York Chiropractic College, purchased in 1989.

Courtesy New York Chiropractic College, Seneca Falls, New York.

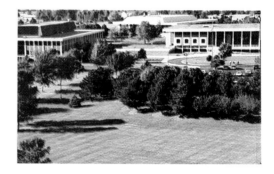

An exterior view of the Seneca Falls campus of New York Chiropractic College, circa 1992.

Courtesy New York Chiropractic College, Seneca Falls, New York.

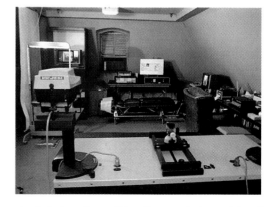

An interior view of the Greenvale Long Island Clinic of New York Chiropractic College, circa 1993.

Courtesy New York Chiropractic College, Seneca Falls, New York.

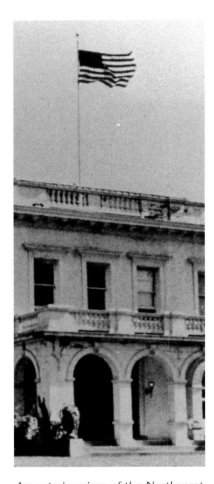

An exterior view of the Northwestern College of Chiropractic Campus on Nicollet Avenue, circa 1950.

Courtesy of Northwestern College of Chiropractic, Bloomington, Minnesota.

alistic self-evaluation led to the introduction of the Giant Stop Program in 1965. This program provided for a new clinic, a 2-year preprofessional requirement for all incoming students, a remodeling of the main building including a library, an all purpose biology teaching laboratory, and the adoption of objectives that would insure the development of a quality educational program designed for the needs of the profession. Northwestern was among the first colleges to adopt the 6-year academic program.

As a result of the successful completion of the Giant Step program, the College was elevated to the status of "Professionally Accredited" in June of 1967 by the Commission on Accreditation of the CCE. With this status came eligibility for educational grants from the Foundation for Chiropractic Education (FCER).

In the 1969 to 1970 school year a new systems-based curriculum was developed. This included seven single-semester basic science courses, including laboratory experiences taught at Saint Thomas College. In 1971 Northwestern was awarded accredited status by the Commission on Accreditation. By 1973 the continuing growth of the college necessitated the search for a new campus, which led to the Upward Bound development program and purchase, in 1974, of a campus in Saint Paul, located on Mississippi River Boulevard. The Saint Paul campus included basic science laboratories. With the addition of some full-time faculty, the association with Saint Thomas was phased out, and all courses were once again taught on the college campus.

Northwestern also introduced the multiple clinic concept and the final trimester off-campus preceptorship for the training of chiropractic interns. Presently, Northwestern owns and operates public clinics located in Saint Paul, Minneapolis, Robinsdale, Burnsville, and Bloomington.

A major development was the purchase in 1983 of a large campus located in Bloomington, Minnesota. The campus consists of 25 acres that include part of a private lake. The new complex itself is complete with

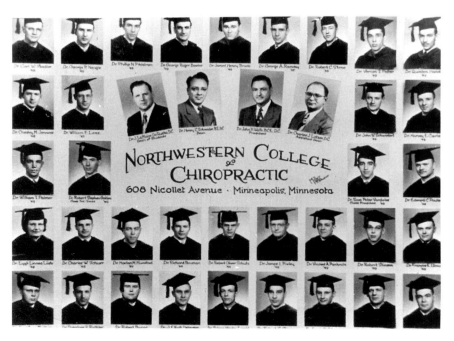

A class composite of the 1960 class of Northwestern College of Chiropractic.

Courtesy Northwestern College of Chiropractic.

laboratories, lecture halls, classrooms, library, public clinic, auditorium, cafeterias, gymnasium, and an indoor swimming pool and fitness center. This campus and its location better serves the students as well as provides a permanent home for the college..

In 1984 Dr. John B. Wolfe retired after 43 years of presidency. Dr. Donald M. Cassata was appointed as the second president of Northwestern College of Chiropractic and served until 1991. The college's third and current president is John F. Allenburg, D.C., a diplomate of the American Board of Chiropractic Orthopedics.

Toward achieving its mission of education, research, and patient care, the college is dedicated to attaining the highest quality in each of these areas. The college will maintain a limited enrollment, foster clinical research, promote individualized instruction, provide faculty development, and establish standards for clinical competencies.

The attainment of these objectives coincides with the college's ongoing postdoctoral and continuing education programs for the community practitioners and the provision of quality care to people in the Twin Cities communities.

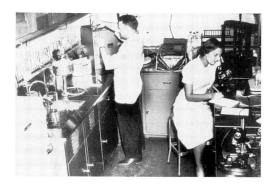

A laboratory at Northwestern College of Chiropractic, circa 1960.

Courtesy Northwestern College of Chiropractic, Bloomington, Minnesota.

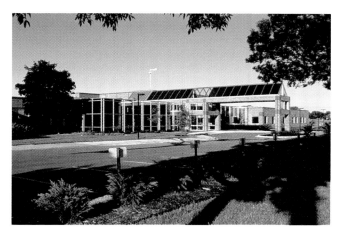

An exterior view of Northwestern College of Chiropractic's Bloomington Campus, circa 1990.

Courtesy Northwestern College of Chiropractic, Bloomington, Minnesota.

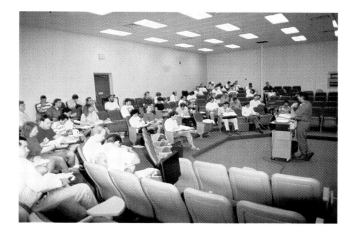

An interior view of a classroom at Northwestern College of Chiropractic, circa 1990.

Courtesy Northwestern College of Chiropractic, Bloomington, Minnesota.

Palmer College of Chiropractic

Palmer College of Chiropractic is the world's first and oldest institution dedicated to teaching chiropractic. The school was started by D.D. Palmer who decided to teach his newly discovered science after narrowly escaping death in a trolley car accident. The date of the school's founding is open to interpretation, depending on whether the year of D.D.'s discovery of chiropractic (1895) is used, whether the year in which he chartered his first school (1896) is used, or whether the year he accepted his first student (1897) is used. Palmer College today officially accepts the 1897 date.

The Palmer School and Cure (PSC), as it was first known, was located in the Ryan Building at the intersection of 2nd and Brady Streets in downtown Davenport. The tuition was $500, and the course consisted of 3 weeks of training in anatomy, physiology, symptomology, pathology, chiropractic philosophy, and adjusting technique. In 1902 B.J. Palmer,

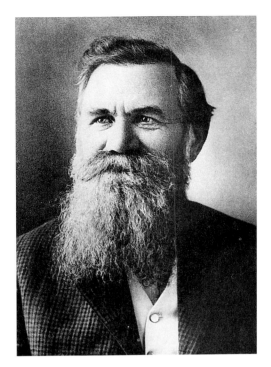

D. D. Palmer, Founder of Chiropractic, and founder and president of the Palmer School and Cure, circa 1904.

Courtesy Logan College of Chiropractic Archives, Chesterfield, Missouri.

D.D.'s son, graduated and worked in the school, which was now called the Palmer Infirmary and Chiropractic Institute. In 1902 D.D. went to California and stayed to start a school there, while B.J. stayed behind and ran the school in Davenport. When D.D. came back in late 1902, he and B.J. established an equal partnership.

In 1905 the Palmer School moved up the hill to 828 Brady Street. During March 1906, D.D. was convicted of practicing medicine without a license. After serving 23 days in the Scott County jail, D.D. paid a $500 fine and was released. On April 30, 1906, B.J. and D.D. signed an agreement in which B.J. purchased D.D.'s half of the school for $2196.79. D.D. then headed West where he would start schools in Oklahoma and Oregon.

From its humble beginnings at 828 Brady Street, where B.J. and his wife Mabel cooked and cleaned for the boarding students as well as taught, the PSC expanded rapidly. The course work was extended from 3 months in 1906 to 12 months in 1909 to 18 months in 1916. Student enrollment grew from 8 students in 1906 to 400 in 1911. D.D. returned to Davenport in 1913, and he and B.J. reconciled. In October D.D. died of typhoid fever in Los Angeles.

During the decade following his father's death, B.J. was the undisputed leader of the profession. The D.D. Palmer Memorial Classroom Building, built in 1916, was the first building erected specifically for chiropractic education. The Administration Building and the B.J. Palmer Classroom Building were built in 1920 and 1921, respectively.

The Palmer School was a leader in the use of the x-ray, installing a unit in 1910 and incorporating it in the classroom by 1911. The osteological museum on campus was praised by an AMA inspection team as being "the best collection of human spines in existence." B.J.'s UCA, with the guidance of attorney Tom Morris, was defending chiropractors all across the country for practicing medicine without a license, and B.J. was one of its most flamboyant witnesses. The printing presses at Palmer produced hundreds of thousands of patient education tracts every year, and his radio station, WOC, was selling the message of chiropractic to the whole country.

In 1924 B.J. introduced the neurocalometer to the profession. The controversy over its high cost and B.J.'s insistence on its use marked the

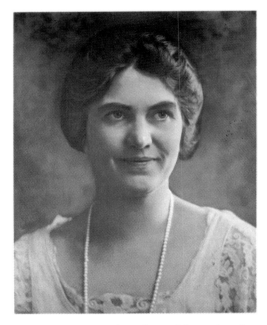

Mabel Palmer, B.J.'s wife, and long-time faculty member in the anatomy department.

Courtesy Palmer College of Chiropractic Archives, Davenport, Iowa.

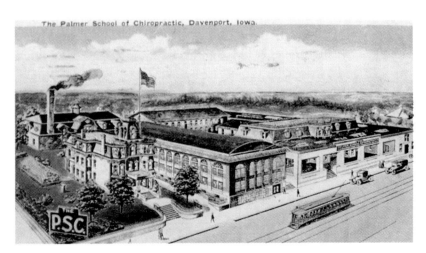

A postcard of the Palmer Campus as it looked, circa 1918.

Courtesy Palmer College of Chiropractic Archives, Davenport, Iowa.

beginning of the decline of B.J. Palmer's influence in the profession. Although he would continue to exert a powerful influence on the profession, no longer would he be its undisputed leader. Partially as a result of the erosion of B.J.'s support, partially as a result of a tougher basic sciences law and a renewed medical assault, and partially as a result of the economic depression, the PSC's enrollment dropped from a high of 3000 in 1924 to 1400 in 1932.

Despite lower student enrollments in the 1930s and 1940s the PSC continued to progress. B.J.'s cooperation with a German medical team in 1934 produced the first wet specimen showing a transparency of the spinal canal. In 1934 B.J. opened the B.J. Palmer Clinic, a facility which received the most difficult of medically diagnosed diseases from referring chiropractors all over the country. His instrument for reading brain wave conduction through the spinal cord, the electroencephaloneuromentimpograph, was a prototype of the EEG used today. B.J. also encouraged research in chiropractic care of mental illness, purchasing the Clear View Sanitarium in 1951. A 36-month curriculum was introduced in 1950 and a 48-month curriculum in 1957.

Upon B.J. Palmer's death in 1961, his son David assumed the presidency of the PSC. Under his presidency, the school was renamed the Palmer College of Chiropractic. He started the Palmer Junior College the Chiropractic Technologists program, and he set the steps in motion for acquiring accreditation by the CCE. David founded the alumni association, which built the Alumni Auditorium in 1972. In addition, the 3-story library/classroom building, built in 1977, was named after him. By 1970 enrollment at the college stood at 1034. Enrollment was 1800 in 1980 and 1700 in 1990.

Upon David Palmer's death in 1978, Dr. Galen Price, a longtime faculty member of Palmer College, was named president. Dr. Jerome McAndrews was appointed president in 1979. During his presidency, Palmer received accreditation by the North Central Accrediting Agency; the bachelor of science degree program was begun; and master of chiropractic science and master of anatomy programs were formulated. Construction was begun on a campus student center; a satellite clinic was opened in Rock Island, Illinois; and a research facility was purchased to facilitate research on the chiropractic principles. After Dr. McAndrew's resignation in 1987, Donald Kern, D.C., a third generation chiropractor, became the college's sixth president in 1988. In 1989, a satellite clinic was opened near Walcott, Iowa, and in 1990 the B.J. Palmer Occupational Health and Trauma Center opened. The college's campus center was also completed in 1990. Vicki Palmer, D.D. Palmer's great-granddaughter, continues the 95 years of Palmer's heritage in chiropractic by serving as a board member since 1979 and as the chairperson of the college's Board of Trustees since 1987. In February 1991, the Board of Directors announced the formation of the Palmer Chiropractic University System. Mr. Michael Crawford was appointed chancellor of Palmer Chiropractic University. The university system oversees the operation of Palmer Chiropractic Colleges, which consist of Palmer College of Chiropractic and Palmer College of Chiropractic—West.

In the nearly 100 years that Palmer College has been in existence as the Palmer School and Cure, Palmer Infirmary and Chiropractic Institute, Palmer School of Chiropractic, Palmer College of Chiropractic, and Palmer Chiropractic University, one principle has remained the same—an unswerving adherence to the principles of chiropractic and a dedication to excellence in chiropractic education.

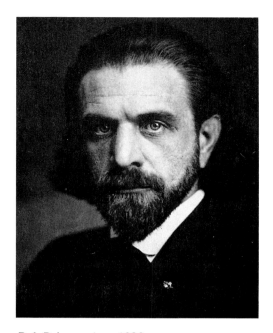

B.J. Palmer, circa 1930.
Courtesy Palmer College of Chiropractic Archives, Davenport, Iowa.

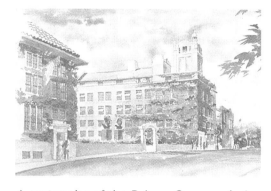

A watercolor of the Palmer Campus during the 1960s, done by Quad-City artist, Paul Norton.
Courtesy Palmer College of Chiropractic Archives, Davenport, Iowa.

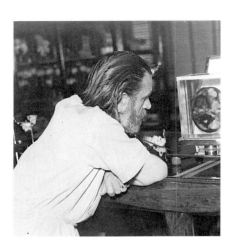

B.J. Palmer observing the "wet specimen" produced by the Spalteholz method, circa 1940. The organic material was removed from the skull, allowing a subluxation to be viewed through the transparent organic material that was left.

Courtesy Palmer College of Chiropractic Archives, Davenport, Iowa.

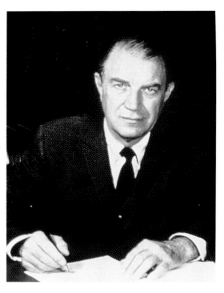

David D. Palmer, third president of the Palmer School of Chiropractic from 1961-1978.

Courtesy Palmer College of Chiropractic Archives, Davenport, Iowa.

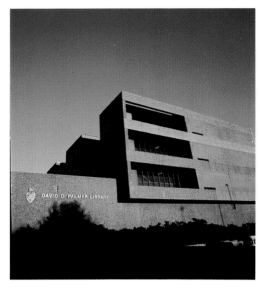

The library building at Palmer College of Chiropractic, named after the College's third president, David D. Palmer, in 1978.

Courtesy Palmer College of Chiropractic, Davenport, Iowa.

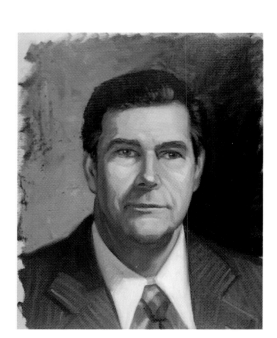

Galen Price, long-time faculty member, fourth president of Palmer College and its first non-Palmer family president.

Courtesy Palmer College of Chiropractic Archives, Davenport, Iowa.

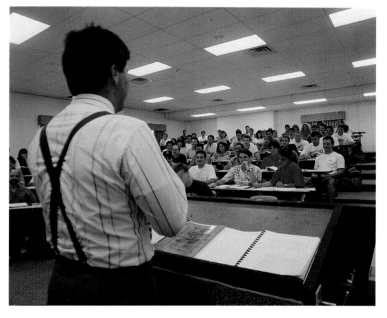

A Palmer College Classroom, circa 1993.

Courtesy Palmer College of Chiropractic, Davenport, Iowa.

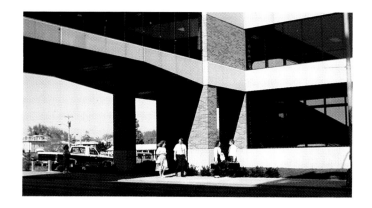

The Palmer College Campus Center was completed in 1990.
Courtesy Palmer College of Chiropractic, Davenport, Iowa.

Palmer College of Chiropractic—West

On July 28, 1978, a number of chiropractic students, educational administrators, and teachers met in San Lorenzo, California, for the purpose of establishing a college of chiropractic. Their goal was to establish a school for chiropractic education dedicated to excellence in instruction and serving as an academic center for chiropractic practitioners of Northern California. They named this new college the Northern California College of Chiropractic (NCCC). Facilities were temporarily secured at Chabot Community College in Hayward, California, and classroom instruction commenced with an enrollment of 62 on August 1, 1978.

In October 1979 a site was acquired in Sunnyvale, California, and classes were held there in the fall quarter. In January 1979 NCCC was granted preliminary membership by the CCE. In December 1979 the college was authorized by the state of California to grant the degree of doctor of chiropractic.

Palmer College had been considering the founding of a sister college on the West Coast. The NCCC, in some financial difficulties wished its students to be able to continue their education without loss of previously completed credits, and Palmer College of Chiropractic wished to establish another campus dedicated to the founder, Dr. Daniel David Palmer.

Negotiations culminated in a transition to a new entity in September 1980. The NCCC Board of Trustees resigned, and a new board was appointed in accordance with the new bylaws. The name of the institution was subsequently changed to Palmer College of Chiropractic—West (Palmer—West, or PCCW), and Dr. John L. Miller became president and chief executive officer. Dr. Miller proceeded to obtain full accreditation status for Palmer-West from the CCE in June 1985. Reaccreditation was renewed in July 1988 and June 1991.

Early in 1989 Palmer—West obtained additional facilities. An auxiliary site was acquired on Santa Clara, approximately 1 mile from the Sunnyvale campus.

In May 1991 Palmer College and Palmer—West strengthened their academic mission with the unification of the two institutions to form Palmer Chiropractic University (PCU). Mr. Michael Crawford, former chief executive officer and chancellor of St. Louis Community College, was named chancellor of PCU. Dr. John Miller was followed as president of Palmer—West by Dr. Peter A. Martin, who became the second president of the college in April 1992.

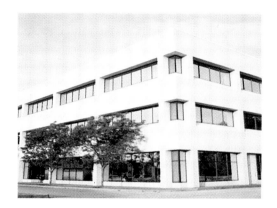

A building purchased in 1993 for use as a clinic facility by Palmer College of Chiropractic.
Courtesy Palmer College of Chiropractic, Davenport, Iowa.

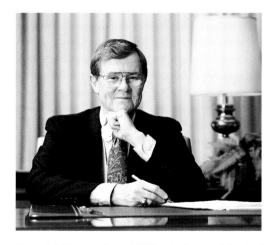

Donald Kern, circa 1993, sixth president of Palmer College of Chiropractic.
Courtesy Palmer College of Chiropractic, Davenport, Iowa.

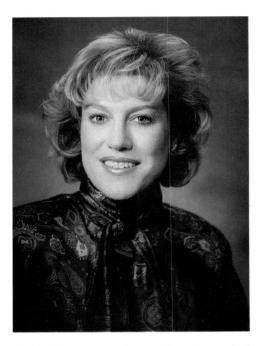

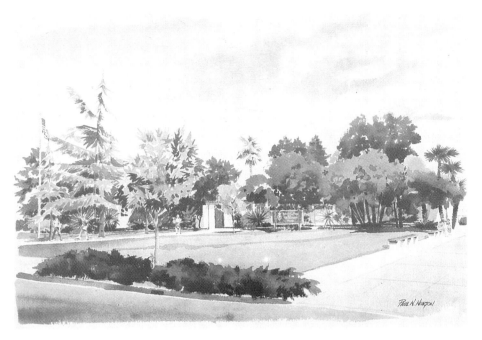

Vicki Palmer, great-granddaughter of the founder of chiropractic and Chairman of the Board of the Palmer Chiropractic University.

Courtesy Palmer Chiropractic University, Davenport, Iowa.

Watercolor by Paul Norton of the Palmer-West Sunnyvale campus, circa 1982, formerly the Northern California College of Chiropractic.

Courtesy Palmer College of Chiropractic Archives, Davenport, Iowa.

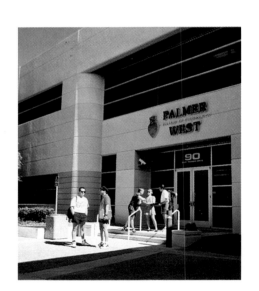

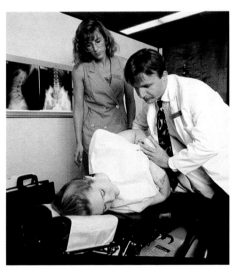

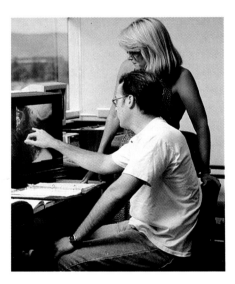

The Palmer College of Chiropractic— West San Jose campus was acquired in 1993.

Courtesy Palmer Chiropractic University, Davenport, Iowa.

A student adjusting under the supervision of a faculty member at Palmer College of Chiropractic—West, circa 1993.

Courtesy Palmer Chiropractic University, Davenport Iowa.

Students analyzing x-rays at the Palmer College of Chiropractic—West San Jose campus, 1993.

Courtesy Palmer Chiropractic University, Davenport, Iowa.

In 1993 Palmer—West acquired a large campus in San Jose, California, in order to accommodate the growing student population, and the academic and administrative requirements necessary for the support of the growing program. This relocation also served to eliminate dual campuses and enhance staff, faculty, and student communication.

Parker College of Chiropractic

The Parker College of Chiropractic is named for Dr. James William Parker, whose consuming interest, effort, skill, and love have been almost totally chiropractic for nearly 5 decades—since the day he began recuperating from childhood illnesses following chiropractic care. Even while a senior in college, Dr. Parker opened two successful practices in Illinois (Rock Island and Geneseo), and upon graduating from Palmer School of Chiropractic in 1946, he developed in Fort Worth, Texas, one of the fastest growing chiropractic practices in the history of chiropractic, followed by the establishment of 18 clinics, one each in almost every major Texas city.

From this, the Parker Chiropractic Resource Foundation (PCRF) was founded in 1951. This organization has held nearly 350 4-day postgraduate chiropractic seminars called the Parker School for Professional Success (PSPS) throughout North America and many parts of the world during the last 4½ decades.

Dr. Parker first consented to lend his name and to help establish and fund the college as a response to strong urging and requests from thousands of doctors and students. These chiropractors came to realize that students should have the benefit of his unique success, his healing and practice consciousness, his philosophy and business training, and his curriculum.

The college was chartered by the state of Texas on March 8, 1978, and received its nonprofit IRS status in October 1978. A 63-acre tract of land was purchased in Dallas, and the college officially opened September 12, 1982, with 27 students at 300 East Irving Boulevard in Irving, Texas. The original campus is now being used to house the Research and Rehabilitation Department, the intern lounge, and a public clinic, where about 1000 patients a week receive chiropractic care.

Parker College achieved recognized candidate status from both the CCE and the Southern Association of Colleges and Schools (SACS) in

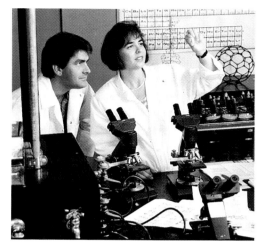

An interior view of the Palmer College of Chiropractic–West San Jose campus in 1993.

Courtesy Palmer Chiropractic University, Davenport, Iowa.

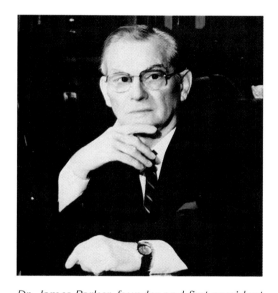

Dr. James Parker, founder and first president of Parker College of Chiropractic.

Courtesy Parker College of Chiropractic, Dallas, Texas.

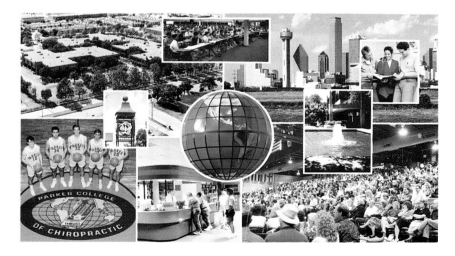

A 1993 composite photo of the Parker College of Chiropractic, which opened in 1982.

Courtesy Parker College of Chiropractic, Dallas, Texas.

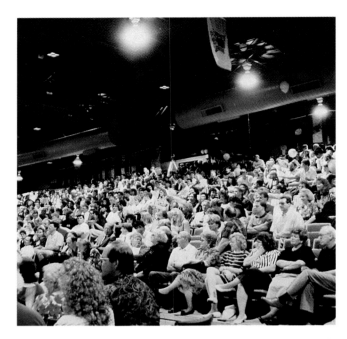

An interior view of Parker College of Chiropractic's auditorium/gymnasium in 1993.
Courtesy Parker College of Chiropractic, Dallas, Texas.

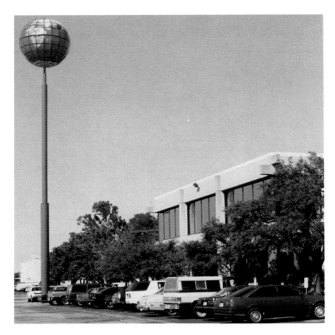

The 109-foot revolving lighted globe at the Parker College of Chiropractic campus is a Dallas landmark, signifying the 79 foreign countries represented among the students and alumni.
Courtesy Parker College of Chiropractic, Dallas, Texas.

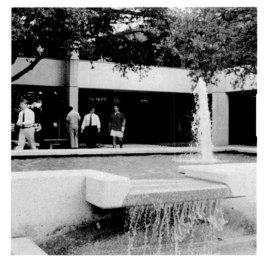

An exterior view of Parker College of Chiropractic's Beta campus, circa 1993.
Courtesy Parker College of Chiropractic, Dallas, Texas.

1985, and attained accreditation status from the Southern Association in January 1987, followed by accreditation from the CCE in June 1988. On January 25, 1991, Parker College was granted authority to award the Bachelor of Science degree with a major in anatomy by the Texas Higher Education Coordinating Board of the Texas College and University System and SACS.

Just seven years after its beginnings, the college moved from Irving to its new campus in Dallas, which commenced operation in September 1989 and is located at 2500 Walnut Hill Lane in Dallas, Texas. The purchase of the new campus provided space for the library and resource center; the center for basic sciences, and its labs, including one of the most advanced gross anatomy labs in any educational facility; the x-ray department; and all amphitheater classrooms. The south building was designated as mainly administrative but also includes the cafeteria, student lounges, x-ray labs, bookstore, and classrooms. Presently, the east building provides newly appointed labs for nine techniques required in the curriculum, student clinic facilities, and offices for faculty and campus support services. In 1992 the college completed the 30,000 square foot gymnasium/auditorium that seats over 1200 and provides complete weight training facilities.

The first Parker College Public Clinic, for the training of interns, was opened in May 1984 and had over 1000 new patients within the first year. By early 1992 it was evident that the increase in numbers of patients receiving care and in enrollment necessitated a second outpatient facility to be constructed on the main campus in Dallas. In 1993 a 3-acre parcel was purchased adjacent to the college as the new site of the public and student clinic complex in 1992. With over 52,000 square feet and 144 additional parking spaces, the existing buildings have been renovated to

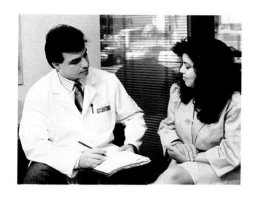

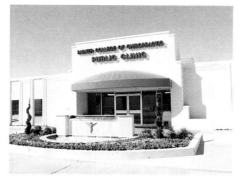

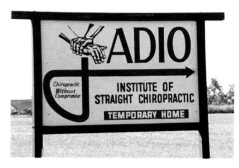

A student at Parker College of Chiropractic conducting a patient history.

Courtesy Parker College of Chiropractic, Dallas, Texas.

The patient clinic on Parker College of Chiropractic BETA campus, circa 1994.

Courtesy Parker College of Chiropractic, Dallas, Texas.

Adio Institute of Straight Chiropractic, which later became the Pennsylvania College of Straight Chiropractic, enrolled its first class in January 1978.

Courtesy Pennsylvania College of Straight Chiropractic, Horsham, Pennsylvania.

achieve a twenty-first century wellness center that keeps all patient services, including lab, x-ray, treatment, and physical modality, totally self-contained for the convenience of the patient and the efficiency of the intern. The student clinic and Rehabilitation Center will soon occupy another of the buildings, and another amphitheater classroom will be constructed where the student clinic is presently located.

Pennsylvania College of Straight Chiropractic

Pennsylvania College of Straight Chiropractic, formerly ADIO Institute of Straight Chiropractic, was incorporated in the Commonwealth of Pennsylvania in July 1977 and enrolled its initial class in January 1978.

On March 3, 1984, the Board of Trustees changed the name of the institution from ADIO Institute of Straight Chiropractic to the Pennsylvania College of Straight Chiropractic (PCSC). On April 10, 1984, the state of Pennsylvania officially recognized the name change.

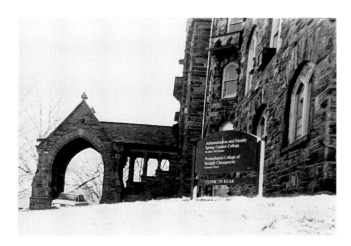

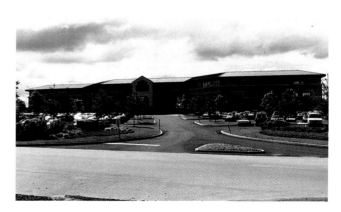

The Levittown campus of Pennsylvania College of Straight Chiropractic, circa 1990.

Courtesy Pennsylvania College of Straight Chiropractic, Horsham, Pennsylvania.

The Horsham campus of Pennsylvania College of Straight Chiropractic, circa 1992.

Courtesy Pennsylvania College of Straight Chiropractic, Horsham, Pennsylvania.

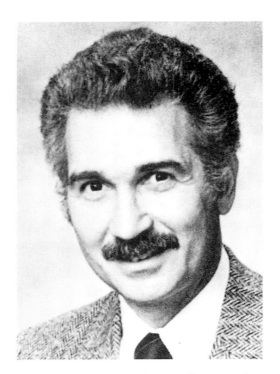

Thomas Gelardi, founder and first president of Sherman College of Straight Chiropractic.

Courtesy Sherman College of Straight Chiropractic, Spartanburg, South Carolina.

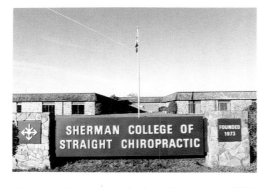

An exterior view of the Mack and Kitty Scallen Building, circa 1992.

Courtesy Sherman College of Straight Chiropractic, Spartanburg, South Carolina.

On March 4, 1981, ADIO received certification as an institution of higher education under the Three Institutional Certification (3IC) program of the United States Department of Education. This approval made ADIO students eligible for federal grants and guaranteed student loans.

Beginning with the December 1983 graduation class, ADIO Institute was awarded the right to grant the degree Doctor of Chiropractic by the commonwealth of Pennsylvania Department of Higher Education.

In Pennsylvania, H.B. 1362 became law on December 16, 1986, as the Pennsylvania Chiropractic Practice Act, which places the college under the Pennsylvania Department of Education and requires the college to attain specialized accreditation within a 5-year period.

On November 15, 1987, PCSC was awarded candidate for accreditation status with the Straight Chiropractic Academic Standards Association. The college was granted renewal of that status in December 1989. The college was granted full accreditation status in November 1991.

In September 1990 the Board of Trustees agreed to a 10-year lease with Hansen Properties. The program was relocated to a newly built facility in Horsham, Pennsylvania, a northern suburb of Philadelphia.

Sherman College of Straight Chiropractic

Sherman College of Straight Chiropractic was established in 1973 by Dr. Thomas A. Gelardi. Gelardi, a doctor of chiropractic, sensed the necessity for an institution that, while possessing an academically and institutionally stimulating environment, remained fully consistent with the goals and objectives of the founder of the chiropractic profession, D.D. Palmer. Sherman College is based on a vitalistic philosophy. Chiropractic is the science and art of correcting vertebral subluxations in accordance with a vitalistic philosophy.

Sherman is a 4-year, private, non-profit institution. It is accredited by the Commission on Accreditation of the Straight Chiropractic Academic Standards Association and the Commission on Colleges of Southern Association of Colleges and Schools. The goal of the college is to prepare its students to be primary health care providers, fully qualified to assume their responsibilities of contributing to patient health (life expression) through the correction of vertebral subluxations.

In order to fulfill its mission, Sherman has assembled a distinguished faculty of highly qualified, highly skilled professionals. It includes respected doctors of chiropractic and basic scientists from throughout the world.

The school's facilities are outstanding. Sherman's campus is located on 80 acres of rolling hills in Spartanburg, South Carolina. The campus is a short drive from the Blue Ridge and Great Smoky Mountains and the nationally famous Grand Strand of Myrtle Beach.

The Mack and Kitty Scallon Building is Sherman's primary facility, housing administrative and faculty offices, classrooms, a specialized library, the computer resource center, and the Sherman bookstore.

The E.C. Taylor Building opened in 1981. This facility contains classrooms, a public lecture room, x-ray rooms, the Research Department, and the Sherman College Chiropractic Health Center, which is the largest of its kind in the world. Students provide chiropractic care to the local community as part of their training in the health center. The Sherman College Research Department offers the finest instruction and equipment to prepare the student for a possible career in research. Sherman also offers

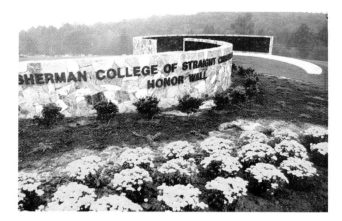

The Wall of Honor on the campus of Sherman College of Straight Chiropractic.

Courtesy Sherman College of Straight Chiropractic, Spartanburg, South Carolina.

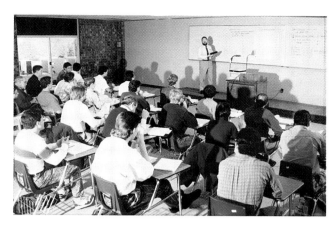

A classroom at Sherman College of Straight Chiropractic, circa 1993.

Courtesy Sherman College of Straight Chiropractic, Spartanburg, South Carolina.

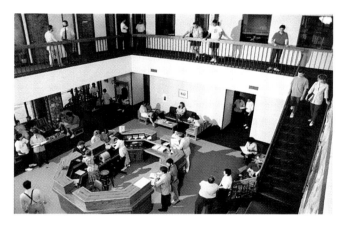

An interior view of the Sherman Health Center, circa 1993.

Courtesy Sherman College of Straight Chiropractic, Spartanburg, South Carolina.

students the opportunity to research methodology skills to advance the chiropractic profession through research.

Also located on the Sherman campus is the We Care Chiropractic Clinic and Research Center. Dr. Walter V. Pierce and Dr. Burl R. Pettibon conduct chiropractic research in their facility and provide care to patients with problem cases from all over the world.

Sherman offers the Doctor of Chiropractic program, which provides students a fresh new perspective on life and natural good health. The basic and clinical science programs not only afford students the opportunity to learn and practice important health care procedures, but also the chance to broaden themselves personally to meet the challenges of the future.

The college is named in honor of the late Dr. Lyle W. Sherman, a pioneer in the development of modern chiropractic and former assistant director of the B.J. Palmer Chiropractic Research Clinic in Davenport, Iowa. Dr. Sherman's commitment to humanity and advancing the state of chiropractic art was frequently recognized by his peers.

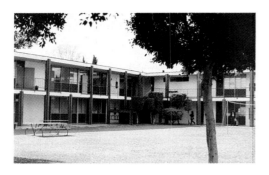

An exterior view of Southern California College of Chiropractic, formerly known as the University of Pasadena, circa 1993.

Southern California College of Chiropractic

Southern California College of Chiropractic (SCCC) was originally incorporated in January 31, 1973, as the International Chiropractic College of Neurovertabrology, located in Pasadena, California. The name was subsequently changed to the University of Pasadena. The college's stated purpose was to "teach persons who desire to be Doctors of Chiropractic." In 1977 it became the Pasadena College of Chiropractic and retained this name until May 1989.

The college received formal approval to conduct its educational program from the California State Board of Chiropractic Examiners in September 1974. In January 1978 it was granted approval to award the doctor of chiropractic degree from the Office of Private Post-Secondary Education in the California State Department of Education.

From 1988 to 1989 was a time of great change for the college. Not only did its name change to Southern California College of Chiropractic, but the school underwent a change in mission, in essence becoming a new institution. A new board of trustees was created by Dr. Daniel Kuhn, who is currently the chairman.

Under the direction of the Board of Trustees, the college continued its new direction, holding candidate for accreditation status with the Straight Chiropractic Academic Standards Association (SCASA). In December 1992 the college was granted accredited status with SCASA.

Dr. William Ralph Boone, Ph.D.,D.C., was inaugurated as college president in March 1991. During his tenure the college has continued its transition as envisioned by the Board of Trustees.

The college is presently located in Pico Rivera, a suburb of Los Angeles, with plans to relocate in the near future to a site more conducive to its growing student body.

Southern California College of Chiropractic is a credit to the profession that Daniel David Palmer founded in 1895. It has a student body that is multicultural with representatives from 20 different countries. A vibrant and dedicated staff, faculty, and administration, led by an inspired president and board of trustees, gives this Southern California College a personality all its own and a uniqueness that would be difficult to find elsewhere.

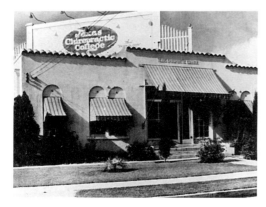

An early exterior view, circa 1925, of the Texas Chiropractic College, San Antonio, Texas.

Texas Chiropractic College

Texas Chiropractic College (TCC), the nation's fourth-oldest chiropractic college, was organized and founded by a pioneer chiropractor, Dr. J.N. Stone, in 1908 in San Antonio. On April 16, 1913, the college received its first charter from the state of Texas, and was known as "The Chiropractic College."

In 1919 the college came under the administration of Dr. J.M. McCleese and his associates. In 1920 the charter and all interests of the chiropractic college were purchased by Dr. B.F. Gurden, Dr. Flora M. Gurden, and Dr. James D. Drain.

In 1924 Dr. B.F. Gurden and Dr. Flora Gurden retired, and their interest in the college was transferred to Dr. H.E. Weiser and Dr. C.B. Loftin.

During its early history, the college moved to various locations in downtown San Antonio. After several reorganizations under proprietary ownerships, the institution was renamed and rechartered as Texas Chiropractic College, Inc., on December 19, 1925. In 1926, while under the administration of Dr. Drain, Dr. Weiser, and Dr. Loftin, the college moved

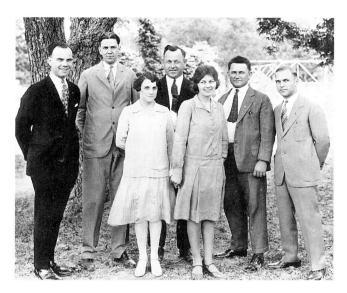

Early administrators at the Texas Chiropractic College.
Courtesy Texas Chiropractic College, Pasadena, Texas.

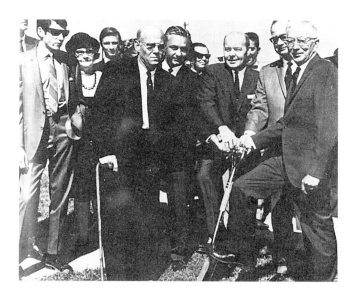

Ground breaking ceremony with Dr. William Harper, (right), *circa 1975.*
Courtesy Texas Chiropractic College, Pasadena, Texas.

into its own newly constructed building opposite San Pedro Park in San Antonio.

The Texas Chiropractic College Foundation, Inc., was established in 1955 as a nonprofit institution. Its bylaws established a board of regents with full responsibility for the college's policies and programs. The policy has proved to be ideal because of the prestige enjoyed by the college throughout the nation.

When the facilities needed restoration and more land was required for expansion, the board of regents sought a new location since a suitable site was not available in San Antonio. In 1965 the college moved to a site in Pasadena, Texas, which was originally developed to be a country club. The physical plant and caretaker quarters, located on an 8-acre tract, allowed for expansion, but only for a limited time. In 1966 an additional 10 acres was purchased to ensure room for continued expansion.

TCC received its accreditation in 1971 from the CCE.

In 1974 an outpatient clinic, the W.D. Harper Chiropractic Clinic and Research Center, was constructed, providing larger facilities for patient consultation, examination, and treatment. A research laboratory, senior classroom, and student lounge were housed in the same facilities.

Completion of the James M. Russell Education Center in 1978 provided larger facilities for classrooms, a library, cafeteria, bookstore, and auditorium. A laboratory building for anatomical studies, the Turley Anatomical Building, was completed in 1979, furthering the expansion of the physical plant to accommodate the trends in chiropractic education.

In 1982 another major expansion of the physical plant was dedicated. This facility, known as the Learning Resource Center, has more than 35,000 square feet of space for a multimedia library, bookstore, and additional classrooms and laboratories to meet the future needs of the college's steady increase in enrollment.

In 1987 ownership of the college was assumed by the United Chiropractic Education Foundation, Inc., a non-profit subsidiary of the Texas Chiropractic Association. By this action, the chiropractic profession in

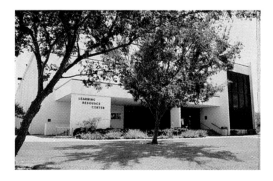

An exterior view of Texas Chiropractic College's Learning Resource Center, circa 1991.
Courtesy Texas Chiropractic College, Pasadena, Texas.

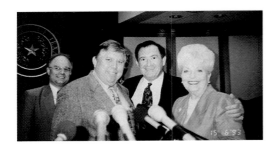

Texas Chiropractic College was instrumental in getting S.B. No. 201 authorizing Texas funding for chiropractic education signed into law in May 1993. Left to right, *Dr. Dan Petrosky, Chairman of the TCC Board of Regents; Texas Senator Carl Parker, TCC President Dr. S.M. Elliott; and Governor Ann Richards.*

Courtesy Texas Chiropractic College, Pasadena, Texas.

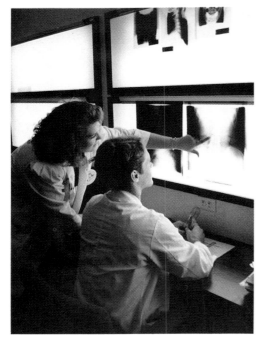

Two students viewing x-rays, circa 1993, at the Texas Chiropractic College.

Courtesy Texas Chiropractic College, Pasadena, Texas.

Texas demonstrated its dedication to continuing the growth and service of Texas Chiropractic College for generations to come.

TCC has continued to grow along with the profession, diversifying its curriculum and adding an impressive selection of postgraduate courses to further educational enrichment of established physicians. The TCC Postgraduate Studies Division offers diplomate courses in clinical neurology, orthopedics, and chiropractic diagnosis and management of internal disorders. Certification courses are also offered in clinical pharmacology, manipulation under anesthesia (MUA), impairment rating, clinical nutrition, and chiropractic sports physician, as well as a wide variety of special offerings. Currently courses are offered by the Postgraduate Studies Division in 24 states.

TCC is also leading the way in forging relationships with the medical community through its visiting faculty exchange program and rotations for student interns at area hospitals.

TCC made major advances both on the behalf of chiropractic education and for recognition of the profession as a whole, when, after three attempts in nearly 7 years, a bill authorizing state funding for chiropractic education was finally signed into law by Texas Governor Anne Richards on May 15, 1993. Senate Bill no. 201 (House of Representative Bill #861) was introduced and championed by Senator Carl Parker and Representative Mike Jackson. Further support for the bill and its lobbying effort were not only provided by a TCC student lobbying and letter writing campaign, but enthusiastically bolstered by support from the Pasadena Chamber of Commerce Legislative Committee, led by its chairman, Jim Kite, who was also a member of TCC's board of regents, and from the Texas Chiropractic Association. This lobbying effort was later joined by Parker College of Chiropractic. The resulting recognition from the rest of the Texas educational community and health care community has been phenomenal.

The college is swiftly approaching its enrollment capacity of 600 students, with the growing acceptance of non-allopathic healing methods and with the growth of the Pasadena area. Plans are under way to address the needs created by new growth.

University of Bridgeport—College of Chiropractic

Opened in 1991, the University of Bridgeport—College of Chiropractic is housed in the renovated nursing building on campus.

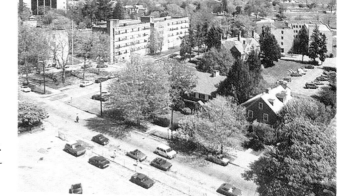

An exterior view of the University of Bridgeport campus, circa 1992. The College of Chiropractic is housed in the renovated nursing building.

Courtesy University of Bridgeport, Bridgeport, Connecticut.

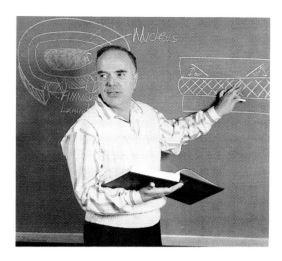

A faculty member lecturing at the University of Bridgeport.

Courtesy University of Bridgeport, Bridgeport, Connecticut.

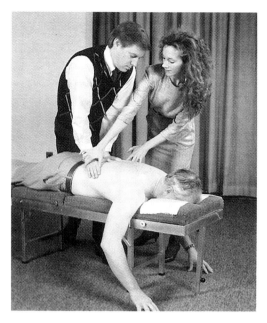

A technique class at the University of Bridgeport's College of Chiropractic.

Courtesy University of Bridgeport, Bridgeport, Connecticut.

Western States Chiropractic College

Western States Chiropractic College (WSCC) traces its historical roots back to 1904 when Drs. John and Eva Marsh opened Marshes' School and Cure, whose graduates included William Powell. Dr. John Marsh and Dr. Powell incorporated and expanded the Marshes' school in 1909 and changed its name to the Pacific College of Chiropractic, located in the Fliedner Building.

A second chiropractic school, the D.D. Palmer College of Chiropractic, was founded in 1908 by Dr. D.D. Palmer and John LaValley. A schism developed between the two men, and in 1911 Dr. LaValley reorganized the college, changing the name to the Oregon Peerless College of Chiropractic—Naturopathy. Its first site was the Buchanan Building. A Peerless College catalogue postmarked 1911 lists the course of study as 12 months. It was here that human dissection was first placed on the curriculum of an Oregon chiropractic school.

In 1913 chiropractic education in Portland was consolidated by a merger of Pacific College of Chiropractic and The Oregon Peerless College of Chiropractic into a single institution called Pacific Chiropractic College, which was located in the Commonwealth Building. In late 1913 the school moved to the Hassalo Church Building in East Portland, near what is the Lloyd Center. Its president was Dr. W.O. Powell, until his death in 1916, when the college was purchased by Dr. Oscar Elliot, who then was president until his death in 1926. His widow Lenore took over the office until she sold the college to Dr. W.A. Budden in 1929. The college moved to several locations in Portland during 1922 to 1938. It was set up as the first 4-year chiropractic college in the country.

In 1932 the Pacific Chiropractic College was reorganized and became Western States College of Chiropractors and Drugless Physicians. In 1937 the Health Research Foundation was formed as a non-profit organization under which Western States College was operated.

In 1939 a 2-story brick building was purchased at S.E. 11th and Clay, where the school remained until 1947.

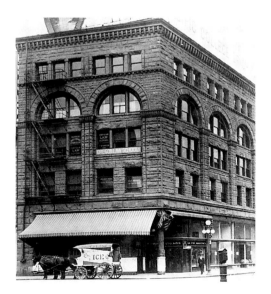

An exterior view of Pacific College of Chiropractic, circa 1910, Portland, Oregon, a forerunner of Western States Chiropractic College.

Courtesy Western States Chiropractic College, Portland, Oregon.

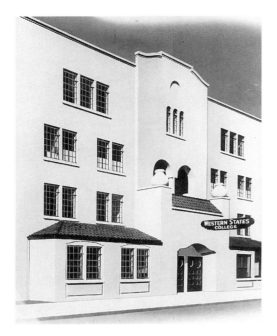

The campus of Western States Chiropractic College, located at Southeast 63rd and Foster from 1947-1973.
Courtesy Western States Chiropractic College, Portland, Oregon.

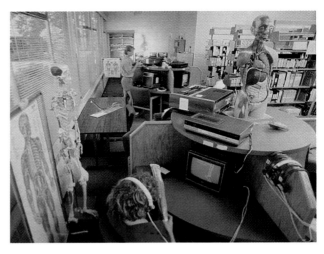

Students at Western States Chiropractic College in the Learning Resource Center, circa 1993.
Courtesy Western States Chiropractic College, Portland, Oregon.

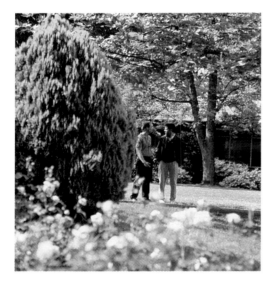

An exterior view of the Western States Chiropractic College in 1993.
Courtesy Western States Chiropractic College, Portland Oregon.

In 1946 the college purchased a former lodge building on Southeast 63rd Avenue in Portland. This marked the site of the school and clinic facilities until its move to a new 22-acre campus in northeast Portland in 1973. The college's name changed to Western States Chiropractic College in 1967.

An increase in student enrollment then made the need for a new and larger clinic obvious. As a result, the college purchased a facility near the campus in July 1976 and began operations that September. It became apparent that it would be desirable to have the clinic located on campus and to have the facility architecturally designed to function as a teaching clinic. During Fall 1986 this goal was achieved with the opening of a new 9000 square foot clinic. This half-million dollar clinic is the largest chiropractic facility in the Northwest and is an outstanding professional setting for interns to develop and perfect their diagnostic and clinical skills.

It should be noted that WSCC has pioneered certain aspects of chiropractic education in the United States. It was the first to set up a 4-year course of study; one of the first to remove itself from private ownership to a non-profit status as a chiropractic college; the very first to require the 2-year preprofessional requirements to enroll in the school; and one of the first to adopt a curriculum inclusive of all the basic sciences. From the mid-1930s until 1956, WSCC offered a course in herbology and a degree in naturopathy.

The presidents of the college since 1927 are Lenore Elliot, 1927 to 1929; W.A. Budden, 1929 to 1954; Ralph Failor, 1954 to 1956; Robert E. Elliot, 1956 to 1974; Samuel G. Warren, 1975 to 1976; Richard H. Timmins, 1976 to 1979; Herbert J. Vear, 1979 to 1986 and William H. Dallas, the current president.

Canadian Memorial Chiropractic College

The Canadian Memorial Chiropractic College (CMCC) is the longest running chiropractic college in Canada. A privately funded educational institution, the college offers a 4-year professional program leading to the

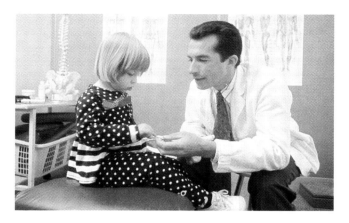

A student at Western States Chiropractic College examining a child, circa 1993.

Courtesy Western States Chiropractic College, Portland, Oregon.

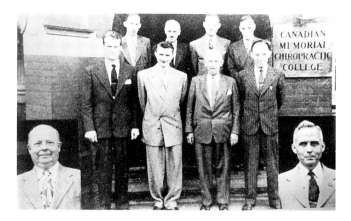

Administrators and Faculty of the newly formed Canadian Memorial Chiropractic College at the Bloor St. campus in Toronto, circa 1947.

Courtesy Canadian Memorial Chiropractic College, Toronto, Ontario.

doctor of chiropractic diploma. The primary purpose of the college is to educate the future chiropractors of Canada and thereby ensure a vibrant and growing chiropractic profession.

Chiropractors have been providing health care to Canadians for almost 100 years. Prior to 1945 Canadians wishing to study chiropractic were required to attend colleges in the United States. The gradual growth of the profession in the 2 decades before World War II eventually underlined the need for an educational institution in Canada, and the desire for a chiropractic college grew within the profession.

The history of the college began in January 1943 when chiropractors representing the Canadian provinces gathered in Ottawa to form the profession's first national chiropractic organization—the Dominion Council of Canadian Chiropractors. The name was later changed to Canadian Chiropractic Association.

The first act of the fledgling association was to establish an educational institution. Accordingly, in January 1945 the Dominion Council established the Canadian Association of Chiropractors, later the Canadian Memorial Chiropractic College, which was granted the authority to establish and conduct schools of chiropractic.

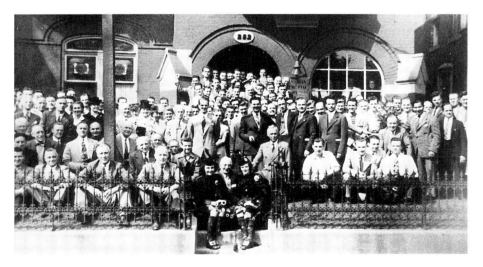

The first class of the Canadian Memorial Chiropractic College in front of the Bloor St. campus in 1945.

Courtesy Canadian Memorial Chiropractic College, Toronto, Ontario.

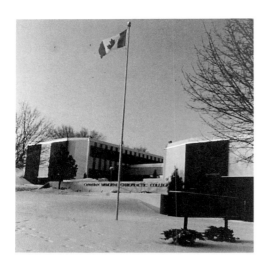

A winter scene on the Canadian Memorial Chiropractic College's Bayview campus, circa 1992.

Courtesy Canadian Memorial Chiropractic College, Toronto, Ontario.

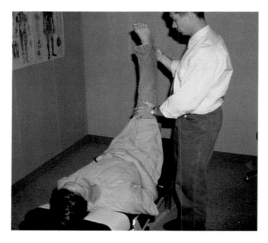

A student adjusting at the Canadian Memorial Chiropractic College, circa 1993.

Courtesy Canadian Memorial Chiropractic College, Toronto, Ontario.

The CMCC was founded on September 18, 1945, on the fiftieth anniversary of the profession's first adjustment. It was located in the former Medonia Hotel on Bloor Street West in downtown Toronto. Its first class of 97 men and women was composed mostly of veterans returning from World War II, whose tuition fees and living expenses were paid by the Department of Veteran Affairs of the government of Canada. Two years later when additional space was required, the 3-story Henderson Building was constructed to the rear of the renovated hotel.

In April 1959 part of the college's land was expropriated by the city of Toronto for subway expansion. Excavation soon began, and at one point a portion of the Henderson Building was suspended in midair, resulting in considerable structural damage. The court case, which lasted until 1968, awarded partial damages to the college.

In 1968 the college moved to a newly constructed campus on Bayview Avenue, which further enhanced the college's academic and clinical image. The first off-campus outpatient clinic was opened on Parliament Street in Toronto's "Cabbagetown" area in 1976. The clinic served the college in two ways: ensuring a positive chiropractic profile in the community and providing a logistical solution to the ever increasing number of interns needing a place to develop their clinical expertise. Presently, the college operates three outpatient clinics in Toronto, located on the Bayview Avenue campus, on Dundas Street West at Bloor Street, and on Eglinton Avenue West near the Allan Expressway.

From the beginning CMCC has been a nonprofit organization, owned by the profession and chartered under the nonprofit section of the Companies Act of Ontario. The college has been accredited by the Council on Chiropractic Education (CCE) (Canada), Inc. The Council is incorporated under the laws of Canada and has adopted similar standards to those of CCE (USA) to establish uniform international standards of accreditation for the profession. Through a reciprocal agreement between the United States CCE, this status is also effective in the United States and allows the college's graduates to apply for licensure in most of the jurisdictions of that country.

Today, CMCC has an enrollment of approximately 600 students, continues to increase in stature as a primary contact, health care, professional, educational institution. Fulfilling its responsibilities to the profession by providing both excellent research and well-qualified graduates, the college remains committed to the development of graduates who possess the necessary knowledge, skills, and attributes to practice chiropractic care effectively and safely.

Université du Québec a Trois-Rivières

Chiropractic was granted legal recognition by the Quebec National Assembly in 1973, when the Chiropractic Act and the Professional Code came into effect, which led to the establishment of corporations for various professionals, including chiropractors in Quebec. At the time, there was consensus among all the political parties that legal recognition would logically lead to the creation of a training program to be offered in Quebec.

For planning purposes, the Ministry of Education launched Operation Health Sciences as a means of gaining an overview of health sciences programs offered by Quebec universities. Following a 4-year review, a moratorium was announced on any new health sciences programs. The

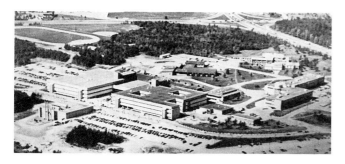

An aerial view of the University of Quebec at Three Rivers, whose first class entered in September 1993.

Courtesy Ordre des Chiropracticiens du Québec, Ville D'Anjou, Quebec.

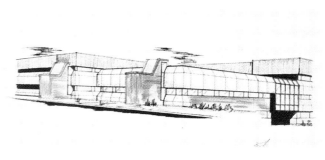

An artist's rendition of the chiropractic science building planned for the University of Quebec at Three Rivers.

Courtesy Ordre des Chiropracticiens du Québec, Ville D'Anjou, Quebec.

report also stated that although no new program in chiropractic was to begin immediately, a financial aid plan modelled on the loans and bursaries program should be set up to help Quebec students pursue their studies outside the province. Over the past 2 decades, 150 students from Quebec have enrolled in colleges in Ontario and the United States every year.

In the spring of 1987, the Université du Québec decided to proceed with plans for a program in chiropractic. Another task force was formed between the Université du Québec and the Order of Chiropractors of Quebec, which resulted in an opinion that favored the opening of a doctoral program in chiropractic. Additionally the study recommended a 5-year course of study on a university campus. With the approval of the university officials, a request was forwarded to the Minister of Education of Higher Education and Science for funding. In November 1992 the Quebec Minister of Education of Higher Education and Science officially announced the opening of a university doctoral program in chiropractic at the Université du Québec a Trois Rivières.

In September 1993, 45 students enrolled in the doctoral program in chiropractic. For this first year, courses were given in existing university buildings, with construction beginning in 1994 on a new building to be dedicated to chiropractic studies. The first Université du Québec a Trois Rivières D.C.s will graduate in 1998.

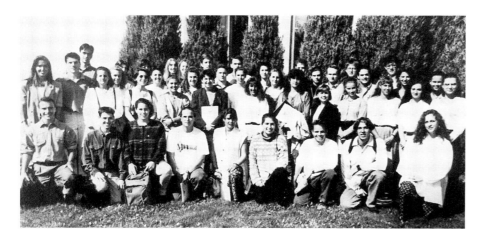

In September 1993, the first class of the College of Chiropractic, University of Quebec at Trois Rivières matriculated.

Courtesy Ordre des Chiropracticiens du Québec, Ville D'Anjou, Quebec.

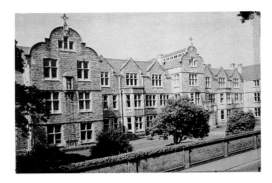

An exterior view circa 1990 of the Anglo-European College of Chiropractic, Bournemouth England.

Courtesy Anglo-European College of Chiropractic, Bournemouth, England.

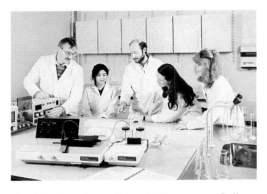

An interior view of Anglo-European College of Chiropractic's physiology lab, circa 1993.

Courtesy Anglo-European College of Chiropractic, Bournemouth, England.

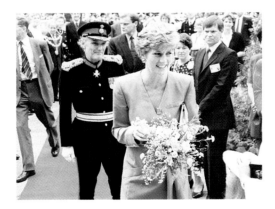

In 1991 Her Royal Highness Princess Diana agreed to become the Patron of the Anglo-European College of Chiropractic.

Courtesy Anglo-European College of Chiropractic, Bournemouth, England.

Anglo-European College of Chiropractic

The Anglo-European College of Chiropractic (AECC) is the only college in Europe offering a university validated 5-year full-time degree course. It is also the only European course accredited by the European CCE and has reciprocity with Australia and the United States of America. It is the flagship of the European Chiropractors' Union and as such has strong links with the profession in Europe.

The college was founded in 1965 in a small house in the centre of Bournemouth, the premier seaside resort in Southern England. At the first graduation ceremony there were only 2 graduates. The college grew rapidly, and the house next door was purchased for future expansion. However, in order to develop the course offerings to degree standards, significant investment in facilities had to be made, and in 1981 AECC moved to its current location, the former Boscombe Convent.

The campus, set in attractive woodland surroundings close to the sea, comprises three buildings: the main building, college clinic, and assembly hall.

The Grade II-listed main building, constructed of Purbeck Stone, dates back to 1888. The character has been carefully preserved—even the ghost remains! It houses college administration, the research department, the Vilhelm Krause Library, faculty, classrooms, laboratories, and lecture theatres. Prosection facilities are presently under construction.

The convent chapel with its outstanding stained glass windows contains the Vilhelm Krause Library. The characteristics of the chapel remain intact and the amalgamation of impressive marble furnishings with the fine collection of library material provides an air of peace and tranquility for the students. Within Europe the library houses a unique collection of material, holding a stock of some 8500 books and periodicals and over 700 items of audiovisual and computer software.

The AECC has one of the finest research units in Europe, and all students are required to develop investigative skills during their undergraduate training. This takes the form of a project that requires critical thinking and the evaluation of scientific evidence.

The college clinic deals with an average of 30,000 outpatient visits per year, and students under close supervision, after passing their clinic entrance examination, put into practice their previous years of training. It contains modern diagnostic and treatment facilities as well as a sophisticated computerized appointment system. It has earned a reputation as a provider of high quality chiropractic care.

From 1987 the college assumed degree status with students qualifying after 4 years with BSc Chiropractic. In September 1993 the course was revalidated, and after successful completion of 4 years students are awarded BSc (Hons) Human Sciences (Chiropractic). However, to become a practicing chiropractor it is essential to complete successfully a fifth year as an intern in the college clinic in order to obtain the postgraduate diploma in chiropractic and to register with the appropriate national chiropractic association.

In 1991, the AECC's twenty-fifth anniversary year, Her Royal Highness the Princess of Wales agreed to become Patron of the AECC. When she visited the campus, she was presented with an honorary fellowship, and she continues to take a keen interest in its fortunes and activities. Almost 400 students attend the college and over half of these are from overseas. The mixture of accents and cultures, together with the campus's picturesque setting, creates an exciting environment in which to work.

Institute Francais de Chiropractic

The French Chiropractic Association established a 1-year precollege course for baccalaureate level students for any of the established chiropractic colleges. In 1983, a 5-year course of study was developed, based on the 4-year course of study in the United States, and graduated its first students in 1987.

Macquarie University—Centre for Chiropractic and Osteopathy

First established in 1959, the Sydney College of Chiropractic was founded by Alfred Kaufman, D.O., D.C., Ph.D., as a private college with a 4-year course curriculum. In 1978 the program was expanded to a 5-year curriculum with a unique university "end-on" model of subject sequencing.

The course was coconducted by 2 institutions, Sydney College of Chiropractic and a local university. During the initial 3 years, students enrolled concurrently in a university working towards a bachelor of science degree, majoring in anatomy, and in the Sydney College of Chiropractic program in Principles of Chiropractic and Technic. With the completion of the initial 3-year program, students were awarded the bachelor of science degree. The final 2 years of study involved diagnostics, therapeutics, and clinical training.

In July 1990 the Sydney College of Chiropractic merged with Macquarie University and became the Centre for Chiropractic Studies within the Macquarie University. Graduates earn the Master of Science with a Specialty in Chiropractic.

Royal Melbourne Institute of Technology—School of Chiropractic and Osteopathy

The Royal Melbourne Institute of Technology (RMIT) is one of Australia's oldest educational institutions and one of its newest universi-

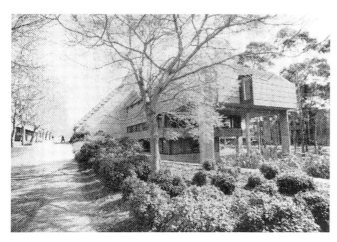

An exterior view of Macquarie University in Summer Hill, New South Wales, where the Centre for Chiropractic Studies is located.

Courtesy Macquarie University, Summerhill, New South Wales, Australia.

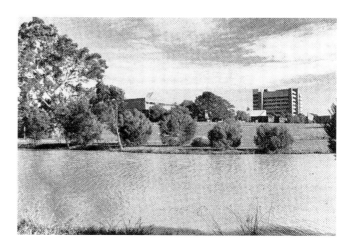

An exterior view of the Philip Institute of Technology, School of Chiropractic and Osteopathy, circa 1992, located in Bundoora, Victoria, Australia.

Courtesy Philip Institute of Technology, Bun doora, Victoria, Australia.

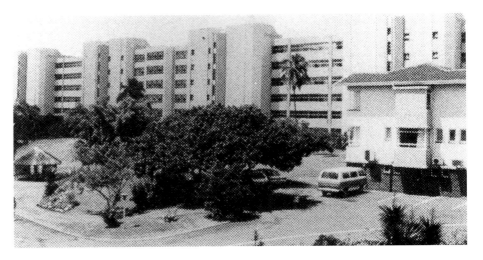

An exterior view, circa 1991, of the Technikon Natal in Durban, South Africa, where a Masters Diploma in Technology with a Specialty in Chiropractic is offered.

Courtesy Technikon Natal, Durban, South Africa.

ties. RMIT first opened its doors to students in 1887, achieving university status in 1992. The School of Chiropractic and Osteopathy was established in 1981 in the then Phillip Institute of Technology.

The School conducts undergraduate programs in both chiropractic and osteopathy and has a range of master programs by coursework, as well as higher degrees by research. The streams available within the Master by Coursework include sports chiropractic, paediatrics, musculoskeletal management, acupuncture, medical acupuncture, clinical rehabilitation, and rehabilitation counselling.

Chiropractic education is broad so that the future chiropractor not only masters this healing art but is also fully cognizant of professional limitations. The student is presented with a holistic view of health care and made aware of the chiropractor's responsibility to other members of the health team and to the community. Following a 4-year course of study, graduates earn a bachelor of applied science, specialty in chiropractic; then following their internship study, they receive a master of science with a specialty in chiropractic.

The school is a member institution fully accredited by the Australian Council on Chiropractic and Osteopathic Education. Graduates are eligible for registration in all Australian states, New Zealand, and many overseas jurisdictions.

Technikon Natal

A 5-year degree course leading to a master's in technology with a specialty in chiropractic was initiated in 1989. The first class contained 33 students.

Chukyo College of Chiropractic

Chukyo College was established in 1974 as Chukyo Chiropractic Research Center with Masanori Murai as director. It was inaugurated as Chukyo Chiropractic Private School in 1976; then in 1979 it was established as Chukyo College of Chiropractic in Nakamura-ku in Nagoya. Shingo Fukinbara, a Palmer College graduate, was appointed president. At this point the course was 2 to 3 years for licensed students.

In 1980 Chukyo College signed a sister-college affiliation with Life Chiropractic College in Georgia, and the following year established its alumni association, the Chukyo Chiropractor's Club, and held the first International Postgraduation Seminar, with Dr. George Goodheart, D.C., as lecturer.

In 1982 Chukyo College began technical cooperation for applied kinesiology between the college and Dr. Goodheart and David Walker, D.C. Contracts were exchanged, and Drs. Goodheart and Walker were installed as Professors Emeritus.

In 1984 Chukyo College began a 5-year chiropractic education for new high school graduates, and Kentaro Takagi, a Professor Emeritus at Nagoya City University assumed the presidency of Chukyo College of Chiropractic. The following year a larger campus was constructed at Tenpaku-ku, Nagoya, and the college moved to its new campus.

In 1987 the fifth-year students of Chukyo College were sent to the United States for short-term study abroad. Since then, study abroad for 3 months has been made every year. The students attended 297 hours of anatomy and dissection courses and obtained credits for the first time in the history of chiropractic colleges in Japan. Chiropractic students must pass an examination given by the All Nippon Chiropractor's Association (ANCA) prior to graduation and licensure. Because Japan does not recognize or regulate chiropractic, all licensure is intraprofessional.

In March 1989 Chukyo College of Chiropractic held its first commencement with five graduates of the 5-year course. Chukyo College has graduated 28 students since then. On September 23, 1990, Kentaro Takagi died and was succeeded as president by the former managing director, Masanori Murai.

Along with 12 other chiropractic organizations, college officials helped form the Chiropractic Federation of Japan (CJF) on November 25, 1992. Some 7000 members now belong to the CJF, including 60 graduates of colleges in the United States. Chukyo College of Chiropractic has proven itself to be dedicated to improving the chiropractic curriculum in Japan and is determined to reach the educational level of chiropractic colleges in the United States.

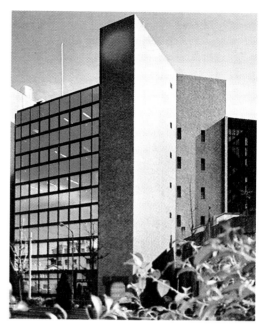

An exterior view of the building in Nagoya, Japan in which classes of Chukyo College of Chiropractic were first held.

Courtesy Chukyo College of Chiropractic, Nagoya, Japan.

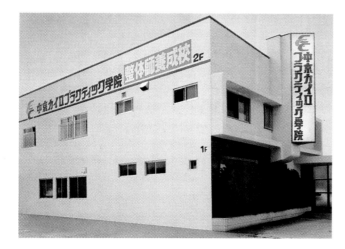

The campus of Chukyo College of Chiropractic, circa 1993.

Courtesy Chukyo College of Chiropractic, Nagoya, Japan.

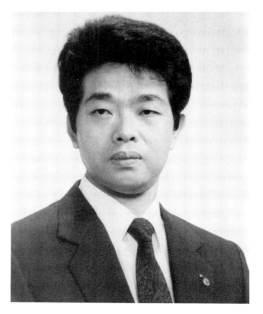

Masanari Murai, President of Chukyo College of Chiropractic.

Courtesy Chukyo College of Chiropractic, Nagoya, Japan.

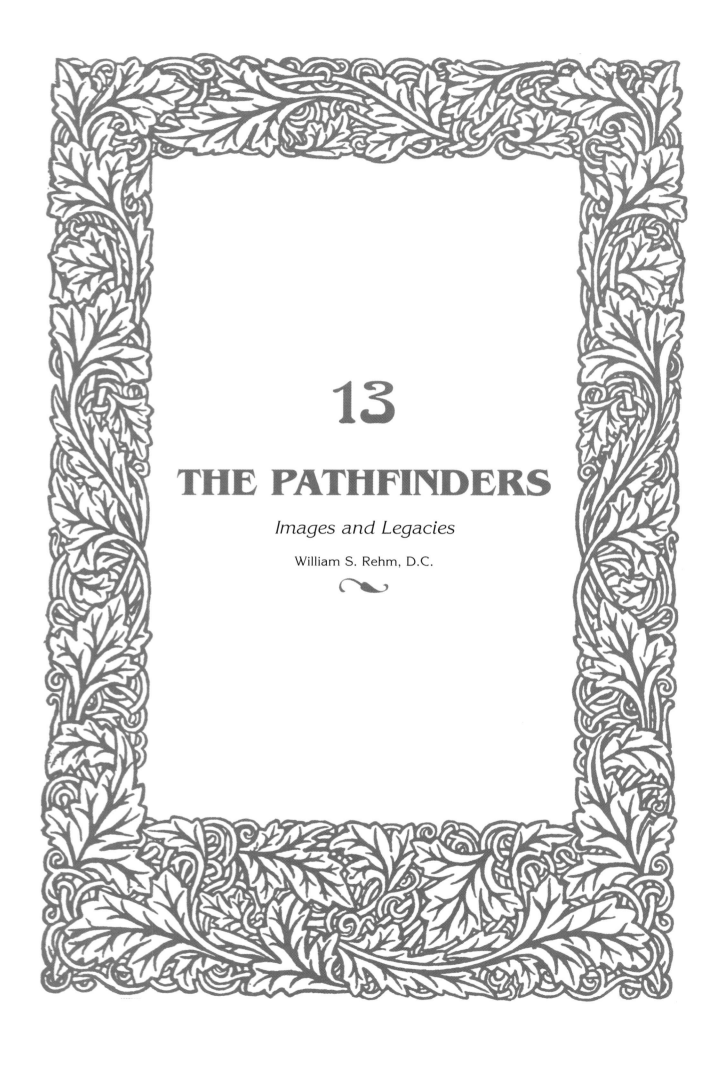

13

THE PATHFINDERS

Images and Legacies

William S. Rehm, D.C.

C hiropractic was under siege. Ad hominem attacks by organized medicine grew in frequency and ferocity: "Chiropractic was a fraud whose adherents preyed on an unsuspecting public . . . . These were self-styled 'doctors' lacking any medical training or ability . . . . Motivated only by greed, they advanced an unproven theory and treatment that was worthless at best, and probably dangerous."

Influenced by steady doses of such ritual condemnation, legislatures were reluctant to grant even limited recognition of the "cult." Eradication was tried in several jurisdictions by jailing the perpetrator for any perceived encroachment into the medical domain, which could be anything. In one extreme case, an offending chiropractor was charged with being "about to practice medicine without a license." The threat of arrest caused many chiropractors to be fearful. In larger cities and towns "quack hunting" was encouraged by an unsympathetic press.

Such was the situation during much of chiropractic's first quarter-century from 1895 to 1920. Organized medicine's boycott, fueled as it would be for years by the pen of the American Medical Association's self-righteous Morris Fishbein, M.D., seemed to be having success.

To survive, chiropractic would need to shed its parochial tendencies and, in fact, follow the lead of its chief tormentor. The profession recognized the imperative to organize, to build measurable financial strength, and to use its ever-increasing public support.

The profession's emerging leadership, far from the "cultist, ignorant lout" perception painted by detractors, would become its source of strength and stability.

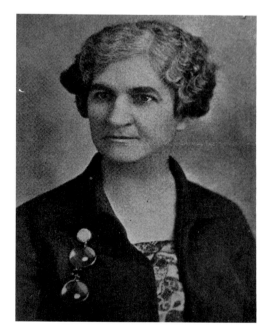

Sylva L. Ashworth, an important early chiropractic leader from Nebraska, was instrumental in passing Nebraska chiropractic legislation. She was an effective leader on the national level also because she effectively bridged the conservative and liberal camps of the profession.

Courtesy Cleveland Chiropractic University, Kansas City, Missouri.

SYLVA L. ASHWORTH (1874-1958)

Anticipating the women's movement of a future generation, Sylva Ashworth achieved prominence as a practitioner, businesswoman, and political activist. In 1910, at age 36 and while a single parent with four children, she took her doctor of chiropractic degree from the Palmer School of Chiropractic (PSC). Although a self-professed "straight," she became an effective bridge between the conservative Palmer faction and the profession's more liberal wing represented by the National Chiropractic Association (NCA). She was the only woman ever elected president of a national chiropractic society in the United States, the Universal Chiropractors' Association (UCA) in 1926. She was a founder of the International Chiropractic Congress (1928), the NCA (1930), and the Chi-

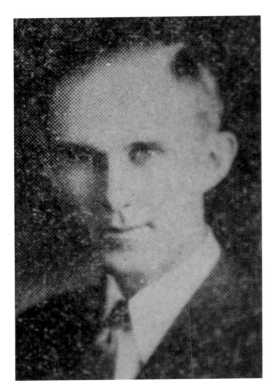

Homer G. Beatty, author of Anatomical Adjustive Technique, *served as president of the University of Natural Healing Arts in Denver, until his death in 1951.*

From *The National Chiropractic Journal,* February 1935.

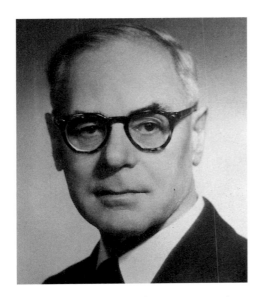

William A. Budden, a former economics professor, purchased and reorganized the Western States Chiropractic College and served as its president until his death in 1954. Dr. Budden also championed broad educational reforms for the chiropractic profession.

Courtesy Western States Chiropractic College, Portland, Oregon.

ropractic Research Foundation (1944). In 1938 she became the first woman to be elected a fellow of the International College of Chiropractors.

Dr. Ashworth enjoyed astonishing success in her Lincoln, Nebraska, practice of 44 years and served as president of the Nebraska Board of Chiropractic Examiners for many years. She was a tireless leader in her state to secure and protect chiropractic legislation and, nationally, to standardize professional education. She was always appreciated for her generous support of charitable causes both within chiropractic and her community. Sylva Ashworth gave stature to women in early chiropractic and was the inspiration for her daughter Ruth to follow her in the profession.

HOMER G. BEATTY (1897-1951)

For a quarter of a century Homer G. Beatty was regarded as one of the profession's foremost masters of diversified technique. He authored his classic text, *Anatomical Adjustive Technique,* in 1939 and was one of chiropractic's most popular lecturers and teachers. Educated at Kansas State University before World War I, he studied under Dr. Willard Carver and graduated from the Carver College of Chiropractic in Oklahoma City in 1922. In 1923 he was named dean and director of technique of Carver's new Colorado Chiropractic University in Denver and became president a year later.

In the mid-1930s, Dr. Beatty led the reorganization of the Denver institution as the non-profit University of Natural Healing Arts, which also granted degrees in naturopathy and physical therapy. He remained as president of the university until his death in 1951. By that time he had initiated discussions with the University of Denver toward academic affiliation, a prospect still 2 decades ahead of its time for chiropractic institutions. The University of Natural Healing Arts, later renamed Rocky Mountain Chiropractic College, was merged with the National College of Chiropractic in 1965.

WILLIAM A. BUDDEN (1884-1954)

A onetime economics professor at the University of Alberta, W.A. Budden changed careers at the age of 38 to become one of the foremost and most progressive educators in chiropractic for 3 decades. During the proprietary school era of the 1930s, he was one of the first to speak out for standards in chiropractic education equal to the other health professions. After receiving his chiropractic degree from the National College of Chiropractic, Chicago, in 1924, his background in higher education became a natural springboard in his new profession. Named academic dean at National College of Chiropractic, he was responsible for expanding the curriculum at that broad-scope institution to 4 collegiate years. In January 1929 Budden purchased the financially troubled Pacific Chiropractic College in Portland. Tracing its roots from 1904, the Pacific College was the profession's second oldest institution. Within 3 years, he guided the reorganization of Pacific as the non-profit Western States Chiropractic College, where he served as president for the rest of his life.

W.A. Budden felt strongly that accreditation of chiropractic education had to become the first priority for the profession. This would mean serious upgrading of standards and divesting of private ownership. It was an unpopular message. He was equally outspoken in his belief that chiropractic colleges should prepare students to meet the challenge instead of mounting opposition to state basic science laws being enacted during the 1920s and 1930s. He was always a strong advocate for the broadest possible training in diagnosis and treatment modalities to best prepare the chiropractic physician.

In 1937 Western States was again reorganized under the trusteeship of the Health Research Foundation, a step Budden felt necessary for continuity and stability. Educational standards at Western States were gradually strengthened. Within a decade, a model 4-year course with 9 months of instruction each year was offered, and in 1953, the college began to require 2 years of college for entrance. Western States became the first college accredited by the NCA's Council on Chiropractic Education. Dr. Budden was president of the Council on Chiropractic Education at the time of his death.

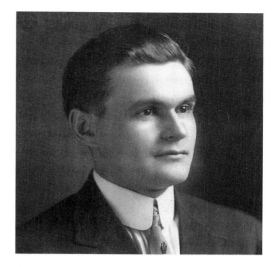

Steven J. Burich, a gifted teacher and administrator, was one of the four founders of Lincoln Chiropractic College in Indianapolis, Indiana.

Courtesy Palmer College of Chiropractic Archives, Davenport, Iowa.

STEVEN J. BURICH (1887-1946)

Serious, scholarly, but affable, he was a born teacher swept into celebrity by some of the most irresistible events in chiropractic history. A high school chemistry instructor in Milwaukee, he applied for a teaching position at the PSC in June 1912. Simultaneously, he taught chemistry and pursued a degree in chiropractic. S.J. Burich's duties at the PSC soon included teaching neurology, and for the next 13 years he seemed comfortably established as a favorite professor and student advisor. He authored one of the early "green book" texts and coauthored a second.

In August 1926 Burich became the last of five bright young professors at the PSC who resigned from the faculty over a period of several months. Four of the five, Burich, J.N. Firth, A.G. Hendricks, and H.E. Vedder, were instrumental in the founding of Lincoln Chiropractic College at Indianapolis, Indiana, during September 1926. Burich served as secretary and as a full-time professor at Lincoln for 20 years.

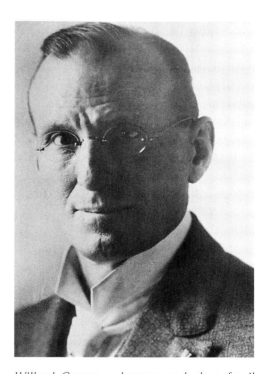

WILLARD CARVER (1866-1943)

Willard Carver, a friend and intimate of D.D. Palmer, was one of the first to learn of the discovery of chiropractic. Iowa-born, Carver graduated in law from Drake University and was a practicing attorney in the state for about 15 years. In 1906, after D.D. had permanently departed from the seat of chiropractic, Carver himself took a doctor of chiropractic degree, not from the PSC but from the Charles Ray Parker School of Chiropractic in Ottumwa. The same year, Carver and his business partner, L.L. Denny, opened a school in Oklahoma City bearing both their names. The Carver-Denny School of Chiropractic was incorporated as

Willard Carver, a lawyer and close family friend of "Old Dad Chiro," was an important figure who influenced a number of early chiropractic leaders. Dr. Carver's lectures and books added a scientific dimension to the new profession. A prolific writer, "The Constructor" established four separate schools of chiropractic in Oklahoma, Colorado, New York, and Washington, DC.

Courtesy Palmer College of Chiropractic Archives, Davenport, Iowa.

Carver Chiropractic College in 1908 and became one of chiropractic's leading broad-scope institutions. He presided over four separate chiropractic schools at the same time in Oklahoma, Colorado, New York, and Washington, D.C. All the schools were eventually merged with other institutions.

In 1907, when the new Oklahoma legislature convened for the first time, Carver and his associates introduced the first bill to legalize chiropractic in the state and provide for a board of examiners. However, the legislature adjourned before the bill could come out of committee. It would be 14 years before chiropractic finally attained legal status in Oklahoma. For years Carver would be called upon to testify in legislative hearings in Oklahoma and other states. He was the author of 18 books, his signature text being *Carver's Chiropractic Analysis,* first published in 1909.

Although he and B.J. Palmer remained polar opposites in almost every respect throughout their careers, they managed a show of personal reconciliation shortly before Carver's death. In 1922 he was acclaimed one of the young state's "ten greatest Oklahomans" by a popular vote.

CARL S. CLEVELAND (1896-1982)

Carl S. Cleveland presided over two colleges for the better part of 60 years, the longest tenure in the history of chiropractic education. C.S., as he was always known to his contemporaries, married Ruth Ashworth, the daughter of chiropractic pioneer Sylva Ashworth, in the year both graduated from the PSC, 1917. In 1922 they founded the Central Chiropractic College in Kansas City, Missouri, 5 years before chiropractic was legalized in Missouri. The college was later renamed Cleveland Chiropractic College.

Dr. Cleveland had also acquired privileges to teach human anatomy by dissection even though chiropractic had not yet been legalized in Missouri. He purchased the Ratledge College of Chiropractic, Los Angeles, in 1950 and renamed it Cleveland Chiropractic College of Los Angeles the following year. Dr. Ruth Ashworth Cleveland (1895 to 1975) who had taught gross anatomy, resigned from the college faculty in 1942 to enter private practice. Their son, Carl S., Jr., and grandson, Carl S., III, followed to the presidency of the Cleveland institutions, which can lay claim to being the fourth oldest continuous chiropractic college, via Ratledge of 1908, and thousands of alumni. The Cleveland Colleges of Kansas City and Los Angeles merged into a single corporate entity in 1992, the Cleveland Chiropractic University.

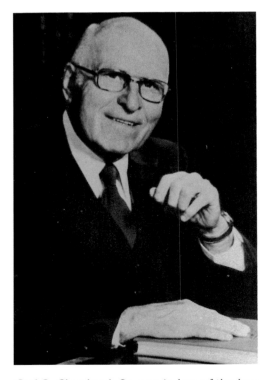

Carl S. Cleveland, Sr., son-in-law of the honored Dr. Sylva Ashworth, founded the Cleveland Chiropractic College in Kansas City, Missouri, in 1922 and in 1951 absorbed the Ratledge Chiropractic College in Los Angeles. He was at the helm of the two institutions for 60 years, the longest tenure in chiropractic education.

Courtesy Cleveland Chiropractic University.

JOHN S. CLUBINE (1884-1956)

Dr. John S. Clubine was a 1919 graduate of the Canadian Chiropractic College, Hamilton, Ontario, Canada. Dr. Clubine was associated with the two chiropractic colleges that were established in Toronto. In 1920, with Dr. J.A. Cudmore, he founded the Toronto Chiropractic College. Then in 1945, after retiring from his 25-year practice in Toronto, he helped organize the Canadian Memorial Chiropractic College and was elected its first director, serving for 1 year.

Dr. Clubine also served as president and secretary of the Ontario Chiropractic Association from 1927 to 1931 and was reelected president in 1936, serving continuously until 1945. As representative to the NCA at its Toronto convention in 1938, he unveiled the plans for the Port Perry monument honoring the founder of the chiropractic profession, Daniel David Palmer. The assembly hall of the Canadian Memorial Chiropractic College is dedicated to his memory.

ANDREW P. DAVIS (1835-1915)

Credentialed in both the allopathic and homeopathic medical schools, A.P. Davis pursued virtually every known alternative healing school and associated himself with the new manipulative schools in their formative years. He went to Kirksville, Missouri, in 1896 to study with the founder of osteopathy, Andrew Taylor Still, and a year later began formal instruction with Daniel David Palmer at the latter's School and Cure in Davenport, Iowa. Palmer listed him among the graduates of 1898.

Retaining his M.D. credentials, Davis continued to advocate both osteopathy and chiropractic even as he would also call himself a "neuro-ophthalmologist" and later a "neuropath." Although his "dabbling" in other therapies would earn the disdain of D.D. Palmer, he issued a notarized affidavit in 1903 stating in effect that Palmer had *not* "stolen" his ideas from Still's osteopathy. This statement would carry considerable weight in later legal battles as the profession fought for political and legislative survival. Davis was an itinerant who set up neuropathic institutes in several locations before World War I. His 1909 text, *Neuropathy,* was a compilation of the various therapeutic methods he had studied and practiced.

FRANK E. DEAN (1891-1958)

Frank E. Dean, a 1917 graduate of New York's Standard Institute of Chiropractic, was president of the Columbia Institute of Chiropractic for 39 years. When he founded the Columbia Institute in New York City in 1919, which is believed to have been the first non-proprietary school in the profession, chiropractic had no legal status in New York. Therefore the school's non-profit charter was granted by the state of Delaware. In 1946 Dean was named director of education and dean of a branch school in Baltimore, soon chartered independently as the Columbia College of Chiropractic. Baltimore's Columbia College was known for its strong emphasis on the basic and clinical sciences and its faculty, which included professors from area colleges and universities. It was among the first chiropractic colleges to require 2 years of college experience for entrance.

Dr. Frank Dean's mild-mannered demeanor was in sharp contrast to the charismatic leadership of many of his contemporaries and almost masked his many impressive accomplishments. Before the age of 28, he had undertaken studies in medicine at Warsaw and Heidelberg universities and at the Imperial Institute of Russia, and had traveled extensively to observe native healing practices. His early background undoubtedly

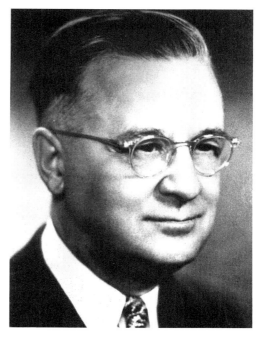

John S. Clubine, a Canadian, founded the Toronto College of Chiropractic and in 1945 was a founding member of Canadian Memorial Chiropractic College, Toronto.

Courtesy Canadian Memorial Chiropractic College, Toronto, Ontario, Canada.

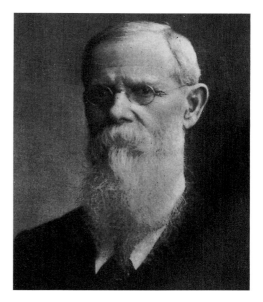

Andrew P. Davis, a homeopath, allopath, and osteopath, studied osteopathy with A.T. Still and chiropractic with D.D. Palmer, graduating in 1898. Dr. Davis' experience in both professions would help establish a crucial legal distinction in a 1907 landmark case. He then established his own system of health and healing that he called neuropathy.

Courtesy Palmer College of Chiropractic Archives, Davenport Iowa.

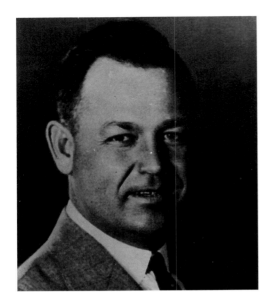

James R. Drain, a native of Kansas and a 1912 graduate of the Palmer School of Chiropractic, was instrumental in ensuring the passage of the first chiropractic legislation in the United States in Kansas. He later was president of Texas Chiropractic College, San Antonio, for 34 years.

Courtesy Palmer College of Chiropractic Archives, Davenport, Iowa.

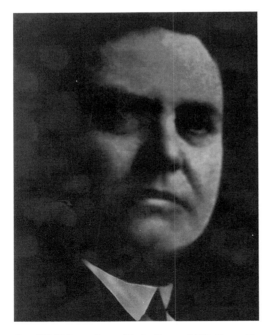

Lee W. Edwards, with both an M.D. from the University of Nebraska and a D.C. from the Palmer School of Chiropractic, served as a chiropractic expert witness in more trials for arrested colleagues than any other chiropractor.

Courtesy Palmer College of Chiropractic Archives, Davenport Iowa.

influenced the curriculum of the Columbia schools, which embraced many styles of adjusting and manipulative techniques. As his schedule permitted, Dean lectured on diagnosis and manual techniques. (He commuted regularly by train between New York and Baltimore.)

In 1954, a time when many chiropractic colleges were experiencing postwar depression after the GI Bill student boon, Columbia College was merged with the Columbia Institute. The New York Chiropractic College of today is a direct descendant of Dr. Frank E. Dean's Columbia Institute of Chiropractic and has legitimate claim as the oldest chiropractic college in the East.

JAMES R. DRAIN (1891-1958)

As a 20-year-old resident of Scott City, Kansas, in 1911, he was one of the curious spectators who watched and listened as pioneer chiropractor I.B. Hall was tried for violating the state's medical practice laws. Dr. Hall's acquittal by the jury was not unexpected as his defense team again and again repelled the state's charges with brilliance. The Hall trial was precedent setting for the profession in Kansas. For young James Riddle Drain, then a college student, it was the expert testimony of Dr. B.J. Palmer that most intrigued and would lead him to the PSC in Davenport, Iowa. Receiving his D.C. in May 1912, he returned to Scott City and practiced there until 1919. He participated actively to help win the first chiropractic law in the country, in Kansas in 1913. In 1919 he became involved with the Texas Chiropractic College (TCC) at San Antonio (founded in 1908), and with others purchased the school's charter in March 1920. Named president of TCC, he remained in the post for 34 years.

Bankruptcy was averted during the early days of the Great Depression because of the extraordinary personal sacrifices of Drs. Drain, C.B. Loftin, and H.E. Weiser, and because of Drain's administrative talents. Texas College became a professionally owned, non-profit corporation in 1948. With his warmth, soothing smile, and supreme self-confidence, it is said that James R. Drain rallied the entire profession through many difficult times. His treatment of chiropractic philosophy made him a favorite convention speaker, and he authored two books on the subject—*Chiropractic Thoughts*, 1927 and 1946, and *Man Tomorrow*, 1949. Twelve members of his immediate family followed him in the profession.

LEE W. EDWARDS (1870-1947)

Lee Edwards successfully combined medical and chiropractic practice in Omaha, Nebraska, for many years. He earned a medical degree from the University of Nebraska in 1902 and his doctor of chiropractic degree from the PSC in 1911. As an expert witness for the UCA, he is believed to have testified at more trials of arrested colleagues than any other individual. He also gave testimony for chiropractic before most of the legislative bodies in the United States and Canada during the pre-World War II period when many chiropractic licensing battles were waged and won. Dr. Edwards was the last president of the UCA when that body merged with the American Chiropractic Association (ACA) in 1930 to form the NCA.

FRANK W. ELLIOTT (1887-1976)

Dr. Frank Elliott was a longtime and trusted associate of Dr. B.J. Palmer. A cousin of Mabel Palmer, he was the first registrar and business manager of the PSC and later a vice president.

Frank Elliott grew up in Kansas and attended Southwestern College. He received his doctor of chiropractic degree from the PSC in 1911 and immediately became connected with the school, where he would remain for 27 years. He was an early leader of the UCA, holding the offices of treasurer and business manager. In 1922 he became general manager of the pioneer Palmer-owned radio station, WOC, in Davenport, and was an organizer of the National Association of Broadcasters (NAB). He was named president of the NAB in 1926 and sat on its first board of directors. He was also vice president and general manager of the Central Broadcasting Company, the operator of radio stations WOC-Davenport and WHO-Des Moines. From 1919 to 1935 he served in the Iowa State Assembly.

Dr. Elliott resigned from the PSC in 1937 and entered private practice in Denver. He was a director of the Colorado Chiropractic Association for 27 years and served as secretary-treasurer for 9 years.

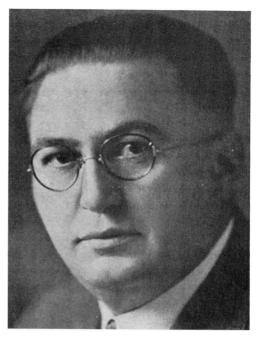

Frank W. Elliott, a native of Kansas, was a trusted associate of B.J. Palmer as registrar and later business manager of PSC. Dr. Elliott was also general manager of Palmer's WOC radio station and an organizer of the National Association of Broadcasters.

Courtesy Palmer College of Chiropractic Archives, Davenport, Iowa.

JAMES N. FIRTH (1886-1964)

Dr. James N. Firth was a popular teacher, author, and lecturer whose disagreements with B.J. Palmer helped spark one of the profession's great early controversies. Having been a public school teacher and principal in Michigan for 3 years, the 23-year-old Firth enrolled at the PSC in 1909 and graduated a year later in August 1911. After a year in practice in Manistee, Michigan, he was persuaded to return to the PSC as a temporary instructor of symptomology, but his association with the school would continue until September 1925. It was Firth who originally expanded the concept of chiropractic diagnosis; his 1914 *Textbook on Chiropractic Symptomology* was later retitled *Chiropractic Diagnosis* and revised five times through 1948.

Faculty unrest had been building since August 1924 when the PSC began marketing a device called the neurocalometer. In August 1925 two popular faculty members, Drs. E.A. Thompson and A.E. Hendricks, resigned to pursue other interests. Dr. Firth submitted his resignation on September 1, 1925, to establish a practice in Chicago and conduct a lecture tour for Dr. Leo Spears of Denver. Two more faculty resignations followed in 1926, Drs. Harry Vedder and Steve Burich.

What had begun as open dissatisfaction with B.J. Palmer resulted in the establishment of a competing school, Lincoln College of Chiropractic. The school opened in Indianapolis, Indiana, in September 1926 as a non-profit institution offering a course of instruction based on "diversity

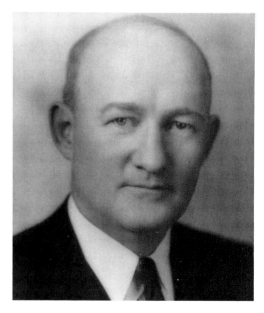

James N. Firth, one of the four founders of Lincoln Chiropractic College, Indianapolis, later served as its president. Dr. Firth authored the Textbook on Chiropractic Symptomology.

Courtesy Palmer College of Chiropractic Archives, Davenport, Iowa.

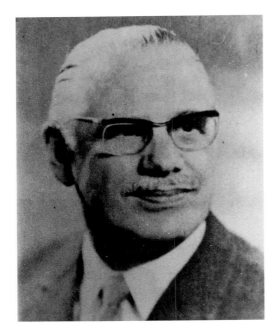

Henri J. Gillet, born in Canada and a 1928 Palmer School of Chiropractic graduate, practiced for 48 years in Brussels, Belgium, when his father was the country's first chiropractor. Dr. Gillet would become one of the most influential chiropractic researchers of his era.
Courtesy William Rehm, Baltimore, Maryland.

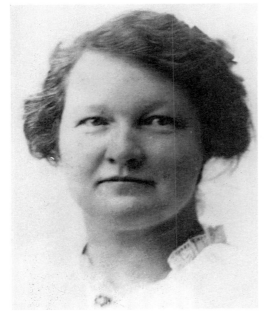

Almeda J. Haldeman, believed to be the first chiropractor to practice in Canada, influenced and inspired son, Joshua Haldeman, D.C., and grandson, Scott Haldeman, D.C, M.D., Ph.D.
Courtesy Scott Haldeman, Santa Ana, California.

in chiropractic technique and philosophy." Its first administration consisted of Harry E. Vedder, president; James N. Firth, vice president; Steven J. Burich, secretary; and Arthur E. Hendricks, treasurer. In 1940 after the retirement of Dr. Vedder, James Firth became the college's second president. Dr. Firth retired in 1954.

ARTHUR L. FORSTER (1884-1931)

Dr. Arthur L. Forster, a graduate in medicine from the University of Illinois, joined the faculty of the National School of Chiropractic about 1912 and organized the first formal instruction in human dissection in any chiropractic institution. For several years he conducted investigations by autopsy into the relationship of the spinal nerves with various pathologies. The result was his 1915 text, *Principles and Practice of Spinal Adjustment,* revised several times and translated into three foreign languages. One of Forster's elaborate spinal dissections was displayed for years at Chicago's Museum of Science and Industry. Forster also wrote *Practice of Chiropractic* (1922) and *The White Mark* (1921), "an editorial history of chiropractic." He edited the *National College Journal* for many years.

About 1916, when Dr. William Schulze purchased the National School, Dr. Forster was named secretary and general manager, but continued to teach courses in diagnosis.

HENRI J. GILLET (1907-1989)

Dr. Henri Gillet, a Canadian-born, American-trained chiropractor who practiced for 48 years in Brussels, Belgium, is noted for his extensive clinical research on vertebral fixations. He graduated from the PSC in 1928 and did postgraduate study at Lincoln Chiropractic College in 1931. Gillet founded the Belgian Chiropractic Association, the European Chiropractors' Union, and the *European Chiropractic Bulletin,* for which he served as longtime editor. He first published *Belgian Notes on Fixation* in 1951 in collaboration with Dr. M. Liekens, which went through ten editions. Dr. Gillet presented his research on fixation of vertebral mobility, its diagnosis, and its correction in lectures throughout the world.

His father, Jules Gillet, was the first chiropractor in Belgium. A brother, Marcel Gillet, also pioneered in the profession in Belgium.

ALMEDA J. HALDEMAN (1877-1948)

Dr. Almeda Haldeman personified the dauntless zeal of the pioneer. She was one of the first women to enter the chiropractic profession and is believed to have been the first chiropractor to practice in Canada. Widowed, she was left with two young children on the wilderness of the western prairie.

Almeda Haldeman received her diploma from one of the first offshoot schools of D.D. Palmer, Dr. E.W. Lynch's Chiropractic School and Cure at Montevideo, Minnesota, in 1905. In 1907 Almeda and John Haldeman moved to Canada to homestead in Herbert, Saskatchewan. Her husband died only months after filing for the homestead. Virtually destitute, Almeda managed to supplement her small income from chiropractic by teaching in the local schools. Later, as conditions improved, she resumed her practice full-time.

Almeda's son, the late Joshua N. Haldeman, D.C., was a prominent and prosperous chiropractor for 40 years in Regina, Saskatchewan, and finally in Pretoria, South Africa. Her grandson, Scott Haldeman, D.C., Ph.D., M.D., has become one of the most prominent chiropractic and medical researchers in the United States.

GEORGE E. HARIMAN (1893-1977)

Dr. George Hariman, born in Greece, emigrated to the United States in 1909 and settled in Chicago. Having studied English in evening classes, he enrolled at the National School of Chiropractic and received his doctor of chiropractic degree in 1914. He practiced in Chicago until 1919, when he moved to North Dakota to take charge of a sanitarium. Dr. Hariman moved to Grand Forks, North Dakota, in 1924, where he established the Hariman Clinic. In 1928, he completed the 4-story Hariman Sanitorium and Hospital, believed to have been the first state-licensed chiropractic hospital.

Dr. Hariman participated in the preparation of the present chiropractic law in North Dakota, enacted in 1933. He served two terms as president of the state association and was delegate to the NCA and later the ACA for many years. As a director of the NCA, he helped negotiate the purchase of *The Journal* from private ownership to become the official journal of the NCA. Later he participated in the purchase of the first national headquarters of the ACA in Des Moines, Iowa. He was a founder of the NCA Council on Hospitals and Sanitariums and served as secretary for many years. He was a longtime member of the North Dakota Board of Chiropractic Examiners and the National Board of Chiropractic Examiners, and was a founder of the National Chiropractic Mutual Insurance Company. Dr. Hariman served as editor of the state association *Bulletin* for 46 years. In 1970 he authored and published *A History of the Evolution of Chiropractic Education*. After his death, the Hariman Hospital property was sold to the University of North Dakota.

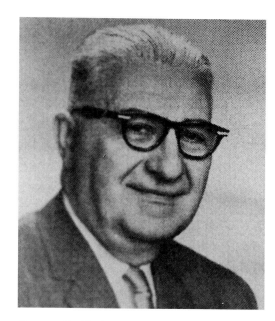

George E. Hariman, born in Greece and a 1914 graduate of National School of Chiropractic, was a hospital founder in North Dakota and a leader of the National Chiropractic Association.

From *The ACA Journal of Chiropractic,* December 1977.

HENRY C. HARRING (1888-1974)

Dr. Henry Harring began teaching when he was only 16, in the same one-room schoolhouse in rural Missouri he had attended as a child. After attending business school in Sedalia, Missouri, he moved to St. Louis where he eventually became interested in chiropractic. He enrolled in the St. Louis College of Chiropractic and graduated in 1918 at the age of 30. Deciding to become a teacher while still a chiropractic student, but feel-

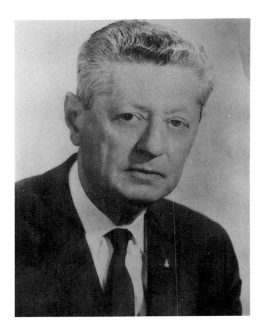

George H. Haynes was a 1936 graduate of Ratledge Chiropractic College and a biochemistry professor with Los Angeles College of Chiropractic. Dr. Haynes later served as president of Los Angeles College of Chiropractic.

Courtesy William Rehm, Baltimore, Maryland.

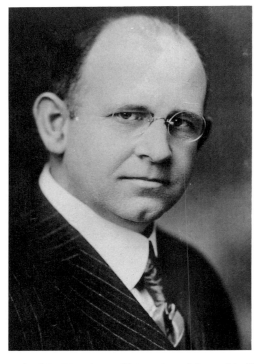

Alfred B. Hender, a University of Iowa Medical School graduate and obstetrician, became dean of the PSC faculty and valued fixture at the Palmer School of Chiropractic for more than 30 years.

Courtesy Palmer College of Chiropractic Archives, Davenport, Iowa.

ing the need for additional background, Harring enrolled at the St. Louis College of Physicians and Surgeons and received his M.D. in 1921.

Dr. Harring, with Drs. Robert Colyer and Oscar Schulte, founded the Missouri Chiropractic College in St. Louis in 1920. A proprietary school, he was its only president until he sold his interest in 1961 and retired from teaching. During those years, he taught anatomy, diagnosis, and technique, and was a popular lecturer at state and national chiropractic conventions.

The Missouri College was merged with the Logan College of Chiropractic, also in St. Louis, in 1964. Dr. Harring maintained a private practice in St. Louis until shortly before his death at the age of 86.

GEORGE H. HAYNES (1911-1979)

Dr. George Haynes, an educator deeply involved in the accreditation process, received his undergraduate degree from Loyola University, Los Angeles, in 1935, and a master of science from University of Southern California in 1938. He earned his D.C. from Ratledge College in Los Angeles in 1936. After several years in private practice, he joined the faculty of the Los Angeles College of Chiropractic (LACC) in 1947 as a biochemistry teacher. In 1950 he was named assistant dean of Los Angeles College of Chiropractic (LACC) and, in 1953, was named chief executive officer of the college. He was named president of LACC in 1974, retiring 2 years later with the title of president emeritus.

During his administration, LACC, then located in Glendale, grew economically and academically. The student body grew as other colleges merged with LACC, more faculty were hired, the clinics expanded, and its graduate school faculty began teaching nationwide. Dr. Haynes also presided over the certification of its library, the granting of a recognized B.A. degree, establishment of a fully functioning research department, and full accreditation by the Council on Chiropractic Education. In 1976 a new classroom building on the campus was dedicated in his honor.

Dr. Haynes was elected president of the NCA's Council on Chiropractic Education in 1954 and was largely responsible for early progress toward recognition by the United States Office of Education. He declined the council's presidency in 1972 but did chair a special advisory committee to the Commission on Accreditation.

ALFRED B. HENDER (1874-1943)

Dr. Alfred Hender was a 1901 graduate of the medical school of the University of Iowa, trained in general surgery and obstetrics. In 1905 he began to lecture on anatomy at the PSC and joined the faculty in 1910, occupying the chair of obstetrics. At the same time, he was granted a doctor of chiropractic degree. By 1912 he was listed as dean of the faculty.

Dr. Hender was credited with delivering more than 3700 babies, about a quarter of them within the Palmer campus community. He gave postgraduate courses in obstetrics, minor surgery, and emergency medical procedures both on campus and at field locations for some 20 years, and frequently testified at legislative hearings on behalf of the profession.

Two sons, two grandsons, and one great-grandson followed him in the chiropractic profession. Retiring in 1943, he was succeeded as dean of the PSC by his son, Dr. Herbert C. Hender.

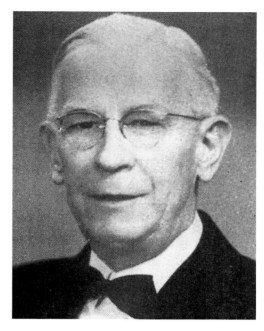

John A. Henderson, a 1911 graduate of the Robbins Chiropractic College, was closely identified with the founding of two chiropractic colleges in Canada and the first law regulating the profession in the province of Ontario.

Courtesy Canadian Memorial Chiropractic College, Toronto, Ontario, Canada.

JOHN A. HENDERSON (1883-1956)

John A. Henderson was closely identified with the founding of two chiropractic colleges in Canada and the first law regulating the profession in the province of Ontario. A 1911 graduate of the Robbins Chiropractic College, Sault Ste. Marie, Ontario, he was one of the first chiropractors in the city of Hamilton, where, in 1913, he helped establish the Canadian Chiropractic College with Dr. Ernest Duval. In 1924 he was elected president of the Drugless Physicians' Association of Ontario and worked to formulate the Drugless Practitioner's Act of 1925. The act provided a regulatory board for the major non-medical classifications—chiropractors, osteopaths, and physical therapists. Dr. Henderson served four terms as a member of the drugless practitioners' board and 20 years as the association's legislative director. (An independent chiropractic board was not established in Ontario until 1929.)

Dr. Henderson discontinued practice temporarily in 1945 to serve as the first registrar and business manager of the new Canadian Memorial Chiropractic College in Toronto, a position he held for 5 years. A new building erected on the campus in 1947 was dedicated in his honor.

ARTHUR G. HENDRICKS (1894-1962)

Dr. Arthur Hendricks, the youngest of the quartet who founded Lincoln Chiropractic College, served as that institution's third president from 1954 until its closing and merger with National College of Chiropractic in 1962. Following service at the U.S. Navy Ensign School in Chicago, he enrolled at the PSC in April 1919 and received his doctor of chiropractic degree a year later. He then accepted a faculty position, which he held for 5 years, teaching anatomy, orthopedy, gynecology, and symptomology. Hendricks resigned in May 1925 to pursue business interests in Florida.

During the summer of 1926, Dr. Hendricks joined his former PSC colleagues, J. Firth, S. Burich, and H. Vedder, as corporate treasurer of Lincoln College of Chiropractic in Indianapolis. In 1948, when fire destroyed one of the college buildings, Dr. Hendricks's administrative resourcefulness kept the school going with a minimum of disruption. In less than 3 months, he managed the purchase and renovation of a vacant school building in suburban Indianapolis, Keystone Hall, as quarters for first and second-year students.

Dr. Hendricks taught diagnosis and x-ray interpretation for many years. With Dr. Earl Rich, he coauthored *X-Ray Technique and Interpretation* in 1947. He succeeded Dr. James Firth as president of Lincoln in July 1954.

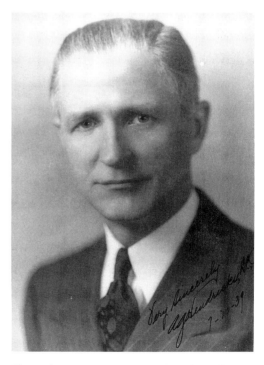

The administrative skills of Arthur G. Hendricks, one of the four founders of Lincoln Chiropractic College, saved the institution after a near-disastrous fire. He served as its last president from 1954 to 1962.

Courtesy Palmer College of Chiropractic Archives, Davenport, Iowa.

A. Earl Homewood, an original faculty member of Canadian Memorial Chiropractic College, was one of chiropractic's most respected and popular educators. As president of CMCC, he is credited with returning that financially struggling institution to solvency and guiding the development of its new campus.

Courtesy William Rehm, Baltimore, Maryland.

John F.A. Howard, founder of the National School of Chiropractic in 1906, was its president until 1914 when he sold his interest in the school to Dr. William Schulze.

Courtesy National College of Chiropractic, Lombard, Illinois.

A. EARL HOMEWOOD (1916-1990)

Dr. A.E. Homewood's retirement from the classroom in 1982 meant an opportunity to pursue his passion for teaching in a new setting, as a columnist and commentator in the chiropractic popular press. For more than 7 years, his by-line regularly observed the "state of the art," culled from his 37 years devoted to education and scholarship.

Born in Toronto, he was a 1942 graduate of Western States Chiropractic College and a Canadian naval veteran of World War II. Dr. Homewood joined the original faculty of the Canadian Memorial Chiropractic College (CMCC) in 1945 as an anatomy instructor. In 1952 he was named dean of faculty at CMCC and, in 1958, promoted to the office of president-dean, serving until illness forced him into retirement in 1961. Dr. Homewood was persuaded to return to the presidency of CMCC from 1967 to 1970, an eventful period which saw the college recover financial stability and construct a new campus. Between 1963 and 1967, he was associated with two other chiropractic institutions as both an administrator and teacher: Lincoln Chiropractic College and the LACC. He returned to LACC in 1970 as assistant dean and was named acting president in 1976. After a brief second retirement, Homewood was persuaded to return to his alma mater in 1979 as a professor by President H.J. Vear of Western States Chiropractic College, a member of CMCC's first graduating class.

Always a prolific writer for numerous professional journals, Dr. Homewood authored two classic books in the profession, *The Neurodynamics of the Vertebral Subluxation* and *The Chiropractor and the Law*. It is a little known fact that Dr. Homewood also earned a law degree in the late 1950s. He was secretary of the Council on Chiropractic Education for several years and had also served on its Commission on Accreditation.

JOHN F.A. HOWARD (1876-1954)

A native of Utah and a graduate of the state university, Dr. Howard was one of the last students to graduate under D.D. Palmer in Davenport. In 1906, with the full approval of the senior Palmer, Howard started the National School of Chiropractic in the same Davenport building where D.D. had begun his School and Cure. Two years later he moved the school to Chicago where he felt the clinical advantages were better. He authored one of the profession's classic early texts, the 6-volume *Encyclopedia of Chiropractic*.

Between 1910 and 1914 Dr. Howard brought onto the National School of Chiropractic faculty six physicians, including, as a business partner, William C. Schulze, M.D. The course of instruction was expanded to include human dissection and laboratory work in chemistry, microbiology, physiology, and pathology. Howard sold his interest in the school to his partner Schulze in 1914. After a brief interlude with another school venture, he returned to Utah and entered private practice.

FRED W. ILLI (1901-1983)

Dr. Fred Illi was a much-honored clinical scientist whose research at his Institute for the Study of the Statics and Dynamics of the Human Body in Geneva, Switzerland, earned acclaim throughout the chiropractic and scientific community.

Dr. Illi graduated from the Universal Chiropractic College, Pittsburgh, Pennsylvania, in 1927 and practiced in Germany for 5 years before going to Geneva in 1932. He began his investigations of spinal biomechanics in 1937. With Joseph Janse, he accelerated his research at the National College of Chiropractic dissection laboratories in Chicago, principally on the sacroiliac mechanism. He authored several books and innumerable articles on his research. Dr. Illi was the first chiropractor to utilize orthogonal radiography of the spinal column, and he pioneered the utilization of cineroentgenography to evaluate spinal and pelvic motion. His studies also produced several inventions to measure and define spinal biomechanics. Dr. Illi's best known work, *The Spinal Column: Lifeline of the Body,* was published by the National College of Chiropractic in 1950.

Dr. Illi participated in the fight for legal recognition in Switzerland, successfully concluding in 1939 and 1947, the first such formal recognition in Europe. He retired in 1975. His son, Claude B. Illi, D.C., continues his work and the institute.

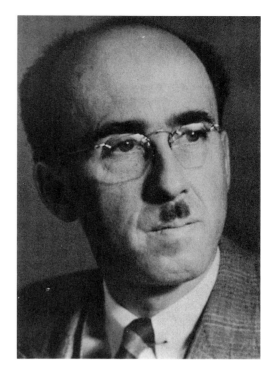

Fred W. Illi, a 1927 Universal Chiropractic College graduate, was a prominent Swiss chiropractor who pioneered research on cineroentgenology and spinal biomechanics at his Geneva Institute.

Courtesy William Rehm, Baltimore, Maryland.

JOSEPH JANSE (1909-1985)

Dr. Joseph Janse, born in Holland, settled in Utah and studied at the state university. Entering the National College of Chiropractic, Chicago, in 1935 and graduating in 1938, he literally bridged the gap from private proprietary to non-profit, professional ownership of that institution. By 1942 he was dean, and in 1945 was named the third president of National College of Chiropractic, which he would guide for the next 38 years.

He worked closely with John Nugent to establish the NCA's Council on Chiropractic Education, on which he served as president from 1959 to 1961. He had also helped organize the National Board of Chiropractic Examiners, the Federation of Chiropractic Licensing Boards, and several scientific councils in the profession. In the 1970s he provided crucial testimony to the Australian government as it considered establishing the world's first federally funded chiropractic institution.

The author of numerous scientific and technical papers, countless articles, and three textbooks, his interest in clinical research led to collaboration with Dr. Fred Illi of Geneva, Switzerland, on pioneering studies of the spine and pelvis. An accomplished anatomist, he instructed in the dissection laboratory at National College of Chiropractic for many years. Janse created the atmosphere for and conception of the *Journal of Manipulative and Physiological Therapeutics,* the profession's first scientific journal to be indexed in the National Library of Medicine's *Index Medicus.*

It was Dr. Janse's visionary leadership that led to construction of National College of Chiropractic's campus in suburban Lombard, Illinois. Occupied in 1963, it was the first all new campus in chiropractic since the early postwar era.

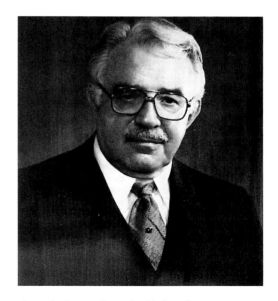

Joseph Janse, born in Holland, was to serve as president of the National School of Chiropractic for 38 years. Dr. Janse was a central figure who brought academic propriety and theoretical perspective to the profession. He became a prominent spokesman for the Council on Chiropractic Education.

Courtesy National College of Chiropractic, Lombard, Illinois.

CRAIG M. KIGHTLINGER (1881-1958)

One of chiropractic's most influential early leaders, Dr. Craig M. Kightlinger was a graduate pharmacist and had also earned a master of education degree from Valparaiso University prior to embarking on his later career. He graduated from the New Jersey College of Chiropractic in Newark, New Jersey, in 1917 and, in 1919, from the PSC with a Ph.C. degree. He founded Eastern Chiropractic College in Newark in 1919. Dr. Kightlinger then moved the school to New York City in 1923, renaming it Eastern Chiropractic Institute.

In 1944 Eastern Chiropractic Institute was merged with the Standard School of Chiropractic and the New York School of Chiropractic to form the non-profit and professionally owned Chiropractic Institute of New York. Dr. Kightlinger was named its first president. Because the institute was functioning in one of the last open, that is unlicensed states, school officials were subjected to occasional harassment. Such was the case in 1947 when Dr. Kightlinger and others were arrested and charged with operating a school of medicine without approval of the Department of Education of New York. A landmark court verdict subsequently ruled on the parameters of schools of medicine and chiropractic, thus allowing the institute to continue undisturbed. Dr. Kightlinger retired from the presidency of the Chiropractic Institute of New York in 1952.

He had been vice president of the UCA in the 1920s. His resignation from that organization is said to have hastened its merger with the ACA. He became a charter member of the newly formed NCA in 1930.

Dr. Kightlinger was responsible for organizing the first known Chiropractic Union, chartered by the American Federation of Labor in 1939. To combat efforts of the New Jersey Medical Association to eliminate the chiropractic profession through legislative pressure, in 1944, he helped organize the Chiropractic Research Foundation and was a longtime member of its executive board.

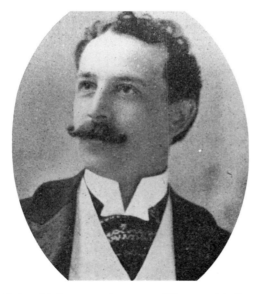

Craig M. Kightlinger, with degrees in law, pharmacy, and education and a D.C. from New Jersey College of Chiropractic, founded the Eastern Chiropractic College that would eventually merge with other schools to become the New York Chiropractic College. He was regarded as one of the profession's finest speakers.

From *The Chiropractic Journal,* June 1933.

SOLON M. LANGWORTHY

Solon Langworthy, the founder of the first important competing school with D.D. Palmer, is considered to be one of the most influential personalities in early chiropractic. One of three graduates under D.D. Palmer in 1901, Langworthy soon established the American School of Chiropractic in Cedar Rapids, Iowa, and was the first to establish a systematized curriculum of lectures and clinical work. He launched the first regular scholarly journal in chiropractic, *The Backbone,* in 1903 and, in 1906, collaborated with Oakley Smith, D.C., and Minora Paxson, D.C., in publishing the profession's first textbook, *Modernized Chiropractic.* In 1905 he established the first organized chiropractic society, the American Chiropractic Association, and was instrumental in passage of chiropractic legislation in Minnesota, although it was vetoed by the governor.

Solon Langworthy was also a pioneer researcher who, in 1903, advanced the concept of intervertebral foramina compression. The following year he published a hypothesis on aging and its relationship to the "spinal windows" theory that he had earlier proposed, and advanced a corrective technique utilizing a specially designed "Anatomical Adjuster," or traction table. The latter brought him into further conflict with the Palmers who disagreed with anything other than hands-only adjustment of ver-

Solon M. Langworthy, one of the most influential of early chiropractors, was a 1901 graduate of D.D. Palmer's. He established the American School of Chiropractic in Cedar Rapids, Iowa, in 1903 and published the first chiropractic textbook, Modernized Chiropractic *in 1906.*

Courtesy Palmer College of Chiropractic Archives, Davenport, Iowa.

tebrae. Langworthy's scholarly writings were decisive in the precedent-setting 1907 defense of Shegataro Morikubo, charged in Wisconsin with illegally practicing medicine and osteopathy.

LYNDON E. LEE (1887-1983)

Except for the first two campaigns of 1913 and 1914, Dr. Lyndon Lee was a central figure in the 50-year struggle of New York state chiropractors to gain the legal right to practice. Educated at Amherst College in Massachusetts and intent on studying law, Lee changed his career direction for personal reasons and received his doctor of chiropractic degree from the PSC in 1915. Immediately entering the fray as legislative chairman of the New York State Chiropractic Society, he quickly established himself as a leader in the profession. As a public speaker and writer, he was appreciated in the profession as quite exceptional, something also recognized by the press in general. The first of Lee's many published defenses of chiropractic rights appeared in *Harper's Weekly,* September 18, 1915. Early in 1933 Lee was himself indicted for practicing in New York state without a license (he held valid licenses in neighboring Connecticut and New Jersey). Although finally acquitted, his case was in and out of the courts 30 times during the next 3 years, attracting considerable attention. The November 1, 1933, issue of *Nation's Commerce* defended Lee editorially.

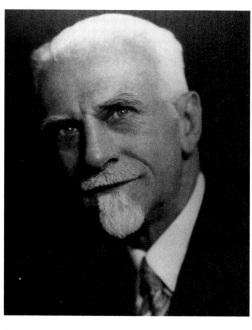

Lyndon E. Lee, a 1915 graduate of the Palmer School of Chiropractic, would play a central role during a 50-year struggle to pass chiropractic legislation in New York state.
Courtesy William Rehm, Baltimore, Maryland.

Lee was among a small group of chiropractors and others who, in 1950, organized the independent, non-profit Foundation for Health Research in New York for the purpose of focusing public attention on the scientific basis of chiropractic. After several years of careful development, the foundation submitted the first proposal for a controlled clinical study of chiropractic to the National Institutes of Health. Although it would be rejected for government funding because of certain design flaws, the proposal merited plaudits from some research scientists.

After the legislative victory of 1963, Lyndon Lee continued occasional speaking engagements before chiropractic groups. He was in active practice for 65 years.

CHARLES C. LEMLY (1892-1970)

Born in 1892 in Texarkana, Texas, Dr. Charles Lemly was a graduate of the high school, preparatory school, and junior college of the Nashville Naturopathic College and of the National College of Drugless Physicians. He earned his doctor of chiropractic degree from the Universal Chiropractic College in Davenport, Iowa, in 1915 and soon set up a practice in Waco, Texas. He also held a B.S. degree from Texarkana College and a Fellow of the International College of Chiropractors (F.I.C.C.) degree. His father, Samuel Lemly, was not only among the first graduate pharmacists in Texas, but also among the first chiropractors in the state of Texas.

Dr. Lemly began his chiropractic career when Texas was still an open (unlicensed) state and where prosecutions occurred with regularity. Lemly himself became something of a phenomenon, arrested 66 times for al-

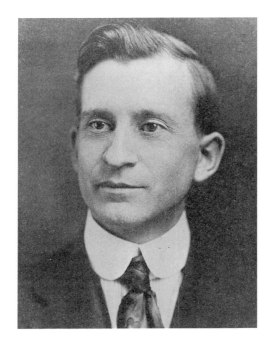

Joy M. Loban, a protege of B.J. Palmer's, was to leave PSC in 1910 and establish Universal Chiropractic College in Davenport, which moved to Pittsburgh, Pennsylvania, in 1918. He also was the author of several textbooks including Textbook of Neurology.

Courtesy Palmer College of Chiropractic Archives, Davenport, Iowa.

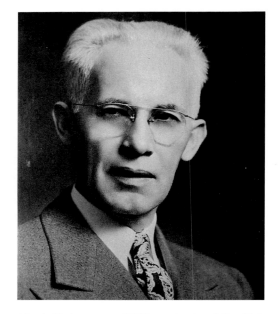

Hugh B. Logan, a 1915 graduate of the Universal Chiropractic College, developed the Logan Basic Technique and founded the Logan Basic College of Chiropractic in St. Louis, Missouri in 1935.

Courtesy Logan College of Chiropractic Archives, Chesterfield, Missouri.

legedly violating the medical practice laws. He lost only one verdict (the first one) and was required to spend 1 hour in jail along with paying a $95 fine.

He was one of seven founders of the Texas State Chiropractic Association in 1915 and served one term as president. He was the association's legislative director until passage of the original chiropractic law in 1943, and was appointed to the first chiropractic board of examiners, which was soon declared unconstitutional by the court. It is generally agreed that Charles Lemly's work was largely responsible for the present chiropractic law, passed in 1949. He was the first Texas delegate to the new NCA, organized in 1930, and was elected permanent chairman of its Committee on Development in 1938. In 1944 he was named a director of the Chiropractic Research Foundation and elected secretary of the board of trustees. He and his brother, F. Lee Lemly, D.C., founded and operated the Bon Aire Sanitarium in Waco for many years. Dr. Charles Lemly was also a founder and former president of the NCA's Council on Hospitals and Sanitaria.

JOY M. LOBAN

Dr. Joy Loban was an enigmatic early teacher, author, and practitioner whose known career spanned only 2 decades but whose influence in the formative years of chiropractic was indisputable. Early Palmer historian August A. Dye wrote that B.J. "discovered Loban in 1908, whom he thought proper material to take his place as Lecturer on the Philosophy of Chiropractic." Less than 2 years later in April 1910, Loban joined a group of rebellious Palmer faculty and students who formed the rival Universal Chiropractic College in Davenport. "Deep philosophical divisions" were cited as the reason for his abandonment of B.J., as Loban became dean of the faculty of Universal College.

Loban left the Universal College and Davenport about 1915 as dean of the Washington (D.C.) College of Chiropractic. His stay there was short-lived. He emerged in 1917 as dean of the Pittsburgh College of Chiropractic, which in 1918 became the new home of the Universal College of Chiropractic. Loban guided Universal as president until 1927 and gave impetus to some of the first clinical research in chiropractic, the radiographic investigations of Steinbach and Garbisch.

A writer of acknowledged competence, he authored *Technic and Practice of Chiropractic,* in 1915, and another volume entitled *Diet and Exercise.* His 550-page *Textbook of Neurology,* published in the 1920s with coauthor C.R. Bunn, D.C., was considered exceptional for its time. Loban also edited two journals—*Chiropractic Progress* and the Universal College *Bulletin.*

HUGH B. LOGAN (1881-1944)

Dr. Hugh Logan was the founder of the Logan College of Chiropractic and developer of his trademark Logan Basic Technique. He was a 1915 graduate of the Universal Chiropractic College in Davenport, Iowa. He practiced for years in Atchison, Kansas, and Los Angeles, and conducted classes in many parts of the United States on the principles of his technique for full-spine correction. He published the original *Logan Basic Technique* in 1936, later revised as the *Textbook of Logan Basic Methods from the Original Manuscript of Hugh B. Logan* in 1950.

With his son Vinton Logan, he established the Logan Chiropractic College of Basic Technique in St. Louis in 1935. A year later the college moved to a newly acquired 17-acre site in the city's suburbs and was renamed Logan Basic College of Chiropractic. It was operated as a nonprofit, 4-year institution from the beginning.

VINTON F. LOGAN (1905-1961)

Dr. Vinton Logan was the son of Dr. Hugh B. Logan. He grew up in Atchison, Kansas, where his father began his practice. While attending St. Benedict's College Seminary in Atchison, studying for the Roman Catholic priesthood, he decided to follow his father in the chiropractic profession. Graduating from the Universal Chiropractic College in Pittsburgh in 1926, he practiced in Los Angeles until 1934.

With the opening of Logan Chiropractic College of Basic Technique in 1935, Vinton served as dean of the college, assuming the presidency on his father's death in 1944. The student body had been depleted by World War II but quickly grew from 60 to more than 500 by war's end. The Memorial Clinic building and modern housing for students planned and built during the 1950s constituted the first large-scale chiropractic college expansion in that period. He was also active in the Missouri State Chiropractic Association and the International Chiropractors' Association. Vinton Logan was succeeded as president of Logan College by Dr. William N. Coggins.

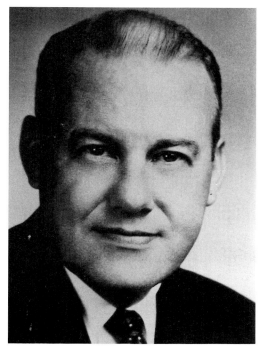

Vinton F. Logan, son of Dr. Hugh Logan, succeeded his father as president of Logan Basic College of Chiropractic and led its postwar expansion.

Courtesy Logan College of Chiropractic Archives, Chesterfield, Missouri.

FRANK R. MARGETTS (1871-1968)

Dr. Frank Margetts, a graduate of the Southern Baptist Theological Seminary and the Chicago College of Law, received his doctor of chiropractic degree from the National School of Chiropractic, Chicago, in 1920 at the age of 49. He was the last president of the old ACA, serving from 1923 to 1929. He was an articulate and persuasive spokesman for chiropractic and argued its case for years before numerous legislatures, especially in the unlicensed states of New York, Louisiana, Pennsylvania, Texas, Indiana, and Massachusetts. His presentation before the New York State Assembly on March 4, 1925, was reprinted by the ACA as a primer for chiropractic legislative committees.

Long supporting efforts to merge the two national organizations— ACA and the older UCA—he resigned the ACA presidency in 1929 to facilitate a smooth transfer of leadership in the newly created NCA. Declining an active role in the NCA, Dr. Margetts returned to his practice in Denver and, finally, in California.

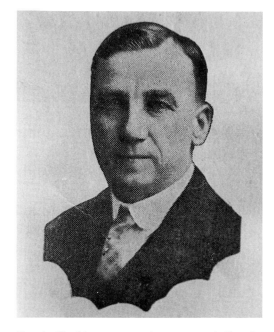

Frank R. Margetts, a lawyer and Baptist seminary graduate, was active during the 1920s with state chiropractic legislation and an early American Chiropractic Association president.

From *The Bulletin of the ACA*, September 1927.

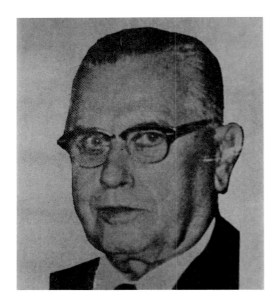

LILLARD T. MARSHALL (1890-1970)

Dr. Lillard Marshall was a 1915 graduate of the PSC who practiced in Lexington, Kentucky, for 55 years. He was a founder and the first president of the NCA, serving four successive terms in that office from 1930 to 1934. In 1944 he was named the first executive director of the Chiropractic Research Foundation and, in 1938, was named the first honorary Fellow of the International College of Chiropractors. He also served two terms as president of the International Congress of Chiropractic Examining Boards, three terms as treasurer of the American Society of Chiropractors, and two terms as executive director of the NCA.

Dr. Marshall was president of the Kentucky Association of Chiropractors for four terms and was its legislative director for 22 years. For nearly as long, he was secretary of the Kentucky Board of Chiropractic Examiners. His *Report of State Supervisor of Chiropractors of Kentucky* in 1932 demonstrated possible utilization of chiropractic care in the rehabilitation of inmates in state prisons. Compiled over 2 years, it was one of the first state-commissioned studies of its kind.

Lillard T. Marshall, a 1915 graduate of the Palmer School of Chiropractic, practiced in Kentucky for 55 years and was prominent with the National Chiropractic Association.
From *The ACA Journal of Chiropractic,* March, 1970.

CHESTER B. MCDONALD (1896-1948)

Dr. Chester McDonald received the degree of doctor of chiropractic and drugless therapeutics from the National School of Chiropractic, Chicago, in 1920 and started his practice as a licensed chiropractor and drugless practitioner in Benton Harbor, Michigan, that same year. In 1933 he moved his busy clinic into a newly constructed building combining inpatient services with the clinic. A year later the McDonald Clinic and Chiropractic Hospital expanded from 24 beds to 40 and became the first chiropractic hospital to offer preceptorships to students.

Dr. McDonald was a former president of the Michigan Naturopathic Society and board member of the American Naturopathic Association. He was a founder of the Council on Hospitals and Sanitaria of the NCA and spoke frequently on the need for chiropractic and non-allopathic hospitals. At the time of his death, he was serving a 4-year term on the Michigan Board of Chiropractic Examiners.

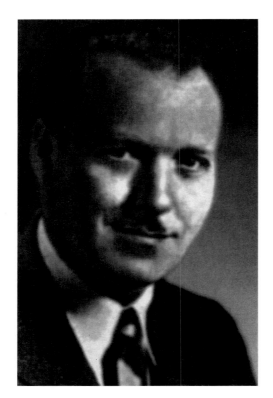

Chester B. McDonald was a 1920 graduate of the National School of Chiropractic. His Benton Harbor, Michigan, McDonald Clinic and Chiropractic Hospital offered preceptorships to chiropractic students.
Courtesy William Rehm, Baltimore, Maryland.

HARRY K. MCILROY (1885-1963)

Dr. Harry McIlroy was a 1919 graduate of the National School of Chiropractic in Chicago, became the first legislative director of the Indiana Chiropractic Association the same year, and led the successful campaign of 1927 amending the Medical Practice Act to permit licensing of chiropractors. He served as the chiropractic member of the Indiana Board of Medical Registration and Examination from 1937 to 1940.

A charter member of the NCA in 1930, he served as state delegate for 9 years and was chairman of the NCA Bureau of Public Information for 6 years. He was elected president of the NCA in 1941. He resigned as president of the Chiropractic Research Foundation in 1947 to become executive director of the NCA. He also served as a director and chairman of the Lincoln Chiropractic College board of trustees.

THOMAS S. MORRIS (1868-1928)

A Wisconsin attorney, Tom Morris designed and executed the first successful courtroom defense of chiropractic in the 1907 trial of Shegataro Morikubo in La Crosse, Wisconsin. As chief counsel for the UCA from 1906 to 1930, Morris's law firm represented thousands of chiropractors across the nation charged with the "illegal practice of medicine." His influence on the profession during much of this period was said to be second only to that of B.J. Palmer himself.

Canadian-born Tom Morris had studied medicine at McGill University before earning his law degree from the University of Wisconsin in 1899. He served as state's attorney in La Crosse for several years. In 1904 he was elected to the state senate and served two terms as speaker. In the senate Morris was instrumental in establishing the state's first teacher's college and the nation's first workmen's compensation law. An ardent progressive and political ally of Robert La Follette, he was elected lieutenant governor in 1907, after the successful Morikubo case, but failed in his bid for the governorship in 1914. Leaving politics, he devoted his full time to law. Morris died suddenly while on a visit to New York City. His former longtime law partner Fred H. Hartwell died earlier the same year.

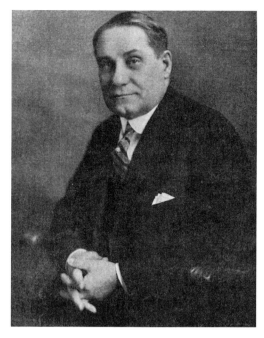

Thomas S. Morris was Canadian born and a former Wisconsin state's attorney and lieutenant governor. Morris was instrumental in defending chiropractors against lawsuits through the United States, including chiropractic's landmark 1907 case of Shegataro Morikubo in LaCrosse, Wisconsin.

Courtesy Palmer College of Chiropractic Archives, Davenport, Iowa.

EMMETT J. MURPHY (1902-1965)

Dr. Emmett Murphy was chiropractic's first lobbyist-at-large and national representative. As labor relations director for the NCA from 1938 to 1964, he functioned chiefly in the public relations area to increase awareness of chiropractic among legislators, the federal bureaucracy, veterans organizations, labor, and other groups equally concerned with the affairs of government. Many of his accomplishments were pioneering efforts; however, all of his work required a day-to-day alertness, particularly to the actions of Congress, to ensure that the best interests of chiropractic were protected.

A native of Iowa, he attended Dubuque College and received his chiropractic education from the PSC, graduating in 1925. He settled permanently in Washington D.C., where, until his office was officially established by the NCA in 1938, he functioned as an informal ad hoc committee of one. His list of accomplishments on behalf of the chiropractic profession was long and impressive. Two of his most notable achievements were deferments from military service for chiropractic students, as were other health-provider students, and inclusion of chiropractors as health professionals in such government publications as the *Directory of Occupational Outlook Handbook.* Outside government, Dr. Murphy was effective in his contacts with labor unions and veterans organizations.

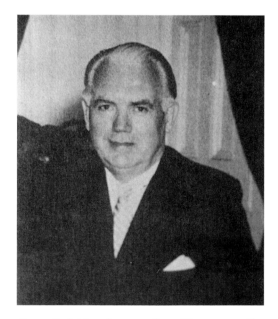

Emmett J. Murphy, a native of Iowa, was the National Chiropractic Association's long-time public-relations director, which gave the profession a needed and familiar presence in national affairs between 1938 and 1964.

Courtesy William Rehm, Baltimore, Maryland.

ERNEST G. NAPOLITANO (1911-1985)

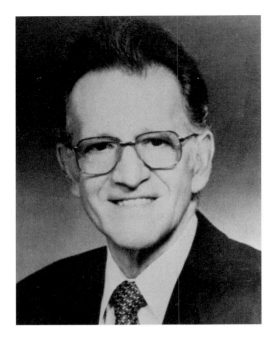

Dr. Ernest Napolitano, an internationally recognized educator, author, and lecturer, was the founder of New York Chiropractic College (NYCC). Chartered by the New York Board of Regents in 1977, NYCC was the first chiropractic college included within the structure of the State University of New York (SUNY). Dr. Napolitano had been president of the Columbia Institute of Chiropractic from 1959 to 1977, prior to its reorganization as NYCC.

Dr. Napolitano received his doctor of chiropractic degree from the PSC in 1942. He profited from his association with Dr. B.J. Palmer, yet maintained his independence of opinion. He served in the United States Army Medical Corps during World War II and was awarded the Purple Heart and Bronze Star.

Dr. Napolitano earned a law degree in 1954 and for some 30 years authored countless articles ranging from educational standards, economics, and ethics to jurisprudence and the principles and practice of chiropractic. He served as president of the Council on Chiropractic Education from 1982 to 1984. In addition to holding positions with numerous professional societies and academies, and many civic organizations, his honors included 13 honorary degrees, 11 fellowships in learned societies, and more than 50 educational, professional, religious, and civic awards.

Dr. Napolitano was a founder of the Association for the History of Chiropractic in 1980 and had been elected its third president on the very eve of his death.

Ernest G. Napolitano, a 1942 graduate of PSC, was an author, educator, a lawyer, a decorated World War II veteran, and a much-honored community leader. He was founder of the present-day New York Chiropractic College.

Courtesy New York Chiropractic College, Seneca Falls, New York.

JOHN J. NUGENT (1891-1979)

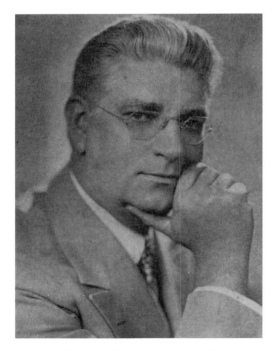

Dr. John Nugent spearheaded early reforms in chiropractic education and the conversion of its institutions from private ownership. Irish-born, he was educated at the University of Dublin, and emigrated about 1914 to settle in Connecticut. At the outset of World War I, he was appointed to the special officers candidate program at the United States Military Academy. After the war he studied at the PSC.

His experiences at the PSC portended the restlessness that characterized his career. Unable to come to terms with the educational objectives of Dr. B.J. Palmer, he was reportedly expelled for "discourtesy to the president" but reinstated at the insistence of faculty members. He later practiced in Connecticut for several years.

Dr. Nugent became a prime mover in organizing chiropractic's first effective committee on professional standards, the National Council of Chiropractic Examining Boards, an independent group of state and Canadian representatives seeking uniformity in education and licensing. The council was formed in 1935. He was elected to head a task force which, by 1938, completed an inspection of every chiropractic college and recommended a code by which standards could be measured. In 1939, at Nugent's urging, the NCA established a Committee on Educational Standards, joining with the Council of Chiropractic Examining Boards to implement an accreditation process. This combined influence would result in the present-day Council on Chiropractic Education. Nugent was named NCA's first director of education in 1941.

Given the authority to supervise the colleges that applied for accredi-

John J. Nugent, Irish born and a University of Dublin graduate, graduated from the Palmer School of Chiropractic in 1922. He is considered by many to be the "Abraham Flexner of chiropractic" for the educational reforms he advocated.

From *The National Chiropractic Journal,* November 1941.

tation, he authored *Chiropractic Education: An Outline of a Standard Course* published by the NCA in 1941. Compliance with these standards was expected by 1943. It was Dr. Nugent, along with Dr. Emmett Murphy, who established contact with the United States Office on Education, which would eventually result in formal recognition of the Council on Chiropractic Education in 1974. Dr. Nugent retired from his position with the NCA in 1961.

BARTLETT JOSHUA PALMER (1882-1961)

The only son of Daniel David Palmer, B.J., as he was known, earned his diploma from the Founder in 1902 and took over operation of the Palmer Institute and Chiropractic Infirmary later that year. B.J. and his father continued in partnership until 1906, when B.J. purchased his father's interest in the school. In 1907 the institution was incorporated as the PSC, with B.J. continuing as president until his death. For the better part of 2 decades the self-styled "Developer" was the undisputed leader of the profession. With the introduction of the neurocalometer in 1924, B.J.'s base of support eroded, although he continued to exert his influence through the International Chiropractors Association.

Although B.J. had little formal education, his obvious genius for organization allowed him to become president of five corporations that included the PSC and a prosperous broadcasting network. He authored at least 37 volumes of varying lengths, some titles of up to 900 pages, and edited two of chiropractic's earliest periodicals, *The Fountainhead News* and *The Chiropractor.* His printery at the PSC annually churned out literally millions of tracts promoting chiropractic.

B.J., the entrepreneur, also provided an environment to advance the science of chiropractic. The x-ray laboratories he established in 1910 were the first in chiropractic and among the finest to be found anywhere. The B.J. Palmer Osteological Collection, which was started by D.D. in the 1880s, was declared in 1928 by an investigating team of the American Medical Association as " . . . without doubt, the best collection of human spines in existence." The B.J. Palmer Research Clinic, established in 1935, received the most difficult of medically diagnosed cases and provided state-of-the-art facilities for diagnosis and chiropractic care and rehabilitation. Clear View Sanitarium in Davenport was purchased by the PSC in 1940 and operated for some 20 years as a chiropractic hospital for psychiatric patients.

For more than half a century, B.J. was a dominant force in three professional organizations, including the UCA, the first such society in chiropractic. It was under the UCA banner that B.J.'s testimony in many courtroom and legislative battles aided chiropractic in its survival years. Millions heard the chiropractic story that B.J. broadcast regularly from WOC, the pioneer radio station he established atop the Palmer School in 1922, and on WHO–Des Moines, a radio station which he acquired in 1930.

B.J. married Mabel Heath of Rock Island, Illinois, in 1904. Their only child, the founder's namesake, Daniel David Palmer II, would eventually assume the leadership role of the PSC and other Palmer enterprises.

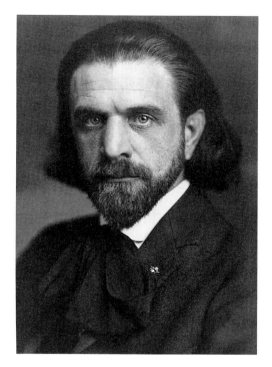

Bartlett Joshua (B.J.) Palmer, the only son of D.D. Palmer, was one of the two or three most influential leaders during the profession's first 100 years. Besides acting as one of its leading spokesmen and defenders, the "Developer" of chiropractic was president of PSC from 1906 until his death in 1961. He also served as president of WOC and WHO radio and television stations in Davenport and Des Moines, Iowa.

Courtesy Palmer College of Chiropractic Archives, Davenport, Iowa.

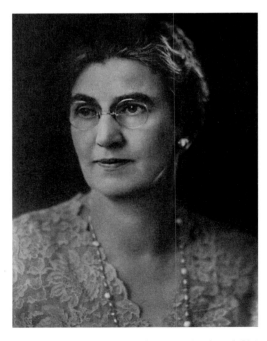

DAVID DANIEL PALMER (1906-1978)

Dr. David D. Palmer was born in 1906 on the PSC campus and raised among the faculty and students of the PSC. His given name was his grandfather's, Daniel David Palmer, but he was referred to throughout his life as David D. Palmer to avoid confusion with his grandfather.

No one in the profession had either as unique a view of chiropractic or as unique a role in chiropractic as did Dr. Dave. He was ideally suited for the reformist role he would play as eventual head of the family and the PSC and for his leadership in the profession.

Having spent the whole of his young life at the very center of the profession, he earned a college degree from the prestigious Wharton School of Business and Finance and was a sophisticated world traveler by the age of 23. David D. Palmer was named vice president and treasurer of Palmer Properties in 1929. He earned his doctor of chiropractic degree from the PSC in 1939, completing the full course.

Following his father's death in 1961, he became president and chief executive officer of the Palmer interests and initiated a succession of dramatic changes, which saw the PSC rechartered as the non-profit Palmer College of Chiropractic, the chiropractic curriculum revised, the entrance and graduation standards raised, the existing facilities enlarged and remodeled, new facilities constructed, the faculty increased in size, and various research programs started. Full accreditation of Palmer College of Chiropractic by the Council on Chiropractic Education was also realized during the administration of Dr. Dave Palmer. Dr. Palmer also founded the Palmer Junior College in 1965 to provide low cost liberal arts education to the people of Scott County. He authored two books: *Three Generations,* in 1967, and *The Palmers,* in 1971.

In community affairs, he was a highly honored citizen of the Quad Cities for his undaunting support of business, higher education, and the arts. In 1967 he was named the Quad Cities B'Nai B'Rith "Man of the Year" and in 1977 named United States Jaycees Ambassador, the highest honor bestowed by the Jaycees.

David D. Palmer, grandson of "Old Dad Chiro" and the only son of B.J. and Mabel Palmer, became the president of PSC and Palmer Enterprises in 1961 with the death of his father. Among many business and community accomplishments during his life, he became known as the "Educator" because of the educational reforms he instituted at Palmer College of Chiropractic.

Courtesy Palmer College of Chiropractic Archives, Davenport, Iowa.

MABEL HEATH PALMER (1881-1949)

The daughter of W.L. Heath, D.C., pioneer graduate of the Palmer Institute and Chiropractic Infirmary and early faculty member of the PSC, Mabel married B.J. Palmer in Davenport on April 30, 1904. She became secretary at the Palmer Institute and Chiropractic Infirmary and business manager for both the school and infirmary. After the school was reorganized in 1906 as the Palmer School of Chiropractic, she enrolled at a medical college in Chicago, and completed a special 1-year course in anatomy and dissection. She returned to the PSC, obtained her doctor of chiropractic degree and became professor of anatomy, a position she held for almost 40 years. In 1918 she authored a well-regarded text, *Textbook on Anatomy.* Dr. Mabel Palmer was charter president of Sigma Phi Chi, founded in 1914 as the first undergraduate chiropractic sorority, and served as its national patron for the rest of her life.

Outside of chiropractic, Dr. Palmer attained prominence in leadership and literary circles, having been elected president of Quota International and the Business and Professional Women's Clubs of America. She also

Mabel Heath Palmer, "The First Lady of Chiropractic," was a key figure in the stability and longevity of the early PSC. Known simply as Mabel, Dr. Palmer was a leader of and inspiration to women in chiropractic and the author of Textbook of Anatomy.

Courtesy Palmer College of Chiropractic Archives, Davenport, Iowa.

authored two books on her travels around the world with B.J. Palmer, one of which was titled *Stepping Stones.* Their child Dave was born in 1906.

MINORA C. PAXSON

Minora Paxson holds the distinction of being not only one of the first two female chiropractors but also the first chiropractor to receive a state license. Graduating from D.D. Palmer's original School and Cure in 1899, she practiced in several Iowa communities until 1904, when she joined two other Palmer graduates, Solon Langworthy and Oakley Smith, in launching the American School of Chiropractic at Cedar Rapids. In the 1906 text *Modernized Chiropractic,* which she coauthored with Smith and Langworthy, Paxson is listed as "Professor of Gynecology and Obstetrics," a title that gives currency to the possibility that she had been a practicing midwife before studying chiropractic. She was also a lecturer on physiology and symptomology and secretary of the school.

It is documented that she was licensed in 1905 under the Illinois Medical Practice Act to "practice obstetrics in accordance with the principles of chiropractic" and granted the "first certificate licensing the treatment of disease by chiropractic." Details of her later life are unknown.

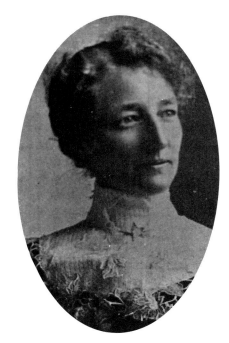

Minora C. Paxson, an 1899 graduate of D.D. Palmer's, in 1905 received the first license in the nation to practice chiropractic and co-authored the 1906 Modernized Chiropractic *with Oakley Smith and Solon Langworthy, then seemed to disappear from the profession.*

Courtesy Palmer College of Chiropractic Archives, Davenport, Iowa.

THURE C. PETERSON (1898-1970)

Dr. Thure Peterson, a lifelong resident of New York City, was active in chiropractic education for 45 years. He graduated from the Carver Chiropractic Institute, New York, in 1920 and joined the faculty of the school. In 1928 he was named dean. When the Carver Institute merged with the New York School of Chiropractic in 1934, Peterson continued as dean. He was instrumental in the 1944 amalgamation of New York's three remaining privately run schools under the single banner of the professionally owned Chiropractic Institute of New York (CINY). Dr. Peterson was named associate dean of the new school, now considerably strengthened in finances, student body, faculty, and course content.

CINY was soon able to purchase a substantial 4-story building once occupied by the New York University School of Medicine. Soon after the establishment of CINY, however, its principal officers, including Peterson, were arrested and charged with illegally operating a medical school without state approval, a charge not sustained by the court.

Dr. Peterson chaired the Council on Education of the NCA for 10 years. In 1953 he was named president of CINY.

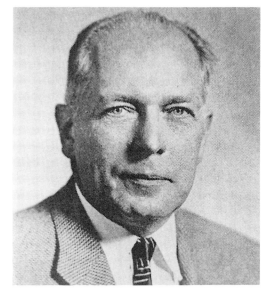

Thure C. Peterson, a 1920 graduate of the Carver Chiropractic Institute of New York, was a respected educator for 45 years and in 1953 became president of the Chiropractic Institute of New York.

From *The ACA Journal of Chiropractic,* November 1970.

GERARD M. POTHOFF (1889-1937)

Dr. Gerard Pothoff was born in Holland and emigrated to the United States in 1907. He earned a degree in civil engineering from Notre Dame University about 1912 and became associated with the Tri-City Railway

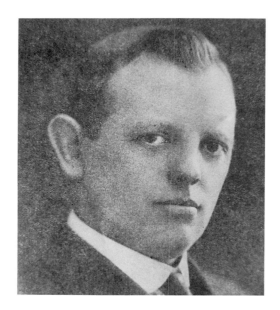

Gerard M. Pothoff, a civil engineer who graduated from PSC in 1922, established and operated the Forest Park Sanitarium in Davenport, Iowa, which provided mental, nervous, and custodial care to its patients for 15 years, until his death in 1937.

From *The National Chiropractic Journal,* February 1937.

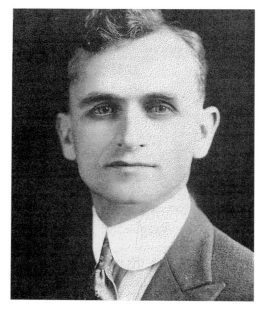

Tullius F. (T.F.) Ratledge was one of the most prominent early leaders of the profession in the west, particularly California. A 1907 graduate of the Carver Chiropractic College in Oklahoma City, T.F. opened a school in Tulsa, then moved to Kansas and eventually to Los Angeles where he was president of the Ratledge Chiropractic College from 1911 to 1945.

Courtesy Paul Smallie, Stockton, California.

Company in Davenport, Iowa. In 1919 he enrolled at the PSC and graduated in 1922. In October of that year, he cofounded the Forest Park Sanitarium in Davenport, incorporated as the Chiropractic Psychopathic Sanitarium, one of the first chiropractic inpatient centers. The institution offered hospital care for mental, nervous, and custodial cases, with both chiropractic and necessary medical treatment, and a 24-hour nursing service. He became secretary of the sanitarium in 1924, vice president and general manager in 1925, and president in 1926, remaining in that post until his death. The institution was later renamed the Davenport Psychiatric Hospital and continued operation until the mid-1950s.

TULLIUS F. RATLEDGE (1881-1967)

Dr. Tullius Ratledge, T.F. as he was known, was one of the first graduates of Dr. Willard Carver's Oklahoma City college, in 1907. Beginning practice in Guthrie, then the capital of Oklahoma, he soon opened a school in Tulsa, later relocating to Kansas, and operating there until he moved to Los Angeles in 1911. There he opened the Ratledge Chiropractic College. The first students of the school had the distinction of hearing lectures by the founder of chiropractic, Dr. D.D. Palmer. A dedicated lobbyist, he was instrumental in gaining licensure for chiropractic in Kansas—which passed the first chiropractic law in 1913—and in California through the successful referendum of 1922. He was once arrested (in California) and went to jail rather than accept guilt for what was alleged to be the practice of medicine. This brought considerable publicity to what chiropractic was trying to gain legislatively.

In 1955, having relinquished the college to Dr. Carl S. Cleveland, Sr., he went to Arkansas where he hoped to continue practice. In 1963, he was admitted to practice through a special exemption granted by the governor, and continued until the age of 89.

EARL A. RICH (1921-1967)

Dr. Earl Rich was the first American D.C. to investigate cineroentgenology (motion picture x-ray), a procedure pioneered by the Swiss chiropractor Dr. Fred Illi.

Earl Rich received his doctor of chiropractic degree from Lincoln College of Chiropractic in 1943, after attending Indiana State University for 2 years. He served in the U.S. Army Medical Corps for 3 years as an x-ray technician and instructor. After his discharge from the service, he returned to Lincoln as head of the x-ray department and clinic supervisor. In 1955 he became secretary of Lincoln College of Chiropractic, advancing to vice president in 1962, and president in 1965, succeeding Dr. Arthur Hendricks, one of the four founders. He was elected a diplomate of the American Board of Chiropractic Roentgenologists in 1958, appointed research consultant to the ACA, and became the cineroentgenological research director of the ACA in 1962. He also fully implemented an ongoing research program at Lincoln, including residency training in radiology. His two texts became classics: *Manual of Radiography and Diagnostic Roentgenology* and *Atlas of Clinical Roentgenology.* An earlier work, *X-Ray Diagnosis and Interpretation,* was published in collaboration with Dr. A.G. Hendricks. He was also a member of the American Chiropractic Council of Education and held a Fellowship in the International College of Chiropractic.

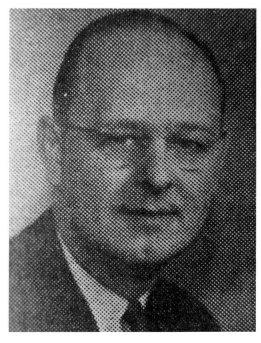

LORAN M. ROGERS (1897-1976)

A 1924 PSC graduate, Dr. L.M. Rogers came out of private practice in Webster City, Iowa, in 1932, and for the next 40 years, served in many ways as the voice and conscience of chiropractic. L.M. Rogers became the second executive secretary of the new NCA and continued as such throughout the history of that organization. He was publisher and editor of the *Journal of the International Chiropractic Congress* from 1928 to 1932, which was later renamed *The Chiropractic Journal* and then *National Chiropractic Journal,* which became the official organ of the NCA. Today's *Journal of Chiropractic,* published by the ACA, is a direct descendant of his first journal.

In addition to his more than 500 published articles in the pages of the journal, Rogers authored several monographs and contributed regularly to various encyclopedias and other references on the subject of chiropractic. After establishment of the ACA in 1963, Dr. Rogers was named executive director and served until his retirement in 1972.

L.M. Rogers was also instrumental in organizing the National Chiropractic Mutual Insurance Company in 1946, the oldest and largest insurer of its kind. He was secretary-treasurer of National Chiropractic Mutual Insurance Company from 1946 to 1972, and from 1950 to 1961 held the same position with the Chiropractic Research Foundation, forerunner of today's Foundation for Chiropractic Education and Research.

Loran M. Rogers, a 1924 graduate of PSC, was editor of the NCA's Journal *and the first executive secretary of the American Chiropractic Association, 1963-1972.*

From *The National Chiropractic Journal,* August 1941.

WILLIAM C. SCHULZE (1870-1936)

Dr. William Schulze, a graduate of Rush Medical College, Chicago, in 1897, was a physician whose influence on chiropractic education contributed favorably on early legislative efforts. He had practiced general medicine in Lornira, Wisconsin, for 3 years before returning to Chicago, where he became medical director of the Zander Institute (for mechanotherapy). Later he specialized in obstetrics and gynecology and authored a textbook on the subject.

Resuming his interest in the field of mechanotherapy, he established the Institute of Physiological Therapeutics, a venture that brought him into contact with Dr. John F.A. Howard, president of the National School of Chiropractic. Initially his involvement with National involved a series of clinical lectures, but he soon discontinued medical practice to devote himself full time to chiropractic education. Dr. Schulze introduced physiological therapeutics, or physiotherapy, and other drugless methods to the curriculum as early as 1912 and inaugurated the first laboratory courses in chiropractic education.

Dr. Schulze became president of the school in 1914, when he purchased ownership from Dr. Howard, and remained in that post until his

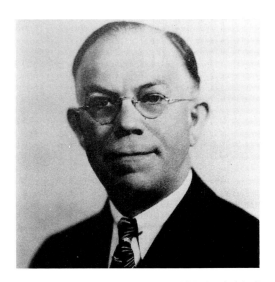

William C. Schulze, M.D., a 1907 Rush Medical College graduate, purchased the National School of Chiropractic from Dr. John Howard in 1914 and served as its president until his death in 1936.

Courtesy National College of Chiropractic, Lombard, Illinois.

413

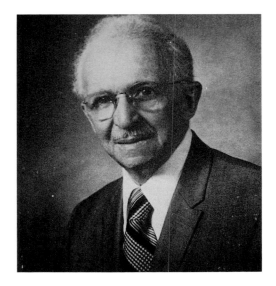

Herman S. Schwartz, born in Russia, was a 1922 graduate of the Carver Chiropractic Institute of New York City and a leader in the utilization of chiropractic care for the mentally ill. He was the author of many articles and two noteworthy books, Mental Health and Chiropractic *and* Home Care for the Mentally Ill.

Courtesy William Rehm, Baltimore, Maryland.

death. He was also responsible for establishing the Chicago General Health Service (the college clinic) in 1927.

HERMAN S. SCHWARTZ (1894-1976)

Dr. Herman Schwartz pioneered the concept of utilizing chiropractic for the mentally ill. In 1924 he organized the first committee on mental health in chiropractic with the New York State Chiropractic Society, and in 1928 he founded the Citizens League for Health Rights. He also founded the Council on Psychotherapy of the NCA in 1950 and was a longtime member of the World Federation on Mental Health. In 1968 he was named president emeritus of the Council on Mental Health of the American Chiropractic Association.

Dr. Schwartz authored two books, *The Art of Relaxation* and *Home Care for the Emotionally Ill,* and more than 200 articles. In 1949 he published the research report, "Nervous and Mental Illness Under Chiropractic Care." His last literary effort was as editor of the text, *Mental Health and Chiropractic* (Sessions, 1973), which included contributions from several recognized scientists and health professionals. He graduated from the Carver Chiropractic Institute, New York City, in 1922, and practiced in New York City and Elmhurst, New York for 54 years.

LYLE W. SHERMAN (1905-1977)

Dr. Lyle Sherman, a graduate of the PSC in 1934, was admitted to the PSC faculty in 1936, where he taught chiropractic philosophy, orthopedy, clinical pathology, and spinography. In 1942 he was named assistant director and chief-of-staff of the B.J. Palmer Chiropractic Research Clinic. His research contributions included development of new instrumentation—the neurotempometer, conturographometer, and neurocalograph, the latter a version of the neurocalometer. He also developed a turntable for taking precision upper cervical x-rays in the sitting position and published several papers on the "physiological effects of the chiropractic adjustment."

Leaving Palmer in 1957, he developed a successful practice in Spartanburg, South Carolina. In the mid-1950s, he was secretary-treasurer of the International Chiropractors' Association and a member of the board of control from 1955 to 1966. A founder of the college that bears his name, Sherman College of Straight Chiropractic, Spartanburg, South Carolina, he was a member of its original board of trustees.

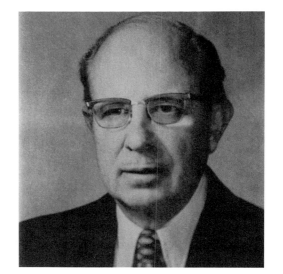

Lyle W. Sherman, a 1934 graduate of the Palmer School of Chiropractic, was on the Palmer faculty from 1936 to 1957. In 1973 the newly founded Sherman College of Straight Chiropractic in South Carolina was named for him.

Courtesy William Rehm, Baltimore, Maryland.

OAKLEY G. SMITH (1880-1967)

Dr. Oakley Smith, born on a farm in Iowa, was weakened by scarlet fever as a child and spent much of his early life seeking out practitioners to restore his health. In 1897 he spent 2 months at the Kirksville, Missouri, infirmary of osteopathic founded by A.T. Still. Later he became both a patient and student of D.D. Palmer and was granted a diploma by the Founder in the spring of 1899. In fall 1899 Smith entered the medical school of the University of Iowa for a 2-year course of study. It is reported that Smith also studied the techniques of Czech folk healers, known as bonesetters.

In 1905 he joined two other early Palmer graduates, Solon Langworthy and Minora Paxson, in launching the rival American School of Chiropractic in Cedar Rapids, Iowa. Smith's lectures before the first class of the American School of Chiropractic were published in 1906 as *Modernized Chiropractic,* with Paxson listed as editor and Langworthy as publisher holding the copyright. It was chiropractic's first textbook. He was issued a drugless practitioner's license by the Illinois Medical Board in May 1904. Leaving his association with the American School sometime during 1905, Oakley Smith moved to Chicago, where he announced his discovery of diseased ligaments from microscopic evidence, and theorized that he had found the real cause of disease. He called his discovery "naprapathy" and developed corrective techniques resembling chiropractic. He founded the Chicago College of Naprapathy in November 1905.

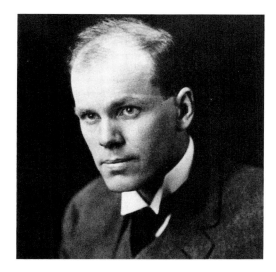

Oakley G. Smith, an 1899 graduate of D.D. Palmer's Chiropractic School and Cure, studied at the University of Iowa Medical School from 1899 to 1901. In 1906, he established the American School of Chiropractic in Cedar Rapids, Iowa, and co-authored Modernized Chiropractic *with colleagues Minora Paxson and Solon Langworthy. In 1907, he moved to Chicago and founded the Chicago College of Naprapathy.*

Courtesy Palmer College of Chiropractic Archives, Davenport, Iowa.

LEO SPEARS (1894-1956)

Leo Spears, a World War I Marine Corps veteran and 1921 graduate of the PSC, became one of the nation's most successful and controversial chiropractors. His non-profit hospital in Denver, the largest of its kind ever built without public funding, was the focus of bitter medical opposition and interminable legal entanglements. His most important legal battle was won on July 1, 1950, after 7 years of litigation. Then the Colorado Supreme Court unanimously ruled that the State Health Department could not deny the hospital proper licensure and ordered the department to issue Spears an unrestricted license retroactive to the original date of application.

Dr. Spears argued tirelessly for the right of veterans of both World Wars to receive chiropractic care on demand. In one celebrated case in the early 1920s, after charging medical monopoly within the Veterans' Bureau, his license to practice was suspended by the Colorado Medical Board for "unprofessional conduct." In 1953 a Senate subcommittee investigating more charges of medical monopoly in veterans affairs convened two hearings at Spears Hospital.

During the depression years of the 1930s, Leo Spears virtually depleted his personal savings to operate free food distribution centers serving thousands of needy citizens, only to be dismissed by one mainline charity as a "meddler." This costly experience, along with ongoing legal hassles and the onset of World War II, delayed construction of the hospital for several years.

The first 236-bed unit of Spears Hospital finally opened on May 1, 1943, and a second, larger unit, was added in 1949, bringing the bed capacity to 600. The master plan also called for a large chiropractic college on the 15-acre site. A hallmark of the hospital was its intern training program, started in the late 1940s. A third major building (a massive 8-story structure) was begun in 1953 but never finished. After the death

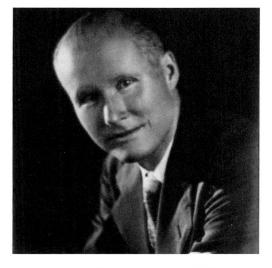

Leo Spears, a 1921 graduate of PSC, settled in Colorado and was one of the state's more active leaders. A dynamic achiever in the face of adversity, he is best known for building the profession's largest hospital complex and his charity work with the poor. He was the author of the 1950 text, Spears Painless System of Chiropractic.

Courtesy William Rehm, Baltimore, Maryland.

of Dr. Spears in May 1956, the uncompleted building was sold for private development.

Spears Chiropractic Hospital continued to flourish another 25 years under the leadership of Drs. Dan and Howard Spears, nephews of the founder. Facing increasingly high operating costs without benefit of public or charitable support, the hospital closed in the spring of 1984. In its history, more than 151,000 patients were admitted, and it is estimated that more than $8 million of free services were dispensed.

LEO J. STEINBACH (1886-1960)

Leo J. Steinbach deserves partial credit for the first serious clinical research in chiropractic. With Dr. Edwin H. Garbisch, their seminal x-ray investigations at Pittsburgh's Universal Chiropractic College demonstrated the mechanical effects of unequal leg lengths and pelvic distortions under the influence of gravity. The first report of their study was published in the Universal College *Bulletin* in 1924. Ultimately, after 10,000 erect-posture radiographs were correlated, Steinbach developed what became known as the Universal Technique, incorporating corrective and prophylactic exercises for optimum spinal health. He presented the technique in its complete form as *spinal balance and spinal hygiene* at the 1936 convention of the European Chiropractors' Union in Geneva.

Dr. Steinbach graduated from the Universal Chiropractic College in Davenport in 1916, then under the direction of its founder, Dr. Joy M. Loban. In 1921, after the college relocated to Pittsburgh, Steinbach was named dean, a position he maintained until 1944. Wartime manpower shortages caused the merger of Universal Chiropractic College with Lincoln Chiropractic College at Indianapolis in 1944. Dr. Steinbach was named as vice president and trustee and twice yearly lectured on his technique.

He entered private practice in Pittsburgh and was instrumental in passage of the chiropractic licensing law in Pennsylvania. He was elected the first president of the Pennsylvania Chiropractic Society in 1945 and continued in that office until 1952.

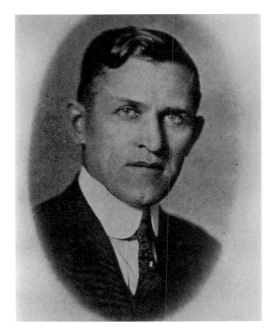

Leo J Steinbach, a 1916 graduate of Universal Chiropractic College, was an early clinical chiropractic researcher who developed a comprehensive system of spinal analysis and care. He and his associates took the first erect posture radiographs of the spine.

From *Annual Catalog,* Universal Chiropractic College, 1924.

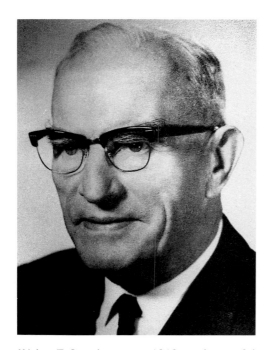

Walter T. Sturdy, was a 1919 graduate of the PSC and a long-time leader of chiropractic in Canada. He was a founding member of the Canadian Memorial Chiropractic College in Toronto.

Courtesy Canadian Memorial Chiropractic College, Toronto, Ontario, Canada.

WALTER T. STURDY (1877-1971)

Dr. Walter Sturdy, one of Canada's most honored chiropractic pioneers, was the acknowledged guiding force behind two historic developments for the profession in that country: formation of the Dominion Council of Canadian Chiropractors in 1943, the forerunner of the Canadian Chiropractic Association, and formation of the organizing committee that established the Canadian Memorial Chiropractic College.

A 1919 graduate of the PSC, Sturdy practiced in Vancouver, British Columbia, where he helped organize the British Columbia Chiropractic Association in 1920. He served continuously as president of that organization from 1922 to 1934. He also spearheaded the long campaign to establish the British Columbia Chiropractic Act and Chiropractic Examining Board.

With the establishment of the professionally owned Canadian Memorial Chiropractic College, he served on its first board of directors from 1945-1946 and was elected college director in the 1946-47 school year. The administrative building on the present campus of Canadian Memorial Chiropractic College is dedicated as the Walter T. Sturdy Building.

ERNEST A. THOMPSON (1891-1976)

Dr. E.A. Thompson, a pioneer in chiropractic radiology, authored the first text on the subject, *Chiropractic Spinography,* in 1918. This classic text was revised three times through 1924. He had received his doctor of chiropractic degree from the PSC in 1914 and immediately accepted an invitation to supervise the newly established x-ray department at PSC.

In May 1925 Thompson resigned from the faculty, the first of a wave of defections during that stormy period that saw the influence of B.J. Palmer weakened. Dr. Thompson went to Baltimore, where he established a commercial x-ray laboratory and private practice. Former fellow PSC faculty members J.N. Firth, S.J. Burich, H.E. Vedder, and A.G. Hendricks founded the Lincoln Chiropractic College in Indianapolis in 1926. Dr. Thompson served for many years on the Lincoln Chiropractic College board of trustees. He was a founder of the Maryland Chiropractic Association in 1925 and later was elected president three times. He was also a founder of the National Council of Chiropractic Roentgenologists in 1947. During the war years of 1944 to 1946, he served as president of the NCA. Dr. Thompson practiced in Maryland for 50 years.

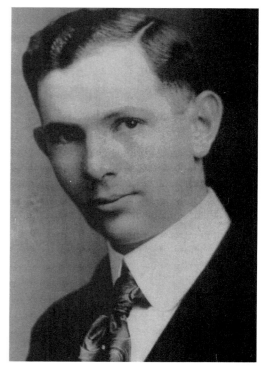

Ernest A. Thompson, a 1914 graduate of PSC, was a leading expert in chiropractic radiography. His 1918 text, Chiropractic Spinography, *is considered an early chiropractic radiographic classic.*

Courtesy Palmer College of Chiropractic Archives, Davenport, Iowa.

HARRY E. VEDDER (1891-1949)

Dr. Harry Vedder enrolled at the PSC in January 1911, after a brief career in banking. Receiving his diploma in January 1912, he joined the faculty as an instructor in physiology. His duties subsequently included supervising the school's printing and advertising. He became editor of the *Chiropractic Educator,* a lay publication which grew to a circulation of more than 3 million. He also authored three textbooks, *Chiropractic Physiology* (1916), *Chiropractic Gynecology* (1919), and *Chiropractic Advertising* (1924).

Dr. Harry Vedder was one of the popular PSC faculty members who resigned during the tumult of 1924 to 1925, following the introduction of the neurocalometer. Dr. Vedder initiated discussions that led to the establishment of the Lincoln College with colleagues S.J. Burich, A.G. Hendricks, and J.N. Firth. He became the first president of the Lincoln Chiropractic College in Indianapolis, Indiana. He also originated the popular *Lincoln Bulletin.*

During his administration, Lincoln grew to rival the Fountain Head itself. By 1941 Lincoln was one of three colleges approved under the new rating system approved by the NCA's Council on Education. Dr. Vedder retired in 1940, but remained a popular lecturer for several years.

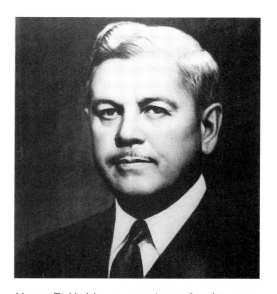

Harry E. Vedder, a prominent faculty member at the early Palmer School of Chiropractic, was a 1912 graduate of PSC; he taught physiology and authored three textbooks. In 1926, he was a founder and first president of Lincoln Chiropractic College, Indianapolis, Indiana.

Courtesy William Rehm, Baltimore, Maryland.

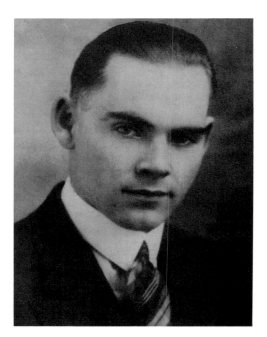

Claude O. Watkins, a 1925 graduate of PSC, was a lifelong advocate of chiropractic clinical research. He authored more than three dozen papers and served as the chairman of the NCA's Committee on Education and on its Committee on Research.

Courtesy Joe Keating, Los Angeles, California.

CLAUDE O. WATKINS (1902-1977)

Claude Watkins, unlike his European colleagues, was virtually a lone voice in his lifelong crusade against indifference to practice-based chiropractic clinical research in America. A 1925 graduate of the PSC who always referred to himself as a "chiropractic physician," Watkins thoroughly rejected dogma which he blamed for the disunity of the profession and lack of full public support. He reasoned that serious clinical research would attract the attention of educators and scientists and could only improve the quantity and quality of scholarly activities in chiropractic. The introduction in 1978 of the *Journal of Manipulative and Physiological Therapeutics,* the first chiropractic journal which would eventually be indexed in the National Library of Medicine's *Index Medicus,* is vindication of C.O. Watkins's years of advocacy.

C.O. Watkins practiced in Sidney, Montana, for 51 years. He was founding editor and publisher of the *Montana Chirolite* and the short-lived *American Chiropractic Journal,* intended for scientific publishing in the profession. He served as the first chairman of the Committee on Education of the NCA (1935 to 1938) and was later a member of the NCA Board of Directors. In 1951 he was chairman of NCA's Committee on Clinical Research. Among more than three dozen published papers, many of which focused on chiropractic education and clinical experimentation, his best known work was self-published in 1944, *The Basic Principles of Chiropractic Government.*

CLARENCE W. WEIANT (1897-1986)

Dr. Clarence Weiant was a giant intellectual presence in chiropractic for some 60 years who, like John Nugent, Earl Homewood, and Joseph Janse, cherished academic integrity. He received his prechiropractic education in chemistry at Rensselaer Polytechnic Institute in Troy, New York, from 1915 to 1918, then took his doctor of chiropractic degree from the PSC in 1921. In 1943 he earned Columbia University's first doctorate of philosophy in anthropology and established an important reputation in that discipline.

During 1921 to 1922, while on an expedition to Mexico City to study Aztec artifacts, the subject of his eventual doctoral thesis, he established the first chiropractic office in the Mexican capital. Returning from Mexico, he began his 60-year career in chiropractic education. He served at Texas Chiropractic College, San Antonio; Eastern Chiropractic Institute, New York City; and eventually at the Chiropractic Institute of New York where he was dean for many years. Dr. Weiant became a leading proponent of professional educational standards and an advocate for basic research within the chiropractic institutions.

Clarence Weiant was fluent in Spanish, French, Italian, and German and was frequently called upon to utilize those talents. After World War II he traveled Europe to reopen dialogue within the profession cut off by the war. He also investigated the growing research of chiropractic by the German medical community after the war and translated much of that literature. His writings on the anatomical and physiological basis of chiropractic were regularly published or reprinted in virtually every chiropractic journal. His 1958 book *Medicine and Chiropractic,* coauthored with Sol Goldschmidt, D.C., remains one of the most compelling presentations of its kind.

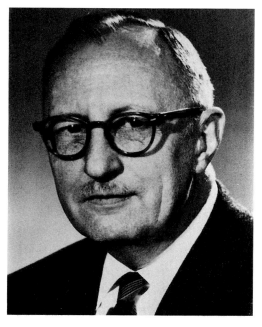

Clarence W. Weiant, a graduate of PSC in 1921, earned a Ph.D. in anthropology from Columbia University in 1943. Dr. Weiant was multilingual and served as dean at the Chiropractic Institute of New York. He was a highly regarded educator who co-authored the 1958 classic chiropractic text, Medicine and Chiropractic.

Courtesy William Rehm, Baltimore, Maryland.

419

14

CHIROPRACTIC PROFESSIONAL ASSOCIATIONS

*The Names and Politics that have Forged
Present Pathways*

Joseph C. Keating, Jr., Ph.D.

Chiropractors began to organize in the early years of the twentieth century in order to obtain licensing laws, to deal with the prosecution of practicing medicine without a license, and to raise public consciousness about the new health care method. The earliest organizations were the faculty and students of the Palmer School of Chiropractic (PSC) and spin-off institutions. The seeds of disagreement among chiropractors were planted at this time by "Old Dad Chiro" and his former pupil, Solon M. Langworthy, D.C. ᖆ

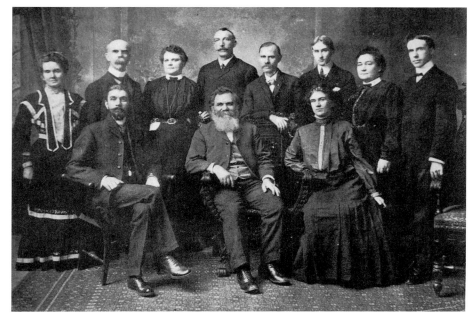

D.D. Palmer and Palmer School and Cure faculty circa 1906.
Courtesy Palmer College of Chiropractic Archives, Davenport, Iowa.

SOLON LANGWORTHY'S AMERICAN CHIROPRACTIC ASSOCIATION

The earliest known professional organization, the National Association of Chiropractic Doctors (NACD), was established in Minnesota in 1904. The NACD's most prominent leader, Daniel W. Reisland, D.C., had been a student of Thomas H. Storey, D.C., who would later teach chiropractic to Charles A. Cale, the founder of the Los Angeles College of Chi-

This work was made possible by the support of the National Institute of Chiropractic Research, Western States Chiropractic College, and Palmer College of Chiropractic, Archives Department.

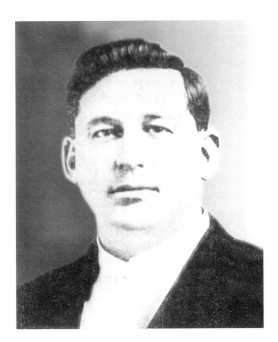

Daniel Riesland, who had been a student of Tom Storey, was a leader in the first chiropractic organization, the National Association of Chiropractic Doctors, established in 1904.
Courtesy Palmer College of Chiropractic, Davenport, Iowa.

ropractic (LACC). Dr. Reisland collaborated with Dr. Langworthy in 1905 to introduce to the Minnesota legislature the first bill to regulate the profession. Langworthy, owner and president of the American School of Chiropractic & Nature Cure (ASC&NC) in Cedar Rapids, Iowa, had established a 2-year broad-scope curriculum in place of the 9-month program offered at the PSC in Davenport. The proposed legislation would have required prospective licensees to have completed the more broad-scope educational program at the ASC&NC to qualify for licensure, which would have left Palmer graduates ineligible for licensure.

D.D. Palmer, founder of chiropractic and head of the PSC, was furious that his former pupil, Langworthy, was competing with him in the school business. He railed against the "mixer" character of Langworthy's disciples: "They have mixed what little they do know of this science with medicinal and mechanical remedies, till today, there is but little, if any, resemblance between what is now called chiropractic in Minnesota and that which is taught at the Palmer School."

With his son, B.J., Old Dad Chiro mounted a vigorous campaign to convince Minnesota legislators to defeat the proposed bill. When the bill nevertheless passed both houses of the legislature, the father of chiropractic paid a personal visit to John A. Johnson, governor of Minnesota, to plead that the governor veto the legislation. Old Dad Chiro's advice to the state's chief executive officer was apparently reinforced by similar recommendations from leaders of organized medicine in the state. The governor refused to sign the legislation. Despite other attempts, it would be 1913 in Kansas before chiropractic legislation would be signed into law.

The year 1905 also saw Langworthy and several of his alumni organize the first of five organizations to call itself the American Chiropractic Association (ACA). The Langworthy ACA organization apparently combined with the Minnesota-based NADC to make it a truly interstate, if not national professional association for chiropractic. Little more is known of Langworthy's first ACA, except that the Minnesota branch lasted into the 1930s as the Minnesota American Chiropractic Association.

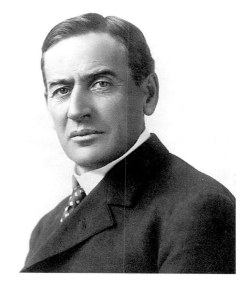

Governor John A. Johnson of Minnesota. At the urging of D.D. Palmer, Governor Johnson vetoed the chiropractic's legislative bill on April 16, 1905.
Courtesy Minnesota Historical Society, St. Paul, Minnesota.

B.J.'S UNIVERSAL CHIROPRACTORS' ASSOCIATION

In 1906, following D.D. Palmer's conviction and jailing for practicing medicine without a license in Scott County, Iowa, B.J. Palmer and a number of Palmer graduates organized the Universal Chiropractors' Association (UCA) in order to provide for the legal defense of chiropractors who were increasingly being charged with practicing medicine without a license. B.J. was elected secretary of the UCA and held this post for 20 years, during which time the organization was headquartered at his Davenport school.

One of the first actions of the UCA was to officially condemn the mixer policies of Langworthy's ACA. Since most early UCA members were Palmer alumni, while most ACA members were aligned with, if not graduated from, Langworthy's ASC&NC, interschool rivalry probably fueled the frictions between these two organizations. Although in later years many Palmer graduates would become members and leaders of various broad-scope (mixer) associations, the tendency of professional societies to align either with so-called straight (Palmer) or with so-called mixer (Langworthy) schools has characterized many of the political disputes among chiropractors ever since.

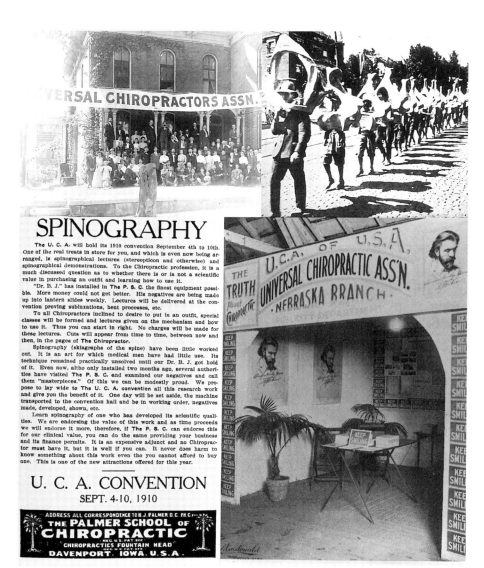

SPINOGRAPHY

The U. C. A. will hold its 1910 convention September 4th to 10th. One of the real treats in store for you, and which is even now being arranged, is spinographical lectures (stereopticon and otherwise) and spinographical demonstrations. To the Chiropractic profession, it is a much discussed question as to whether there is or is not a scientific value in purchasing an outfit and learning how to use it.

"Dr. B. J." has installed in The P. S. C. the finest equipment possible. More money could not get better. His negatives are being made up into lantern slides weekly. Lectures will be delivered at the convention proving subluxations, bent processes, etc.

To all Chiropractors inclined to desire to put in an outfit, special classes will be formed and lectures given on the mechanism and how to use it. Thus you can start in right. No charges will be made for these lectures. Cuts will appear from time to time, between now and then, in the pages of The Chiropractor.

Spinography (skiagraphs of the spine) have been little worked out. It is an art for which medical men have had little use. Its technique remained practically unsolved until our Dr. B. J. got hold of it. Even now, altho only installed two months ago, several authorities have visited The P. S. C. and examined our negatives and call them "masterpieces." Of this we can be modestly proud. We propose to lay wide to The U. C. A. convention all this research work and give you the benefit of it. One day will be set aside, the machine transported to the convention hall and be in working order, negatives made, developed, shown, etc.

Learn spinography of one who has developed its scientific qualities. We are endorsing the value of this work and as time proceeds we will endorse it more, therefore, if The P. S. C. can endorse this for our clinical value, you can do the same providing your business and its finance permits. It is an expensive adjunct and no Chiropractor must have it, but it is well if you can. It never does harm to know something about this work even tho you cannot afford to buy one. This is one of the new attractions offered for this year.

U. C. A. CONVENTION
SEPT. 4-10, 1910

ADDRESS ALL CORRESPONDENCE TO B. J. PALMER D. C. PH. C.
THE PALMER SCHOOL of CHIROPRACTIC
REG. U.S. PAT. OFF.
"CHIROPRACTICS FOUNTAIN HEAD"
DAVENPORT, IOWA, U.S.A.

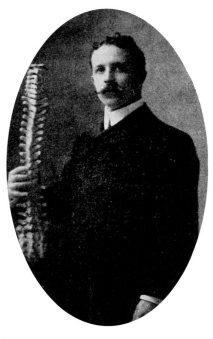

Solon Langworthy organized the first American Chiropractic Association in 1905.

Courtesy Palmer College of Chiropractic Archives, Davenport, Iowa.

Photo montage of the early Universal Chiropractor's Association, organized by B.J. Palmer in 1906.

Courtesy Palmer College of Chiropractic Archives, Davenport, Iowa.

Elective Officers of the Universal Chiropractor's Association

B. J. Palmer, D. C., Ph. C.
Secretary
Davenport, Iowa

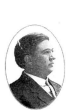

Frank W. Elliott, D. C.
Treasurer
Davenport, Iowa

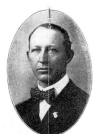

Geo. A. Newsalt, D. C.
President
Fargo, N. D.

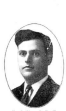

Paul Strand, D. C.
Vice President
Youngstown, Ohio

O. F. Strand, D. C.
Director
Minneapolis, Minn.

S. C. Scharnhorst, D. C.
Director
Milwaukee, Wis.

G. G. Wood, D. C.
Director
Kenmore, N. D.

J. W. Daugherty, D. C.
Chairman of Board
Mason City, Iowa

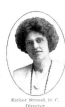

Esther Strand, D. C.
Director
Minneapolis, Minn.

Photo montage of the Elective Officers of the Universal Chiropractor's Association in 1913.
From *The Chiropractor*, August 1913.

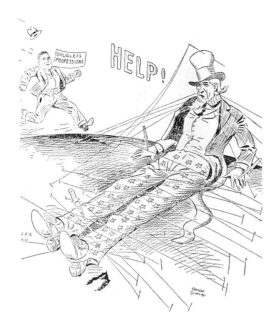

A cartoon in which drugless professionals are depicted as the hero, rescuing an Uncle Sam restricted by knives and needles.

Courtesy Palmer College of Chiropractic Archives, Davenport, Iowa.

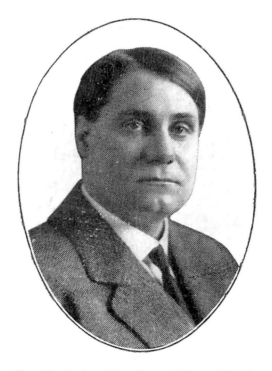

Tom Morris, long-time General Counsel for the Universal Chiropractors Association.

Courtesy Palmer College of Chiropractic Archives, Davenport, Iowa.

However, the UCA was first and foremost a legal protection organization in a time when only a few chiropractors were licensed, not as chiropractors, but under the drugless practitioner (DP) laws available in a few American states. In Illinois, for example, Oakley G. Smith, D.C., dean of Langworthy's ASC&NC and Minora Paxson, D.C., chair of the Department of Obstetrics for ASC&NC, were licensed to practice as DPs in 1905. Similarly, Carl V. Schultz, M.D., N.D., LL.B., remembered as the "father of naturopathy in California," was successful in 1908 in having a naturopathic law passed in California, under which members of the state naturopathic society were licensed by the Board of Medical Examiners. This law lasted less than 2 years, but during this time a number of chiropractors, including several of D.D. Palmer's early West Coast graduates obtained the legal right to practice the healing arts without the use of drugs and surgery. These chiropractors included Charles A. Cale, D.C., who was later to found the LACC.

However, in other states chiropractors were not so fortunate. Since its formation in 1846 the American Medical Association (AMA) had sought to prevent non-medical doctors and "irregulars," such as homeopathic and eclectic medical physicians, from competing with the "regular" medical doctors. By the turn of the nineteeth century, organized medicine was well on the way to suppressing all medical sects, that is, irregular practitioners. The new professions of chiropractic, naturopathy, and osteopathy soon became targets of organized medicine's efforts to control, contain, or eliminate rival health care professions.

An important turning point for chiropractic came in 1907 when a chiropractor arrested for unlicensed practice of medicine, surgery, and osteopathy was acquitted of these charges in La Crosse, Wisconsin. Shegatoro Morikubo, D.C., a 1901 graduate of the PSC, was exonerated when UCA defense counsel, Tom Morris, LL.B., convinced a jury that chiropractic was "separate and distinct" from other healing arts, and therefore ought not to be under the regulatory control of the state's medical board. Morris first asked that charges of medical and surgical practice be dismissed on the grounds that Dr. Morikubo had used only his hands to heal the sick. Morris next entered into evidence the textbook authored by Drs. Smith, Paxson, and Langworthy of the ASC&NC, presented letters from the deans of several osteopathic schools indicating that there was nothing similar between osteopathy and chiropractic, and placed on the stand several expert witnesses who held degrees in both disciplines and stated that chiropractic theory and practice was separate and distinct from osteopathy. Morris argued that the people of Wisconsin ought to have the right to choose the new health science of chiropractic.

Although the legal strategy in the Morikubo case did not set a strong legal precedent (a Massachusetts court ruled in 1915 that the practice of chiropractic was the practice of medicine and therefore required licensure), it did provide a model for other successful defenses of chiropractors in the years to come. Time and time again Morris and the UCA legal defense team would argue the separate and distinct character of chiropractic and would paint organized medicine as a monopoly-seeking bully who sought to block the people's right to choose their own type of doctor. Such images helped to persuade many juries to find on behalf of defendant chiropractors in thousands of cases. Palmer graduates such as Lee W. Edwards, M.D., D.C., came to prominence in the profession for their role in aiding in the acquittals of many chiropractors.

OTHER EARLY CHIROPRACTIC PROFESSIONAL ASSOCIATIONS

Chiropractors' legal defense needs and the frequent success of the Morris defense team helped to swell the ranks of the early UCA. However, many chiropractors were already rejecting B.J. Palmer's leadership and his insistence upon "pure, straight, and unadulterated chiropractic." Several rival organizations were formed to provide an alternative to the UCA. One such was the International Chiropractic Association (ICA), no relation to today's International Chiropractors' Association (ICA). This early ICA was affiliated with Joy Loban's Universal Chiropractic College in Davenport, published an *International Chiropractic Journal,* and drew membership from throughout the United States and Canada.

Another UCA rival organization was a second American Chiropractic Association (ACA), which was organized in Oklahoma by a number of graduates of Willard Carver's Carver Chiropractic College and of the Palmer-Gregory College of Chiropractic, which D.D. Palmer initially supported but abandoned in 1907 or 1908. This second ACA was philosophically in the tradition established by Andrew P. Davis, M.D., N.D., D.O., D.C., Oph. D., who had published one of the first textbooks on osteopathy and had subsequently studied under D.D. Palmer. Davis's ACA may have had no ties to Langworthy's earlier organization, but it clearly paralleled them in terms of the broad scope of practice methods advocated. Within its orbits were such notorious mixers as Joe Shelby Riley, M.D., Ph.D., D.O., D.C., N.D., who would subsequently establish chiropractic schools in Massachusetts and Washington, D.C.; George D. Gillespie, M.D., D.C., N.D., a leader in the naturopathic community in Southern California; Charles A. Cale, N.D., D.C., founder and president of the LACC; Albert W. Richardson, D.C., founder and president of the California Chiropractic College; John L. Hively, D.O., D.C., an early Palmer graduate who practiced in Illinois; Frederick W. Collins, D.O., D.C., of the Mecca College of Chiropractic in New Jersey; and C. Sterling Cooley, D.C., of Enid, Oklahoma, later a prime leader for the reorganized NCA of the 1930s.

Davis's ACA, formed circa 1910, clearly had strong naturopathic influences and looked to Alva Gregory, M.D., D.C., for leadership. Gregory, who was D.D. Palmer's former business partner in the Palmer-Gregory school gave seminars in chiropractic throughout the United States. Gregory also edited and published the ACA journal, *The American Drugless Healer.* Gregory's influence continued at least until 1913, when Gregory merged his school with the St. Louis School of Chiropractic in Missouri. The ACA led by Davis and Gregory declared that its purpose was ". . . to secure recognition by obtaining representation upon the medical examining boards in the different states, where we cannot get separate legislation, so that by examination upon the branches studied and used in the practice of this science, those wishing to practice Chiropractic may be determined."

CHIROPRACTIC LEGISLATIVE DILEMMAS

The ACA's resolve was a reflection of the initiative already displayed by chiropractors in various jurisdictions. By 1908 chiropractors were actively pursuing legislation in Oklahoma, Virginia, and Washington, D.C.,

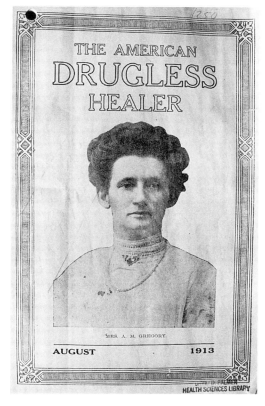

A cover of the American Drugless Healer *featuring a photo of Mrs. Alva Gregory.*

From *The American Drugless Healer,* August 1913.

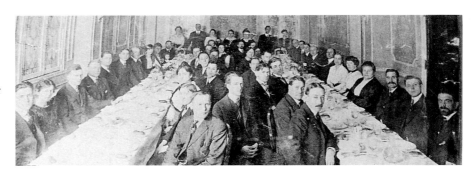

Photograph from the Wisconsin Chiropractic Association banquet of 1916, including B.J. Palmer, Frank Logic, Tom Morris, and F.G. Lundy.

From *Chiropractic in Wisconsin,* by Robert Mawhiney, 1984.

among others. However, "separate and distinct" legislation was not at first a goal of the Palmers.

In his 1914 posthumously published volume, *The Chiropractor,* Old Dad Chiro suggested that the practice of his theories and methods was a "religious duty," and thereby exempted from legal regulation under the religious freedom clauses in states such as California, Illinois, Kansas, Virginia, and Washington. B.J. Palmer and Tom Morris argued for a "law of survival;" they suggested that incompetent chiropractors would weed themselves out by their inability to satisfy patients. The UCA's secretary suggested that "only the people could and should determine the fate of chiropractic." B.J. insisted that he was not against the "right kind" of legislation but was not optimistic that chiropractic would remain "pure" once it became legally institutionalized. He particularly resisted the passage of laws requiring more than the 18 months of chiropractic education offered by the PSC. Morris, the UCA's chief legal counsel, believed that legislation would cause the profession to drift away from straight chiropractic principles.

However, by 1927 several dozen states had legalized the practice of chiropractic, and the UCA, bowing to the inevitable, had long since become involved in seeking to influence such laws. Kansas had been first, in 1913, to pass such a law, but owing to the governor's refusal to appoint a chiropractic board of examiners, Arkansas was first, in 1915, to issue a chiropractic license. True to expectations, many chiropractic laws were not consistent with B.J.'s hands-only, subluxation-only version of chiropractic. The state of Oregon for example, which had been influenced by the broad curriculum offered at the D.D. Palmer College of Chiropractic in Portland from 1908 to 1910, permitted the practice of obstetrics, minor surgery, and physiotherapy by chiropractors. B.J. Palmer and the UCA sought to prevent such broad-scope legislation, supported chiropractors who pressed for more narrow scopes of practice, and sought the revision of laws which did not suit them. The preexisting tensions between broad-scope and narrow-scope chiropractors could only be aggravated by such disputes.

In Nebraska, for instance, a schism between narrow-scope and broad-scope factions of the state association was precipitated by legislation which required 27 months of instruction, rather than the 18 months offered at the PSC. H.C. Crabtree, M.D., D.C., who operated the Nebraska Chiropractic College in Lincoln, the state's capital, offered the required minimum 27-month curriculum. Crabtree allied himself with O.G. Clark, D.C., in pressing for prosecution of the state's then unlicensed Palmer graduates, who were not even qualified to take the licensing examination. Such hostilities continued through 1923, when Nebraska reduced its educational requirements to 18 months of chiropractic education.

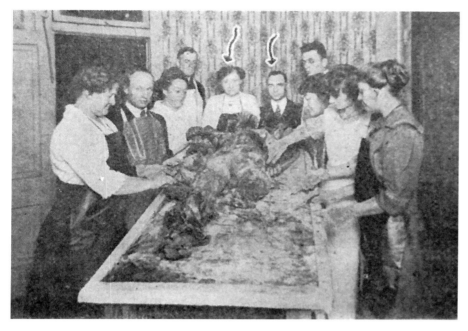

Dissecting Room of the Nebraska Chiropractic College, Drs. Crabtree and Crabtree instructing circa 1920.

From the Nebraska Chiropractic College's Contact, September 1921.

The Palmer-UCA victory in Nebraska would be short-lived, however. In 1927 Nebraska passed a basic science law which prevented any new chiropractic licenses from 1929 to 1951. Basic science legislation requiring chiropractors and other healing arts professionals to pass examinations in fundamental topics such as anatomy, physiology, pathology, and diagnosis was introduced by organized medicine in many states to prevent the licensing of chiropractors, naturopaths, osteopaths, and other irregular practitioners. Such laws were part of a nationwide campaign to contain and eliminate all healing arts competition, but they were perhaps most pointedly directed at chiropractors.

Go-To-Jail Strategies

Organized medicine's political efforts to prevent the licensing of chiropractors sometimes backfired, however, because of the go-to-jail strategy adopted by the UCA. The policy was modeled partly after the successful methods of men like O.L. Brown, D.C., and T.F. Ratledge, D.C. Ratledge, who had been convicted in 1916 of unlicensed practice of medicine, had served 90 days in Los Angeles County jail. His incarceration made him a martyr.

California newspapers, which had formerly given little positive press to the chiropractors, suddenly took an interest in a doctor who would rather serve time in jail than receive a pardon from the governor on the condition that he accept a license from the state's medical board. Ratledge had argued that licensure by the Board of Medical Examiners would be fraud against the people of California, since the medical board knew nothing about chiropractic and were not qualified to judge his competence. The go-to-jail policy, which required chiropractors to accept imprisonment rather than pay a fine when convicted of unlicensed practice, became a badge of courage among chiropractors.

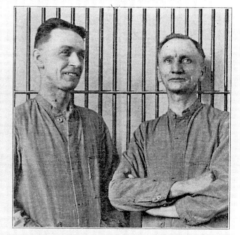

KEEP SMILING

A. G. ECKOLS, D. C.   F. D. IRISH, D. C.

We're in jail for doing good, not by the protest of any San Diego citizen, but by the medics themselves.

WHY?

If you want medical freedom protest Now!

ECKOLS and IRISH

Chiropractors used their incarceration to gain the public's support against medical monopoly.

Courtesy Palmer College of Chiropractic Archives, Davenport, Iowa.

427

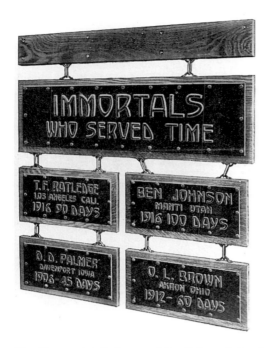

The "Immortals" plaque at the Palmer School of Chiropractic, which commemorates chiropractors who went to jail for their beliefs. From *The Fountain Head News,* February 1917.

In California prior to passage of the 1922 Chiropractic Act, organized medicine adopted a policy of keeping at least one chiropractor in jail in each county of the state at all times. It was rumored that the Los Angeles County Sheriff's Office had more chiropractic adjusting couches than all the chiropractors in the state. When a chiropractor was arrested, his table was also confiscated. The Alameda County Chiropractic Society adopted the UCA's go-to-jail strategy and established a fund to support the families of jailed doctors. The public came to think of chiropractors as a bullied minority who were willing to sacrifice their freedom in defense of their beliefs. When the issue of licensing was placed on the ballot in the 1922 elections, the people of California expressed their approval by voting to legalize chiropractic. Many other chiropractors followed Ratledge's example. In Ohio in 1923 future UCA president Charles E. Schillig, D.C., served a 6-month term in the Huron County jail and gained national attention from his jail cell by collecting 100,000 petitions to legalize chiropractic.

Universal Chiropractors' Association Model Bill Legislation

As success in securing legislation in several states grew, Palmer and the UCA increasingly sought to direct the shape of these laws. The organization adopted a model bill, which could be introduced in those states that did not yet have a law. The model bill called for 18 months of training for chiropractic doctors, a hands-only scope of practice, that is no mixing, and a board of examiners composed exclusively of chiropractors. At about the same time, 1921, the UCA formed an early National Board of Chiropractic Examiners (NBCE), which is of no relation to today's NBCE, to attempt to standardize licensing examinations and to inspect the various chiropractic colleges. Prominent among the members of this board were Sylva L. Ashworth, D.C., of Nebraska; Lillard T. Marshall, D.C., of Kentucky; and Anna Foy, D.C., of Kansas, all of whom served on their respective state boards. This early NBCE did not last long, owing to the unwillingness of many school leaders to submit to any supervision and to the great variation in opinion among the profession about what standards of education and scope of practice should be adopted.

Much of this disagreement can also be traced to the UCA's simultaneously introduced house cleaning policy, which required the various state associations affiliated with the UCA to purge all mixers from their ranks. The UCA threatened to organize competing, straight-only chiropractic organizations in those states where the existing chiropractic society failed to comply.

Many chiropractors were outraged by the UCA's heavy-handed tactics. Exemplary was Harry K. McIlroy, D.C., of Indianapolis, who would later become a leader in the National Chiropractic Association (NCA). A 1919 graduate of the broad-scope National School of Chiropractic, McIlroy resigned in protest from the Indiana Chiropractic Association's board of directors in 1922 when the state society voted to affiliate with the UCA and to comply with UCA's straight chiropractic policies. Along with Willard Carver, LL.B., D.C., and A.B. Cochrane, D.C., McIlroy was instrumental during 1922 in establishing a third American Chiropractic Association (ACA), a group which would compete with the UCA for membership.

THE THIRD AMERICAN CHIROPRACTIC ASSOCIATION

This third ACA may have been a reorganization of a former, weaker society known as the National Federation of Chiropractors (NFC). The NFC had been established during the first World War in order to "obtain recognition for D.C.'s in the armed services." N.C. Ross, D.C., founder-president of the Ross Chiropractic College in Fort Wayne, Indiana, had served as the first president of the NFC. He was succeeded in 1919 by Albert B. Cochrane, D.C., a Ross College graduate. Cochrane became one of the ACA's vice presidents in 1922 and later served as president of the ACA from 1928 to 1930. The NFC's efforts to obtain commissions for chiropractors in the United States Army Medical Corps were continued throughout the 1920s by Leo L. Spears, D.C., an early supporter of the ACA.

The ACA's membership grew in proportion to the UCA's decline, which was attributable not only to dissatisfaction with the restrictive policies emanating from B.J. Palmer and the UCA, but also to the tireless efforts of Frank R. Margetts, LL.B., D.D., D.C. Margetts graduated from the Chicago College of Law circa 1893 and from the National School of Chiropractic in 1920, then served as president of the Colorado Chiropractic Association in 1922. At the 1923 ACA convention in Chicago, he was elected president and served in this post until 1929. During this period Margetts toured the country, spoke to thousands of chiropractors and laymen, participated in various court cases and in campaigns to either establish or amend chiropractic legislation, and played a role within the profession that paralleled that of the UCA's Palmer and Morris. His oratorical skills, honed by his training as an ordained Baptist minister, served the ACA very well. When he stepped down from the presidency in 1929, the membership of the broad-scope ACA matched that of the narrow-scope UCA: each had about 1500 chiropractors.

Margetts was instrumental in establishing the ACA's Public Lecture Bureau, through which nationwide lecture tours were arranged. He also oversaw the development of the ACA's patient magazine, *Life Line,* which began publication in 1929, and rivaled the PSC's lay magazine, *The Chiropractic Educator.* In April 1930, *Life Line* magazine was reinforced by a weekly *Life Line* radio program, which aired over KOA in Denver, WJR in Detroit, KYW in Chicago, WOV in New York, WSYR in Syracuse, WGR in Buffalo, WTNT in Nashville, KGIR in Butte, KOH in Reno, and KFI in Los Angeles.

Margetts's campaign throughout the profession expressed the association's desire to develop a democratic organization providing legal protection, promoting broad-scope chiropractic legislation, and pressing for higher standards of education. However, the ACA's major selling point among chiropractors was its independence from the influence of the chiropractic colleges.

School versus field control of the profession was clearly the bone of contention among chiropractors in the 1920s, and this at a time when the mounting assault from organized medicine made such internal divisiveness especially troublesome. In 1924 Morris Fishbein, M.D., succeeded G.H. Simmons, M.D., as editor of the *Journal of the American Medical Association,* and the AMA redoubled its efforts to have chiropractors prosecuted in states both with and without chiropractic legal regulation. Fishbein would come to be known as the chiropractors' arch nemesis. His many articles and books on quackery, chiropractic, and other drugless healing arts earned the wrath of chiropractors of all persuasions.

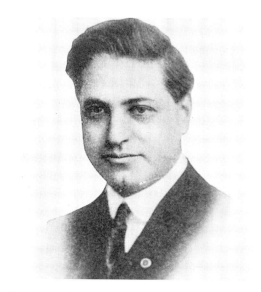

N.C. Ross, founder and president of the Ross Chiropractic College in Fort Wayne, Indiana, served as the first president of the American Chiropractors Association in 1922.
From the *Catalog,* Ross Chiropractic College, 1916.

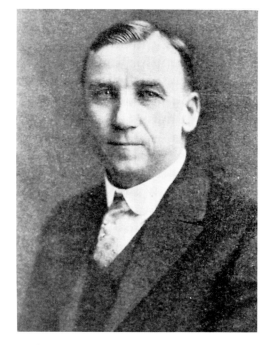

Frank Margetts, an attorney and 1920 National School graduate, was the president of the ACA from 1923 to 1929.
From the *Bulletin of the ACA,* July 1924.

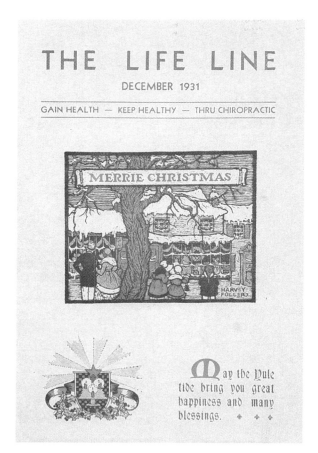

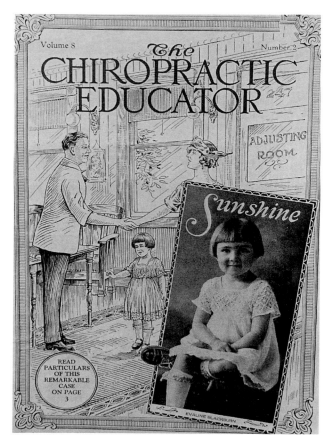

Covers of The Life Line *(left), the ACA's patient magazine, and* The Chiropractic Educator, *the UCA's lay magazine.*

Courtesy Palmer College of Chiropractic Archives, Davenport, Iowa.

It was clear the profession was besieged both from within and from outside its own ranks. Fishbein wrote in 1925,

> It has been said that osteopathy is essentially a method of entering the practice of medicine by the back door. Chiropractic, by contrast, is an attempt to arrive through the cellar. The man who applies at the back door at least makes himself presentable. The one who comes through the cellar is besmirched with dust and grime; he carries a crowbar and he may wear a mask.

THE CHIROPRACTIC HEALTH BUREAU

It was at this most inopportune time that B.J. Palmer chose to introduce the neurocalometer (NCM). The two-pronged device detected side-to-side differences in the temperature of the spine, theoretically caused by nerve pinching as the spinal nerve roots exited the spine, that is, subluxation. Palmer claimed that no chiropractor, no matter how skilled in palpation and x-ray, could detect these classic chiropractic lesions as accurately as the NCM.

Palmer characterized the NCM's introduction as a means of forcing mixer chiropractors back to a straight focus on subluxation detection and adjustment. When criticized for the cost of renting an NCM, Palmer likened the chiropractic profession to a cow, which he had fed for 20 years while the mixers took all the cream.

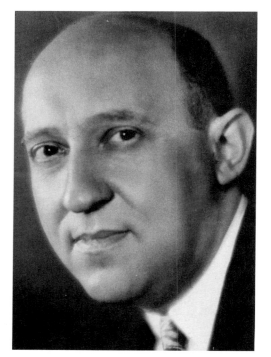

As editor of the Journal of the American Medical Association, *Morris Fishbein, M.D., would earn the wrath of chiropractors of all persuasions with his many articles and books on quackery, chiropractic, and other drugless healing arts.*

Courtesy the National Library of Medicine, Bethesda, Maryland.

Membership recruitment flyers of the Chiropractic Health Bureau.

Courtesy Palmer College of Chiropractic Archives, Davenport, Iowa.

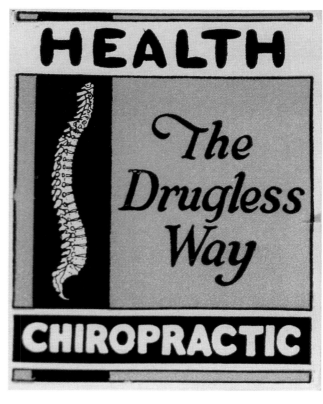

Decal from the 1930's advertising health through chiropractic.

Courtesy Logan College of Chiropractic Archives, Chesterfield, Missouri.

Chiropractors were outraged, including many who had previously accepted Palmer as chiropractic's "Maximum Leader." At the UCA convention in 1925, Tom Morris, UCA Chief Legal Counsel since 1906, tendered his resignation and suggested that the marketing of a $30 device for $2200 was unconscionable. When Palmer promptly resigned as UCA secretary, Morris was reinstated. Hard-core Palmer loyalists worked furiously, but unsuccessfully, behind the scenes to have Palmer returned to the UCA secretariat at the association's next convention in August 1926.

On September 4, 1926, having failed to return to the UCA, Palmer founded the Chiropractic Health Bureau (CHB), forerunner of today's International Chiropractors' Association (ICA). Attorney George Rinier took over the legal defense activities with the CHB, while Morris continued with the UCA. Both Morris and Rinier traveled extensively throughout the nation on behalf of their clients. The CHB remained as a protective organization for chiropractors until 1941 when it was rechartered to become the ICA.

INTERNATIONAL CONGRESS OF CHIROPRACTIC EXAMINING BOARDS

Now there were three national professional associations of chiropractors: the ACA, the CHB, and the remaining UCA. Soon, there would be a fourth, though of a somewhat different character. In September 1926 rep-

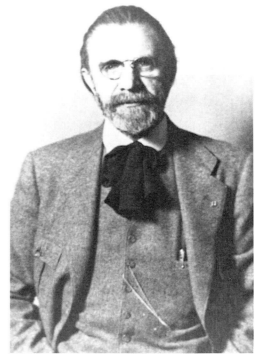

B.J. Palmer, circa 1935, after the time of upheaval in the Universal Chiropractor's Association.

Courtesy Palmer College of Chiropractic Archives, Davenport, Iowa.

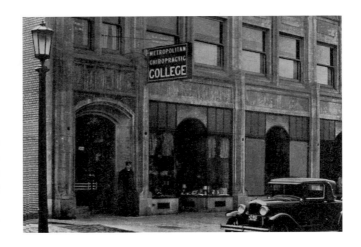

Metropolitan Chiropractic College in Cleveland, Ohio, was a member of the International Chiropractic Congress, as were a combination of both narrow- and broad-scope schools.

Courtesy Palmer College of Chiropractic Archives, Davenport, Iowa.

resentatives of the licensing boards of 16 states met in Kansas City to organize the International Congress of Chiropractic Examining Boards (ICCEB). Called by Harry Gallaher, D.C., of Oklahoma, this first meeting of the ICCEB elected Eugene Cox, D.C., of North Carolina as its first president. Other officers included Anna Foy, D.C., of the Kansas board; Sylva Ashworth, D.C., president of the Nebraska board; C. Sterling Cooley, D.C., of the Oklahoma board; and J. Ralph John, D.C., of the Maryland board.

The ICCEB was conceived as a potential authority for the regulation of chiropractic education and licensing that would be independent of the feuding national professional associations and the warring schools. There was such delight at the success of this amicable effort that a number of state associations and chiropractic colleges sent delegates to the 1927 meeting in Memphis. The following year two divisions were added to the Congress: one for state associations and another for the colleges. Today's Congress of Chiropractic State Associations may be viewed as a continuation of the second division of this expanded International Chiropractic Congress (ICC).

The ICC's wide acceptance throughout the profession derived in part from the fact that it did not compete with the ACA, CHB, and UCA to provide malpractice insurance and legal defense services. Moreover, the chiropractic schools, most of which were private, for-profit business ventures that competed vigorously with one another for students, finally found a neutral arena in which they could meet to discuss the thorny problems they all confronted. No one school leader had any authority greater than any other, and the wider ICC nurtured the hope that the schools could improve themselves and end their battles.

Included within the Educational Institutions Division of the ICC were not only such broad-scope leaders as William C. Schulze, M.D., D.C., of the National College in Chicago, and Ernest J. Smith, D.C., of the Metropolitan Chiropractic College in Cleveland, Ohio, but also leaders from narrow-scope schools, such as B.J.'s PSC, Carl Cleveland, Sr.'s Kansas City school, T.F. Ratledge's ultra-straight Los Angeles institution, and the Texas Chiropractic College. All found an organizational home, at least temporarily, within the ICC. The various successful meetings of the state association delegates also lent credibility to the idea that chiropractors of divergent views, even leaders of influential schools, could indeed work together harmoniously.

THE EMERGENCE OF THE NATIONAL CHIROPRACTIC ASSOCIATION

The year 1928 also saw the early death, at age 60, of Tom Morris, who was succeeded as general counsel of the UCA by Arthur T. Holmes, LL.B. Morris's departure from the political scene may have opened the way for the merger of the ACA and UCA. Despite the widely held wish that the two largest professional bodies would amalgamate, Morris had been skeptical. Now Frank Margetts, D.C., of the ACA and Charles E. Schillig, D.C., of the UCA each stepped down as president of their respective organizations and worked behind the scenes to bring the two groups together. With the assistance of Lillard T. Marshall, D.C., president of the Kentucky Board of Chiropractic Examiners, these men quietly worked out the details for a new professional society, the National Chiropractic Association (NCA), forerunner of the current American Chiropractic Association (ACA), which was established in 1963. At a meeting in Chicago's LaSalle Hotel during October 1930, the boards of directors of the ACA and UCA agreed to the merger.

The following month the NCA was chartered with Marshall as its first president; Cecil E. Foster, D.C., of Jacksonville, Florida, as vice president; and Benjamin A. Sauer, D.C., of Syracuse, New York, as secretary-treasurer, a position Dr. Sauer had held with the ACA.

Although the success of the ICC seems to have encouraged the formation of the NCA, the ICC itself did not survive in its original form. The ICCEB continues today as the Federation of Chiropractic Licensing Boards, and the ICC's division of state organizations continues as the Congress of Chiropractic State Associations.

By 1934, as the NCA grew, parallel councils within this national body were formed to match or replace the ICC divisions. The NCA joined with the ICC in 1932 to cosponsor the *Journal of the International Chiroprac-*

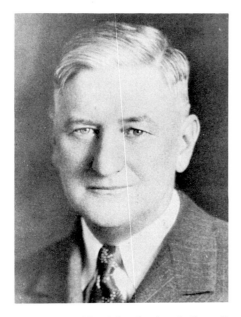

After Tom Morris's death, Arthur T. Holmes became the Chief Legal Counsel of the UCA and later of the NCA.
From *The Chiropractic Journal,* October 1939.

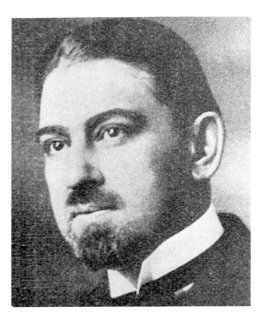

Charles Schillig, president of the UCS in 1928, worked behind the scenes with ACA president Frank Margetts to bring the two groups together.
From *The U.C.A. News,* December 1927.

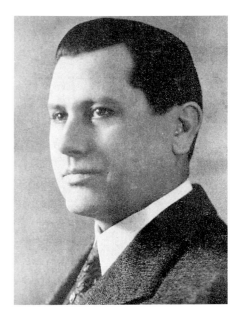

Lillard T. Marshall, circa 1943, first president (1930-1934) of the National Chiropractic Association.
From the *Journal of the NCA,* April 1943.

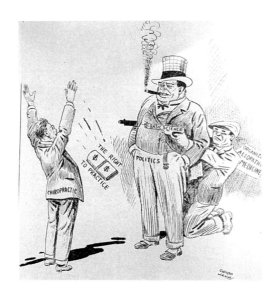

Cartoon reflecting the chiropractor's view of the basic science legislation. The original caption stated, "Medical monopolist is a modern highwayman."

From the *Chiropractic Journal,* April 1936.

tic Congress, which was renamed *The Chiropractic Journal.* This magazine would go through a number of title changes, but until the 1960s was always edited by one man, Loran Meredith Rogers, D.C. Rogers became as prominent within the NCA's orbit as was B.J. Palmer in narrow-scope chiropractic and the CHB. By 1934, however, the ICC had ceased to function, and many of its officers had become officials of the NCA.

The early years of the NCA were exhilarating but strenuous. Political activity was stressed, given the mounting two-pronged campaign by organized medicine to eliminate the chiropractic profession. While efforts to prosecute chiropractors in the remaining states without chiropractic legislation continued, medicine's campaign to broaden basic science legislation was expanded. In states where basic science laws had been enacted, the examinations were usually administered by biologists with Ph.D.s associated with the state university–based medical schools.

Basic science legislation forced a number of chiropractic schools to close and made recruitment of students difficult. In Indiana, for example, where the Lincoln Chiropractic College was located, administrators explained to students that it was unlikely that they would be able to obtain licensure unless they moved out of state after graduation. Chiropractors complained bitterly to the various state legislatures but to no avail. Basic science laws appeared to lawmakers and the public to be fair, in that all healing arts license applicants were required to take the same exam, a test supposedly intended to ensure minimum competency to diagnose human illness. In many states such laws would remain on the books until after the 1974 federal recognition of the Council on Chiropractic Education as the official accrediting body for chiropractic schools. In the meanwhile, chiropractors pioneered license renewal credits, and the NCA organized a traveling "National Chiropractic Clinics" program to bring quality educational programs to various state chiropractic conventions.

The stress on chiropractors was aggravated by the economic hard times throughout the nation brought about by the stock market crash of 1929 and the subsequent economic depression. Added to this were the continuing battles within the profession over scope of practice. For example, B.J. Palmer worked strenuously in California to restrict the right of chiropractors to use electrical modalities, colonic irrigation, and naturopathic remedies. Similarly, Palmer continued to insist that chiropractic education be limited to an 18-month curriculum and decried instruction in such medical topics as diagnosis and physiotherapy. Oregon chiropractors' bid to place their basic science examinations under the control of a Board of Chiropractic Examiners was defeated when Palmer added his voice to the opposition of organized medicine in the state; the president of the CHB would tolerate no form of legal relief that condoned the broad-scope expansion of chiropractic education and the inclusion of adjunctive therapies.

It was against this background that the profession moved towards the fortieth anniversary of chiropractic. Despite the economic hard times, the NCA planned a gala convention at the Hollywood Roosevelt Hotel in Los Angeles. It was the first national chiropractic convention held on the West Coast, and it attracted nearly 2000 chiropractors, or about 15% of the entire chiropractic population of the United States. More importantly, the NCA's 1935 convention marked a turning point for chiropractic education and set the stage for the disagreement between broad-scope and narrow-scope educational standards for the next 50 years.

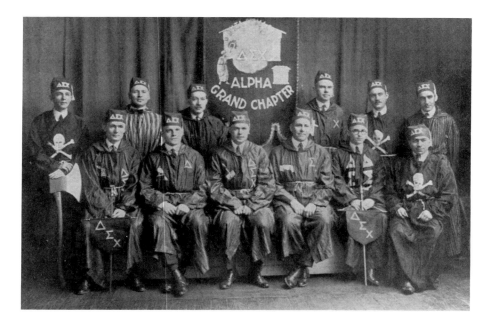

Members of Delta Sigma Chi, circa 1922. This fraternal organization was founded to protect the principles of narrow-scope chiropractic in 1913.

From *Classmates,* by Palmer School of Chiropractic, 1922.

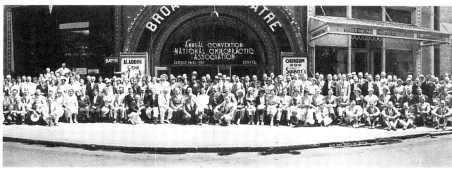

The annual NCA convention, held in Denver, Colorado, in August 1933.

Courtesy Logan College of Chiropractic Archives, Chesterfield, Missouri.

REGULATION OF SCHOOLS AND COLLEGES

The Council on State Chiropractic Examining Boards, led by Wayne Crider, D.C., of Maryland, collaborated with the NCA's Council on Chiropractic Schools to organize the NCA Committee on Educational Standards. The Educational Standards committee, headed first by C.O. Watkins, D.C., of Montana and later by Gordon M. Goodfellow, D.C., N.D., of Los Angeles, would require some 6 years to establish its authority and develop a plan for the accreditation of chiropractic colleges. The appointment of John J. Nugent, D.C., in 1939 to prepare the first formal college accreditation standards and his appointment in 1941 as the first NCA Director of Education would hasten the process of improvement and upgrading of the colleges.

Seven years would pass before Nugent released the NCA's first official list of accredited schools, during which time he inspected many of the chiropractic institutions. Nugent earned the respect of those NCA leaders and those college leaders such as Janse of National, Budden of Western States, and Smith of Metropolitan who favored the broad-scope educational upgrade. Among many in the profession who advocated a narrow-scope of practice or who owned for-profit schools, Nugent was a

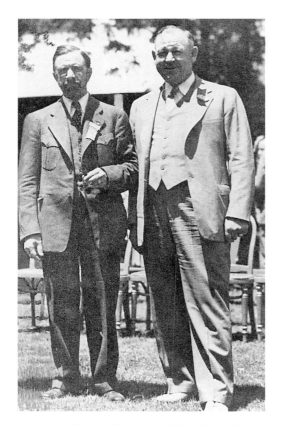

James R. Drain, President of the Texas Chiropractic College in San Antonio with B.J. Palmer. Drain was a founding member of the Associated Chiropractic Colleges of America and the Allied Chiropractic Educational Institutions.

Courtesy Palmer College of Chiropractic Archives, Davenport, Iowa.

threat, and some considered the NCA education director a villain. B.J. Palmer would have nothing to do with NCA's broad-scope educational reform efforts.

But the handwriting was on the proverbial wall even before Nugent's appointment. Sensing this, school leaders Carl S. Cleveland, D.C., of Cleveland Chiropractic College, T.F. Ratledge, D.C., of Ratledge Chiropractic College, James R. Drain, D.C., of the Texas Chiropractic College, and Craig M. Kightlinger, D.C., of the Eastern Chiropractic Institute in New York City banded together in 1938 to form the Associated Chiropractic Colleges of America to resist the NCA's reform efforts. By 1940 this group had been joined by B.J. and the PSC, and was reorganized as the Allied Chiropractic Educational Institutions (ACEI).

The NCA was undeterred by the ACEI, believing that tolerance for the broader scope of practice was actually desired by a majority of the profession and worthy of the greater educational demands it sought. Moreover, the NCA believed that increased standards of training in such preclinical subjects as anatomy, physiology, biochemistry, and pathology was the only means available to block the spread of and eventually to roll back the hated basic science laws. *The National College Journal of Chiropractic* expressed the view that "only chiropractors can define chiropractic," noting that "when chiropractic definitions were written into state laws, chiropractors themselves wrote those definitions. Chiropractors alone could say what was chiropractic."

The disagreements between the factions of chiropractors would soon be eclipsed by world events. In December 1941 the United States entered World War II officially, and the repercussions for the chiropractic profession would be significant. Unable to obtain commissions for chiropractors in the armed forces' medical departments, and unsuccessful in having chiropractors deferred from the draft as essential personnel on the home front, thousands of chiropractors served as enlisted men in all branches and occupations within the military. Many schools were forced to close. It looked as though the war might accomplish what the AMA had not been able to: decimation of the chiropractic ranks.

The war had other profound effects on the profession. Many chiropractors volunteered for service in the Medical Corps of the Army and Navy and received extensive training in physiotherapies and rehabilitation methods for disabled soldiers. Exemplary were men such as A.C. Johnson, D.C., N.D.; Robert W. Dishman, D.C., N.D; and J.G. Anderson, D.C., N.D., who would influence chiropractic education and practice for decades as authors and school leaders. Frank O. Logic, D.C., of Iron Mountain, Michigan, a veteran of World War I and a member of the NCA's

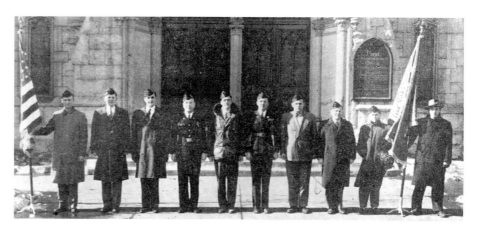

Officers of the American Society of Military Chiropractors, circa 1947.

From the *National Chiropractic Journal,* May 1947.

executive board, helped to organize the American Society of Military Chiropractors (ASMC), which published a regular monthly column in the NCA's *National Chiropractic Journal* entitled "The Chiron Call" devoted to chiropractors in the armed services.

Chiropractic Research Foundation

Other important wartime developments included the establishment of Canada's Dominion Chiropractic Council and the incorporation of the Chiropractic Research Foundation (CRF).

Discussions concerning the organization of a non-profit corporation intended to raise and receive funds for research, education, and the development of chiropractic hospitals had begun within the executive board of the NCA during 1943, while C.O. Watkins, D.C., served as chair. Watkins's successor, Gordon M. Goodfellow, D.C., N.D., of Los Angeles, presented the tentative Articles of Incorporation to the NCA's Council of Past Executives for their approval on July 26, 1944, and the following day the CRF Articles were notarized in Cook County, Illinois, and filed with the secretary of state in Delaware. Longtime NCA leader, Arthur W. Schwietert, D.C., is remembered as the father of the CRF, and served as its first president until his death in 1947.

The CRF got off to a somewhat shaky start. Its earliest efforts were directed to mounting a nationwide fund-raising campaign. Modeled after the successful March of Dimes, the chiropractic initiative involved hiring an expensive marketing firm, which was apparently unable to overcome the often negative image of chiropractic. Several hundreds of thousands of dollars were spent during the late 1940s and early 1950s, with meager results outside the profession itself. The campaign came near to bankrupting the CRF, and pledges from NCA members were reconsidered. Research became something of a dirty word during this period, and the exuberance and drive with which the professional leaders had approached chiropractic's research gap at the end of the war soon lost its momentum.

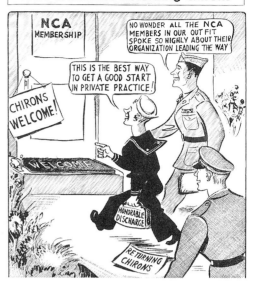

NCA Welcomes Returning Chirons

Cartoon of DCs returning from World War II; legend says, "NCA welcomes returning chirons."

From the *National Chiropractic Journal,* January 1946.

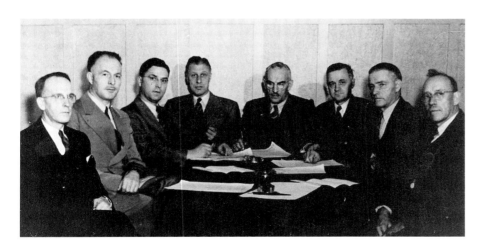

A 1943 photo of the new Canadian organization; caption reads, "Pictured above are Directors of the recently organized Dominion Chiropractic Council, representing all Provinces in Canada. (Left to Right) Dr. Gaudet, Montreal; Dr. Haldeman, Regina; J.S. Burton, Vancouver; Dr. J.A. Schnick, Hamilton; Dr. Sturdy, Vancouver; Dr. J.S. Clubine, Toronto; Dr. McElrea, Winnipeg; Dr. Messenger, Calgary."

From the *National Chiropractic Journal,* March 1943.

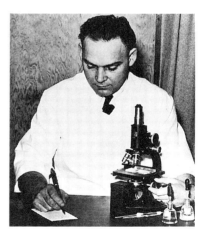

C.O. Watkins, first chairman of the NCA's Committee on Educational Standards and later a member of the NCA Board of Directors, 1938-1943.

Courtesy Palmer College of Chiropractic Archives, Davenport, Iowa.

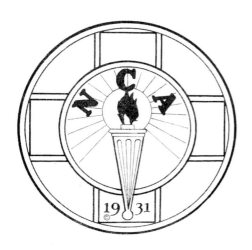

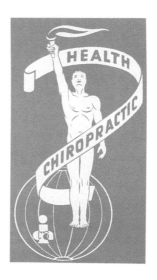

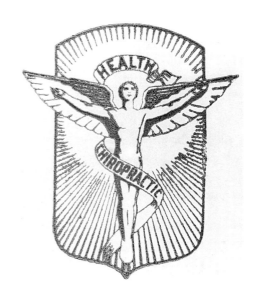

Although the NCA Torch and the ICA figure holding a torch were used, the most popuar logo depicting chiropractic has been the winged angel.

Courtesy Palmer College of Chiropractic Archives, Davenport, Iowa.

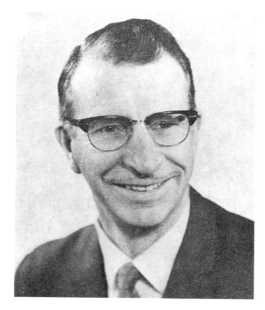

Ralph J. Martin, D.C., N.D., President of the non-profit Southern California College of Chiropractic, who collaborated with John J. Nugent, D.C, in 1946 and 1947 to lead his school into a merger with the Los Angeles College of Chiropractic, then owned by Wilma Churchill Wood, D.C.

Courtesy Los Angeles College of Chiropractic, Whittier, California.

A more conservative program followed a reorganization of the CRF at this time, and the locus of interest in clinical research seems to have shifted from the CRF to college leaders such as John B. Wolfe, D.C., of Northwestern College of Chiropractic in Minnesota; George Haynes, D.C., N.D., M.A.; and Henry Higley, D.C., N.D., M.S., of the LACC, as well as C.O. Watkins, D.C., of Montana, who chaired the NCA's Committee on Research. In the late 1950s the CRF was renamed the Foundation for Accredited Chiropractic Education (FACE), and in this capacity funneled block grants to those NCA-affiliated chiropractic colleges that were attempting to upgrade their basic science instructional facilities.

In its early years the CRF also played a supporting role in NCA Director of Education John Nugent's efforts to consolidate small, proprietary schools into larger, more fiscally sound, non-profit and professionally controlled schools, much as Abraham Flexner had helped to reform medical education in the first 2 decades of this century.

Nugent first established a non-profit holding corporation, the California Chiropractic Educational Foundation (CCEF), which was controlled partly by the NCA, partly by the broad-scope California Chiropractic Association, and partly by the state branch of the CRF. In 1946 the CCEF received the entire property of the Southern California College of Chiropractic (SCCC), no relation to today's straight chiropractic institution by the same name. The SCCC had been probably the first non-profit chiropractic school in the state, having been established as such in 1929, and was among the broadest scope institutions in the profession. The war had shriveled SCCC's student ranks, as it had most of the schools throughout the nation. On May 8, 1947, with funds contributed by the CRF, the CCEF purchased LACC from its owner and secretary, Wilma Churchill Wood, D.C., and merged the two institutions to create today's non-profit LACC. The reborn LACC-CCEF would eventually absorb a number of other, smaller chiropractic institutions in California, including the California Chiropractic Colleges, the Hollywood College of Chiropractic and Naturopathy, the San Francisco College of Chiropractic and Drugless Physicians, and the California College of Natural Healing Arts. Nugent's success in California would be repeated throughout the nation in order to both standardize and upgrade chiropractic education with an eye toward eventual federal recognition of the chiropractic colleges.

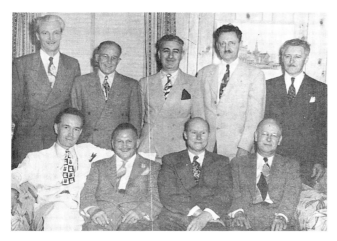

Leaders of the Chiropractic Research Foundation (CRF) meeting with Leo Spears, D.C., August 22 and 23, 1947; caption reads, "Denver conference committee: Front row (left to right) *Drs. O.A. Ohlson of Denver; Frank O. Logic of Iron Mountain, Michigan; Leo L. Spears of Denver; L.M. Rogers, of Webster City, Iowa.* Back row (left to right) *Drs. Neal Bishop of Denver, F. Lorne Wheaton of New Haven, Conn.; George E. Hariman of Gland Forks, N.D.; W.H. McNichols of Omaha and Gordon M. Goodfellow of Los Angeles, Calif."*

From the *National Chiropractic Journal,* October 1947.

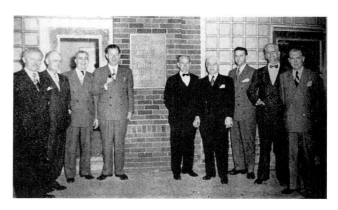

A 1950 photo of the NCA in Webster City, Iowa, reads, "Executive Officers in front of new headquarters." Left to right: *Gordon Goodfellow, Executive Director; L.M. Rogers, Executive Secretary; George Harriman; Justin Wood; John Prosser; Harry McIleroy, Executive Director; Robert Johns, Legal Counsel; John Nugent, Director of Education; Dr. Emmett Murphy, Director of Public Relations.*

From the *Journal of the National Chiropractic Association,* February 1950.

Yet another major initiative on the part of the CRF was its attempt to acquire the Spears Hospital in Denver, Colorado, as a research and postgraduate teaching facility for the profession. The initial plans, to which Leo L. Spears, D.C., the hospital's founder and president had agreed, called for the creation of a board of management composed of chiropractors familiar with the operation of inpatient facilities. The new board could then manage the facilty and "relieve Dr. Spears so that he may devote his entire time and skill to the relief of the suffering thousands who clamor for his professional attention." The arrangements between Spears and the CRF apparently fell through when Dr. Spears became dissatisfied with the operation of the facility.

Nugent's efforts toward consolidated, non-profit education put many of the proprietary and fiscally weaker schools at a great disadvantage. Although the end of the war had created a pool of veterans whose GI benefits could repopulate the student bodies of the chiropractic colleges, some schools could not attract sufficient students owing to the NCA's increasing success in raising school standards. In California, for example, the NCA's educational reform efforts paralleled the broad-scope state association's actions to raise the legally mandated minimal number of hours of chiropractic instruction from the 2400 required in the 1922 Chiropractic Act to 4000 hours, including instruction in diagnosis and physiotherapy. T.F. Ratledge's narrow-scope school, the Ratledge Chiropractic College of Los Angeles, which had operated since 1911, lost its approval by the Veterans' Administration owing to its resistance to these new standards. Meanwhile, Nugent sought to amplify the prestige of the NCA-affiliated colleges and to cultivate the interest of returning soldiers.

In fact, many schools that had barely survived the lean years of the depression and the severe drop in enrollment during the war, with the war's end, suddenly found themselves strained to capacity with the influx of veterans. Unfortunately and ironically, although the national professional associations were successful during President Harry Truman's term of office in having chiropractors deferred from military service, they were unable to have chiropractic services authorized for reimbursement under federal programs for veterans' rehabilitation.

North American Association of Chiropractic Schools and Colleges

Meanwhile, the strongest of the ICA-affiliated institutions, including the PSC, Carver College in Oklahoma City, Columbia Institute in New York City, and Cleveland Chiropractic College of Kansas City, formed the North American Association of Chiropractic Schools and Colleges (NAACSC) to counter the Nugent-led NCA Council on Education.

In the 1950s and 1960s the NAACSC filled the role that had been played by the ICA-affiliated Allied Chiropractic Educational Institutions of the 1940s. The NAACSC accredited its member institutions, the leaders of which met at least annually at the PSC homecoming to discuss mutual problems. As GI benefits for veterans' education began to expire in the 1950s, the pressing need of all chiropractic colleges became the recruitment of new students. Many in chiropractic felt that organizational unity was the only way that the profession could hope to accomplish its multiple goals.

But collaboration among the various factions within the profession was limited at best. From Davenport and the PSC, B.J. Palmer exerted his influence until his death at age 79 in 1961, and while he lived there was little chance that the ICA-affiliated PSC, the largest chiropractic school, would accept any organizational or educational terms not in accordance with B.J. With B.J.'s death, however, and with the appointment of his son, David D. Palmer, D.C., as the third president of the PSC, many believed there was once again a real opportunity for discussion of the creation of a single unified national political chiropractic organization.

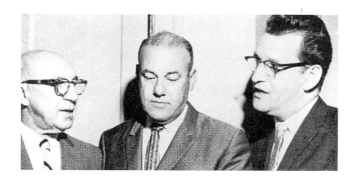

A campaign to "Fill the colleges" was initiated by the NAASC leadership, in response to the dipping enrollments as the G.I. benefits expired. Left to right: *O.D. Adams, Educational Consultant; Vinton Logan; and Ernest Napolitano.*
From the ICA International Review of Chiropractic, October 1960.

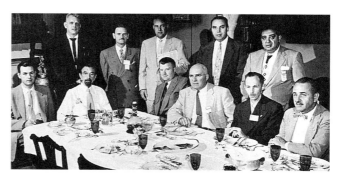

Members of the ICA's President's cabinet are shown during a 1950's breakfast meeting. Included are B.J. Palmer; Hugh Chance; Carl Cleveland, Sr.; Carl Cleveland, Jr.; Leonard Griffin; Vinton Logan; and A. Earl Homewood.
Courtesy Palmer College of Chiropractic Archives, Davenport, Iowa.

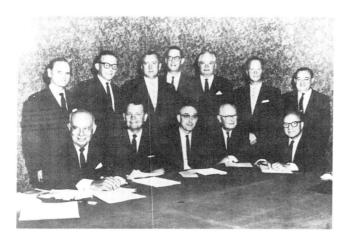

Photo of the NCA-ICA merger committee in 1963. Back row, from left: *Leonard K. Griffin, R.T. Leiter, Claire O'Dell, James Bunker, Devere Biser, and Harold Russell, and Hiliary Pruitt.* Front row, from left: *Cecil Martin, Richard Tyer, Arthur Schierholz, L.M. Rogers, and A.A. Adams.*

From *Chiropractic History,* December 1988.

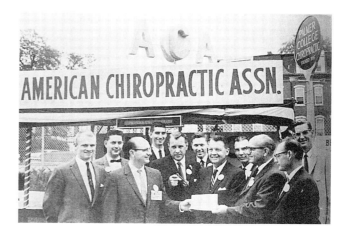

The ACA exhibit booth at the 1963 Palmer College Homecoming attracted many visitors who signed ACA membership applications. The booth was manned by such stalwarts as Drs. Leland Chance, J.J. Kehoe, J. Clay Thompson, W. Heath Quigley, Robert Griffin, A.A. Adams, Richard Tyer, and Clair O'Dell. Paul Mendy and a number of Palmer students gave their assistance by distributing literature and lapel buttons reading "I'm for unity—it's ACA all the way!"

From the *Journal of National Chiropractic Association,* September 1963.

THE MODERN AMERICAN CHIROPRACTIC ASSOCIATION

Plans for yet another single unified national organization had been initiated as early as 1958 by Claire O'Dell, D.C., of Wyandotte, Michigan. However, despite the shared interest in the plan from among the NCA Board of Directors and at least five members of the ICA's Board of Control, the 1963 attempt to merge the NCA and ICA to form the new American Chiropractic Association (ACA) was not acceptable to the majority of the ICA's leadership. In language with the flavor of the international cold war between the Soviet Union and the United States, dire predictions about the effects of this new ACA emanated from the ICA.

But the tide had finally turned. Paul Smallie, D.C., longtime editor of *World-Wide Reports,* sought to emphasize the interests that narrow-scope and broad-scope chiropractors shared. Frank W. Elliott, D.C., a 1909 graduate of the PSC, longtime business manager of his alma mater, and former secretary of the old UCA, urged all chiropractors to join the new organization. Many other previously narrow-scope chiropractors similarly believed that professional unity was more important than ideological purity. In April 1964 Ernest Napolitano, D.C., who had succeeded Frank Dean, D.C., as president of the Columbia Institute of Chiropractic in 1959, resigned from the ICA's Board of Control and announced that his New York City school, which would merge with the Atlantic States Chiropractic Institute of Brooklyn later that year, would seek accreditation from the ACA. Logan College of Chiropractic in St. Louis also joined the ranks of the ACA-accredited schools.

Late in 1963 the ACA was chartered, and in November and December the first two special editions of the *ACA Journal of Chiropractic* overlapped the final issues of the *Journal of the National Chiropractic Association (JNCA).* Longtime editor of the *JNCA* and executive secretary of

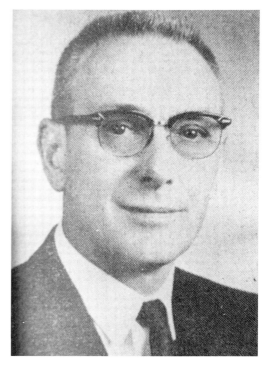

Arthur Schierholz, the chairman of the ACA's first Board of Governors.

From *The ACA Journal of Chiropractic,* January 1964.

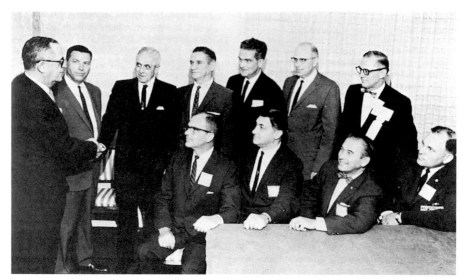

The newly elected ICA Board of Control of 1963, including John Q. Thaxton (president), Leonard W. Rutherford, Walter Gingerich, Homer V. York, Ben O. Evans, Lyle W. Sherman, Roy E. LeMond, W.E. Vanderstolp, Charles P. Miller, Gerard L. Bellavance, and William S. Day.

From the *ICA International Review of Chiropractic*, October 1963.

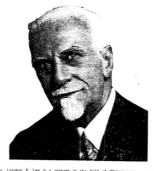

Poster with a photograph of Lyndon E. Lee, entitled, "should chiropractors be licensed in New York State?" Dr. Lee waged a campaign from 1915 to 1963 to have chiropractic legislation enacted in the Empire State.

Courtesy Palmer College of Chiropractic Archives, Davenport, Iowa.

the NCA, Loran M. Rogers, D.C., served for a few months in similar capacity in the new organization. Arthur M. Schierholz, D.C., who would serve the new ACA and its agencies for the next several decades, was appointed chairman of the ACA's first board of governors. Dewey Anderson Ph.D., who had replaced John J. Nugent, D.C., as NCA Director of Education following Dr. Nugent's retirement in 1961, was succeeded in 1964 by John Fisher, Ph.D., as ACA Director of Education. The ACA began a concerted effort to enable the ACA-accredited colleges to achieve federal recognition. Soon after taking over L.M. Rogers's role as executive director of the ACA in October 1964, Dr. Schierholz announced that "40 per cent of ACA dues will be budgeted each year to ACA colleges for education and research . . . . [and] $100,000 annually from ACA reserves to the upgrading program."

CONTINUED POLITICAL STRUGGLES FOR RECOGNITION

In June 1963 the present day National Board of Chiropractic Examiners was founded and provided an organizational platform for unifying the licensing process among the various state boards. In April 1963, after nearly 50 years of effort, chiropractors in New York finally succeeded in winning licensing legislation when Governor Nelson A. Rockefeller signed the Chiropractic Act. Chiropractors then practicing in the Empire State were grandfathered in, but new licentiates were required to have graduated from a chiropractic college accredited by an agency recognized by the United States Office of Education.

Federal recognition of the chiropractic colleges was still a decade off, however, and in the meantime the ACA and the profession would have to contend with organized medicine's renewed campaign to eradicate chiropractic. On November 2-3, 1963, the AMA's Committee on Quackery was formed, and set as its primary mission "first to contain, and then to eliminate" the chiropractic profession. The ACA Education Director,

Dewey Anderson, had warned the profession of organized medicine's plans as early as 1961, when he suggested that the AMA Department of Investigation "has a definite program to destroy chiropractic, root and branch, by 1970." Another 15 years would pass before chiropractors Chester Wilk, D.C., Michael Pedigo, D.C., and others would file suit in federal court charging the AMA and a number of other medical organizations with conspiracy to restrain trade by their efforts to eradicate the chiropractic profession. Not until the late 1980s would this Wilk's case find legal resolution, when the AMA et al. were found to have violated the Sherman Anti-Trust laws by their boycott of chiropractors.

In the hostile political climate of the 1960s and later, any and all criticisms of chiropractic were likely to be viewed as threats of professional annihilation, whether they came from within or outside the chiropractic profession. Coming on the heels of the Stanford Research Institute's negative review in 1960 of chiropractic in California, Samuel Homola, D.C.'s 1963 *Bonesetting, Chiropractic & Cultism* would earn him a 30-year exile from his own profession. Homola, a second generation chiropractor and 1956 graduate of the Lincoln Chiropractic College of Indianapolis, challenged the notion that chiropractors should and could seriously compete with allopathic physicians in the care of anything other than musculoskeletal conditions. The book lays out in great detail the foibles and shortcomings of chiropractic professional associations and colleges as they existed in the period between B.J. Palmer's death and the ACA's formation. Homola would be denied membership in the ACA until the early 1990s.

The first 70 years of organizational history within chiropractic set the stage in the early 1960s for the struggles and successes of the past 30 years. The final third of the chiropractic century would see the achievement of federal recognition of chiropractic education, the inclusion of chiropractic services in federal reimbursement programs, the beginnings of substantive scientific research bearing on the effectiveness of chiropractic care and yet another attempt to form one political voice for the profession when a proposed ACA-ICA merger failed in the mid-1980s. However, these victories would take place during a period of increased hostility between organized medicine and chiropractic, and despite the continuing disagreements within the chiropractic ranks. How the chiropractic profession accomplished so much in the face of such adversity is a remarkable testimony to the determination of the leaders of the profession.

I wish to thank Fred H. Barge, D.C.; Carl S. Cleveland, Jr., D.C.; and William S. Rehm, D.C.; for their assistance in locating sourceworks.

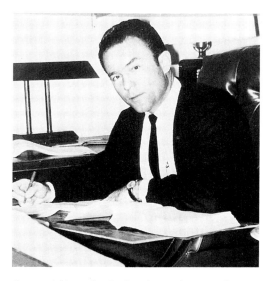

Samuel Homola, D.C., about the time he authored Bonesetting, Chiropractic Cultism, *which detailed Homala's view of the foibles and shortcomings of the profession in 1963.*
Courtesy Samuel Homola, Panama City, Florida.

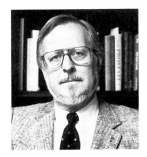

Fred Barge, author and lecturer, served as President of the ICA from 1988 to 1991.
Courtesy Fred Barge, La Crosse, Wisconsin.

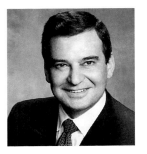

Louis Sportelli, author and often featured spokesman for the profession, served as the ACA's chairman in 1989.
Courtesy Louis Sportelli, Palmerton, Pennsylvania.

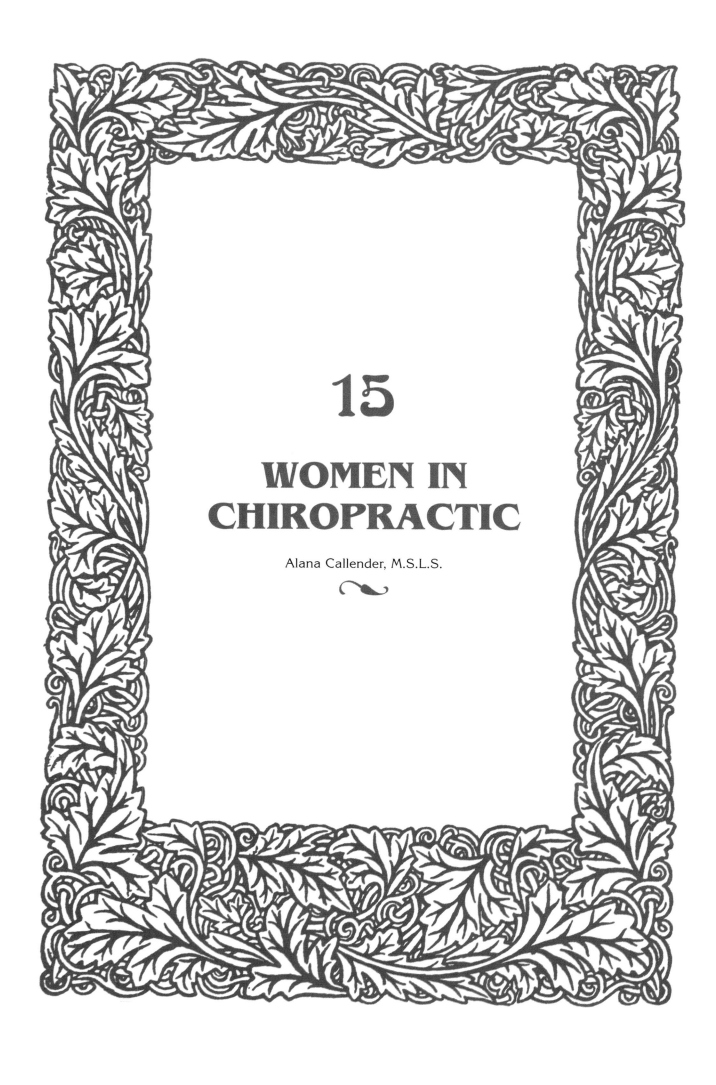

15

WOMEN IN CHIROPRACTIC

Alana Callender, M.S.L.S.

C hiropractic has no Elizabeth Blackwell or Susan B. Anthony. Regardless of whether D.D. Palmer was enlightened by his five wives, a shrewd businessman, or an early feminist, he held the chiropractic door open for women from the beginning. Women have been consistently recruited as students for chiropractic colleges. ∿

CHIROPRACTIC: THE PROFESSION FOR WOMEN

The percentage of women in chiropractic practice has varied over the years. In the earliest years of chiropractic through World War I, women chiropractors were much more in evidence than women in any other profession. Between the world wars the number of women entering the schools lessened and the women in practice were graying. After a slight revival during the early 1940s, the number of women in practice seriously declined immediately after World War II and women chiropractors became a novelty until the 1970s.

Although women were recruited and accepted as colleagues, nowhere throughout the history of the profession in America is there evidence of

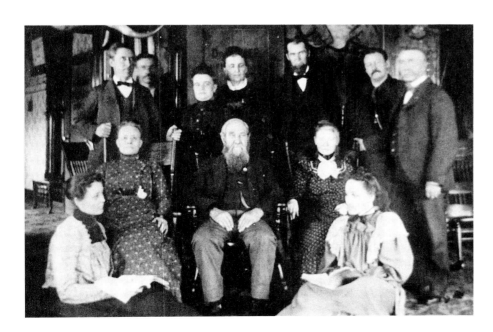

Twelve of the first fifteen graduates of D.D. Palmer's School, pictured in his offices on the fourth floor of the Ryan Building. Note that six of the twelve are women.

Courtesy Logan College of Chiropractic Archives, Chesterfield, Missouri.

445

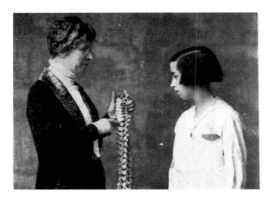

An advertisement placed by an early woman chiropractor, Cora Jacobson, circa 1910.

Courtesy Palmer College of Chiropractic Archives, Davenport, Iowa.

women playing a major political role. When the few exceptions crossed the gender barrier, the state or national association office held by a woman was almost always that of secretary.

Nevertheless, women chiropractors have been successful and found happiness in solo practices, as partners in wife-and-husband practices, and as associates in larger operations. Many patients seek out women doctors for the very qualities that seem to be considered stereotypical in today's society—intuition, compassion, and a gentle touch.

The Early Twentieth Century to the 1930s

The history of the earliest years of chiropractic is made up of the history of the leading individuals. Associations, which would keep records in later years, were not yet formed, and publications were concerned with defining the profession, rather than recording its progress. Chiropractic historian J. Stuart Moore, however, has examined the history of women in chiropractic. Moore reports that 40% of the practicing chiropractors in Kansas from 1910 to 1920 were women. In the District of Columbia, the number reached 50%.

In 1911 Mabel Palmer founded the chiropractic sorority, Sigma Phi Chi, to promote a social, mental, and spiritual culture at the Palmer School of Chiropractic (PSC) and to strengthen the bonds between women in chiropractic. Incorporated in 1914, Sigma Phi Chi has the distinction of being the oldest chiropractic organization and has had over 1000 members involved in its activities. Chapters have been organized at Life College and Texas Chiropractic College. The Life chapter was reorganized as Alpha Delta Upsilon in 1989.

In 3 different eras women have been surveyed about their experience as chiropractors. The first survey was from 1917 to 1920, when at least

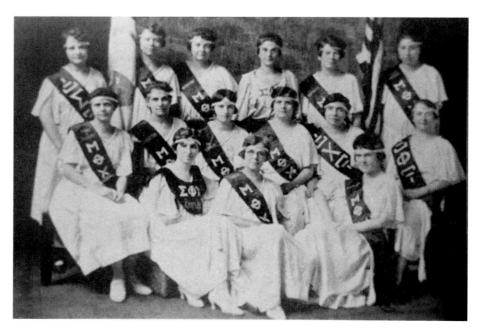

Mabel Palmer formed the Sigma Phi Chi in 1911, the first organization in chiropractic specifically for women.

From Palmer School of Chiropractic: *The Recoil,* October Davenport, Iowa, 1927.-

three colleges used testimonials from women chiropractors as recruiting tools. B.J. Palmer explained his method in the foreword to *Chiropractic for Women*. Hoping to fill the classes at the PSC with women when 25% of his enrollment faced military conscription, he sent a form letter in May 1917 to all Palmer women graduates. B.J. appealed for letters from practicing women chiropractors to present chiropractic from a "woman-chiropractor's" viewpoint. The letters were to cover their date and reason for enrolling at Palmer, their graduation date, their total number of patients seen, and their approximate average annual income. Further, they were asked whether study in school was hard and whether adjusting was hard manual labor. Ross College of Chiropractic of Ft. Wayne, Indiana and National School of Chiropractic in Chicago also produced similar documents at about the same time and probably gathered the information in much the same way.

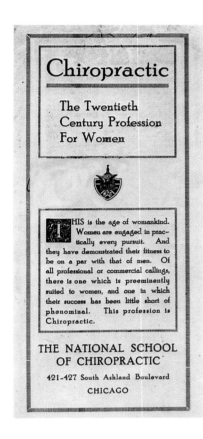
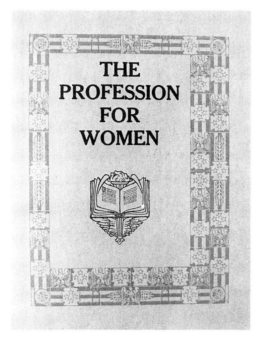
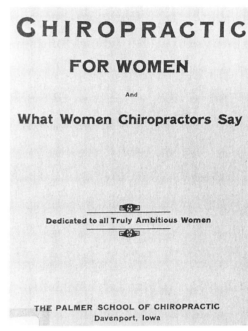

Three brochures intended to boost enrollment in chiropractic colleges during World War I. From left to right are brochures from the National School of Chiropractic, Ross College of Chiropractic, and the Palmer School of Chiropractic.
Courtesy Palmer College of Chiropractic Archives, Davenport, Iowa.

From the brochures of the three schools, we are able to piece together a composite woman chiropractor of that era. She became a chiropractor because chiropractic care had either helped her or someone close to her after allopathic medicine had failed them. She found that women patients were very receptive to a female physician. Adjusting called more upon skill than upon strength, and so was suitable for a woman's more delicate constitution. She generally had a solo practice and felt that the decision to enter chiropractic had been the right one.

Tuition breaks offered by the various schools for husband-wife teams were surely a factor in the decision of many women to attend, although their effect is not well documented. Between 1895 and 1925 when 5% to 11% of all professional or technical jobs were held by women, 25% to 33% of practicing chiropractors were women.

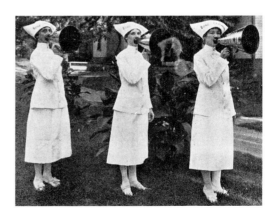

The three women are labeled Lady Bone-Cracker Trio in an early Carver catalog.
Courtesy Palmer College of Chiropractic Archives, Davenport, Iowa.

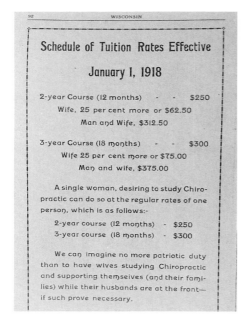

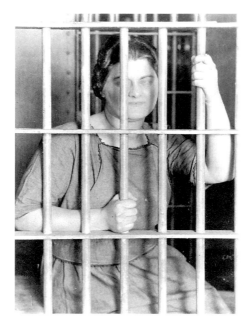

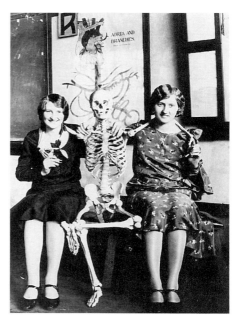

A schedule of tuition rates for women at the PSC in 1918. Although husband-wife teams got a break, single women were required to pay the same tuition.

From Palmer School of Chiropractic: *Chiropractic for Women and What Women Chiropractors Say* 1918.

Dr. Mildred Creveling in the Mahoning County Jail, circa 1930.

Courtesy Palmer College of Chiropractic Archives, Davenport, Iowa.

PSC student, Esther Mork and a friend, circa 1935. Later Dr. Mork and her husband, Arthur Mork, would be arrested in Wisconsin for practicing medicine without a license.

Courtesy Dr. Esther Mork, Janesville, Wisconsin.

Moore has proposed that women in the 1920s may have been attracted to chiropractic because of its connection with restoring proper nerve flow "when common wisdom charged women with particular susceptibility to nerve weakness or 'neurasthenia.' " Although Moore presents this as a well-reasoned explanation for chiropractic's attractiveness, it is not substantiated by writings of the women of that period.

Writing in 1953, Dr. Viola Lancaster described the pioneer women chiropractors of 1923. They were more likely to be middle-aged and in school with their husbands. Practically all the women had secured their health through chiropractic, and their paramount desire was to "help suffering humanity." They practiced in more or less constant fear of arrest, with no license available to them. "The worry, heart-break, and apparent disgrace inflicted on these pioneers could not be conceived."

The 1930s to the 1950s

The 1930 census listed 11,916 chiropractors in the United States. Throughout the decade, women were actively recruited as potential students and seem to have reached an early peak in their acceptance as professionals.

The most successful of the professional women's organizations was the National Chiropractic Association Council on Women Chiropractors. As early as 1935 tentative plans for a national organization for practicing women chiropractors were drawn. At the 1936 National Chiropractic Association (NCA) convention, an association was formed that became the National Council of Women Chiropractors (NCWC) and held a seat in the

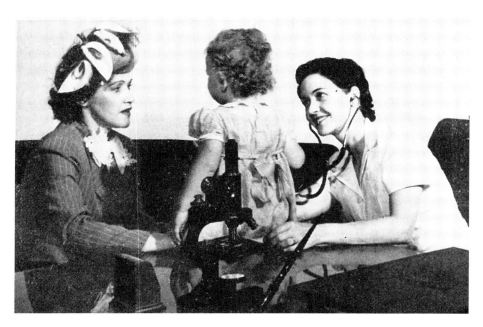

Chiropractic was pictured as a desirable career for women in John Nugent's 1954 pamphlet Chiropractic: a Career.

From Nugent J: *Chiropractic: a career,* 1954.

NCA's House of Counselors. The objectives of the council called for women to carry their share of the work, while receiving just representation in the NCA to solve the problems unique to women in the profession. Dr. Edna Smith of Johnson City, Tennessee, led the drive for organization, and Dr. Gladys Ingram of Chillicothe, Missouri, was elected first president of the council.

Other than the council officers, it does not appear that any woman held an office in the NCA at that time, even at the state director level. Because of the liberal use of initials instead of first names, it is hard to determine—although all the women on the council are clearly listed by name.

During that 1936 convention only one woman was a program speaker in any of the meetings. A photograph of the 1940 NCA convention is captioned, "600 doctors and their wives."

World War II and its concomitant shortage of young men (for the schools) made women students attractive. Twelve women and sixty men graduated from the PSC in the spring 1942 class. In 1944, when the NCA was recruiting "10,000 chiropractic students," the advertisement made it clear that women were as welcome as men.

In March 1943, 25.3% of American chiropractors were women, but only 15% of the American chiropractors under the age of 45 were women. In 1946 the NCA reported that women made up 18% of the chiropractors in practice, which was 13% more women than in medicine, 16% more than in dentistry, 8% more than in optometry, and 15% more than in law.

Moore cites this decade as the time when domesticity came to the women of chiropractic. By the late 1940s women had all but disappeared

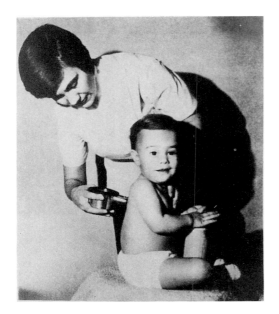

A woman chiropractor doing a neurocalometer reading on a young patient, circa 1960.
Courtesy Life Chiropractic College, Marietta, Georgia.

from the pictures, rosters, and ranks of practicing chiropractors. The early pioneers were retiring, and younger women were under social pressure to stay home and leave the jobs to the men.

In 1950 the president of the NCA, Dr. Harry R. Bybee, wrote a salute to the women of chiropractic:

> In no other profession in which men are dominant is there so much welcome to women colleagues and associates as in chiropractic. This is a healing profession in which there is truly and genuinely no discrimination. Women students study side by side with men students; they graduate and go into practice without any deprecation of their abilities. That there exists within the National Chiropractic Association the Council of Women Chiropractors is not any effort to differentiate, but is only a recognition of the fact that women are pre-eminent in some fields.

In 1951, Dr. George Smyrl, president of the NCA reminded readers of the *NCA Journal* that "chiropractic offers a wonderful career for women." He continued, "Many young men who would become chiropractic students are either in the armed services or expect to be soon, so we must make a special effort to enroll more women than we have in the past. A little more effort by each chiropractor would soon fill our colleges with women."

Dr. Margaret Schmidt, president of the National Chiropractic Association Council of Women Chiropractors, was featured on the December 1950 cover of the *Journal of the National Chiropractic Association*. Her editorials reflect the ambivalence of the period toward the working woman. While promoting the improved outlook and mentality of the woman who has moved beyond the bridge club to the study club and thrilling for the woman who has distinguished herself in one of the professions, Dr. Schmidt is very careful to remind the reader that homemaking and motherhood are the greatest career of all. In 1951 she wrote, "The role of woman in this world is plain. It is clearly defined. She is always the helpmate, the moderator and she likes it this way. Hers is the glory, if her menfolk excel."

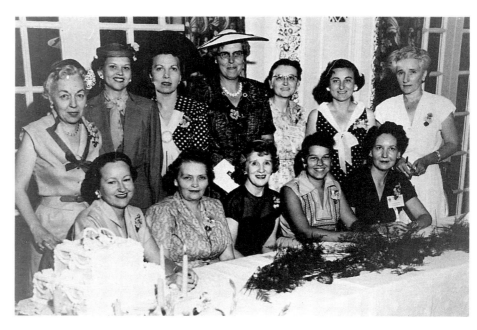

The women's auxiliary of the International Chiropractor's Association in the 1950s.
Courtesy Palmer College of Chiropractic Archives, Davenport, Iowa.

The 1960s to the 1970s

The women's auxiliaries and fraternity wives clubs were in their heyday in the early 1960s. The governor of National Chiropractic Auxiliary District 4, Mrs. Howard Spears, speaks to the new liberation of women:

> We no longer stand behind our husbands, we walk side by side and shoulder to shoulder with our men. In countries like Russia, women are proud to do men's work and we appreciate them for it. Here our women have become social arbitrators, sales managers, trouble shooters, general counselors, mothers and housekeepers. The chiropractor's wife must remember that she personifies the chiropractic ideal.

At the 1961 National Chiropractic Convention, only one woman, Dr. Myrna Schultz, appeared on the program. As president of the NCA–CWC for the past three years, her monthly columns had gradually moved away from women's issues to clinical or professional unity themes. In 1962, when the American Chiropractic Association (ACA) surveyed its members, only 3.3% of the doctors responding were women. Women's names and women's pictures all but disappeared from the journals of chiropractic.

In spite of lip service, such as the 1962 PSC yearbook photo of the old smokestack emblazoned with "Votes 4 Women" and "Equal Rights," the 1960s saw a diminished role for women chiropractors. Dr. Catherine Miller, Dean of Women, the only woman on the faculty at the PSC between 1953 and 1973, left the school after 1 year.

In 1966 the ACA welcomed 513 new members, including 24 women. Posture queens were a regular feature at state conventions. In 1967, the ACA, studying the chiropractor in depth, found that about 7% of the students enrolled were women, but only slightly more than half of these women continued in active practice. Also, by this time the American Chiropractic Association–Council of Women Chiropractors (ACA-CWC) no longer had its own column and its activities were limited to awarding an annual scholarship at the national convention luncheon.

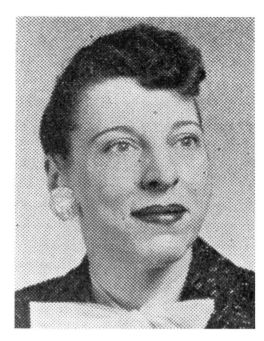

Dr. Myrna Schultz of Mitchell, South Dakota, the President of the National Council of Women Chiropractors in the late 1950s and early 1960s had a monthly column in The Journal of the National Chiropractic Association.

From *The Journal of the National Chiropractic Association,* January 1959.

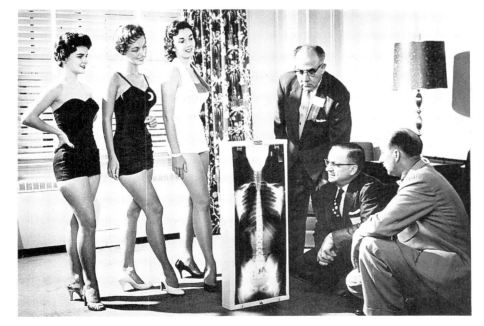

Although this photo may appear to be "cheesecake," the contestants of the Posture Queen contest were eliminated if x-rays showed a problem with their spines.

Courtesy of Logan College of Chiropractic Archives, Chesterfield, Missouri.

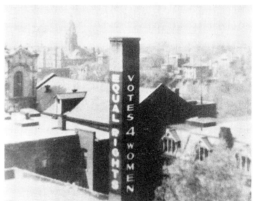

The smokestack at PSC in the 1950s. A 1920s yearbook proudly proclaimed, "Dr. [B.J.] Palmer is a suffragette and believes in the equality of women."

Courtesy Palmer College of Chiropractic Archives, Davenport, Iowa.

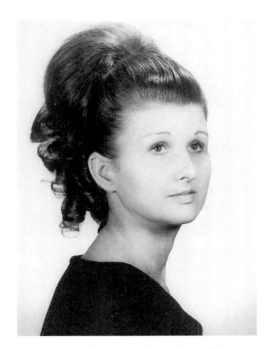

Bernice Brinkman authored a 1972 study The Professional Female Chiropractor.
From *Today's Chiropractic*, October-November 1973.

Dr. Bernice Brinkman's study of the professional female chiropractor found that in 1972 only between 3% and 9% of chiropractors were women. The most frequent reason for choosing chiropractic as a career was the same as in 1918, because of its results. Women patients were still receptive to female physicians. Most of the doctors Brinkman surveyed were married and had an office-home combination, which was a full-time solo practice. They agreed with their counterparts of 50 years earlier that chiropractic had been the right choice.

The same year, Palmer College of Chiropractic appointed its first full-time female faculty members since the early 1960s. Dr. Maxine McMullen and Dr. Marjorie Johnson were named instructors in the diagnosis and technique departments, respectively.

By 1979 the ACA's survey of its membership reported a growth in the percentage of women practicing throughout the decade to 5% of chiropractors surveyed. At that same time, over 15% of Canadian chiropractors were women. The Canadian Congress of Women Chiropractors was formed in 1978 with a mandate to serve as a role model for women students. The congress continues today, providing financial assistance for women wanting to attend Canadian Memorial Chiropractic College, and among other services, teaching adaptations of adjusting techniques to their pregnant colleagues.

The 1980s to the 1990s

A decade after Brinkman's study, Dr. Teresa Gromala again surveyed women chiropractors. Dr. Gromala's survey was done with Sigma Phi Chi chiropractic sorority members. In the 1980s, 60% of the women chiropractors surveyed had turned to chiropractic for their own or a family member's health problems. In her report, Gromala chronicled the overall social change in women's experiences over the past decades. Although the women chiropractors' experiences do not change, women chiropractors' expectations have increased. Community acceptance was reported as "A-1 to good," and the theme of chiropractor as clubwoman was still predominant.

During the 1980s the percentage of women practicing grew steadily, starting the decade at 6% and finishing with a reported 13.2% by 1989. Chiropractic women students rose from 18% of total enrollment in 1982 to 22% by 1985.

The Council of Women Chiropractors was disbanded 50 years after its creation, at its own request, during the 1986 ACA convention in Toronto. It was felt that women chiropractors had become equal and that they were consistently treated fairly. Their involvement in the ACA was representative of their involvement in the profession. The former Council of Women Chiropractors had met the special needs of women in the profession, and future councils would focus on clinical issues.

That same year, 1986, the International Network of Women Chiropractors was formed "to recognize the needs of women chiropractors and chiropractic students and to approach these needs from a feminist perspective." The network disbanded in 1988.

In the 1992 ACA professional survey of its members, 13.8% of the respondents were women, even though the best estimate of the percentage of women students in all the chiropractic colleges was 30%. Perhaps the rest followed in the footsteps of Dorothy Peaslee, D.C. Dr. Peaslee had attended every class reunion for over 50 years. When interviewed for her story of the trials and struggles in the pioneering age of chiropractic, she recalled, "I just kept house for my husband."

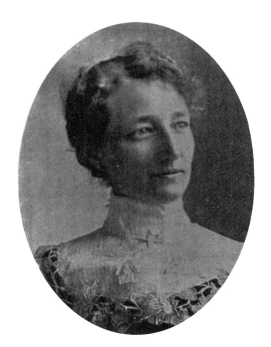

THE PIONEERS

In most professions women have faced a long and oftentimes bitter struggle to be accepted. Women in chiropractic had a different start. At the PSC Helen DeLendrecice was a member of the class of 1899, Mrs. J.C. Bowman was a member of the class of 1899, and Minora C. Paxson was a member of the class of 1900. These three women were among the first 15 students that D.D. Palmer accepted.

Although Mrs. Bowman and Ms. DeLendrecice faded into obscurity, Minora Paxson maintained a high profile in chiropractic for a number of years. With two other early graduates of D.D. Palmer's course, Solon M. Langworthy and Oakley G. Smith, Dr. Paxson founded the American School of Chiropractic in Cedar Rapids, Iowa. There she was professor of gynecology and obstetrics, the first to take chairs on these subjects in any chiropractic school. She was also lecturer on physiology and symptomatology and the secretary of the school.

Most likely a midwife or nurse-midwife before studying chiropractic, Dr. Paxson claimed to be the first chiropractor to pass a state board examination in chiropractic obstetrics. She possibly became the first licensed chiropractor in any jurisdiction when she passed the Illinois state board examination and received license 438 to practice obstetrics in accordance with the principles of chiropractic. The same account states that she was granted the first certificate licensing the treatment of disease by chiropractic. Since she received her license before publication of the text *Modernized Chiropractic* with Langworthy and Smith in 1906, it can be assumed that Paxson took the two state board examinations under the Illinois Medical Practice Act, which at that time provided for non-allopathic drugless practitioners as well as midwives. Accordingly, she may have undisputed claim to being the first licensed chiropractor as well as the first licensed chiropractic obstetrician.

One of the early graduates of the American School of Chiropractic was Alma C. Arnold, a member of the 1902 class. Dr. Arnold was a pioneer chiropractor in New York and became the president of Columbia College of Chiropractic. Clara Barton was one of her patients.

The next major female force to come out of D.D. Palmer's classroom was his daughter-in-law, Mabel Heath Palmer. Rather than be lost in a sea of Doctor Palmers, Mabel was known throughout the profession simply as "Mabel." To this day, there is no need to clarify to any Palmer graduate or most any other chiropractor who is meant by "Mabel."

Mabel Heath was born in 1881 and worked in the post office in Milan, Illinois, until her marriage to D.D.'s son, B.J., in 1904. She graduated from the PSC in 1905 in a class of two. Her father was to become a faculty member of the school.

In 1909 when her son, Dave, was 3 years old, Mabel spent a year in Chicago, where she studied anatomy. On her return, she wrote *Chiropractic Anatomy,* first published by the PSC in 1918 and revised in 1920. As an author and teacher, "she anticipated the feminist movement in the professions by a half-century, giving stature to women in chiropractic in its early years." She was a professor of anatomy for almost 40 years and, in

Minora Paxson, a 1900 graduate of D.D. Palmer's School and Cure, went on to become a faculty member at two chiropractic colleges and co-authored the first textbook on chiropractic.

Courtesy of Palmer College of Chiropractic Archives, Davenport, Iowa.

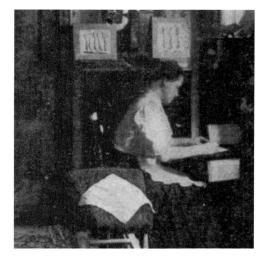

Alice Smaltz, an early woman chiropractor, in her office in Traverse City, Michigan, circa 1915.

Courtesy of Palmer College of Chiropractic Archives, Davenport, Iowa.

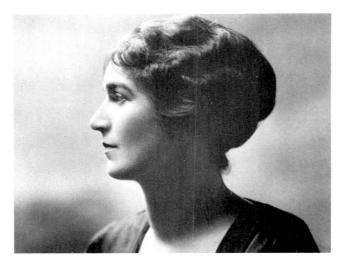

An early portrait of Mabel Palmer.
Courtesy Palmer College of Chiropractic Archives, Davenport, Iowa.

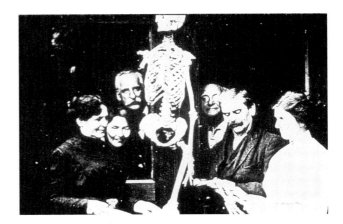

One of the few photos of Mabel Palmer (far right) in the classroom.
Courtesy Palmer College of Chiropractic Archives, Davenport, Iowa.

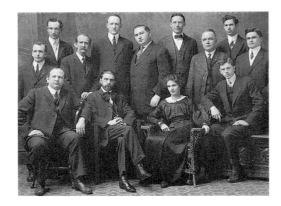

Mabel Palmer with other PSC faculty, circa 1918.
Courtesy Palmer College of Chiropractic Archives, Davenport, Iowa.

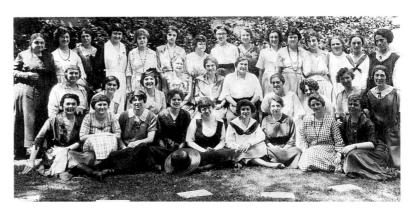

Mabel (center, middle row) and the women in the senior class on the campus of the PSC,
Courtesy Palmer College of Chiropractic Archives, Davenport, Iowa.

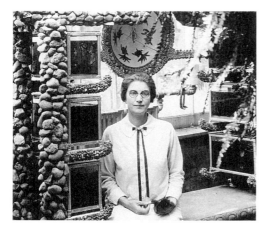

Mabel Palmer seated in A Little Bit O' Heaven, circa 1930.
Courtesy Palmer College of Chiropractic Archives, Davenport, Iowa.

the early years, carried the heaviest teaching load of any faculty member.

Mabel was a world traveler, as she, B.J., and Dave made many trips to temporarily escape the taxing leadership demands of an evolving profession. Her national and international trips were also made to spread the concept of chiropractic throughout the world. From these journeys came the experiences for two more books, *Stepping Stones,* which she wrote herself, and *Around the World with B.J.,* which she worked on with her husband. Their journeys also provided material for B.J.'s radio talk shows.

Mabel earned the sobriquet, "First Lady of Chiropractic," most probably for her diplomatic skills. Married for 41 years to the brilliant, but often eccentric, self-styled leader of chiropractic, Mabel was often the oil upon troubled waters. She took over as secretary-treasurer of the school when imminent litigation threatened the school's resources, and they were transferred into her name for safekeeping. Where B.J. was the fire, she was the ice.

Sylva L. Ashworth graduated from the PSC and started practice in Nebraska in 1910. She was a founder of the Universal Chiropractors' As-

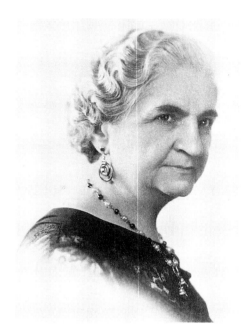
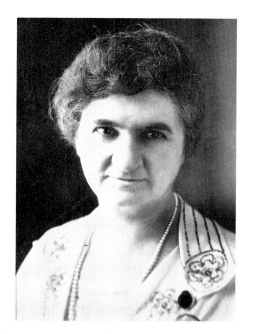
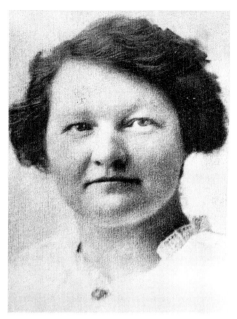

Sylva Ashworth was a powerful political figure in the state of Nebraska and through her daughter, Ruth Ashworth Cleveland, the matriarch of a famous chiropractic family, the Clevelands.

Courtesy Cleveland Chiropractic College—Kansas City, Kansas City, Missouri.

Almeda Haldeman is believed to be the first chiropractor in Canada and was the matriarch of another famous family of chiropractors.

Courtesy Scott Haldeman, Santa Ana, California.

sociation and later its president. Dr. Ashworth was a member of the first Board of Chiropractic Examiners in Nebraska and served as its president for many years. She was also a charter member of the NCA in 1930. "She was a natural politician and . . . a powerful Democrat. . . . They counted on her for 40,000 votes." She still found the time to raise four children by herself. Through her daughter, Rose Ruth Ashworth Cleveland, Sylva became the matriarch of one of chiropractic's most notable families, the Clevelands.

Other women took the practice of chiropractic into new territory. Almeda Haldeman, (Chiropractic School and Cure, Minnesota, 1905) originally trained as a schoolteacher and nurse, and later studied chiropractic under Dr. E.W. Lynch after he restored her husband to health. She homesteaded in Saskatchewan in 1907, making her most likely the first chiropractor in Canada. She strongly opposed the use of vaccines and fed her family only natural foods.

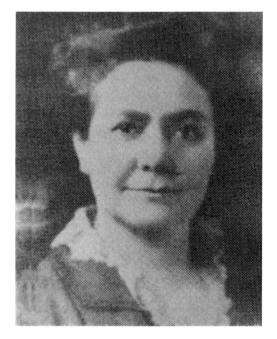

THE GROUNDBREAKERS

Dr. Anna K. Gregoreus was a 1907 PSC graduate. She was the first chiropractor in Delaware, opening her Dover office in 1908. In 1911 Dr. Frances Julander was among the first graduates of the Davenport College of Chiropractic. She had the distinction of receiving the first Iowa chiropractic license in 1921. Dr. Helen McKenzie was the first woman known to practice chiropractic in Australia.

Dr. Anna Foy was a crusader for legal recognition in Kansas. When the International Congress of Chiropractic Examiners elected its first slate of officers in 1926, Dr. Foy became first vice-president. The five-member

Anna Foy crusaded for chiropractic licensure in Kansas and was an officer of the first International Congress of Chiropractic Examiners in 1926.

From Chiropractic History, June 1992.

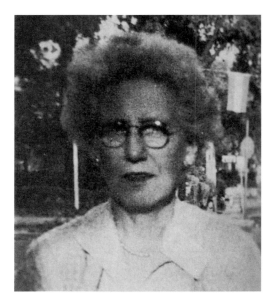

Kathryn "Kitty" Scallon (1926 graduate of PSC) served 6 months in a women's house of detention and returned to practice immediately on her release.

From Today's Chiropractic, October-November, 1973.

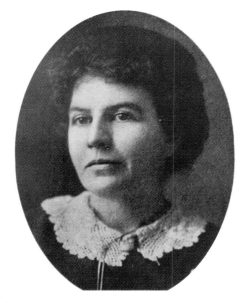

Elizabeth Ross and her husband founded Ross College of Chiropractic in Fort Wayne, Indiana in 1911.

From The Profession for Women, Ross College of Chiropractic, 1918.

board included Dr. Maude Hastings of Tennessee and Dr. Myrtle Long of Iowa.

During the 1917 battle for legal recognition of chiropractic in Alameda County, California, chiropractors who were charged with practicing medicine without a license were instructed by the county chiropractic society to go to jail rather than pay fines. The sacrifices of two women who were among the incarcerated are particularly memorable. When Dr. Minnie Leach collapsed in jail after a 10-day hunger strike, public opinion turned against the California medical practice act. After the arrest of Dr. Reba I. Willis and her husband, they were sentenced to 100 days in jail, leaving their 3-year-old twin daughters to the care of others. As far as is known, this was the first time a mother had been jailed and separated from her young children. Again, public sentiment quickly rose and was definitely in her favor. Dr. Willis was released after serving 65 days when her daughters became ill. Her husband was also released, but for only 3 days to treat his daughters, and then he was returned to prison to complete his sentence.

THE EDUCATORS

Women have always taken an active role in chiropractic education. From Minora Paxson to Nell Williams, they have helped found and manage chiropractic colleges. From Mabel Palmer to Jean Moss, they have been leaders in education.

Many wife and husband teams have founded chiropractic colleges. It seemed that the absolute dedication and teamwork of at least two people was necessary to generate enough energy to start a school, and two workers for the price of one was an advantage in keeping a school open during the proprietary years. Mabel Palmer was as much an asset to the PSC as was her husband, B.J. As a team, they kept it going during chiropractic's most turbulent years.

Linnie A. Cale, D.C., D.O., graduated in 1912, the first class of the Los Angeles Chiropractic College (LACC). Her husband, Charles, had started the school in 1911. She went on to not only teach at LACC, but also become vice-president and then president of the college from 1916 to 1924.

Ruth R. Ashworth Cleveland was a 1917 PSC graduate, who with her husband Carl, founded Central Chiropractic College, later to be renamed Cleveland Chiropractic College, in Kansas City, Missouri, in 1922. She taught gross anatomy and was director of the clinic. Dr. Ruth resigned from the college in 1942 and had a large private practice in Kansas City where she became well-known for her care of children. One of her own children, Carl II, took over the family business and is still chancellor of Cleveland Chiropractic University, while her grandson, Carl III is president of Cleveland Chiropractic College—Kansas City, and —Los Angeles.

The first state chapter of the NCA-CWC was formed in Oregon in 1953. It was named for Dr. Nellie Byrd, a Pacific Chiropractic College graduate of 1917. Dr. Byrd had held teaching positions at Pacific Chiropractic College, Universal Sanipractic College, the Northwest School of Physical Therapy, and the Seattle Chiropractic College.

Although she was only a prospective student at the time, Dorothy Clark was responsible for the founding of a college in 1944. With the en-

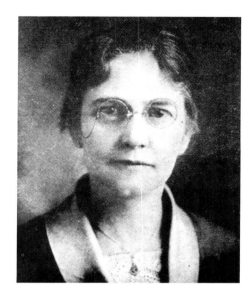

Linnie Cale graduated from the Los Angeles Chiropractic College, which her husband started in 1912. She was president of the school from 1916-1924.

Courtesy Los Angeles Chiropractic College, Whittier, California.

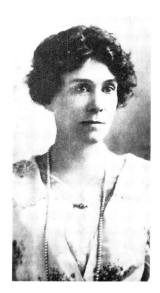

Nellie Gearheart Byrd graduated from the Pacific Chiropractic College in 1917 and held teaching positions at several Northwestern chiropractic colleges.

Courtesy Western States Chiropractic College, Portland, Oregon.

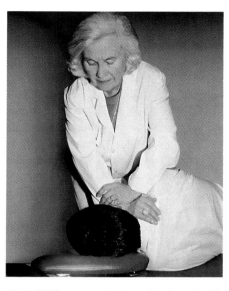

Nell Williams and her husband, Sid, founded Life Chiropractic College in 1974 in Marietta, Georgia.

Courtesy Life Chiropractic College, Marietta, Georgia.

couragement of her field doctor, Dr. Clarence E. Reaver, a 1941 PSC graduate, Ms. Clark applied for admission to the PSC and was turned down as a result of a vote taken at a student assembly. The Southern bloc of students threatened a mass walkout if Ms. Clark, an African-American, was admitted. In response, Dr. Reaver founded Reaver School of Chiropractic, a fully integrated school, in Dayton, Ohio.

When it was time to pioneer the first chiropractic college outside of North America, Elizabeth F. Bennett, D.C., a 1948 PSC graduate, and her husband started the Anglo-European College of Chiropractic in Bournemouth, England. Marcia Cerutty, D.C., became the first lecturer at the International College of Chiropractic in Melbourne, Australia, the school which first took chiropractic education in Australia into the tertiary education system.

The most recent of the chiropractic colleges to be cofounded by a wife and husband team is Life College in Marietta, Georgia. Nell K. Williams, D.C., and her husband, Sid, both 1956 PSC graduates, founded the Life Chiropractic College in 1974 after many years of successful private practice and chiropractic publishing. Together they have established 20 associate clinics and sent numerous students to chiropractic college. In 1958 they established Si-Nel Publishing and Sales Company. Later they established the Life Foundation, a non-profit research, education, and service organization that published a newspaper for laymen.

One of the most influential women in chiropractic education retired in 1992. Dr. Beatrice B. Hagen, a 1940 Logan Basic College of Chiropractic graduate, taught at her alma mater for 8 years after graduation, during which time she met her husband. Together, they had the dubious distinction of being the final cases tried in New York State for practicing medicine without a license. They were arrested individually toward the end of 1953, but it was 2 years before they were acquitted by juries. Their "crimes of diagnosis" were committed by the mere possession of medical equipment, including otoscopes, stethoscopes, x-ray equipment, and

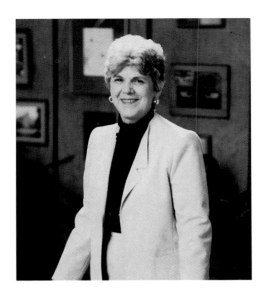

Beatrice Hagen served as President of Logan College of Chiropractic from 1980 to 1992.
Courtesy Logan College of Chiropractic Archives, Chesterfield, Missouri.

baumonometers (blood pressure cuffs), at a time when you could "get your blood pressure taken at Coney Island for 25¢."

In 1977 Dr. Hagen's educational leadership was never so prominent as when she was elected chair of the Logan College Board of Trustees. She served as trustees chair until she was named president of Logan College in 1980. While president of Logan, she also served as secretary-treasurer, vice president, and finally president of the Council on Chiropractic Education.

Two women have made names for themselves in post graduate education. Marianne Gengenbach, D.C., a 1983 Logan College of Chiropractic graduate, has actively served on the ACA Council on Sports Injuries since 1985 and has completed two terms as the president of the American Chiropractic Board of Sports Physicians.

Maxine McMullen, R.N., D.C., is a 1971 Palmer College of Chiropractic graduate. Dr. McMullen has been dean of chiropractic sciences at Palmer College of Chiropractic since 1990 and is one of the few women to hold an honorary membership in the Delta Delta Pi professional fraternity. A long-recognized authority on chiropractic pediatrics, she was one of the first three members of the International Chiropractors' Association Diplomate in Pediatrics program and was the first president of the program.

Women have also taken an active part in chiropractic research, the complement to education. Dr. Mary C. Hibbard, a 1920 PSC, graduate, was the secretary-treasurer of the Cleveland, Ohio, Metropolitan Chiropractic College for 20 years. She taught anatomy and chiropractic orthopedy and conducted research in postural correction and spinal balance.

Dr. Eleanor S. Ridgway, a 1930 PSC graduate, was invited by B.J. Palmer to join the staff of his Research Clinic. She was in charge of the audiometer and visual department until she transferred to the student clinic.

Dr. Helen DeLue, a 1947 Lincoln Chiropractic College graduate, designed in 1965 the Trapezius Scale and Distortion Analyzer used with the sacro-occipital technique (SOT). She was president of the Sacro-Occipital Research Society International (SORSI), from 1965 to 1970. Dr. DeLue also wrote the curriculum and served as director of teacher training for SORSI during those years.

Following B.J. Palmer's early lead in using the broadcast media to promote chiropractic, Dr. Virginia Boydjieff took the opportunity of explaining chiropractic on numerous television shows in the 1950s, including *What's My Line?* Named the "Most Beautiful Doctor in the United States" at the NCA convention in 1954, Dr. Boydjieff presented a gracious image of chiropractic.

When a chiropractor was needed to represent chiropractic on national television talk shows during the 1960s, Dorothea Towne, D.C., Ph.C., B.A., B.S., F.I.C.A., a 1954 Cleveland Chiropractic College—Los Angeles graduate, was often called on. As a researcher and educator, she also addressed many educational seminars, state associations, and civic clubs.

Not all women who supported education did so in the laboratory or the classroom. Dr. Tena Murphy, president of the Arkansas Chiropractic Association (1947 to 1948) raised over $65,000 during World War II toward the building of a Fountain Head Hospital at the PSC. The result was the purchase of Clear View Sanitarium, which gave the Iowa-Illinois area another chiropractic hospital for mental illness.

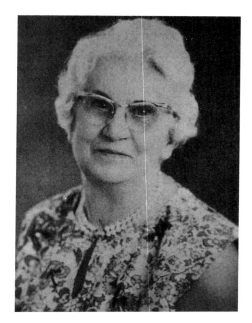

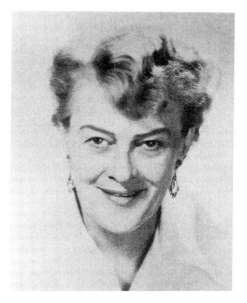

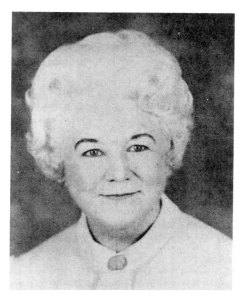

Dr. Eleanor Ridgeway (Palmer class of 1930) was on the staff of the B.J. Palmer Clinic and in charge of the audiometer and visual department and later was in the student clinic.

From *Today's Chiropractic*, October/November 1973. Courtesy SORSI, Prairie Village, Kansas.

During the 1960s, Dorothea Towne represented the profession on national television talk shows.

From *Today's Chiropractic*, October/November 1973.

Dr. Tena Murphy, president of the Arkansas Chiropractic Association in 1947-1948, raised over $65,000 to help build a Fountainhead Hospital at PSC. Instead, Clear View Sanitarium was purchased.

From *Today's Chiropractic*, October/November 1973.

THE COMPASSIONATE

Many student recruiting materials in the 1920s were targeted at women. The colleges' purpose may have been to fill classes depleted by a world war, but the message was that chiropractic was eminently suited for "her peculiar sympathetic disposition" and "her finer sensibilities and generous sympathies."

Chiropractic has indeed attracted a few women who truly fit these lofty ideals. Dr. Lorraine Golden, a 1942 PSC graduate, is the founder of Kentuckiana, an institution that provides free educational and rehabilitation services, psychological and family counseling, audiological and dental referrals, and special education to indigent multihandicapped children. Her clinic is established on property obtained through the first federal grant, from the United States Department of Health, Education and Welfare, to an organization rendering chiropractic services. Dr. Golden was honored as the first Kentucky Chiropractor of the Year, and a Kentucky Colonel in 1958. Dr. Golden was the first woman to receive an Outstanding Service Award for the Betterment of Humanity of the Greater Louisville Central Labor Council in 1972. She was awarded a doctor of humanities degree by the Columbia Institute of Chiropractic.

Assisting Dr. Golden at Kentuckiana is Dr. Joan Partridge, a 1960 Lincoln Chiropractic College graduate, who was resident staff doctor from 1962 to 1965 and is now director of health services. Dr. Partridge has also been honored as a Kentucky Colonel.

In Oklahoma City stands another chiropractic children's center. Oaklahaven was established as a non-profit organization in August 1962 and was originally staffed by six volunteer chiropractors. Dr. Bobby Callahan

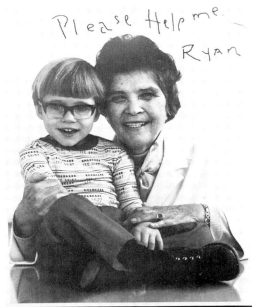

Dr. Lorraine Golden (Palmer graduate in 1942) founded Kentuckiana, an institution that provides free educational and rehabilitation services to indigent multi-handicapped children.

Courtesy Kentuckiana Children's Center, Louisville, Kentucky.

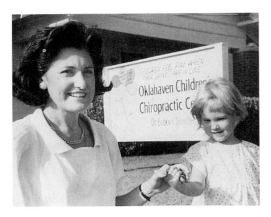

Since 1977, Bobby Doscher (Palmer graduate of 1977) has been president and chief executive of Oklahaven, an institution that earned national and international recognition for success in treating severely handicapped children.

Courtesy Oklahaven, Oklahoma City, Oklahoma.

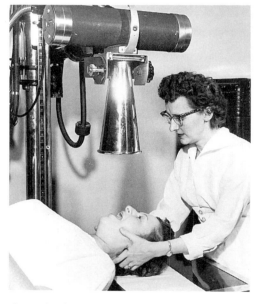

Appa Anderson (Western States) was the first woman to earn a diplomate in radiology.

Courtesy Western States Chiropractic College, Portland, Oregon.

Doscher, a 1977 Palmer College of Chiropractic graduate, has been president and chief executive since 1977. She also has treated children at a shelter for abused women. Oaklahaven has earned national and international recognition for success in treating severely handicapped children. Its mission is to promote the importance of drug-free health care for children.

Dr. Zella M. Muilenburg, a 1917 PSC graduate, was a member of the first postgraduate class of Lincoln Chiropractic College. She performed free rehabilitation work on veteran missionaries.

The first woman to earn a diplomate from the American Chiropractic Board of Radiology was Dr. Appa L. Anderson, a 1953 graduate of Western States Chiropractic College. Dr. Anderson is a professor, author, lecturer, and x-ray consultant. Her practice is limited to birth-injured and handicapped children and earned her the Oregon Chiropractor of the Year award in 1976.

From 1943 to 1958, Dr. Hazel Thompson, a 1939 PSC graduate, and her husband served with the Ethiopian government and the Sudan Interior Mission. She dedicated herself to aiding the underprivileged. A mother of eight children and the foster mother to seven Ethiopian children, Dr. Thompson was elected Chiropractor of the Year in 1965 by the Christian Chiropractic Association.

THE CLUBWOMEN

Women's clubs became a social force in the United States after the Civil War. Women's clubs served two major purposes: they were a means of furthering women's education without formal college experience, and they were a way for middle class women to spread their perception of social correctness to lower class women. With the introduction of each labor-saving device in the home, women had an increased amount of time to devote to themselves, their peers, and their society. Clubs became an outlet for these energies.

Passing references to chiropractic sororities other than Sigma Phi Chi appear in women's individual biographies. Lambda Chi sorority at National College of Chiropractic claimed four chapters and 409 sisters by 1937. At many of the colleges today, women join "Little Sisters" of Delta Sigma Chi fraternity, instead of having a separate organization.

After becoming chiropractors, women continued their club activities. Civic, social, and religious club memberships and honors abound

Members of the Alpha Chi Sorority, Universal Chiropractic College, Pittsburgh, Pennsylvania, circa 1918.

Courtesy Palmer College of Chiropractic Archives, Davenport, Iowa.

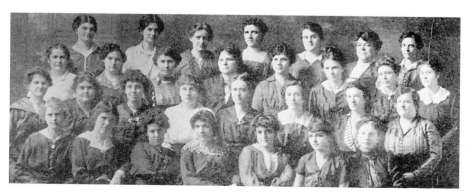

throughout any list of women chiropractors. In the 1960s, many women chiropractors joined chiropractic auxiliaries.

Dr. Gladys Ingram was president of the Women's Chiropractic Association, which merged with the ACA Council on Women Chiropractors. Because of her work and professional contributions, Dr. Ingram was the twenty-fourth chiropractor given the honorary title of fellow of the International College of Chiropractors.

A charter member of the ACA, Dr. Faye B. Eagles, a 1953 graduate of Logan College of Chiropractic, was the first woman to be president of North Carolina Chiropractic Association (1971 to 1972). In 1971 she was one of the three doctors of chiropractic appointed by President Nixon to serve as a delegate to the White House Conference on Aging. She was elected president of the Women's Council in 1976, serving until 1982.

Women have not easily achieved status in other parts of the profession. Cynthia E. Preiss, D.C., a 1967 LACC graduate, was the first woman to become president of the California State Board of Chiropractic examiners, the third woman ever appointed to that board, and the first in 30 years. Dr. Preiss was eminently qualified, having served on the ACA Councils on both mental health and sports injuries.

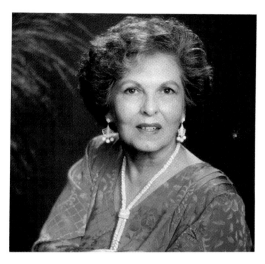

Faye Eagles (Logan graduate in 1953) was appointed by President Nixon in 1971 to serve on the White House Conference on Aging.

Courtesy Faye Eagles, Rocky Mount, North Carolina.

SUMMARY

The official stance of chiropractic has always been open to women who wanted to practice chiropractic. How that translated to the individual experience is a product of the individual's region, time, and male peers. Women may not have been on as many boards, held as many offices, or been given due recognition by their fellow doctors, but chiropractic, from its founder on, has never closed the door on women. There are so many now serving in leadership positions throughout the profession that to begin to enumerate their contributions would only lead to error of omission, so it is left to the chronicler of the second century of chiropractic to recall the leaders of the final decade of this century.

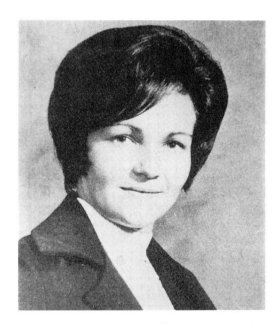

Cynthia Priess was the first woman to become president of the California State Board of Chiropractic Examiners and served on the ACA Council on Mental Health and Sports Injuries.

From *Today's Chiropractic*, October/November 1973.

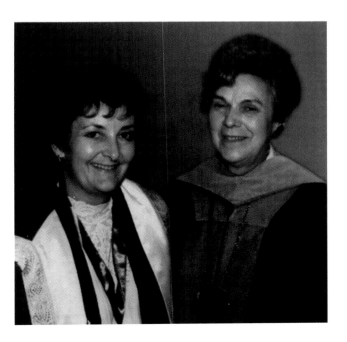

Dr. Jean Moss (left) *and Dr. Beatrice Hagen at Dr. Moss' inauguration as president of Canadian Memorial Chiropractic in 1991.*

Courtesy Logan College of Chiropractic Archives, Chesterfield, Missouri.

16

CHIROPRACTIC AROUND THE WORLD

Herbert J. Vear, D.C.
Pierre-Louis Gaucher-Peslherbe, D.C., PH.D, LITT. D(H.C.)
Rolf Eduard Peters, B.Sc., D.C., F.I.C.C.
Mary Ann Chance, D.C., F.I.C.C.
Glenda Wiese, M.A.

Although chiropractic has made the greatest inroads in English-speaking countries and in Western Europe, chiropractic does exist outside of these areas. The worldwide interests of chiropractic are represented by the World Federation of Chiropractic, an international body representing all national chiropractic associations. Chiropractors are found in 49 countries, with the largest number in the United States (49,000), followed by Canada (3700), Australia (2050), Great Britain (405), and France (400).

A BRIEF HISTORY OF CANADIAN CHIROPRACTIC

Herbert J. Vear

The birth of Daniel David Palmer, the founder of chiropractic, on March 7, 1845, at Port Perry, Ontario, Canada, is cause alone for celebrating the history of chiropractic in Canada. Unfortunately, the origins of chiropractic practice in Canada are vague and not amply recorded at this time. Nevertheless, it is believed that Almeda Jane Haldeman was not only the first person to practice chiropractic in Canada, circa 1907, but also the first woman to practice it. In fact, her grandson, Scott Haldeman, suggests that she was the third woman in the world to graduate as

Three generations of a prominent Canadian chiropractic family. Left to right, Almeda, Joshua, and Scott Haldeman. Almeda is believed to have been the first chiropractor in Canada.

Courtesy Scott Haldeman, Santa Ana, California.

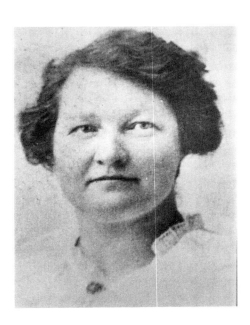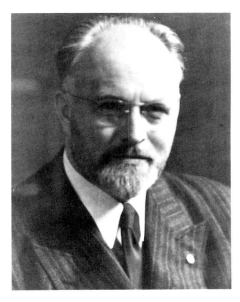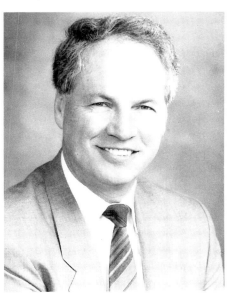

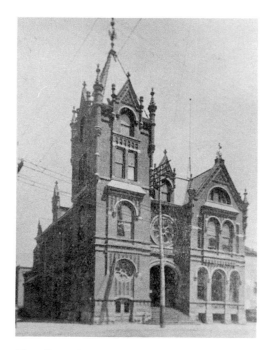

The Canadian Chiropractic College was located in Hamilton, Ontario from 1913-1923. Its beginning and closing dates are uncertain.

From the *Prospectus,* Canadian Chiropractic College, 1919.

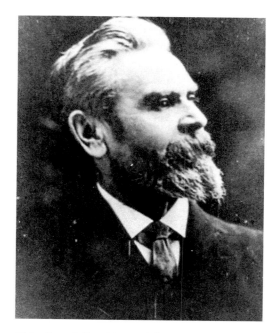

E.A. Duval, President of the Canadian Chiropractic College, circa 1915-1919.

From the *Prospectus,* Canadian Chiropractic College, 1919.

a chiropractor. Although a graduate of 1905, she did not settle in Herbert, Saskatchewan, until 1907. It is not clear to what extent she practiced chiropractic. Nevertheless, her children remember having regular adjustments. Her eldest son, Joshua Norman Haldeman, graduated in 1926 from the PSC in Davenport, Iowa. He became very active in Regina with the Saskatchewan association and was responsible for the chiropractic act passed in 1943. Dr. Haldeman was on the first board of directors of Canadian Memorial Chiropractic College (CMCC) from 1944 to 1950.

It is generally accepted that the practice of chiropractic began in other provinces of Canada in 1908. Unfortunately at this writing, there is no definitive history of chiropractic in Canada other than brief historical notes in Briefs submitted to various royal commissions and provincial health committees from 1961 to 1973. All 10 Canadian provinces have chiropractic acts that legalize and define the practice of chiropractic in each jurisdiction. It is significant that, like the United States, there is little agreement among the practice acts about scope of practice, key chiropractic definitions, and regulations governing the practice.

Canada's Early Educational Programs

Legislation and education are the chief ingredients for the history of Canadian chiropractic. Education preceded all attempts by legislation to regulate practice in the provinces. Although there is evidence that a few chiropractic colleges existed outside of Ontario between 1910 and 1920, there is no record of their activities. Prior to the opening of the CMCC in Toronto in 1945, five colleges are known to have existed in the province: the Robbins Chiropractic College in Sault Sainte Marie, Ontario, circa 1910-1912; the Canadian Chiropractic College in Hamilton, Ontario, circa 1913-1923; the Toronto Chiropractic College, circa 1920-1926; and the Imperial Chiropractic College, circa 1922-1923. Significantly, one 1911 graduate of the Robbins Chiropractic College, John A. Henderson (1883-1956), and two graduates of the Canadian Chiropractic College, John S. Clubine (1884-1956) and J.A. Cudmore, were prominent in the establishment of the CMCC. Dr. J.S. Clubine became the first CMCC president, and Dr. J. Henderson the first registrar.

At the time of the Royal Commission on Medical Education, also known as the Hodgins Report, 1915 to 1918, there were 82 chiropractors practicing in Ontario. Unbelievably, the 82 represented three associations: the Canadian Chiropractors' Association with 24 members, all but eight of whom were graduates of the PSC; the Ontario Chiropractors' Association with 25 members, all but two of whom were graduates of the Universal School of Chiropractic; and the Dominion Chiropractors' Association with a membership of 18, all but five of whom were graduates of the PSC. This division among chiropractors, given such small numbers, has been puzzling to sociologists studying the profession but is probably related to the ubiquitous and persistent philosophical division in the profession. During these early years chiropractic education averaged 1 to 2 years with no prerequisites for matriculation required.

Provincial Legislative Acts

The first chiropractic practice act was passed in Alberta in 1923. Ontario was next in 1925 with the Drugless Practitioners Act, an umbrella law to regulate chiropractic, osteopathic, and drugless practitioners. British Columbia, followed in 1934; Saskatchewan, in 1943; Manitoba, in 1945; New Brunswick, in 1958; Nova Scotia, in 1972; Prince Edward Island, in 1974; Newfoundland, in 1991; Quebec, in 1973; and the Yukon, in 1958.

For 20 years before September 18, 1945, young people desiring to pursue the study of this young, virile profession were required to enroll in colleges in the United States. The cost of education and living in another country prohibited many who wished to study chiropractic from doing so, resulting in a substantial loss to the Canadian economy and an even greater loss in the availability of chiropractic health services.

In January 1943, chiropractic representatives from all provinces gathered in Ottawa to formulate one sociopolitical organization of chiropractors devoted to the benefit of the public and the profession. The Dominion Council of Canadian Chiropractors was thus organized, later incorporated under federal charter on December 10, 1953, as the Canadian Chiropractic Association. The elder statesmen of the council quickly visualized the need for a Canadian college to embody the precepts of Canadian education, principles, and culture.

Founding of Canadian Memorial Chiropractic College

On January 3, 1945, the Canadian Association of Chiropractors was incorporated under the laws of the province of Ontario. The purpose and objects were to establish the CMCC, which was destined to become the hub of Canadian chiropractic education and research and the focal point for unity, cooperation, and professional growth.

The college, thus established in Toronto, was named as a memorial to the founder of the profession, Daniel David Palmer, himself a native son of Port Perry, Ontario. The basic principles of chiropractic, as formu-

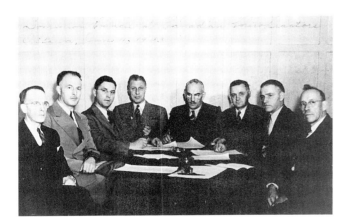

The Dominion Council of Canadian Chiropractors, Ottawa, January 11, 1943. Left to right, *John Gaudet, Quebec; Joshua Haldeman, Saskatchewan; John Burton, lawyer, British Columbia; Jack Schnick, Ontario; Walter Sturdy, British Columbia; John Clubine, Ontario; C.E. Messenger, Alberta; F.B. McElrea, Manitoba.*
Courtesy Herbert Vear, Pickering, Ontario, Canada.

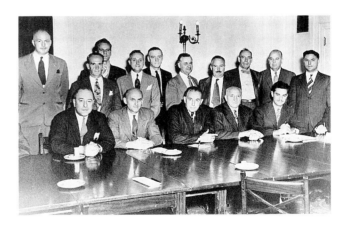

The Board of Governors of CMCC, 1946. Among them are *Joshua Haldeman; Rudy Mueller, dean; Douglas Hoskins; C.C. Messenger; John Clubine, President; Herbert Hill; F.B. McElrea; Gil Young; John Burton, lawyer; and Harry Yates.*
Courtesy Herbert Vear, Pickering, Ontario, Canada.

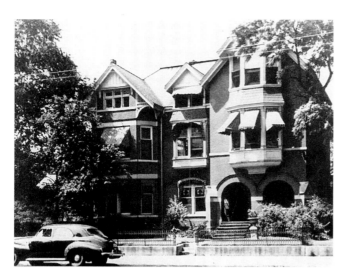

The first campus of CMCC, located at 252 Bloor Street West.
The building had housed a private hotel for several years.
Courtesy Herbert Vear, Pickering, Ontario, Canada.

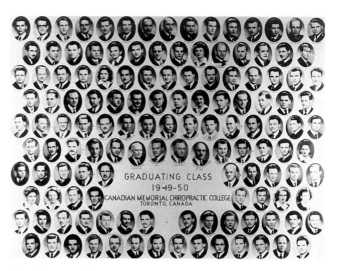

The first graduating class of Canadian Memorial Chiropractic College, May 20, 1949. The first class was identified as the Class of 1949-1950, because about one third started their studies at the end of the first semester and graduated 6 months later in January, 1950. The class started with 150 students and 118 graduated, 90% were World War II veterans.
Courtesy Herbert Vear, Pickering, Ontario, Canada.

lated by D.D. Palmer, were to be the cornerstone of the teachings within the college. This policy continues to be adhered to by the present governing board. In addition, the CMCC adopted a policy to teach all acceptable adjustive technique procedures and to avoid being supportive of any particular one. This policy was unique among chiropractic colleges in 1945. Since then most colleges have adopted a similar policy.

The first undergraduate class, composed almost exclusively of veterans of World War II, commenced studies on September 18, 1945, 50 years to the day from the rediscovery by D.D. Palmer of the merits of Hippocrates' "brachio-therapy" under the new name of chiropractic. The reputation of the college spread so widely that students were attracted, not only from every Canadian province, but also from many states in the United States, Europe, South Africa, Great Britain, Australia, New Zealand, the Bahamas, and South America. On Friday, May 20, 1949, a milestone was passed with the first CMCC graduation at the prestigious Eaton Auditorium in Toronto. Significantly, the graduation address was given by the Honorable D.R. Michener, who became a respected governor general of Canada and a living example for maintaining good health through natural means, which he practiced throughout his lifetime.

Royal Commission Reviews of Chiropractic in Canada

Although CMCC has made major contributions to the recognition of chiropractic health care in Canada through quality education, chiropractic research, scholarship, and graduates with leadership skills, it would be a mistake not to recognize the political leadership provided by the Canadian Chiropractic Association and its provincial affiliates. Two Ontario Royal Commissions have had an impact on the chiropractic profession.

The first was the Royal Commission on Medical Education formed in 1915 and to which the profession made an enthusiastic but unimpressive presentation. The commission reported in 1917 that there was value in physical methods of care like chiropractic, but recommended that they be developed as part of medicine rather than as a separate profession. Chiropractic history may have been much different if medicine had pursued this recommendation. In 1950 the second Royal Commission to affect chiropractic was formed to study the operation of the Ontario Workmen's Compensation Act. Against medical opposition, chiropractic care was retained and became well utilized by injured workers. Chiropractic care was first included in the Ontario act in 1937.

In 1961 the profession entered a decade of Royal Commissions or committees of inquiry prompted by growing public support for a national health insurance plan. There can be little doubt that the self-examination these commissions forced on the profession contributed to the growing strength and maturity of the profession in matters of legislation, scope of practice, education, research, and the importance of interprofessional cooperation with other health care professions.

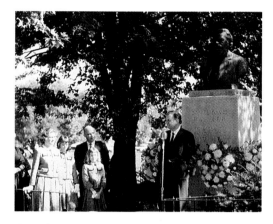

David and Agnes Palmer and their daughters visiting the Port Perry Memorial of D.D. Palmer in the early 1960s.
Courtesy Herbert Lee, Toronto, Ontario, Canada.

The major source and stimulus to develop these strengths came from three Royal Commissions:

1. The federal government's 1961 Royal Commission on Health Services, under the Honorable Mr. Justice Emmett M. Hall;
2. The 1966 Ontario Committee on the Healing Arts, under Mr. I.R. Dowie; and
3. The Ontario Council of Health's Task Force on Chiropractic, 1973, chaired by Dr. Oswald Hall.

The scope of this section does not permit serious discussion of the events and outcomes of each, other than to state that the scholarship and depth of the study of the submissions remain as a monument to the Canadian profession and as a resource to others. For example, the first scientific literature database in chiropractic was developed by the faculty and students of the CMCC in 1975 and published in 1976 as the *Archives,* with almost worldwide acceptance. It has continued as the *Chiropractic Research Archives Collection (CRAC)* with published editions in 1984, 1985, 1986, and 1990. Needless to say the Canadian profession has benefited by such progress, which continues to this day.

Canada's Contemporary Chiropractic Vitality

The CMCC has been the focal point for the political acceptance and expansion of chiropractic practice in Canada. As the first professionally owned, non-profit, chiropractic college in the world it has always placed heavy emphasis on the vix medicatrix naturae and the role of the chiropractor to assist an individual's natural curative process. This approach includes care directed towards maintaining, improving, restoring, or enhancing a patient's health through spinal adjustment, and the associated therapies of nutrition, counseling, and physiological therapeutics. To accomplish this goal, the CMCC employs faculty from many health care disciplines with academic qualifications to teach at the highest level of professional education.

In 1974 CMCC established a resident postgraduate program to train and educate the chiropractor according to the scientist-teacher model and, thereby, to perpetuate the science of chiropractic. From this model, a residency program was developed at University Hospital, University of

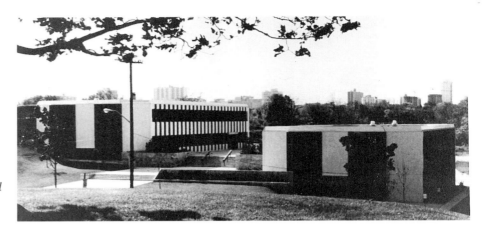

The Bayview campus of Canadian Memorial Chiropractic College, circa 1990.
Courtesy Herbert Vear, Pickering, Ontario, Canada.

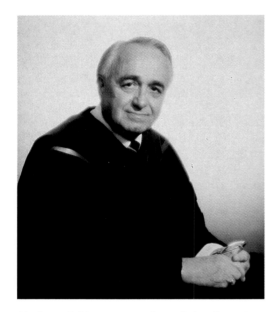

Herbert J. Vear, a member of the Canadian Standards of Practice Committee and past president of CMCC and Western States Chiropractic College.
Courtesy Herbert Vear, Pickering, Ontario, Canada.

Saskatchewan, Saskatoon, Saskatchewan, with the remarkable cooperation of Professor William Kirkaldy-Willis. The opportunity for residents to interact with medical orthopedic researchers and clinicians for several months resulted in a unique collection of research papers and a positive impact on undergraduate education that continues. This leadership provided by CMCC scholars in resident postgraduate education has been adopted by several other colleges with similar research outcomes.

In September 1993 the Université du Québec à Trois Riviéres inaugurated its first class into the new School of Chiropractic, which is taught entirely in the French language. It is the first chiropractic educational facility in North America to be totally funded and accredited by a state-operated university, and only one of two in the world. The fact that the first chiropractic act was not passed until 1973 makes this an even more profound development.

To conclude this succinct overview of Canadian chiropractic history, it is appropriate to mention the research, development, and agreement of practice guidelines for Canada. The process began in 1991 with selection of a Standards of Practice Committee by the Canadian Chiropractic Association. After the involvement of 23 organizations and the preparation of 20 chapters reflecting on the scope of clinical chiropractic, a 4-day conference was conducted in Toronto, beginning on April 4, 1993, and named the Glenerin Conference after the Glenerin Inn site. Over 300 items were considered by 35 panel members before reaching a consensus. As one spokesperson said after the conference, "The Glenerin Conference is the voice of the chiropractic profession in Canada."

There should be no doubt that Canadian chiropractic is prepared to enter the next century, not only with strength for the future but also with respect for its pioneering past.

CHIROPRACTIC IN EUROPE

Pierre-Louis Gaucher-Peslherbe

Chiropractic first appeared in Europe through England before World War I. But there is growing evidence that the old continent truly discovered chiropractic during the war itself, when a number of early chiropractors were drafted into the United States Army and were in a position to act professionally while on trench duty or behind the lines. It is a fact that the war and its aftermath implied important movements of population; people and ideas were traveling fast, and chiropractic looked like too good an idea in health care to remain confined to any single part of the world. A few European individuals had emigrated with their parents or had come as refugees because of the war. Some decided to study and to return home after graduation, believing implicitly in the early teachings of the science. As a result, the number of practitioners rapidly increased.

Beliefs were already divided among them. C.E.R. Bannister, first president of the European Chiropractors' Union (ECU) was to recall once: "In 1920, when I started to practice in Ireland, there were hardly a handful of chiropractors in the whole of Europe (or rather what you could count on the fingers of one hand) and the field was already split up." Among these handful were S. Larsen, in Denmark; A.L. Jester, in Germany; Mrs. Albina Michaelova-Capova, in Czechoslovakia; E.H. Schwing, in France; and A.E. Lundh, in Norway. It can thus be considered that it is only from 1924 to 1926 that the profession was truly established in most European countries. It was certainly the case in Belgium with J. Gillet, a 1922 Palmer graduate, who returned from Canada to Brussels in 1924.

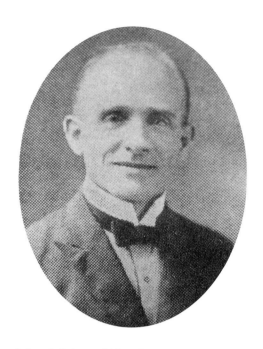

Jules Gillet, a 1922 Palmer graduate, was a chiropractic pioneer in Belgium.

From *The Pisiform,* Palmer School of Chiropractic, October 1922.

Medical Legislation and Chiropractic

In most continental countries, medical laws were of an archaic nature, as in Denmark, whose laws dated back to 1794. This situation contrasted with that in the United States of America, where medicine had just evolved from sects to science and where medical laws were quite recent. Whatever date the laws were issued, as in France in 1892, they were all devised to have the same effect. Namely, they gave doctors of medicine the sole rights to prescribe and to treat or order different treatments for the sick. The only way a chiropractor could avoid being condemned for practicing without a license was to practice under referral by a medical doctor, a common practice for awhile in most European countries and still the usual mode in Italy.

European medical circles and societies were quite aware of the type of challenge chiropractic practice represented. They had the American example to reflect upon. For example, A. Abrams had a widely known method of spine percussion devised, as early as 1910, as a medical riposte to both osteopathy and chiropractic, but, due to the war, it required nearly 15 more years for medical societies in Europe to contrive their own similar devices. Their attacks were drafted along the lines that had been widely rehearsed at the time of F.A. Mesmer and his revolutionary mode of magnetic healing. Either an expert committee was gathered to investigate and report on chiropractic or academic societies merely reported without even a proper investigation. Whichever was the case, the report resulted in a scathing condemnation. Expert commissions of that nature existed in 1923 in Denmark and in 1936 in Switzerland, and they advised against chiropractic recognition.

One of the oldest European references to publish a medical policy statement on the issue dates back to 1925. Both chiropractic and osteopathy were condemned and branded as cults that, according to conventional medicine, considered as basic facts conditions that had been declared scientifically untenable. In Europe the dispute about chiropractic tenets was biased from the onset.

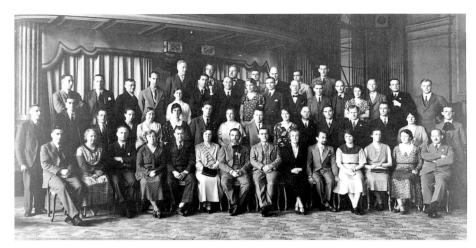

The British Chiropractors' Association Conference, May 19, 1934. Guests B.J. and Mabel Palmer are seated in the front row.

Courtesy Palmer College of Chiropractic Archives, Davenport, Iowa.

Establishment of the European Chiropractors' Union

Medical antagonism had grown so ruthless and malicious that it was even stated that the chiropractor might do a considerable amount of good to the patient, but that he had done so unconsciously and "perhaps even unwillingly"! From now on the stage was set and the issue from a legal standpoint was how to transform a practitioner labeled as an irregular operator into a fully recognized professional. Medical laws no longer authorized the development of a new profession, and chiropractors were faced with long and protracted legal battles. Legislation was different in the various European countries, but prejudices were the same. The need to unite forces became prevalent and resulted in the creation of the ECU in 1931. There were possibly 100 practitioners in Europe then. Only a third of them decided to join on a personal basis. Seven years later, practicing chiropractors numbered about 240 in Europe and 70 had joined the ECU.

The spirit pervading the first meetings is perhaps best expressed in the following: "Numbers of chiropractors do not influence or change basic policies or needs . . . whether we are numerous or whether we are but a few, we have needs in common, which can perhaps be better met and satisfied by common effort . . . however varied in members, however meager in numbers it may for the moment be." These European pioneers were convinced that "big things are bound to happen, and if the

Henri Gillet (left) *edited the first European chiropractic journal as a news-letter in 1931. With his brother Marcel Gillet* (right) *and Marcel Liekens they developed motion palpation to the level of an art.*

Courtesy John Gillet, Brussels, Belgium.

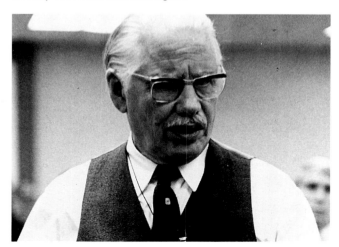

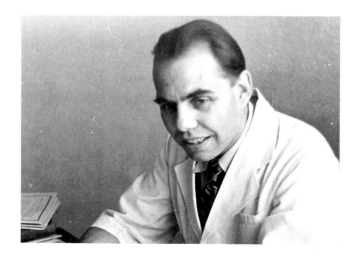

fight was bitter in the early days in the U.S., it will be all the more so here. . . . Our battles will necessitate, we think, less sheer daring and more actual brains and work in law courts. Here is where an organization employing all its resources and trained men can be of great use."

It should be remembered that all this organizing was started in the midst of a severe economic depression, the worst the modern world had known so far. Nonetheless the early members chose to consider the crisis as a warning to chiropractors and to chiropractic associations in Europe not to start building barriers around themselves. They believed that "chiropractic is international and not to be cramped by any local barriers." This attitude is to the credit of the men who stood at that time and in those circumstances with such clear heads. These attempts toward organizing lasted until the outbreak of World War II: "Shortly after the advent of the war in 1939, composed as it was by individual members, contacts were lost because of Europe's division between allied and enemy countries; communication was cut off and the old ECU was forced to cease to function."

World War II and Post-War Effects on Chiropractic

The war gave the medical world new ways and means to curb chiropractic growth in Europe. Some of these were of an unavoidable nature. The years of bitter warfare and the lean years between 1945 and 1951 had taken their toll, and the number of practitioners was greatly reduced: a number had died, some retired, while others had left and gone to live outside the war area. Some other means were of a less unavoidable nature, which can be documented by what occurred in France with the creation of a French Medical Council by the French government in Vichy, whereas only medical syndicates had existed before. The main concern of that council, according to what was published at the time, was to encourage informers against "alien" doctors of medicine, namely the Jews! This example led to informing against "alien medicines" as well.

It took 5 years after the war to lick the wounds so brought about. From that moment onward, chiropractic, as a professional body, and not simply because of a few exceptional individuals (Illi, Gillet, Rames, Bannister, etc.), turned to realize its full scientific potential and steer a course due in time to bring full recognition to all qualified practitioners in the field. From that moment onward, too, the Founder's idea that a subluxation was a state of functional discontinuity that had to be corrected to restore the conditions for continuity of being came to be scientifically documented. A subluxation was not, and could not be, described as an entity, but rather as a convergence of differential elements. Each of these elements and their eventual contradictions could therefore be specifically and scientifically described.

On the other hand, medical awareness about chiropractic tenets and accomplishments was also instrumental in bringing this new awareness to chiropractors themselves. For example, in the case of the 1953 official recognition of chiropractic in France, the decree recognized chiropractic, but banned chiropractors from practicing their art under the pretense that their diploma was alien, limiting the practice to medical doctors even though they could not have learned it. In other words, it was an illegality designed for medical expediency's sake. In complete opposition to it, the recognition of the right to practice was obtained in Switzerland by chiropractors through popular votes. This experience showed that people would, as a rule, refuse to accept abusive medical edicts.

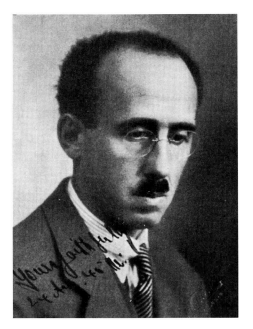

Fred Illi graduated from Universal College, headed by Loban and Steinbach, in 1927. He was to win chiropractic recognition in the first Swiss Cantons almost single-handed, supported by much patients' lobbying.

From *Nation College Chiropractic Journal* December 1940.

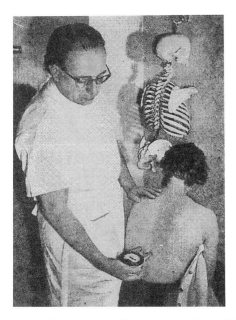

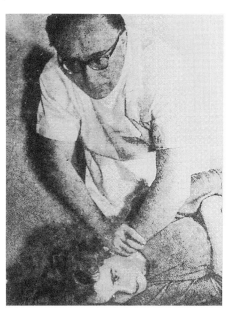

The "German Issue" was created in 1955, when German medical doctors invited B.J. Palmer to lecture on chiropractic, much to the dismay of his European colleagues. After a heated exchange of letters, Palmer declined the invitation.
From *Chiropractic History,* 1982.

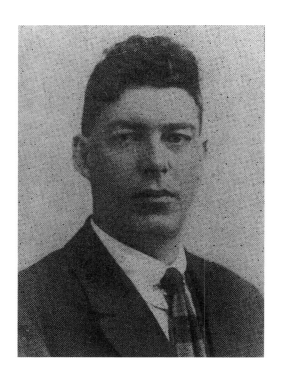

C.E.R. Bannister, the leader of the European Union before World War II.
From *The Chiroprator,* May 1924.

In another instance of how the medical field's attacks on chiropractic forced chiropractors to define themselves, much discussion was generated when German medical doctors invited B.J. Palmer to deliver a lecture to them. Weiant, Janse, and Illi had refused to comply with what they considered to be little short of a baited trap. There was a very heated exchange of letters, and, finally, Palmer declined the invitation. It came to be known and recorded in chiropractic history as "the German issue." The combined action of these momentous issues spurred the profession in Europe to put its house in order and to present a more united and coherent front than ever before. If anything, the German issue had helped to sever the umbilical cord of devotion to B.J. Palmer's person. Hence it helped to state professional issues in terms more appropriate to European mentalities. It was also instrumental in bringing the problem of a European college to the forefront.

Led by Bannister from Belfast, the pre-World War II European Union had defined itself as a self-governing body with power to grant diplomas and examine candidates based upon the claim that "any qualified person who adjusted the spinal column is a chiropractor." The ECU even considered starting a school. O. Melanson, an English chiropractor, thought a college should be established in England and wondered about continental support. The chiropractic college was to graduate prospective individuals "with a social status to which they have been accustomed according to the standards of European life."

The chiropractic profession in Europe had to face an upsurge of nonqualified practitioners: Quite a number of field practitioners considered themselves qualified to *practice and teach,* according to the early D.D. Palmer's injunctions! Parnell Bradbury, the author of the 1957 *Healing by Hand,* was one of the few to be granted such a European diploma with no real schooling.

Establishment of a European Chiropractic College

A college was almost started in 1939 in Geneva by Dr. Fred Illi. It would have opened its doors had it not been for the outbreak of World War II. The college was to have a 4-year course of studies plus a compulsory 6-month assistantship. The curriculum proposed over 3000 hours of instruction. A number of subjects were to be taught in Geneva University. At the time, the PSC was still awarding a D.C. after 18 months! This point was frequently brought to the fore by prospective students. There were not enough qualified practitioners in Geneva alone to fill all the teaching positions required: Marcel Gillet from Brussels, Joseph Janse from Chicago, and Clarence Weiant from New York had accepted invitations to join the professional body. Support from the field was quasi-unanimous especially since Illi had said he would refuse to build up a school "in any other way than a morally high standing one, beyond all critics."

World War II meant that most prospective students would be enlisted to fight. Besides, most governments would forbid any currency exchanges. Hence, all plans about a chiropractic college in Europe had to be shelved. To save the project until after the war, in October 1942, Illi opened the Chiropractic Research Institute that still exists today. At the same time, he organized the International College of Research, so that, as he said, "at least, there is going to be the necessary research." When the war was over, the project was still very much alive. The clinic was to operate right away but only postgraduate courses were to be taught at first, to organize a proper teaching body. Plans to that effect, though, were thwarted by other Swiss chiropractors.

Recognizing that the need for a European chiropractic college still existed, the Danes acted on plans of their own. They launched the short-

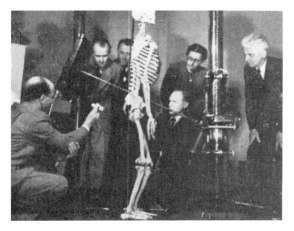

Fred Illi (left) was one of the foremost chiropractic researchers of his time. Together with lifelong friend Joseph Janse from National College, they studied the neuropathological reflexes induced by subluxation and/or poor locomotion. Illi's work is carried on at the Institute for the Study of Statics and Dynamics of the Human Body in Geneva, Switzerland, created by Illi in 1942.

From *The National Chiropractic Journal,* January 1946.

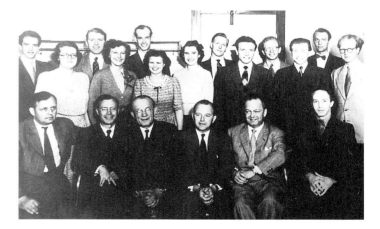

The first graduating class of the Dansk Kiroprakto Kuzsus, which ran from 1948 to 1951. Included are F. Christensen, D.C., E.O. Rames, M.D., D.C., A. Pedersen D.C., and H.A. Simonsen, D.C.

Courtesy Aase and Henning Hviid, D.C.

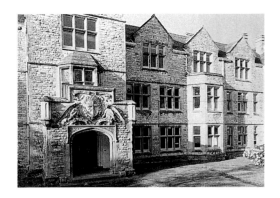

The Parkwood Road campus, circa 1990, of Anglo-European College of Chiropractic, established in 1965. Her Royal Highness, the Princess of Wales is its Royal Patron.

Courtesy Anglo-European College of Chiropractic, Bournemouth, England.

lived *Dansk Kiroprakto Kuzsus,* which was run from 1948 to 1951 by a chiropractor, Finn Christensen, and a medical doctor, E.O. Rames. Reasons for such a short existence have yet to be told. But the fact that it existed at all clearly indicates that a chiropractic college in Europe had become an urgent professional necessity. These failed attempts led individuals from Great Britain to go ahead alone and to launch in 1965 the Anglo-European College of Chiropractic in Bournemouth. The location had a number of advantages, if only for language and teaching purposes. The importance of this institution cannot be overstated because it affected the evolution of the profession in Europe.

Whereas most European practitioners considered themselves as alumni of their American alma mater before anything else, the new college had, by sheer necessity, to be staffed by teachers who had themselves graduated from various American colleges. Hence, students were exposed to the full spectrum of chiropractic doctrines. Their approach to the tenets of their future profession was therefore of a more ecumenical nature than it could have been dreamed of anywhere else. It is never easy to give such factors their proper weight, but taken as they existed, it might explain why in the 1970s chiropractic in Europe came to be approached in a more scientific way than was possible before. Even though the reasons for a similar evolution in America might be of a different nature, the end result is that on either side of the Atlantic Ocean, this trend was present. Chiropractic professionals, both on the American and on the European continents were in step with it and in step with each other.

It has always been of utmost importance to chiropractic to assume the responsibility for its own professional training, defining, and implementing of the conditions of access; the contents of the formation; the types of examination; and so on. These responsibilities represent a professional as well as a political necessity, since no real identity could be preserved otherwise. But resolution of these issues for the profession in Europe has had to be learned the hard way, since the profession was not always prepared to assume them the way that Illi had before World War II. For example, the creation of a Council on European Chiropractic Education was deferred for a number of reasons that did not relate strictly to the educational sphere. This was also the case with the French college. It was started in 1983, more as the result of the personal involvement of a few chiropractors than as the outcome of a clear policy from the European profession. The fact that the profession is young enough in Europe that it has no legal definition in many countries should be to the advantage of chiropractic, not the contrary.

In most European countries, the right to practice or to claim specific titles is strictly limited to appropriate diplomates. Besides, neither a diploma nor other recognized qualification is sufficient to practice according to the law. The practitioner must also be registered by a proper authority. However, because non-conventional medicines are not usually legally defined, the law does not specify the required education nor its peculiarities, which implies that there is no university or other school to provide the required training. The end result for chiropractors is the absence of proper registration, defined qualifications, and professional designation, which could be used for the guidance and the safeguarding of the patient. This, with but few exceptions, is the actual situation for chiropractors in a number of European countries. At the present time, the legislative situation can be described as a patchwork of differing qualifications, which does not foster a strong sense of professional identity.

Chiropractic and Contemporary Europe

There is no way to predict where chiropractors may turn when trapped with licensure regulations. The European Economic Community and its rulings, which concern most countries in which proper legislation is still lacking, do not seem to offer a ready solution to all such cares. As in most federally organized states, each of the constituent countries will more than likely retain its full rights over legislative enactment on both educational and health fields. Therefore, the decisions about the registration of the various health professionals allowed to practice will be made within each country's rules and code specifications. In the past, chiropractic gained a status as an independent branch of medicine and saw its practice regulated because of public involvement. This process is exactly what happened in Switzerland, and it implied full professional rights regarding patient management, x-ray, physiotherapy and laboratory privileges, and insurance coverage.

The report on the regulation of non-conventional methods of health care issued by the Council of Europe in 1984 acknowledges that chiropractic differs from other forms of nonconventional medicines by its standardized and well-structured training. It also states that it equates with medical education, with the proviso that although training in surgery and pharmacology is not required, other more appropriate subjects are very extensively taught. Similarly, the French *Conseil d'Etat* stated in 1985 that the value of chiropractic diplomas is established beyond all questions.

However, at present in Belgium, France, Italy, Portugal, and other countries, chiropractic is not a registered profession. Professionals still have to face lawsuits on the basis of practicing without a license. The situation there amounts to one of "tolerated illegality." It follows that chiropractic treatments are not reimbursed by national security systems. Yet some private companies may have plans to cover the treatment costs. In some other countries, chiropractic is not even supposed to exist as such and is in limbo. In Greece, chiropractors formed a common national organization together with osteopaths, which lasted until recently, and they are practicing under a physiotherapist's license. The situation was similar in Germany, where chiropractors were allowed to practice under the *Heilpraktiker* statute, which still provides for many different types of lay therapies. It is only lately that the specificity of the chiropractic diploma has been recognized by the courts in this country.

On the other hand, chiropractic is fully recognized and chiropractors hold full professional rights in Switzerland, Liechtenstein, Sweden, Norway, and Denmark. The Odense University in Denmark has a prechiropractic curriculum that has received accreditation from the United States Council on Chiropractic Education. In Great Britain, though, the Common

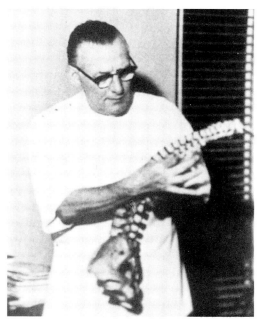

Marcel Trenton was instrumental in establishing chiropractic in Italy.
Courtesy Associazione Italiana Chiropratici.

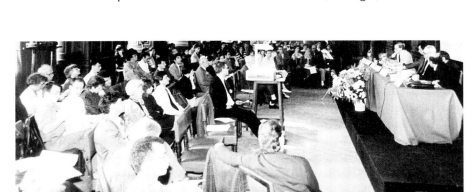

The Walter Wardwell Conference, held in Paris, April 1992, was the first international and interdisciplinary conference held in a University setting in France. It was organized by the Chiropractic Research Information Center (CRIC), France; the European Institute of Biomechanics (IEB), Belgium; and the Institute for the Study of Statics and Dynamics of the Human Body (IESDCH), Switzerland.
Courtesy Pierre-Louis Gaucher-Peslherbe, Vouvray Sur Loir, France.

Law provides for independent and undisturbed practice, but chiropractors cannot yet be registered with the National Health Service.

The World Health Organization (WHO) divides the world into six regions, Europe being one of them. It is clear that the European experience with chiropractic is not a uniform one. The right to practice is granted "under one of two legal environments: those countries governed by common law allow the practice as long as there is no specific law against it, while countries governed by Roman Dutch Law deem that any professional practice not legislated is, in fact, illegal. As a general rule, Northern European countries are governed by common law, while Central and Southern European countries are legislated by Roman Dutch Law."

CHIROPRACTIC IN AUSTRALIA

Rolf Eduard Peters
Mary Ann Chance

Australia, the "island continent," comprises approximately the same land mass as the contiguous United States, and its eastern seaboard lies some 7500 nautical miles southwest of the California coast. Historically the two nations have much in common: both were settled by the British during the great wave of European expansionism of the sixteenth to eighteenth centuries, inheriting the same language and traditions, and a similar form of government and notions of justice. However, the extreme remoteness of Australia from centers of Western civilization, as well as differences in terrain, climate, early immigration patterns, and response to British rule, led to marked variations in population distribution, national characteristics, and legal systems. Both the similarities and the contrasts have had a significant impact on the development of the chiropractic profession in the two countries.

At the time of D.D. Palmer's discovery of chiropractic in 1895, Australia, then still composed of British colonies, boasted a mere 3,000,000 inhabitants, most of whom lived in the major cities of the southeastern coastal region. Australia's wealth and population had grown dramatically over the previous four decades, largely because of discovery of gold in the colony of Victoria just 2 years after the beginning of California's gold rush. The colony's capital, Melbourne, had become a distant outpost of European culture and opulence.

Early Practitioners

It was through a Victorian family of considerable wealth and influence that chiropractic was introduced to Australia. Barbara Brake, wife of James Brake, MLA, suffered from congenitally dislocated hips, and, though money was no object, had never found satisfactory relief through conventional medicine. When they heard of cures through chiropractic, the Brakes decided that she should seek Dr. Palmer's help. Mrs. Brake arrived in Davenport in late 1904, accompanied by her widowed sister-in-law, Martha Brake Thompson. She was apparently impressed by the results, for she completed 3 months of the course at the Palmer School and Infirmary of Chiropractic. There is no evidence that she undertook the additional 6 months of study and examinations necessary to obtain a

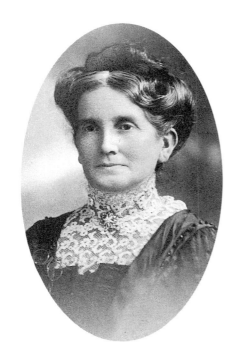

Mrs. Barbara Brake, the first known chiropractic patient and practitioner from Australia.

Courtesy Archives of the Association for the History of Chiropractic, Australia.

476

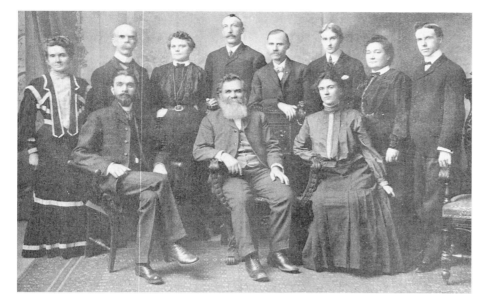

Barbara Brake (far left) *with her class at the Palmer School of Chiropractic, February 1905. Seated* left to right: *B.J. Palmer, D.D. Palmer, and Mabel Palmer. Standing* left to right: *Brake, Darnel, Oas, Hananska, Evans, Danelz, Doeltz, and Parker.*
From *Chiropractor*, February 1905.

legitimate qualification; however, on her return to Melbourne, she established what is believed to be the first chiropractic practice in Australia. In March 1906, her sister-in-law Martha Brake listed her own practice, which was located in the Temperance Building in Melbourne, in the journal *The Chiropractor*. In 1908 two of Barbara's children, a son and a daughter, graduated from the Still College of Osteopathy at Kirksville, Missouri, returning to Melbourne in 1909 to establish what was probably Australia's first osteopathic practice. The development and fortunes of chiropractic and osteopathy in Australia have been closely interwoven ever since, but it is doubtful that this is linked more than coincidentally with the Brake family's early association with both professions.

Sydney has always been the traditional port of entry into Australia,

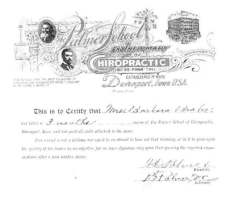

The certificate of attendance, Palmer School and Infirmary of Chiropractic, for Mrs. Barbara Brake, circa 1905. It appears she never completed the full course to earn her doctor of chiropractic degree.
Courtesy Archives of the Association for the History of Chiropractic, Australia.

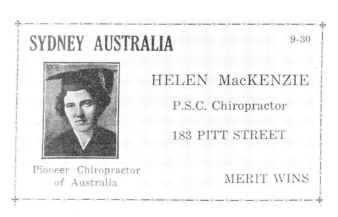

Early professional advertising of Helen MacKenzie, a 1923 Palmer graduate. MacKenzie was the third chiropractor to start practicing in Sydney, Australia, and the first woman graduate to practice in Australia.
From *The Chiropractor*, May 1931.

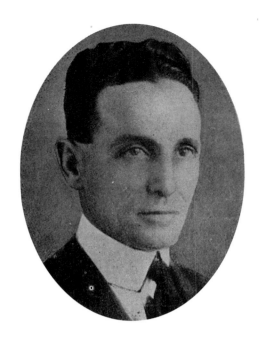

Hector McBeath, a 1920 Palmer graduate, was the first chiropractor to earn an x-ray certificate (at that time an optional course) to practice in Australia.

Courtesy Archives of the Association for the History of Chiropractic, Australia.

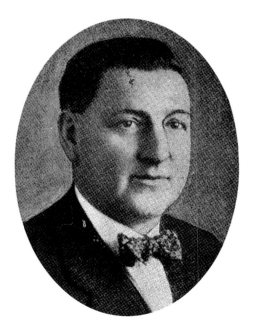

John G. Yerkey, a 1914 Palmer graduate, joined the practice of Hector McBeath in Adelaide in 1925.

Courtesy Archives of the Association for the History of Chiropractic, Australia.

so it is not surprising that it was the first Australian city to attract a substantial number of chiropractors. The first evidence of a chiropractic practice in Sydney is a 1918 telephone directory listing for A.E.P. Summerbell, who was apparently qualified in both chiropractic and osteopathy. He was followed by Harold W. Williams in 1921, then Helen MacKenzie, a 1923 Palmer graduate who set up practice within the year in Sydney. MacKenzie, a former nurse, had been a patient of Henry Otterholt, the first Palmer graduate to set up practice in New Zealand in 1914. In 1928 there were at least seven chiropractors in Sydney, and the number had nearly doubled by 1932. Until the 1940s, Australian chiropractors were predominantly New Zealand-born and overwhelmingly Palmer graduates.

South Australia's first chiropractor was New Zealander Hector McBeath, who was also introduced to chiropractic by Otterholt, and who commenced practice in Adelaide in 1922. He and his wife, Janet, entered the PSC in 1918, graduated in 1920, and practiced briefly in Wellington, New Zealand, before coming to Australia. He is the first chiropractor with qualifications in x-ray, then still an optional course to have practiced in Australia. John G. Yerkey from Dersailles, Pennsylvania, a 1914 Palmer graduate, joined the practice in 1925, and George Theroux from Spokane, Washington, established a practice in Adelaide soon after his graduation in 1923.

Chiropractic was introduced to Tasmania by New Zealanders Leslie Henry Moses (a 1922 Palmer graduate), Cecil H. Wells (a 1926 Palmer graduate), and Frederick C. Wells (a 1930 Palmer graduate), all of whom practiced in Hobart. They were joined later by Michael Atkinson. In 1951, without warning, chiropractic was effectively outlawed by passage of the Physiotherapists Registration Act. At that time only Atkinson and the younger Wells remained in Tasmania, and when their appeals against the act's provisions failed, they too, left for the mainland. It was several years before Richard LeBreton succeeded in reintroducing chiropractic to Tasmania and, through a court challenge, won the right for the state's chiropractors to use x-ray.

The first chiropractors known to have practiced in Western Australia were New Zealander Andrew Martin (a 1920 Palmer graduate), who had practiced in Macon, Georgia, after graduation, then in Sydney in 1924, and thereafter briefly in Kuala Lumpur, arriving in Perth in January 1926, and South Australian S. Bernard Dawson, a 1926 Palmer graduate who spent a short time in Adelaide before moving on to Perth. It was largely through Martin's efforts that the first Australian legislation allowing chiropractors to continue using x-rays was enacted, in an amendment to the Medical Act of Western Australia (1945).

The history of chiropractic in Victoria between 1905 and 1934 is obscure; however, New Zealander Charles Henry Mathieson (a 1921 Palmer graduate) is said to have been the first United States–trained graduate chiropractor to practice in that state. In 1934 Cecil Wells relocated to Melbourne after 7 years in Hobart, and in 1938, Robert and Rita Hart, also Palmer graduates, arrived from Napier, New Zealand, to take over the Mathieson practice.

New Zealander John Pickles was the first formally trained chiropractor to establish a practice in Queensland. He arrived in Brisbane shortly after his graduation from the Palmer school in 1937, but his practice was interrupted by 5 years of military service during World War II. He was followed by James Heggie, a 1941 graduate who, upon his return to Australia, joined the army medical corps, and in 1948 returned to Brisbane, where he practiced for 12 years before moving to Sydney.

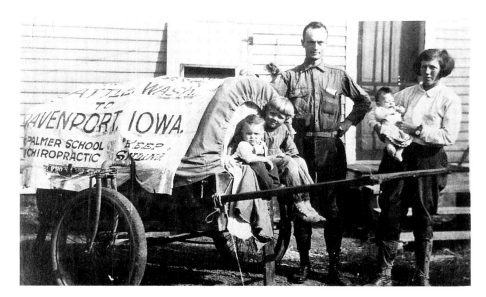

Dorothy Searby and family on their way to the Palmer School. She graduated in 1929 and practiced in Sydney and Wollongong. Her husband, Robert Charles Searby, attended Palmer and practiced in Sydney and Melbourne.

Courtesy Palmer College of Chiropractic Archives, Davenport, Iowa.

Until the early 1960s, when Arthur Paley settled in Canberra, residents of the Australian Capital Territory had to travel to neighboring Queanbeyan and Goulburn in New South Wales for chiropractic care. The Northern Territory was also slow to attract chiropractors. Dorothy Searby, a 1929 Palmer graduate who had previously practiced in Sydney and Wollongong, was in Darwin by the mid-1960s, while Adelaide chiropractor Roy Breen visited Alice Springs on a bimonthly basis from 1969 to 1982.

Expansion of Services

Demand for chiropractic services in Australia increased much more rapidly than growth of practitioner numbers, which was severely impeded by the necessity to travel halfway around the world to obtain a qualification. The increase in chiropractors ground to a complete halt during the 1940s, when the region was isolated by World War II. Because foreign students in the United States were seldom granted work permits, financial difficulties became a greater obstacle after the war when the chiropractic course was lengthened to 4 years. Attempts to meet these challenges have been a powerful influence in shaping the history of chiropractic in Australia and have included circuit and multicenter practices, student recruitment, loans and scholarships, emergence of practitioners without formal qualifications, and establishment of local training facilities.

Perhaps the first, and certainly the most extensive, of the circuit practices was established in the 1930s by Stanley and Mariette Bolton of Sydney, eventually covering most major provincial centers in New South Wales and as far north as Toowoomba in Queensland. During the 1960s most of these centers were taken over by resident chiropractors. Meanwhile, in Victoria and South Australia, Frank McLeod, Mary Ann (Chance) McLeod, and Maxwell McLeod established more than 20 practices, which were staffed, and eventually purchased, by new graduates. In the Northern Territory, where distances are great and the population sparse, two flying chiropractor services were established during the 1970s. Robert Hackett traveled by commercial flights from Darwin east to Nhulumbuy (650 km), west to Kununurra and Wyndham (475 km), and south to

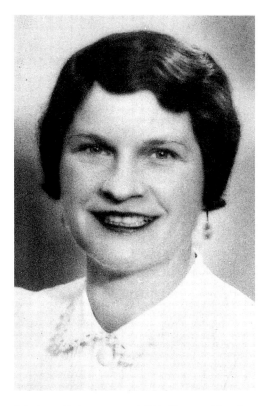

Mariette Bolton, circa 1934. She and her husband Stanley operated a circuit practice in the 1930s.

Courtesy Bolton Archives, Sydney, Australia.

479

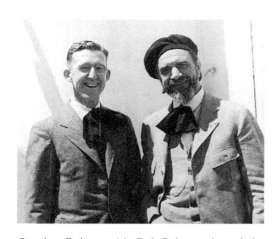

Stanley Bolton with B.J. Palmer aboard the S.S. Bremen on their way to Germany in 1934, where at the Spalteholz laboratories the "wet specimen" showing the relationship of the spinal cord to the spinal canal at the time of death was being prepared.
Courtesy Bolton Archives, Sydney, Australia.

Katherine (275 km)—the largest area ever covered by a single practitioner by air—and Paul Pringle by light aircraft from Alice Springs north to Tennant Creek (475 km) and south to Coober Pedy (625 km). During the 1960s and 1970s, multicenter practices were more the rule than the exception. Even today about one Australian chiropractor in four practices in more than one location.

Student recruitment began in earnest during the 1950s, and to assist students in meeting the high costs of travel and tuition, student trust funds were established, first by the Chiropractors' Association of Victoria, and later by the Australian Chiropractors' Association (ACA). At least one of the colleges offered special scholarships to Australian students. During the 1960s and 1970s there was also a substantial influx of chiropractors from overseas.

Meanwhile a sizeable number of practitioners emerged who lacked formal qualifications in chiropractic but manipulated the spine and called themselves chiropractors, often in conjunction with other therapies and titles such as osteopath, naturopath, and homeopath. Most had been apprenticed to established practitioners, only a few of whom had formal qualifications themselves, and some were apparently self-taught.

Among the large numbers of immigrants from Europe after the two world wars were people with medical backgrounds who were unable to obtain licensure in Australia. Some turned to manipulation and other natural therapies that were not regulated by law at that time in order to remain in the health care field, and a few identified with chiropractic. Another, Ernst Kjellberg, practiced a unique form of manipulation, massage, and hydrotherapy, and although never calling himself a chiropractor, trained several practitioners who were eventually to be not only registered, but highly respected, as chiropractors.

Chiropractic Education in Australia

Establishment of local training facilities contributed yet another stream to chiropractic in Australia. The first institution known to have included chiropractic subjects was the Pax College, which was established in 1933 and appears to have been identified more strongly with osteopathy than with chiropractic. The most important were the Chiropractic College of Australasia, founded in 1960 by F.G. Roberts; the Chiropractic and Osteopathic College of South Australia; and the Sydney College of Osteopathy, later renamed the Sydney College of Chiropractic (SCC), founded in 1959 by Alfred Kaufman. However none of these programs was at a standard acceptable to any chiropractic licensing authority in the world, nor to the ACA, formed in 1938. What formal qualifications their founders and early lecturers may have had remains unclear.

Though chiropractic has been fairly well accepted by the Australian public almost since its introduction, the wide disparity in levels of practitioner education, standards, discipline, and practice procedures remained a serious obstacle to government legitimation and regulation until the late 1970s. Following a Royal Commission, the Western Australian government registered chiropractors in 1964, limiting eligibility to graduates of certain overseas colleges and to persons who had been established in chiropractic practice in the state before the law came into effect. Most other states, however, were reluctant to demand a qualification that could be obtained only overseas or to take any action that might limit practice under common law.

The North American graduates represented by the ACA saw the need for suitable practitioner training courses within Australia and feared that acceptance of a lower educational standard as the basis for registration would not only curtail the role of chiropractic within the Australian health care system, but also become a barrier to reciprocal relationships with the profession in other parts of the world.

To overcome these problems, they supported development of the International College of Chiropractic (ICC), in Melbourne, which would provide practitioner education at an internationally recognized standard. Eventually both the Chiropractic College of Australasia and the Chiropractic and Osteopathic College of South Australia merged with the ICC, which, headed by Marcia Cerutty (daughter of Robert and Rita Hart), accepted its first students in 1975. The following year, under the leadership of the newly appointed principal, Andries M. Kleynhans, ICC moved to the campus of Preston Institute of Technology, later to become the Phillip Institute of Technology (PIT).

The ICC and the PIT presented the chiropractic undergraduate program jointly until 1981, when the course, by then fully accredited and funded by the government, was taken over completely by the institute. In 1992, when PIT merged with the Royal Melbourne Institute of Technology to form RMIT University, Kleynhans was granted a full professorship, the first such appointment in chiropractic by a university. RMIT University now also offers an undergraduate program in osteopathy, as well as a number of postgraduate and specialty programs, and supports a Centre for Chiropractic Research.

Meanwhile, the SCC was upgrading its program, in part by presenting the professional component of the course end-on to a bachelor's degree in anatomy from the University of New South Wales. Under pressure of the Australian government's policy of unified tertiary education whereby colleges of advanced education and freestanding institutions were encouraged to amalgamate with existing universities, SCC linked with Macquarie University in 1990, becoming the Centre for the Study of Chiropractic within the university's school of biological sciences. This was the first such university development in chiropractic in Australia and was also believed at the time to be a world first. The head of Sydney College, Rodney Bonello, was appointed associate professor. A 2-year master's degree program in chiropractic science is now offered by the university as the professional component of a 5-year, double-degree course, a registrable qualification in chiropractic.

Educational standards appropriate to Australia and consistent with those governing accreditation by the Council on Chiropractic Education in the United States were developed during the 1970s by the Australasian Council on Chiropractic Education, a multidisciplinary body initially sponsored by the ACA. Its role was eventually expanded to accredit osteopathic and postgraduate programs. This body has recently been superseded by the Australian Council for Chiropractic and Osteopathy, which has closer links with the state registration boards and other government bodies.

Use of X-Ray by Chiropractors

X-ray was first used in chiropractic practices in Australia during the 1920s, and in 1932 chiropractors were advertising both x-ray and neurocalometer facilities in the Sydney classified telephone directory. By

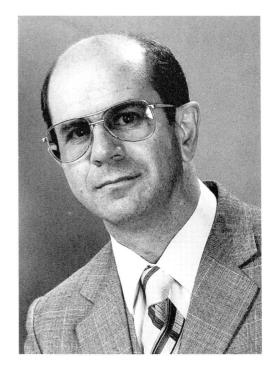

Professor Andries Kleynhans, head of the School of Chiropractic and Osteopathy at the Royal Melbourne Institute of Technology. Dr. Kleynhans is the principal of the first chiropractic college in the world to be fully accredited and funded by any government and the first chiropractor to be granted a full professorship in a multidisciplinary university.

Courtesy The Chance-Peters Archive, Wagga Wagga, New South Wales, Australia.

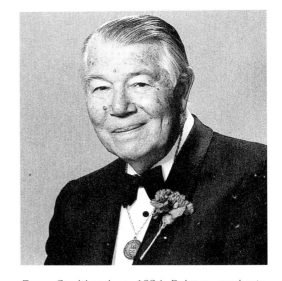

Ross Coulthard, a 1934 Palmer graduate, was the first Australian chiropractor to complete 50 years of service. He was also the first recipient of the Golden Anniversary Award of the Australian Chiropractors' Association and the Palmer College 50 year medallion.

Courtesy The Chance-Peters Archive, Wagga Wagga, New South Wales, Australia.

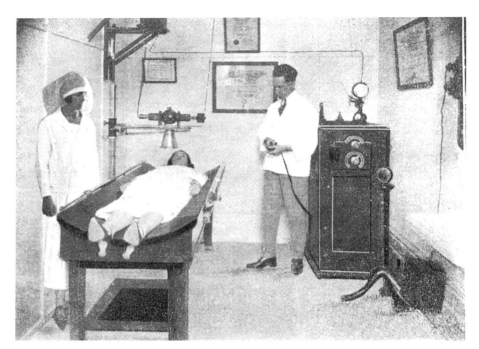

The McBeath and Yerkey spinograph laboratory, Adelaide, South Australia, circa 1928.

Courtesy Archives of the Association for the History of Chiropractic, Australia.

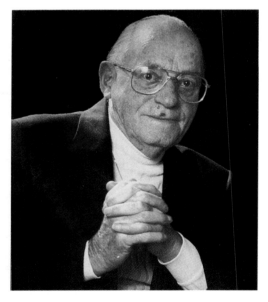

While interning at the B.J. Palmer Chiropractic Clinic in 1937, Felix Bauer developed the base posterior view to image the relationship of the atlas vertebra and the occipital condyles. Author of the textbook, X-ray Expertise from A to X, *he also invented radiographic density equalization filters and the bilateral compression band. He received the Daniel David Palmer Scientific Award in 1987.*

Courtesy The Chance-Peters Archive, Wagga Wagga, New South Wales.

1938 all Sydney-based foundation members of the ACA operated x-ray equipment in their practices.

The legal right of chiropractors to use x-ray was first established in Western Australia in 1945, in South Australia in 1949, and in New South Wales in 1956. From 1954 to 1959, various states passed legislation restricting the use of ionizing radiation and required persons other than registered medical practitioners to be licensed to use x-ray for diagnostic purposes. Most states included chiropractors among those eligible to be licensed; the exceptions were Tasmania, where in 1960 the district court ordered the Minister for Health to reverse his decision to refuse to license a chiropractor who had applied, and Queensland, where chiropractors were not licensed to use x-ray until 1970.

The right to use x-ray has been further enhanced by Australian chiropractors' impressive safety record over the past 25 years, achieved largely as a result of the pioneering work of Felix Bauer as chairman of the ACA's Council on Chiropractic Roentgenology. Bauer's filtration and gonad shielding systems, compression devices, exposure tables, and refined darkroom procedures have enabled chiropractors to produce high diagnostic quality with the lowest possible radiation dose.

Professional Registration

During the 1970s, the chiropractic profession came under the close scrutiny of several government inquiries. The Committee of Inquiry into Chiropractic, Osteopathy, Homoeopathy, and Naturopathy, also known as the Webb Committee, reported to the Australian Parliament in April 1977. This committee was the last to be appointed and its report exerted the widest influence on the chiropractic legislation that emerged over the next few years. All states except Western Australia, which had legislated during the previous decade, registered chiropractors and osteopaths under one law, and all states followed the British common law convention of providing for initial registration of practitioners without prescribed qualifications who were established before the law came into effect. By September 1985 there were registration laws in all Australian states and territories.

Insurance and Compensation Coverage

Chiropractic is included in state laws governing motor accident and worker's compensation as well as private health insurance schemes, but not under the federal government's Medicare system, which refunds 85% of the scheduled fee for approved medical procedures and public hospital charges.

Present Practitioners

There are now nearly 2000 chiropractors registered in Australia (about 1:10,000 population), with the greatest concentration in capital cities and larger provincial centers. Most of them are members of the Chiropractors' Association of Australia, formed in 1991 when the two largest national associations, the Australian Chiropractors' Association and the United Chiropractors Association of Australasia, merged.

NEW ZEALAND

Glenda Wiese

The New Zealand Chiropractors' Association was incorporated in 1920, and 40 years later the Chiropractors' Act was passed. In 1978 a petition to include chiropractic in social security and accident compensation plans led to a government commission of inquiry. Although the report recommended that in the public's interest chiropractic should be accepted as part of the health care system, chiropractic is still subject to medical referral.

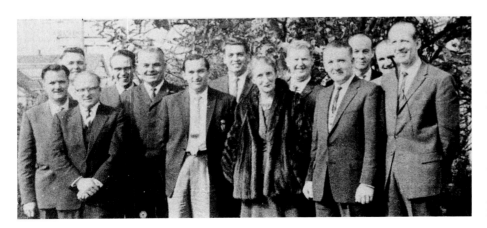

Members of the New Zealand Chiropractic Association at a meeting in 1962. They would influence the New Zealand government to appoint a three-member Commission in the 1970s, which resulted in Chiropractic in New Zealand, *one of the most exhaustive and detailed studies of the profession ever published.*

From *Chiropractic History,* June 1989.

483

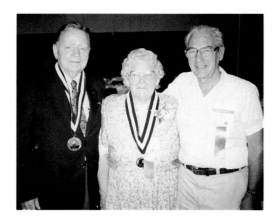

Robert Thompson (left) and his wife Hazel (center) practiced in Ethiopia during the 1950s as missionaries, sponsored in part by the Christian Chiropractor's Association.

Courtesy Christian Chiropractor's Association.

Similar to the introduction of chiropractic into Australia, it was a patient who brought chiropractic to New Zealand. Thomas Giles attended Dr. Robert Skerritt (a 1910 Palmer graduate) during July 1910 in Belfast, Ireland. According to the early dictum in chiropractic ("to practice and teach"), Giles must have learned a great deal. After his arrival in Dunedin, New Zealand, on December 29, 1910, he set up practice as a manipulator and soon established a forty-patient-per-day practice.

He realized from his talks with Robert Skerritt that he would need formal training and, through John Good, a student he had referred to the Palmer School in 1913, actively looked for someone to manage his practice while he would study at Palmer. John Good apparently asked James Firth, Dr. Alfred Hender, and probably others, but they all declined. Henry Otteholt of Wisconsin, who graduated March 30, 1914, decided to take up the offer and thus became the first formally qualified chiropractor to practice in Australasia if not in the Southern Hemisphere.

AFRICA

Although Africa is the second largest continent after Asia, covering almost 12,000,000 square miles, there are scarcely 200 chiropractors on the entire continent. Only South Africa and Zimbabwe have national chiropractic associations, and the profession is registered in both nations. Some of these practices are operated by Christian missionaries. The Congo has at least one chiropractor, Father Félix Pérel, from France, a National College graduate who is practicing in Brazzaville. Palmer school graduates Drs. Robert and Hazel Thompson practiced in Ethiopia during the 1950s with the aid of the Christian Chiropractors' Association. The Christian Chiropractors Association has also placed one chiropractor in Kenya, for a total of five chiropractors in that country.

Chiropractic has had a checkered career in South Africa since the early 1900s. Although chiropractic was not included in the 1928 Medical and Dental Act, chiropractors did manage to pass a chiropractors act in 1971, which would not allow for the registration of any new chiropractors. In 1982 chiropractic was included in the Associated Health Profes-

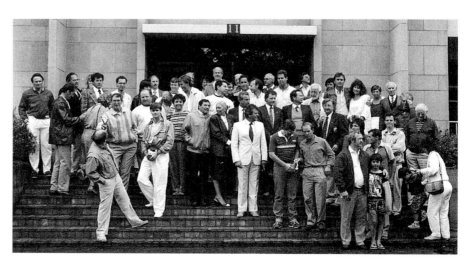

South African Chiropractors Association at the opening of the chiropractic clinic on the campus of Technikon Natal in 1993.

Courtesy G.B. Tasker, East London, South Africa.

sions Board, and in 1985 the Chiropractic Registers were reopened. An associated health professions program that includes chiropractic was established at the Technikon Natal in Durban, where the first class matriculated in 1989.

Chiropractic was introduced to the colony of Rhodesia, now Zimbabwe, in 1932 by Palmer School graduate, Dr. A. Scott. Although there were as many as 17 chiropractors in Rhodesia at one time, with the country's independence, that number has dwindled to five. Chiropractic is recognized in Zimbabwe and is governed by the Chiropractic Council.

CENTRAL AND SOUTH AMERICA

In general, the countries in Central and South America have a low ratio of chiropractors to population. Panama and Mexico are the only countries with chiropractic licensure. Although chiropractic is unrecognized in most countries, chiropractors practice, for the most part, unhampered.

Severe devaluation in these countries' currencies in relation to the U.S. dollar have made the cost of a chiropractic education in the United States prohibitive. Since there is no chiropractic college in a Latin American nation, the self-perpetuation of the profession is at risk.

Chiropractic in Brazil has a long and unusual history. Chiropractic was introduced by William Fipps in the 1920s. In 1945 a chiropractic course was offered by the Association of Biological Renovation and the University of Natural Healing Arts based in Denver, Colorado. The course was offered in Curitiba from 1958 through 1964, with 28 students receiving a chiropractic diploma. In 1972 chiropractic was declared illegal, causing most practitioners to leave the country or change professions. The one lone chiropractor remaining in 1985 was jailed for 8 days by the Board of Health. Since 1987 chiropractors have been authorized to practice under the supervision of a medical doctor or physiotherapist.

The first chiropractor in Mexico was Palmer school graduate Dr. Francisco Montano, who established a practice in 1922. Registration was initially provided for in 1955, but lasted only 1 year. The registry was again opened in 1975, then closed again in 1982, and reopened in 1988. Mexico City was the site of the Daniel David Palmer Spanish-American School of Chiropractic, which operated from 1927 until 1933.

THE MIDDLE EAST

Chiropractic has barely established itself in the Arab World, although in many nations bonesetters are commonplace. Jordan is the only country in the Eastern Mediterranean to recognize chiropractic. Chiropractic was introduced to Jordan in 1979 by CMCC graduate, Dr. Yousef Meshki, its sole chiropractor. Through his work at Jordan's prestigious King Hussein Medical Center, he was able to demonstrate the benefits of chiropractic to high-level government officials.

Chiropractors have been in Greece since the early part of the twentieth century, but have failed to receive legislation, repeatedly requested

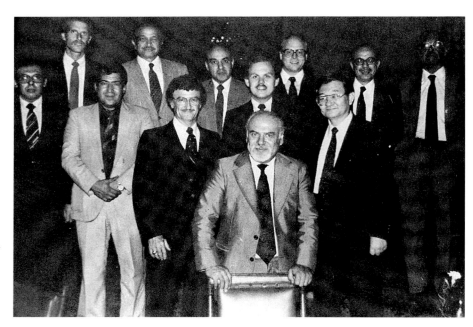

Officials of Palmer, Life, and Cleveland Colleges, and the ICA with officials in the Egyptian ministry and insurance sectors, circa 1982. In 1983 a double-blind study on the effects of chiropractic treatment of on-the-job injuries was completed, showing results favorable to chiropractic. From left are Osami Ghali, M.D., resident in orthopedic surgery; Gary Auerbach, ICA Egyptian Symposium chairman; Hassan Bilal, M.D., chief of information, Egypt's Ministry of Health; Moh Sayed, M.D., vice president of Egypt's General Health Insurance Authority; Virgil Strang, professor at Palmer College; Dr. Samir, chairman of Egyptian Health Insurance Organization; Carl Cleveland III, president of Cleveland College at Kansas City. Front center, Moh Talaat Ezzeldin, M.D., chief of orthopedic surgery at Manchiet El Bakry Ministry of Health Hospital; John Stump, member, World Health Development Committee and conference lecturer; Chung-Ha Suh, Ph.D., chiropractic researcher at the University of Colorado; Dr. Diaez, chief of Cairo clinics, National Health Insurance Organization; and Joseph Myers, chairman of research at Life College.

From PCC Alumni News, July 1982.

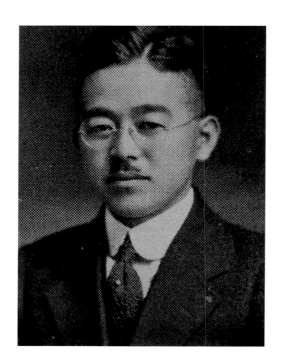

Hataya Kuzan, a 1923 Palmer graduate from Yokohama, Japan.

From The Pisiform, Palmer School of Chiropractic, 1923.

since the 1920s. Although much has been written about the use of manipulation by ancient Greek healers, after the decline of Greece, manipulative therapists, referred to as *practicos iatros,* or makeshift physicians, were not held in as high esteem. Because both employ manipulation, Greeks associate chiropractors with practicos iatros, to chiropractic's detriment.

Although Egypt does not have chiropractic legislation, government contacts have been made and research work has been done as a prelude to requesting legislation. In 1983 the ICA, in conjunction with three chiropractic colleges, completed a 3-week double-blind study on the effects of chiropractic treatment of on-the-job injuries. The results indicated chiropractic's greater effectiveness than drugs, bed rest, and sham manipulations. Impressed with the results of the trial, Dr. Medhad Alattar enrolled at Life Chiropractic College, becoming the first Egyptian to qualify in chiropractic.

When the Shah was deposed in Iran, many chiropractors left the country. The five who are left are allowed to practice with no medical hostility, as there is a shortage of medical doctors.

Israel has a 30-year history of chiropractic, beginning with Robert Small of Tel Aviv. Currently allowed to treat "defects of the body" under the medical practice act, chiroprators are attempting to obtain separate legislation. Because of the lax restrictions, many untrained manipulators are allowed to practice, with many trying to pass as chiropractors. Chiropractic is officially recognized by the Israeli Army. The Israel Chiropractic Society represents the estimated seventeen chiropractors in Israel today.

ASIA

Because there is a strong tradition of folk medicine that includes manipulation, there is confusion in Asia as to what constitutes chiropractic. There are thousands of folk healers in Korea claiming to practice chiropractic, but none appear to have any training in chiropractic per se. Life Chiropractic College established a program at Taegu University in November 1986 to try to remedy the problem.

Chiropractic was first introduced to Japan in 1918 by Palmer school graduate Saburo Kawaguchi, one of a dozen American-educated chiropractors practicing in Japan through the 1930s. Although more than 2000 practitioners claim to be chiropractors, only 50 hold internationally recognized chiropractic qualifications. In the 1980s several chiropractic organizations were started, as well as a dozen private chiropractic schools offering programs of 1 to 3 years. The Chiropractic Council of Japan was formed in 1992, and efforts are underway to form a coalition of all the chiropractic associations in Japan.

Chiropractic has been practiced in Hong Kong for over 50 years, following the arrival of the first chiropractors Dr. Frank J. and Ruth Molthen, in the 1930s. The Hong Kong Chiropractic Association was formed in 1968 and represents the colony's thirty-five chiropractors. The association's efforts to attain registration for chiropractic has resulted in hostility from the medical community, but the Chiropractors Registration Ordinance was finally gazetted in February 1993.

Although mainland China has no Western-style chiropractors, there exists a chiropractic division within the Chinese Herb Physicians' Association. Life College established a program at the Beijing Institute of Traditional Chinese Medicine in 1988.

Singapore has two chiropractors who have practiced since 1978. There is no chiropractic law, but Singapore's chiropractors are allowed to practice as long as they abide by the medical regulations concerning professional conduct. Singapore has approximatley 1000 traditional healers called *sensei,* who use manipulative techniques handed down from generation to generation.

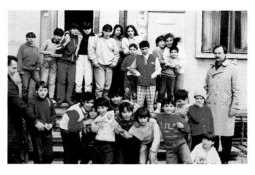

An ICA delegation was met by a group of excited children from the Casa de Copii Orphanage in 1992. Later that year a program was developed by the ICA whereby chiropractic students would be offered a preceptorship in Romania, giving them a chance to treat some of the thousands of orphans in that country.

From *The ICA Review,* March/April 1992.

EASTERN EUROPE AND RUSSIA

In Eastern Europe there is no distinction between medicine and chiropractic, and some chiropractic concepts have been incorporated into health care. Czechoslovakia has a strong manipulative faculty, with Dr. Karel Lewit the dominant figure. In Yugoslavia a chiropractic health center has been established at Dubrovnik, and a number of students have been sent to America to study chiropractic. In the former Soviet Union negotiations have been underway to bring a chiropractic program to Moscow.

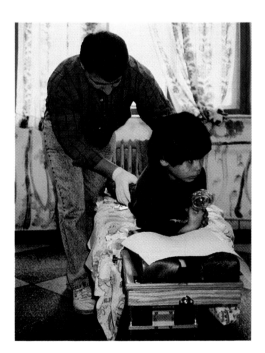

Gary Street, a member of the ICA delegation, adjusting a child in Romania in 1993.

Courtesy Gary Street, Olney, Illinois.

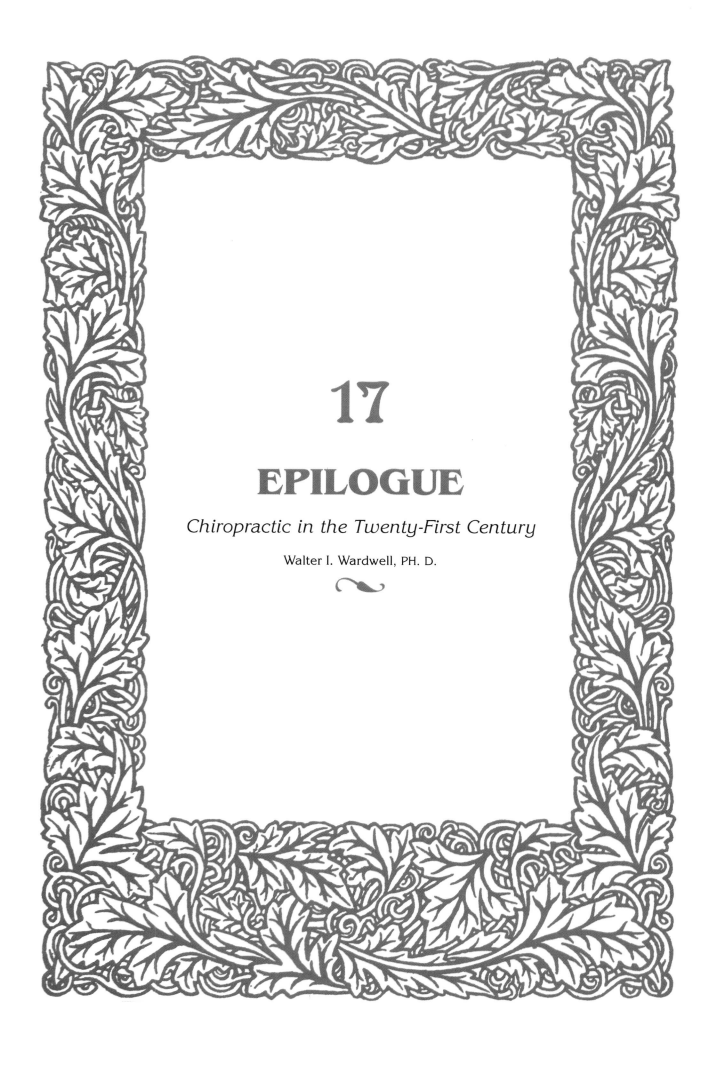

17

EPILOGUE

Chiropractic in the Twenty-First Century

Walter I. Wardwell, PH. D.

hiropractic survived its first century despite the concerted efforts of organized medicine to contain and then eliminate it. Why did it survive? And what is likely to happen to it in the future? Several prognosticators predicted its early demise. For example, in 1932 Stephen Rushmore wrote in the *New England Journal of Medicine:* "Chiropractic is going the way of all sects. . . . No medical sect has ever staged a comeback. . . . The hand of death is already visible." And in that same year a misinformed British barrister, Leonard Minty, wrote: "In most of the states of the union chiropractic has already died a natural death." Both were wrong. Chiropractic continued to grow.

In 1932, Louis Reed estimated that there were 16,000 chiropractors in the United States. By 1980 there were 25,000 and by 1990 over 45,000. Overseas, chiropractic is strongest in English-speaking countries and in northwestern Europe, France, Switzerland, and Italy. Estimates by the 1990 Bureau of Health Professions for the future are 52,500 by 2000, 60,600 by 2010, and 66,600 by 2020.

Chiropractors first achieved licensure in Kansas in 1913. Most states had licensed chiropractors by 1950 and all states by 1974. Chiropractic education became more comprehensive as the years passed, requiring by the late 1960s a minimum of 2 years of preprofessional college credits in the basic health sciences followed by a 4-year, 9-month curriculum

GROWTH IN CHIROPRACTORS

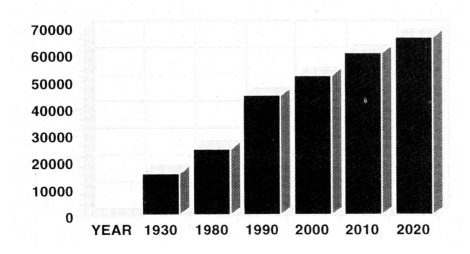

The growth in the number of chiropractors from 1930 to 1990 and projections of their numbers to 2020.

Courtesy Palmer College of Chiropractic Archives.

in a chiropractic college. Today, more than half of chiropractic students have a baccalaureate degree by the time they obtain their doctor of chiropractic (D.C.) degree. Maryland, North Carolina, and Florida have mandated a 4-year preprofessional requirement for all future licensure applicants. Most chiropractic colleges have been accredited by the Commission on Chiropractic Education (CCE) as well as by regional academic accrediting organizations. Most also offer students baccalaureate degrees in human biology or nutrition after appropriate course work.

Chiropractic practice has also greatly improved. Reimbursements of fees are paid by almost all third-party payers—Medicare, Medicaid, Workers' Compensation, and private insurance companies such as Blue Cross/Blue Shield. Chiropractors have served as mayors, as legislators, and as congressmen. One, Clinton A. Clauson, was elected governor of Maine. Many chiropractors have been elected or appointed to offices or committees for health planning or regulation. Chiropractors are now accepted in the best social circles if not in all medical circles. And they are on medical turf more and more as students attend rounds in medical or osteopathic hospitals and later obtain staff appointments, admit patients, and treat them there. If that is not yet true for all hospitals, it soon should be.

During the past decade public opinion surveys have found that the percentage of citizens treated by a chiropractor ranges from 30% in some states to about 50% in California and 58% in Oklahoma. About 90% of those visiting a chiropractor were satisfied with the result and, compared with visiting an M.D., were more satisfied with the amount of personal attention they received and the cost of their visit. In 1980 a randomized survey of 837 members of the American Chiropractic Association revealed that 49% of chiropractors had M.D.s as patients; a similar 1989 survey of 534 members found that 79% had received referrals of patients from M.D.s. In Toronto, Abdu Patel-Christopher reported in a 1990 survey that 62% of the 99 M.D.s she questioned had referred patients to chiropractors. By 1990 at least 60 medical or osteopathic hospitals and ambulatory surgical centers in the United States had appointed chiropractors on staff.

In 1988, *Job Related Almanac* rated chiropractic as tenth best of 250 jobs in the United States, while the student-oriented periodical *Moving Up* named chiropractic as one of the top professions for the 1990s; the fourth highest paying profession and eleventh highest paying career, exclusive of sports it ranked seventh.

CHIROPRACTIC'S UNIQUE IDENTITY

Why did chiropractic survive organized medicine's aggressive campaign to prevent *The Rise of Chiropractic,* which was the title of Chittenden Turner's 1931 book. A bit of history is required to answer this question. In 1895 when chiropractic was begun by Daniel David Palmer, medical education was in a sorry state. Abraham Flexner's famous 1910 report, *Medical Education in the United States and Canada,* led to the closing, merging, or upgrading of many inferior medical schools, so that by the 1920s there were fewer medical schools but they were much improved. However, physico-medicalist colleges lasted until 1911, eclectic colleges until 1939, and homeopathic colleges until the 1950s. During this period osteopathic colleges changed from teaching mainly Andrew Taylor Still's manipulative therapy to teaching a standard medical course. By 1929 accreditation requirements for osteopathic colleges mandated the inclusion of the medical pharmacopoeia and major surgery in the curriculum. By the 1960s, U.S. osteopaths (D.O.) were being accepted into mainstream medical residencies, sitting for specialty board examinations, being accepted onto hospital staffs, and being given commissions in the military. They were in effect becoming allopathic and surgical M.D.s, which they cannot do in any other country. Chiropractors, on the other hand, resisted pressures to follow in osteopathy's footsteps, and maintained their stance to become the largest nonmedical profession in the world.

Chiropractors were led initially by inspired charismatic leaders who were convinced that the old ways of medicine were wrong and that chiropractic was a new science that would cure nearly all diseases. They successfully recruited and trained students to go forth and teach the new therapy to others. After B.J. Palmer developed the Palmer School of Chiropractic into a flourishing enterprise, he united nearly all chiropractors in the Universal Chiropractors' Association, which struggled against the medical monopoly from 1906 to 1930 for separate licensure. He began holding annual Lyceums, homecomings of alumni, in 1906 so that chiropractors could affirm their unique identity and their determination to continue to practice and to defend chiropractic against its oppressors. B.J. maintained contact with the field through marketing millions of tracts, and bulletins and writing 26 books. The leaders of other chiropractic colleges followed suit.

Over 100 chiropractic colleges were established by the 1930s, of which a dozen have persevered to the present day; several new schools have been added since 1974. In 1934 the distinguished medical historian Henry Sigerist offered his judgment: "Chiropractic has held fast to its original faith and so far has resisted every temptation to make concessions, and thanks to this alone it is today the most powerful medical sect in America." One of the characteristics of chiropractic that kept members involved and active in its support was its division into straights and mixers. Every chiropractor could find another chiropractor with whom to ally and others to be against. Chiropractic has had a lively history.

CHIROPRACTIC'S FUTURE

What is chiropractic's future likely to be? No one can be sure what will be until it happens, but the possibilities are fairly easy to see. Since there is little likelihood that chiropractors will follow the path of osteopaths toward fusion with medicine or will simply disappear, there are three conceivable outcomes for chiropractors: (1) they could remain as they are today, marginally accepted by organized medicine and struggling against medical opposition in legislatures and the marketplace; (2) they could become *ancillary* to M.D.s, accepting patients only when an M.D. or D.O. refers them, something which even physical therapists have already succeeded in eliminating in more than 30 states; or (3) they could become another *limited medical profession* like dentistry, podiatry, optometry, psychology, speech therapy, and audiology. These independent professions all see patients without medical referral but limit their practices in two ways—in the parts of the human body they treat, and in the restricted range of techniques, instruments, or therapies they use from among all those available to M.D.s.

Although many chiropractors believe that chiropractic is unlimited in the range of benefits it can provide, they nevertheless do not administer controlled drugs or major surgery. And chiropractors continue to differ from other limited medical professions in that they reject some of medicine's principal theories of illness and treatment. Chiropractors place greater emphasis on lifestyle; natural living; nutrition; avoiding environmental pollutants; homeostasis or the healing power of nature (vix medicatrix naturae), which is the body's tendency to heal itself; and the greater importance of a healthy host. This view contrasts with the usual medical view of health care, which focuses on germs and bacteria in maintaining health and preventing illness. Furthermore, instead of treating the symptoms of disease, chiropractors treat the *causes* of disease, among which they consider vertebral impairment of the neuromusculoskeletal system the most important.

What are the pressures pushing chiropractic toward becoming a limited medical profession? Chiropractors have always offered independent access to patients. And they have reduced the range of illnesses from those they treated in chiropractic's earliest days, not just to musculoskeletal complaints but to the closely related illnesses chiropractic is also known to help, such as headaches, hypertension, asthma, certain gastrointestinal conditions, and so on. It is probably unfortunate that chiropractic colleges, clinical practice, and third-party reimbursement now focus mostly on musculoskeletal conditions. That could change if additional research on treatment outcomes scientifically demonstrates chiropractic's benefits for non-musculoskeletal conditions. In 1989 Daniel Cherkin and medical researchers found that the proportion of chiroprac-

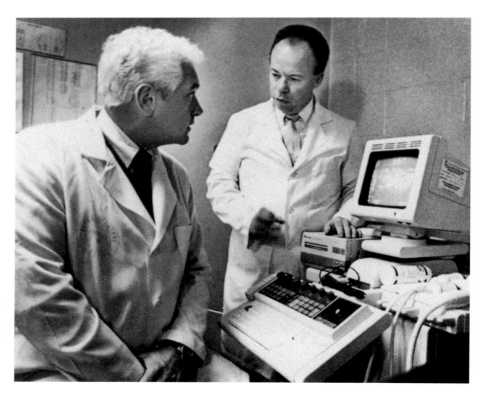

In the 1980s, some hospitals slowly began allowing chiropractors to have staff privileges. Shown here are chiropractor R. James Gregg (right) *and surgeon Earle W. Spohn, 1990.*

From *The Digest of Chiropractic Economics*, January/February, 1991.

tic patients seen with non-musculoskeletal problems in Washington state decreased from 21% in 1979 to 13% in 1985 and concluded, "If the trend continues, . . . physicians and chiropractors may reach a point of peaceful coexistence."

Although not all chiropractors would relish seeing chiropractic become a limited medical profession, that seems to be what is most likely to happen in the long run. When chiropractors are accepted on hospital staffs, they tend to follow the pattern already established for dentists and podiatrists; that is, they coadmit with either an M.D. or D.O., who becomes responsible for medical management of the patient. If a chiropractor performs manipulation under anesthesia (MUA), either an M.D. or D.O. must administer the anesthesia. Although the chiropractor can perform chiropractic adjustments and order diets, diagnostic tests, and physical therapy, a chiropractor is limited in the range of ministrations that can either be done or ordered. Although many chiropractors will not want to be appointed to a hospital staff, those chiropractors who gain hospital privileges and work within the mainstream medical model can be expected to eventually expand the opportunities available to the profession.

The pressures pushing chiropractic toward becoming a limited medical profession can be summarized as follows:

1. *Interdisciplinary research,* which will reduce the knowledge gap separating medicine and chiropractic and will also achieve one of the goals of the 1976 Wilk antitrust suit—"a common lexicon"— which was intended to promote interprofessional scientific exchanges.
2. *Standardized curriculum,* a current strong trend in the colleges that are incorporating both improved skills in differential diagnosis and a hospital clinical experience.
3. *Scope of chiropractic practice,* the pressures from third-party payers for agreement within the profession on the proper scope of chiropractic practice.
4. *Standards of care,* being established by concerted efforts within the profession, which should help unify the profession concerning its scope of practice.
5. *National health care system,* the political pressures for chiropractic to fit into the national health care system and the plans for its reorganization.
6. *Enlightened chiropractic leadership,* the continuing efforts by a more sophisticated leadership aware of these pressures and trends and able to make better decisions regarding chiropractic's future.

David Chapman-Smith, secretary of the World Federation of Chiropractic, who was the attorney who represented chiropractors in the 1979 *Chiropractic in New Zealand* study, listed the following three requirements for chiropractors to become fully successful in the next 10 to 20 years:

1. Continued leadership in skilled manipulative care for neuromusculoskeletal disorders.
2. Become a part of the accepted basic health care team, cooperating with medicine rather than acting as an alternative and adversary.
3. Acceptance of a model similar to dentistry and optometry, functioning as a major profession, with responsibility for primary care, diagnostic rights and duties, but with acknowledged limitations in scope.

If organized medicine should decide that a limited medical status is appropriate for chiropractors, it could help bring it about in the following three important ways:

1. Organized medicine could collaborate more with chiropractors in research on all types of illnesses that chiropractors habitually treat, not just on the musculoskeletal and biomechanical ones. If carefully controlled research is not done on these diseases, it will never be known how effective chiropractic is in treating them.

2. Organized medicine could help improve chiropractic education by allowing more students to attend hospital rounds, especially with medical students, and graduate chiropractors to attend workshops in various specialties such as diagnostic imaging, neurology, internal disorders, and sports medicine.

3. Organized medicine's ultimate goal should be full professional collaboration in patient treatment: consultations, referrals, and shared management both in and out of hospitals.

For the American Medical Association to admit a rival group of practitioners into its sacred medical fold would be a supreme act of good judgment, not an unselfish but a wise one. In the long run a decision for full professional cooperation would be beneficial for all concerned, especially for patients.

If organized medicine should decide to change its policies and accept chiropractors as professional equals, that would improve M.D.s relations with patients who have conditions that medicine and surgery do not handle well. It would remove the documented frustration many M.D.s feel when treating back problems, and it might also prevent much unneeded back surgery. M.D.s would receive more referrals and consultation requests from chiropractors willing to collaborate and share responsibility for patient care. Chronic pain clinics, for example, would seem to be an especially promising area for future collaboration. In general, patient care would improve and be less costly because the best of both chiropractic and medicine would be readily available to every patient. Hence the goal of all health professions could be achieved: optimum care for everyone.

The overall result of the history of chiropractic's enforced isolation and of the barriers between chiropractic and medicine was to embed chiropractic in our legal, economic, political, and social institutions as a separate system of healing. Now that the barriers to interprofessional communication and cooperation have been reduced, it remains to be seen what the effect of future changes in the health care system will be on chiropractic. Although many chiropractors have expressed fear that medicine will take over chiropractic once it discovers how effective it is, it seems unlikely that general medical practitioners, orthopedists, neurologists, or physiatrists will adopt spinal manipulation into their practices to an extent great enough to become truly skilled manipulators.

The best conclusions therefore seem to be that chiropractors' roles in the health care system will continue to change, that they will not remain as marginalized as they have been for a century, that they will not follow osteopaths into the medical mainstream, and that they will most likely evolve into a limited medical profession comparable with dentists, podiatrists, optometrists, and psychologists. When the United States adopts a national health care system, the current social realities will continue to govern the position of chiropractors in it.

Thus the future of chiropractic depends on what four different groups do:

1. *The government,* which holds ultimate responsibility for the national health care system;

2. *Organized medicine,* which has yet to embrace chiropractic and chiropractors;
3. *Chiropractors* themselves, who need to learn better how to unite in order to speak politically with one voice; and
4. *The public, especially chiropractic patients,* who hold the ultimate keys in our democratic political system.

As chiropractors interact more with M.D.s and D.O.s and become familiar with hospital treatment through training as students, coadmitting and consulting on seriously ill patients, they may become more medicalized in their thinking and in their practices. But they will also learn to appreciate what an M.D. can and cannot do for such patients. Similarly, M.D.s will learn to appreciate more than they do now what chiropractors can and cannot do to alleviate pain, achieve cures, and rehabilitate patients suffering from long-standing conditions or handicaps. In this way both medical and chiropractic progress will occur.

BIBLIOGRAPHY

A. Earl Homewood: doing honor to a pioneer, *Chiropractic History* 1(1):4, 1981.

Baer HA: Divergence and convergence in two systems of manual medicine: osteopathy and chiropractic in the United States, *Medical Anthropology Quarterly (New Series)* 1:176-193, 1989.

Baer HA: The divergent evolution of osteopathy in America and Britain. In Roth JA, ed: *Research in the Sociology of Health Care,* vol 5, Greenwich, Conn, 1987, JAI Press.

Baker WJ: A clinical transformation in chiropractic: the research of Dr. Fred Illi, *Chiropractic History* 5(1):59-62, 1985.

Baker WJ: A clinical transformation in chiropractic: the research of Dr. Fred Illi, *Chiropractic History* 5(1):59-62, 1985.

Baltzell LB: *Firth's Technique Notes,* Indianapolis, Ind, 1967, Lincoln College of Chiropractic.

Bartol KM: Algorithm for the categorization of chiropractic technique procedures, *Chiropractic Technique* 4(1):8-14, 1992.

Beideman RP: Seeking the rational alternative: the National College of Chiropractic from 1906 to 1982, *Chiropractic History* 3(1):16-22, 1983.

Bell DL: Blacks in chiropractic—a portrait in history, Speech presented at 16 Institute Consortium, Roanoke, Va, Feb 27, 1993.

Bergmann TF, Peterson DH, Lawrence DJ: *Chiropractic Technique: Principles and Procedures,* New York, 1993, Churchill Livingstone.

Blackstone EA: The AMA and the osteopaths: a study of the power of organized medicine, *Anti-Trust Bulletin* 22:405-440, 1977.

Bolton SP: Women in Chiropractic, *Journal of the Australian Chiropractors Association* 20(2):53-55, 1990.

Brennan MJ: *Demographic and Professional Characteristics of ACA Membership: Annual Survey and Statistical Study,* Arlington, Va, 1989, American Chiropractic Association.

Brennan MJ: *Opinion Survey II: Advertising, Education, Referrals, Insurance Equality, and Other,* Des Moines, Iowa, 1980, American Chiropractic Association.

Brinkman B: *The professional female chiropractor: a clinic research paper,* St Louis, 1972, Logan College of Chiropractic.

Broome RT: The influence of Henri Gillet on the chiropractic profession, *European Journal of Chiropractic* Sept 1989, p 37.

Bureau of Health Professions: *Seventh Report to the President and Congress on the Status of Health Personnel in the United States,* Washington, DC, 1990, Department of Health and Human Services.

Canterbury R, Krakos G: Thirteen years after Roentgen: the origins of chiropractic radiology, *Chiropractic History* 6(1):24-29, 1986.

Carver W: *Carver's Chiropractic Analysis,* ed 3, vol 1, Oklahoma City, Okla, 1921, Seneca Color Press.

Carver W: *Carver's Chiropractic Analysis,* vol 2, East Aurora, NY, 1922, Roycrofters.

Chapman-Smith D: Introduction and review of the 1990 Concensus Conference, *Chiropractic Technique* 4(1):3-4, 1992.

Chapman-Smith D: Perspectives on the future of chiropractic, *California Chiropractic Association Journal* 16(2):31, 49-50, 1991.

Cherkin DC, McCornack F, Berg AO: Family physicians' views of chiropractors: hostile or hospitable? *American Journal of Public Health* 79:636-637, 1989.

Clarence WW, D.C., Ph.D.: "a pioneer chiropractor who cut a path for the profession . . . toward the sciences," *Chiropractic History* 7(1):45, 1987.

Cleveland CS Jr: Recording the 80-year history of one family, *Chiropractic History* 8(1):4, 1988.

Cohen JH, Schneider M: Receptor-tonus technique: an overview. *Chiropractic Technique* 2:13, 1990.

Cox J: Personal correspondence, Fort Wayne, Ind, 1993.

Cox JM: *Low Back Pain: Mechanism, Diagnosis, Treatment,* Baltimore, 1985, Williams & Wilkins.

C.S. Cleveland, 1896-1982, *Chiropractic History* 2(1):4, 1982.

Dr. Willard Carver, 1966-1943, tribute by Oklahoma State Board of Chiropractic Examiners, *Journal of the National Chiropractic Association* Feb 1944, p 4.

Dye AA: *The Evolution of Chiropractic: Its discovery and Development,* Philadelphia, 1939, AA Dye.

Dzaman F, ed: *Who's Who in Chiropractic International, 1976-1978,* Littleton, Colo, 1977, Who's Who in Chiropractic International Publishing.

Dzaman F, ed: *Who's Who in Chiropractic International,* ed 2, Littleton, Colo, 1980, Who's Who in Chiropractic International Publishing.

Dzaman F, ed: *Who's Who in Chiropractic International,* Littleton, Colo, 1976, Who's Who in Chiropractic International Publishing.

Editor: Report of inspections of schools of chiropractic and naturopathy in the United States, *Journal of the American Medical Association* 90:1733-1738, 1928.

Eilbert L, Spector B: The Moire contourographic analysis controversy: a question of validity in present-day clinical practice, *Journal of Manipulative & Physiological Therapeutics* 2(2):85, 1979.

Ernest G. Napolitano, 1911-1985, *Chiropractic History* 5(1):5, 1985.

Etzel SI et al: Graduate medical education in the United States, *Journal of the American Medical Association* 262:1029-1037, 1990.

Fay LE: 1986 Lee-Homewood Award, John B. Wolfe, *Chiropractic History* 6(1):84-86, 1986.

Fay LE: Tribute to Joseph Janse, D.C., Sc.D., *Chiropractic History* 3(1):80-82, 1983.

Fay LE: Tribute to William N. Coggins, D.C., LL.D., *Chiropractic History* 7(1):42-42, 1987.

Faye LJ: *The Subluxation Complex, Lecture Notes.* Huntington Beach, Calif, 1986, Motion Palpation Institute.

Ferguson A, Wiese G: How many chiropractic schools? An analysis of institutions that offered the D.C. degree, *Chiropractic History* 8(1):26-31, 1988.

Ferguson AC: Mabel Heath Palmer—out of the myths, *PCC Research Forum* 1(2):54-56, 1985.

Ferguson AC: "The sweetheart of the PSC"—Mabel Heath Palmer: the early years, *Chiropractic History* 4(1):24-27, 1984.

Fishbein M: *Morris Fishbein, M.D.: an Autobiography,* Garden City, NY, 1969, Doubleday & Company.

Fishbein M: *The Medical Follies: An Analysis of the Foibles of Some Healing Cults Including Osteopathy, Homeopathy, Chiropractic and the Electronic Reactions of Abrams, with Essays on the Antivivisectionists, Health Legislation, Physical Culture, Birth Control and Rejuvenation,* New York, 1925, Boni & Liveright.

Flexner A: *Medical Education in the United States and Canada: a Report of the Carnegie Foundation for the Advancement of Teaching,* Washington, DC, 1910, 1972, Science and Health Publications.

Forester AL: *Principles and Practice of Chiropractic,* ed 3, Chicago, 1923, National Publishing Association.

Forester AL: *Principles and Practice of Spinal Adjustment: for the Use of Students and Practitioners,* Chicago, 1915, National School of Chiropractic.

Fosse M: Dr. Henri Gillet, 1907-1989, *European Journal of Chiropractic* Dec 1989, p 37.

Free RV: Spinal analysis utilizing Moire topography, *Digest of Chiropractic Economics* 17(4):26, 1975.

Gatterman MI: *Chiropractic Management of Spine Related Disorders,* Baltimore, 1990, Williams & Wilkins.

Gatterman MI: Indications for spinal manipulation in the treatment of back pain, *ACA Journal of Chiropractic* 19:51, 1982.

Gatterman MI: WA Budden: the transition through proprietary education, 1924-1954, *Chiropractic History* 2(1):20-25, 1982.

Gatterman MI, Hansen D: Development of chiropractic nomenclature through consensus, *Journal of Manipulative & Physiological Therapeutics* 1993 (in press).

Gibbons RW: Assessing the oracle at the fountain head: B.J. Palmer and his times, 1902-1961, *Chiropractic History* 7(1):8-14, 1987.

Gibbons RW: Chiropractic's Abraham Flexner: the lonely journey of John J. Nugent, *Chiropractic History* 5(1):44-51, 1985.

Gibbons RW: Chiropractors as interns, residents and staff: hospital experience 1910-1960, *Chiropractic History* 3:50-57, 1983.

Gibbons RW: The evolution of chiropractic: medical and social protest in America. In Haldeman S, ed: *Modern Developments in the Principles and Practices of Chiropractic,* New York, 1980, Appleton-Century-Crofts.

Gibbons RW: Forgotten parameters of general practice, *Chiropractic History,* 2:22-34, 1982.

Gibbons RW: Francis Kohlar and chromotherapy, *Chiropractic History* 10:1, 10-11, 1991.

Gibbons RW: Joy Loban and Andrew P. Davis: itinerant healers and "schoolmen," 1910-1923, *Chiropractic History* 11(1):22-28, 1991.

Gibbons RW: Medical and social protest as a part of hidden American history. In Haldeman S, ed: *Principles and Practice of Chiropractic,* Norwalk, Conn, 1980, Appleton & Lange, pp 15-28.

Gibbons RW: Physician-chiropractors: medical presence in the evolution of chiropractic, *Bulletin of the History of Medicine* 55(2):233-245, 1981.

Gibbons RW: Rise of the chiropractic educational establishment. In Dzaman F, ed: *Who's Who in Chiropractic International, 1976-1978,* Littleton, Colo, 1977, Who's Who in Chiropractic International Publishing.

Gibbons RW: Solon Massey Langworthy: keeper of the flame during the "lost years" of chiropractic, *Chiropractic History* 1(1):15-21, 1981.

Gibbons RW: Vision to action: a history of ICA, the first 60 years, *ICA Review* 42(2):33-64, 1986.

Gielow V: Daniel David Palmer: rediscovering the frontier years, 1845-1887, *Chiropractic History* 1:10-13, 1981.

Gielow V: *Old Dad Chiro,* Davenport, Iowa, 1981, Bawden Bros.

Gillett H: The anatomy and physiology of spinal fixations, *Journal of the National Chiropractic Association* 33:22 1963.

Gittleman R: A Chiropractic approach to biomechanical disorders of the lumbar spine and pelvis. In Haldeman S, ed: *Modern Developments in the Principles and Practice of Chiropractic,* New York, 1980, Appleton-Century-Crofts.

Gittleman R, Fligg B. Diversified technique. In Haldeman S, ed: *Principles and Practice of Chiropractic,* ed 2, Norwalk, Conn, 1992, Appleton and Lange.

Gregory AA: *Spinal Treatment,* Oklahoma City, Okla, 1912, Palmer School of Chiropractic.

Grevitz N: *The D.O.s: Osteopathic Medicine in America,* Baltimore, Md, 1982, Johns Hopkins University Press.

Grice A: A biomechanical approach to cervical and dorsal adjusting. In Haldeman S, ed: *Modern Developments in the Principles and Practice of Chiropractic,* New York, 1980, Appleton-Century-Crofts.

The Griffin Files, *Chiropractic History* 10(1):10, 1990.

Griffin LK: Merger almost: ICA unity efforts and formation of the American Chiropractic Association, *Chiropractic History* 8(2):18-22, 1988.

Gromala T: "Bees in his bonnet": D.D. Palmer's students and their early impact, *Chiropractic History* 6:57, 1986.

Gromala T: Women in chiropractic: exploring a tradition of equity in healing, *Chiropractic History* 3:59-63, 1983.

Grostic JD: The origins of the Grostic Procedure, *International Review of Chiropractic* 32(2):33, 1978.

Haldeman S: Almeda Haldeman, Canada's first chiropractor: pioneering the prairie provinces, 1907-1917, *Chiropractic History* 3:65-67, 1983.

Haldeman S: *Principles and practice of chiropractic,* ed 2, Norwalk, Conn, 1992, Appleton & Lange.

Haldeman S, Chapman-Smith D, Peterson DM: *Guidelines for Chiropractic Quality Assurance and Practice Parameters: Proceedings of the Mercy Center Consensus Conference,* Gaithersburg, Md, 1993, Aspen Publishers.

Hansen D: Searching for the common authority in validation and standardization of chiropractic methods, *Chiropractic Technique* 2(3):72-74, 1990.

Harrison DD: Personal correspondence, Alabama, 1993.

Himes HM et al: *Segmental Neuropathy,* Toronto, 1966, Canadian Memorial Chiropractic College.

Chiropractic in New Zealand: Report of the Commission of Inquiry, New Zealand, 1979, PD Hasselberg.

Janse JJ, Houser RH, Wells BF: *Chiropractic Principles and Technic,* Chicago, 1947, National College of Chiropractic.

Jobs Related Almanac, Chicago, 1988, American References.

Joseph Janse, D.C., 1909-1985: academic integrity, a sense of history, *Chiropractic History* 6(1):5, 1986.

Kaminski M et al: A model for the evaluation of chiropractic methods, *Journal of Manipulative & Physiological Therapeutics* 10(2):61-64, 1987.

Keating JC: Clause O. Watkins: pioneer advocate for clinical scientific chiropractic, *Chiropractic History* 7(2):10-15, 1987.

Keating JC: C.O. Watkins, D.C., F.I.C.C., Doctor of Humanities, *Journal of the Canadian Chiropractic Association* 32(4):199-202, 1992.

Keating JC: Paul Smallie, D.C., H.C.D., a man of letters, *Chiropractic History* 12(2):44-48, 1992.

Keating JC, Brown RA, Smallie P: T.F. Ratledge, the missionary of straight chiropractic in California, *Chiropractic History* 11(2):26-38, 1991.

Keating JC, Cleveland CS: Sylva L. Ashworth, D.C., the "Grand Old Lady of Chiropractic," *Chiropractic History* 12(2):14-23, 1992.

Keating JC, Rehm WS: The origins and early history of the National Chiropractic Association, *Journal of the Canadian Chiropractic Association* 37(1):27-51, 1993.

Kightliner C: Natural law, *Bulletin of the American Chiropractic Association* 1:9-10, 1928.

Kimmell EH: Electro-analytical instrumentation, *ACA Journal of Chiropractic* 3(6):11, 1966.

Kyneur JS, Bolton SP: Chiropractic instrumentation: an update for the 90's, *Chiropractic Journal of Australia* Sept 1991, pp 82-94.

Kyneur JS, Bolton SP: Lost technology: the rise and fall of chiropractic instrumentation, *Chiropractic History* 12(1):31-35, 1992.

Lake TT: *Treatment by Neuropathy and The Encyclopedia of Physical and Manipulative Therapeutics,* Philadelphia, 1946, TT Lake.

Lee HK: Albert Earl Homewood, *Chiropractic History* 2(1):66-68, 1982.

Loban JM: *Technic and Practice of Chiropractic,* ed 3, Pittsburgh, 1922, Loban Publishing.

Logan College of Chiropractic: *The Tower,* Fall 1992.

Lombardo DM: William H. Werner and the American Bureau of Chiropractic: organizing a lay constituency, *Chiropractic History* 10(1):24-29, 1990.

Maynard JE: *Healing Hands: The Story of the Palmer Family Discovers and Developers of Chiropractic,* Freeport Long Island, NY, 1959, Jonorm.

Mertz M: *Fifty Years of Chiropractic in Kansas,* 1965.

Minty M: *The Legal and Ethical Aspects of Medical Quackery,* London, 1932, William Heinemann.

Mom & Pop chiropractic schools in Kansas, *Chiropractic History* 12(1):12, 1992.

Moore JS: "The Great Backward State": the 50-year struggle in New York, 1913-1963, *Chiropractic History* 12(1):14-21, 1992.

Moore JS: *Chiropractic in America: the History of a Medical Alternative,* Baltimore, 1993, Johns Hopkins University Press.

Moving Up, Burbank, Calif, 1988, Communications, Inc.

Murphy EJ: U.S. Congress gives chiropractic full recognition in new draft act, *Journal of the National Chiropractic Association* 21(4):18, 1951.

Naef JP: Obituary: Frederic WH Illi, *European Journal of Chiropractic* 32(3): 1984.

National School of Chiropractic: *Chiropractic: the Twentieth Century Profession for Women,* Chicago, 1918, National School of Chiropractic.

Nimmo RL: Receptors, effectors and tonus . . .an approach, *Journal of the National Chiropractic Association* 27:21, 1957.

Outstanding women in Chiropractic, *Today's Chiropractic* Oct/Nov 1973, pp 12-32.

Palmer BJ: *An Exposition of Old Moves,* Davenport, Iowa, 1911-1916, Palmer School of Chiropractic.

Palmer College of Chiropractic Alumni News, Winter 1993.

Palmer DD: *The Palmers: Memoirs of David D. Palmer,* Davenport, Iowa, 1976, Bawden Brothers.

Palmer DD: *The Science, Art and Philosophy of Chiropractic,* Portland, Ore, 1910, Portland Printing House.

Palmer DD: *Three Generations: A Brief History of Chiropractic,* Davenport, Iowa, 1967, Palmer College of Chiropractic.

Palmer School of Chiropractic: *Chiropractic for Women and What Women Chiropractors Say,* Davenport, Iowa, 1917, Palmer School of Chiropractic.

Palmer School of Chiropractic: *Chiropractic for Women,* Davenport, Iowa, 1918, Palmer School of Chiropractic.

Parrott E: Interview, Mar 2, 1993.

The passing of Tom Morris, *The Chiropractor* Sept 1928.

Patel-Christopher A: *Family Physicians and Chiropractors: A Need for Better Communication and Cooperation,* Unpublished thesis, Toronto, Ont, 1990, University of Toronto.

Peters RE, Chance-Peters MA: Milestones in spinography: an Australian perspective, *Chiropractic Journal of Australia* Mar 1993, pp 15-28.

Plaugher G: *Textbook of Clinical Chiropractic: A Specific Biomechanical Approach,* Baltimore, Md, 1993, Williams & Wilkins.

Port Perry revisited, *Chiropractic History* 5:42-43, 1985.

Quigley WH: Early days at Palmer: Lyceums, *Dynamic Chiropractic* 7(1):15-16, 1989.

Ransom JF: Origins of chiropractic physiological therapeutics: Howard, Forester and Schulze, *Chiropractic History* 4(1):46-52, 1984.

Reed L: Chiropractic. In Committee on the Costs of Medical Care: *The Healing Cults,* Pub No 16, Chicago, 1932, University of Chicago Press.

Reed L: *The Healing Cults: a Study of Sectarian Medical Practice: Its Extent, Causes and Control,* Chicago, 1932, University of Chicago Press.

Rehm WS: " . . .of achievements and contributions of a legendary chiropractic name," 1988 Lee-Homewood Award to Dan C. Spears, D.C., *Chiropractic History* 8(1):42-52, 1989.

Rehm WS: Honoring the living pioneer: the Lee-Homewood chiropractic heritage award, 1981-1990, *Journal of Chiropractic* 28(4):29-35, 1991.

Rehm WS: Legally defensible: 1907, chiropractic in the courtroom, *Chiropractic History* 6(1):50-55, 1985.

Rehm WS: Tribute to a living pioneer: Dr. Lyndon Edmund Lee, *Chiropractic History* 1(1):45-50, 1981.

Rehm WS: Who was who in chiropractic: a necrology. In Dzaman F, ed: *Who's Who in Chiropractic International,* ed 2, Littleton, Colo, 1980, Who's Who in Chiropractic International Publishing, pp 265-335.

Reinert OC: Merging with honor: a history of the Missouri Chiropractic College, *Chiropractic History* 12(2):38-42, 1982.

Rex E: *The Lengthening Shadow,* Denver, Colo, 1962, Golden Bell Press.

Rhodes W: *The Official History of Chiropractic in Texas,* Austin, Tex, 1978, Texas Chiropractic Association.

Robinson KC: *The Chiropractic Methods of Dr. Willard Carver,* Greenwich, Conn, 1946, KC Robinson.

Rolf IP: *Rolfing,* Santa Monica, Calif, 1977, Dennis-Landman Publishers.

Rosenthai MJ: Structural approach to chiropractic: from Willard Carver to present practice, *Chiropractic History* 1(1):25-28, 1981.

Ross College of Chiropractic: *The Profession for Women,* Fort Wayne, Ind, 1918, Ross College of Chiropractic.

Rothstein W: *American Physicians in the Nineteenth Century: From Sects to Science,* Baltimore, Md, 1972, Johns Hopkins University Press.

Rubens D: The legitimization of chiropractic, *Chiropractic History* 6:17-25, 1987.

Rushmore S: The bill to register chiropractors, *New England Journal of Medicine* 206:614-615, 1932.

Sigerist HE: *American Medicine,* New York, 1934, Norton.

Smith O, Langworthy S, Paxon M: *Modernized Chiropractic,* vol II, Cedar Rapids, Iowa, 1906, Laurence Press.

Spears L, Spears D: Spears painless system of adjustment. In Kfoury PW, ed: *Catalog of Chiropractic Techniques,* St Louis, 1977, Logan College of Chiropractic.

Starr P: *The Social Transformation of American Medicine,* New York, 1982, Basic Books.

States AZ: *Spinal and Pelvic Techniques,* Lombard, Ill, 1967, National College of Chiropractic.

Stowell CC: Lincoln College and the "big four": a chiropractic protest, 1926-1962, *Chiropractic History* 3(1):74-78, 1983.

Sweat R: Personal correspondence, Marietta, Ga, 1993.

Thompson JC: Thompson terminal point technique. In Kfoury PW, ed: *Catalog of Chiropractic Techniques,* St Louis, 1977, Logan College of Chiropractic.

Travell JG, Simons DG: *Myofascial Pain and Dysfunction: the Trigger Point Manual,* Baltimore, Md, 1983, Williams & Wilkins.

Trever W: *In the Public Interest,* Los Angeles, 1972, Scripture Unlimited.

Triano J: The use of instrumentation and laboratory examination procedures by the chiropractor. In Haldeman S, ed: *Modern Developments in the Principles and Practices of Chiropractic,* New York, 1980, Appleton-Century-Crofts.

A tribute to Thure C. Peterson, *Journal of the American Chiropractic Association* Jan 1971, p 47.

Turbulent (& tranquil) thirties, *Chiropractic History* 10(2):33, 1990.

Turner C: *The Rise of Chiropractic,* Los Angeles, 1931, Powell Publishing.

Wardwell WI: *Chiropractic: History and Evolution of a New Profession,* St Louis, 1993, Mosby.

Wardwell WI: Tribute to Clarence W. Weiant, *Chiropractic History* 4(1):62-65, 1984.

Wells D: From workbench to high tech: the evolution of the adjusting table, *Chiropractic History* 7:2, 35-39, 1987.

Wiese G: Beyond the "Jim Crow" experience: Blacks in chiropractic education (in press).

Wiese G, Ferguson A: How many schools? *Chiropractic History,* 7:2, 1988.

Wilk CA et al vs AMA et al. Complaint #76C3777 filed Oct 12, 1976 in the United States District Court for the Northern District of Illinois, Eastern Division.

Witnesses in Davenport: was Brady and Third Chiropractic's "Dealey Plaza" in August 1913? *Chiropractic History* 12(2):10, 1992.

Vision to action: a history of ICA, the first 60 years, *ICA Review* 42(suppl):33-64, 1986.

Yesterday's man led a varied professional life, *Chiropractic History* 10(1):44, 1990.

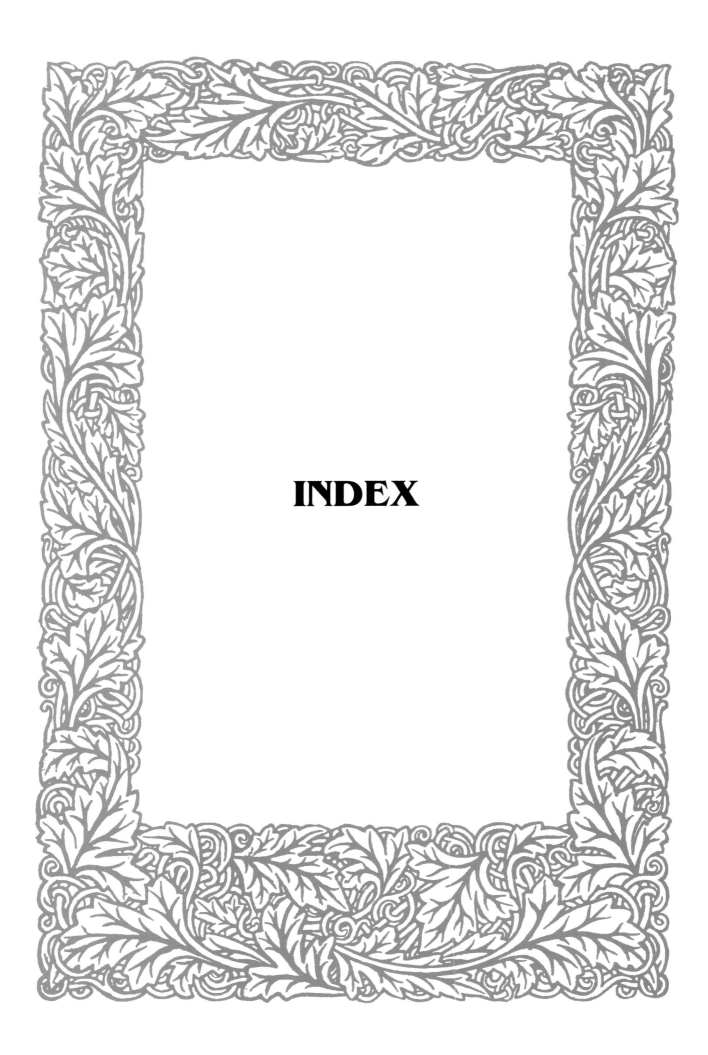

INDEX

A

Activator adjusting instrument (AAI), 275-276
Activator method of chiropractic analysis, 251
Adjusting technique(s), 240-261
    activator, 251
    applied kinesiology, 251
    at centennial, 258
    designed to restore motion, 249-251
    evolution of, 248-249
    Gonstead, 252-253
    Grostic, 254
    Logan basic, 249-250
    low force, 249
    mechanically assisted, 257
    named, developers of, 260-261t
    reflex, 249
    sacro-occipital, 250-251
    soft tissue techniques and, 255-256
    specific contact thrust, 252-253
    teaching, 242-248
    upper cervical, 253-255
Africa, chiropractic in, 484-485
African medicine, traditional, 6-7
Alchemy, Arabic medicine and, 13-14
Allied Chiropractic Education Institutions, 186
Alternative healers, 53-54
American Chiropractic Association (ACA)
    Davis', 425
    Langworthy's, 421-422
    modern, 441-442
    Ross's, 429-430
American Medical Association (AMA)
    antitrust lawsuit against, 219-227
    boycott against chiropractic
        adoption of, 224-227
        origins of, 223-224
    chiropractic and, 193-196
    official chiropractic position of, before antitrust
        lawsuit, 220-223
American School of Chiropractic, 341
Andean societies, traditional, disease in, 5
Anderson, Appa L., 460
Angio-European College of Chiropractic (AECC), 384
Annals of the Swiss Chiropractors Association, 207
Antecedents, 1-25
Applied Kinesiology Technique, 251
Apprenticeship training in medical education, 36-38
Arabic medicine, 13-14
Arnold, Alma C., 453
Ashworth, Ruth R., 456
Ashworth, Sylva L., 121-122, 389-390, 454-455
Asia, chiropractic in, 486-487
Associated Chiropractic Colleges of America (ACCA), 186
Atkinson, Michael, 478

Australia, chiropractic in, 476-483
    early practitioners, 476-479
    education, 480-481
    expansion of services, 479-480
    insurance and compensation coverage, 483
    present practitioners, 483
    professional registration, 482-483
    x-ray use, 481-482
Aztecs
    medicine of, 8-9
    mythical notions of, 2

B

B. J. Palmer Chiropractic Research Clinic, 170-171
"Baby Boomer" generation, 216
Bacteriology, 50-53
Beatty, Homer G., 390
Bellevue Chiropractic Hospital, 169
Bennett, Elizabeth F., 457
Bioelectrical instrumentation, 280
Bloodless surgery, Kolar and, 166-167
Board of Counselors of Chiropractic Spinographers
    and X-ray Operators, 308
Body weight scales in postural analysis, 265
Bolton, Stanley and Mariette, 479
Bonesetting, 21-23
    in African medicine, 6-7
Boydjieff, Virginia, 458
Brake, Barbara, 476-477
Brazil, chiropractic in, 485
Breen, Roy, 479
Budden, William A., 390-391
Buddhism, Tibetan medicine and, 10
Burich, Steven J., 391
Byrd, Nellie, 456

C

Cale, Linnie A., 456
California, prosecutions in, 144-146
Canadian chiropractic, 463-468
    Canadian Memorial Chiropractic College, founding
        of, 465-466
    early education programs of, 464
    provincial legislative acts, 464-465
    Royal Commission reviews of, 466-467
    vitality of, contemporary, 467-468
Canadian Memorial Chiropractic College (CMCC),
    380-382, 465-466
Carver, Willard, 109-110, 391-392
    technique of, 244-245
Central America, chiropractic in, 485
Certification of radiologist in chiropractic, 312-314
    requirements for, 313-314
Cervical techniques, upper, 253-255
Chance, Frank and Mary Ann, 479

Chinese medicine, 10-12
Chiropractic
    in early twentieth century, 90-123
    evolution of, D.D. Palmer in, 70-74
    evolution of magnetic healing into, 92-96
    maturation of (1910-1929), 124-151
    metamorphoses of, 96-100
    1963 to 1993, 214-239
    practice of, early, of D.D. Palmer, 74-76
    renaissance of, 214-239
Chiropractic College of Australia, 480
Chiropractic education, D.D. Palmer in, 76-81
Chiropractic Health Bureau (CHB), 176-178, 430-
        431
Chiropractic Research Foundation (CRF), 181-182,
        183, 437-440
    research and, 205-206
Chiropractic Spinography, 332-333
Christian Science, 53-54
Chukyo College of Chiropractic, 386-387
Cinchona bark, 33
Cineradiography, 326-329
Civil War, medical care after, 43-53
Clark, Dorothy, 456-457
Cleveland, Carl S., 392
Cleveland Chiropractic College
    Kansas City, 347-349
    Los Angeles, 350-352
Clubine, John S., 392-393
Clubwomen, 460-461
College of Chiropractic Physicians and Surgeons,
        168-169
Colleges, 338-387; *see also* Schools/colleges
Council on Chiropractic Education (CCE)
    as college curriculum accrediting agency, 216-217
    educational reform and, 343, 345
    United States Commissioner of Education and, 205
Council on Roentgenology of the American
        Chiropractic Association, 308-309, *311*
Cox-McManus table, 274, *275*

D

Davis, Andrew P., 393
Davis, A.P., 246
Dawson, S. Bernard, 478
Dean, Frank E., 393-394
DeLue, Helen, 458
Depression, chiropractic during, 153-178
Dermathermograph (DTG), 283, *284*
Diphtheria antitoxin, 52
Dispensaries
    hospital movement and, 49-50
    medical care through, 46
Distraction technique, 257
Diversified technique, 252

Doscher, Bobby Callahan, 459-460
Drain, James R., 394

E

Eagles, Faye B., 461
Eastern Europe, chiropractic in, 487
Eastern medicine, 9-13
Eclectic chiropractic, 165-169
Eclectic movement, 42
Education
    chiropractic; *see also* Schools/colleges
        in Australia, 480-481
        in Canada, early programs for, 464
        D.D. Palmer in, 76-81
        early, on radiography, 300-305
        at National School of Chiropractic, 135-139
        1963-1993, 216-218
        at Palmer School of Chiropractic, 132-133
        postgraduate, radiography in, 305-307
        reform of, 156-158, 184-192
            expansion and, 343-345
            length of training program and, 190
        at Universal Chiropractic College, 139-143
    medical
        bacteriology and, 52-53
        early, on radiography, 291-293
        evolution of, 127-131
        in nineteenth century North American, 36-40
Edwards, Lee W., 107-108, 394-395
Egypt, chiropractic in, 486
Egyptians, mythical notions of, 2
Electroencephalogram (EEG), 285
Elliott, Frank W., 395
Ellis microdynameter (MDM), 280
England, Jerry, case of, 200
English professional medicine, 32
Enlightened Age, spinal manipulation in, 17-21
Equipment, 262-287
    adjusting instruments as, 275-277
    adjusting tables as, 265-274
    for postural analysis, 263-265
    radiography, 278-279
    thermoelectrical, 281-285
Essentials in Skeletal Radiology, 334
Europe
    chiropractic in, 468-476
        contemporary, 475-476
        post-war effects on, 471-472
        World War II and, 471-472
    Eastern, chiropractic in, 487
European Chiropractic College, establishment of,
        473-474
European Chiropractors' Union (ECU), 469
    establishment of, 470-471
European folk medicine in 1800, 31-32

European professional medicine, 32
Evins, Dossa, neurocalometer and, 281-282

F

Federation of Chiropractic Licensing Boards (FCLB), 203
Film, radiographic, developments in, 317-322
Filtration systems for radiography, developments in, 322-324
Fipps, William, 485
Firth, James N., 395-396
Flexner Report, 131
Folk medicine, European, in 1800, 31-32
Forster, Arthur L., 396
Foundation for Accredited Chiropractic Education (FACE), research and, 205-206
Foy, Anna, 455
Future, 488-496
    chiropractic's unique identity and, 491-492
    as limited medical profession, 493-494

G

Gengenbach, Marianne, 458
Gillet, Henri J., 396
Golden, Lorraine, 459
Grahamism, 41
Greece
    ancient, spinal manipulation in, 14-15
    chiropractic in, 485-486
Gregoreus, Anna K., 455
Gregory, Alva, 112-113
    technique of, 245
Grostic procedure, 254

H

Hackett, Robert, 479-480
Hagen, Beatrice B., 457-458
Hahnemann, Samuel, homeopathy and, 41-42
Haldeman, Almeda J., 120, 396-397, 455
Hariman, George E., 397
Harring, Henry C., 397-398
Hart, Robert and Rita, 478
Haynes, George H., 398
Health Education Assistance Loan (HEAL) program, eligibility for, 218
Heggie, James, 478
Hender, Alfred B., 398-399
Henderson, John A., 399
Hendricks, Arthur G., 399
Heroic therapy, 39-40
    rebellion against, 40-42
Hibbard, Mary C., 458
Hodgins Report, 464
Hole-in-One (HIO) technique, 248
Homeopathic movement, 40-42

Homewood, A. Earl, 400
Hong Kong, chiropractic in, 487
Hospitals, growth of, after Civil War, 46-50
Howard, John F.A., 106, 400
Hydropathy, 41
Hy-Lo tables, 267-272

I

Illi, Fred W., 401
Incan populations, traditional beliefs in, 5
Indian medicine, 12-13
Institute Francais de Chiropractic, 385
Instruments, 275-277
    bioelectrical, 280
    photoelectrical, 280
    thermoelectrical, 281-285
International Association of Chiropractic Schools and Colleges (IACSC), 184-186
International Chiropractic Association (ICA), 425
International Chiropractors' Association (ICA), 178
    National Chiropractic Association and, 181
International College of Chiropractic (ICC), 481
International Congress of Chiropractic Examining Boards (ICCEB), 431-434

J

Janse, Joseph, 200, 401
Japan, chiropractic in, 487
Journal of Clinical Chiropractic (JCC), 207
Journal of Manipulative & Physiological Therapeutics (JMPT), 207

K

Kanaka medicine, 9
Kightlinger, Craig M., 402
Koch, Robert, bacteriology and, 50-51
Kolar, Francis, bloodless surgery and, 166-167

L

Lambda Chi sorority, 460
Langworthy, Solon M., 401-402
    American Chiropractic Association and, 421-422
    school of, 102-104
Leach, Minnie, 456
LeBreton, Richard, 478
Lee, Lyndon E., 403
Legal actions
    AMA antitrust lawsuit, 219-227
    go-to-jail strategies, 427-428
Legal challenges to chiropractic, 118-119
Legislation
    Canadian, 464-465
    chiropractic, 143-147, 159-160
        in New York, 146
    dilemmas in, 425-428

Legislation—cont'd
  European, medical, chiropractic and, 469
  federal, chiropractic recognition through, 219
  model bill, of UCA, 428
Lemly, Charles C., 403-404
Licensure, state, 196-202
Life Chiropractic College, 352-353
Life Chiropractic College West, 353-355
Lister, Joseph, bacteriology and, 51
Loban, Joy M., 108-109, 404
  technique of, 246
Logan, Hugh B, 404-405
Logan, Vinton F., 405
Logan basic technique, 249-250
Logan College of Chiropractic, 355-356
Los Angeles College of Chiropractic (LACC), 188,
    357-359

M

Macquarie University - Centre for Chiropractic and
    Osteopathy, 385
Magnetic healing
  D.D. Palmer and, 68-70
  evolution into chiropractic, 92-96
Margetts, Frank R., 405
Marshall, Lillard T., 406
Martin, Andrew, 478
Massachusetts, prosecutions in, 146-147
Matheson, C.H., 478
McBeath, Hector, 478
McDonald, Chester B., 406
McIlroy, Harry K., 406-407
McKenzie, Helen, 455
McLeod, Maxwell, 479
McMullen, Maxine, 458, *459*
Medical care in 1800, 31-32
Medical dissent, age of, 23-25
Medical establishment, enlightenment of, Wilk suit and,
    227-236
Medical schools, 38
Medicare, chiropractic and, 195-196
Medicine, primitive, 3-9
Medieval period, spinal manipulation in, 17
Meric system, development of, 247, *248*
Meric theory of subluxation, 116
Meshki, Yousef, 485
Mexico
  chiropractic in, 485
  mythical notions of, 2
Middle East, chiropractic in, 485-486
Modern X-ray Practice and Chiropractic Spinography,
    333
Moire contourography in postural analysis, 265
Montano, Francisco, 485
Morris, Thomas S., 407

Moses, Henry, 478
Muilengurg, Zella M., 460
Murphy, Emmett J., 407
Murphy, Tena, 458, *459*

N

Nahuati medicine, 8-9
Napolitano, Ernest G., 408
National Board of Chiropractic Examiners, 204-205
National Chiropractic Association (NCA), 161-165
  emergence of, 433-434
  International Chiropractors' Association and, 181
  New Deal and, 172-175
National College of Chiropractic, 359-361
National Council on Chiropractic Roentgenology
    (NCCR), 308
National Institute of Neurological Disorders and Stroke
    (NINDS) conference, chiropractic research
    and, 209-211
National School of Chiropractic, 135-139
National Upper Cervical Chiropractic Association
    (NUCCA), 254-255
Native American Indian medicine in 1800, 32
Nervoscope, 282-283
Nervous system in chiropractic, 97-99
Neurocalometer, 247
  Dossa Evins and, 281-282
  introduction of, 149-151
Neurocalometer and Spinographic Society, 307-308
Neuropathy, 102
Neuropyrometer (NPM), 283
New Deal, 171-176
New York, prosecutions in, 146-147
New York Chiropractic College (NYCC), 361-363
New Zealand, chiropractic in, 483
Nineteenth century
  American medicine in, 30-54
  early, changes in medical care in, 34-40
North American Association of Chiropractic Schools
    and Colleges (NAACSC), 192-193, 440
Northwestern College of Chiropractic (NWCC),
    363-365
Nugent, John J., 408-409
  educational reforms and, 156-158
Nurses, trained, hospital movement and, 49-50

O

Opium, early use of, 33
Osteopathy, 54
  chiropractic compared with, 96-97
Otterhalt, Dr., 483

P

Paley, Arthur, 479
Palmer, Bartlett Joshua, 409

Palmer, Bartlett Joshua—cont'd
  declining influence of, 147-151
  as "developer" of chiropractic, 114-118
  techniques developed by, 247-248
  Universal Chiropractors' Association of, 422-424
Palmer, Daniel David, 56-89
  as businessman, 59-62
  early chiropractic practice of, 74-76
  evolution of chiropractic and, 70-74
  family history of, 57-59
  as horticulturalist farmer, 59-62
  leaving Davenport, 83-88
  magnetic healing and, 63-64
  magnetic healing practice of, 68-70
  move to Davenport, 64-67
  in 1905, 81-83
  retrospective on, 88-89
  as schoolmaster, 59
  spiritualism and, 62-63
Palmer, David Daniel, 410
Palmer, Mabel Heath, 410-411, 453-454, 456
Palmer College (School) of Chiropractic, 76-79, 83-89,
    125, *128, 129,* 132-133, 365-368
  West, 369-371
Palmer Infirmary and Chiropractic Institute, 339-340
Palmer Recoil technique, 247
Palmer School and Cure (PSC), 339, 365-367
Palmer School and Infirmary of Chiropractic, opening
    of, 243
Palmer upper cervical technique, 254
Palpation in spinal analysis, 263
Paraprofessional radiological technologists, 336-337
Parker College of Chiropractic, 371-373
Pasteur, Louis, bacteriology and, 50-51
Pathfinders, 388-419
  Ashworth, Sylva L., 389-390
  Beatty, Homer G., 390
  Budden, William A., 390-391
  Burich, Steven J., 391
  Carver, Willard, 391-392
  Cleveland, Carl S., 392
  Clubine, John S., 392-393
  Davis, Andrew P., 393
  Dean, Frank E., 393-394
  Drain, James R., 394
  Edwards, Lee W., 394-395
  Elliott, Frank W., 395
  Firth, James N., 395-396
  Forster, Arthur L., 396
  Gillet, Henri J., 396
  Haldeman, Almeda J., 396-397
  Hariman, George E., 397
  Harring, Henry C., 397-398
  Haynes, George H., 398
  Hender, Alfred B., 398-399

Pathfinders—cont'd
  Henderson, John A., 399
  Hendricks, Arthur G., 399
  Homewood, A. Earl, 400
  Howard, John F.A., 400
  Illi, Fred W., 401
  Janse, Joseph, 401
  Kightlinger, Craig M., 402
  Langworthy, Solon M., 401-402
  Lee, Lyndon E., 403
  Lemly, Charles C., 403-404
  Loban, Joy M., 404
  Logan, Hugh B., 404-405
  Logan, Vinton F., 405
  Margetts, Frank R., 405
  Marshall, Lillard T., 406
  McDonald, Chester B., 406
  McIlroy, Harry K., 406-407
  Morris, Thomas S., 407
  Murphy, Emmett J., 407
  Napolitano, Ernest G., 408
  Nugent, John J., 408-409
  Palmer, Bartlett Joshua, 409
  Palmer, David Daniel, 410
  Palmer, Mabel Heath, 410-411
  Paxson, Minora C., 411
  Peterson, Thure C., 411
  Pothoff, Gerard M., 411-412
  Ratledge, Tullius F., 412
  Rich, Earl A., 412-413
  Rogers, Loran M., 413
  Schulze, William C., 413-414
  Schwartz, Herman S., 414
  Sherman, Lyle W., 414
  Smith, Oakley G., 414-415
  Spears, Leo, 415-416
  Steinbach, Leo J., 416
  Sturdy, Walter T., 416-417
  Thompson, Ernest A., 417
  Vedder, Harry E., 417
  Watkins, Claude O., 418
  Weiant, Clarence W., 419
Patient stabilizing/positioning devices for radiography,
    developments in, 324-326
Pax College, chiropractic education in, 480
Paxson, Minora C., 411, 453
Pennsylvania College of Straight Chiropractic, 373-374
Peterson, Thure C., 411
Pharmacopoeia, traditional, 4-5
Phillip Institute of Technology (PIT), 481
Photoelectrical instrumentation, 280
Physical culture movement, 54
Pickles, John, 478
Plumblines in spinal analysis, 263, *264*
Political struggles for recognition, 442-443

Politics, practice, chiropractic theory and, 118-119
Postural analysis, equipment for, 263-265
Postwar development, 180-212
Pothoff, Gerard M., 411-412
Practical Applied Roentgenology, 334
Preceptor, 36-38
Precision spinal adjustor, 276
Preiss, Cynthia E., 461
Primitive medicines, 3-9
Pringle, Paul, 480
Professional associations, 420-443
  American Chiropractic Association
    Davis', 425
    Langworthy's, 421-422
    modern, 441-442
  International Chiropractic Association, 425
  Universal Chiropractors' Association, 422-424
Prosecutions
  in California, 144-146
  in Massachusetts, 146-147
  in New York, 146-147
Publications, radiological, chiropractic, 332-334

R

Radiography, 288-337
  chiropractic organizations dedicated to, 307-313
  devices and procedures in, developments in,
    316-329
  early chiropractic education on, 300-305
  early chiropractic use of, 293-300
  early medical education on, 291-293
  early use of, 291-293
  equipment for, 278-279
  examinations of specialists in, 315-316
  film for, developments in, 317-322
  filtrations systems for, developments in, 322-324
  paraprofessional technologists in, 336-337
  patient stabilizing/positioning devices for, 324-326
  postgraduate education on, 305-307
  publications on, chiropractic, 332-334
  regulations on, 334-336
  upright, controversy over, 329-332
RAND report, 237-239
Ratledge, Tullius deFlorence, 111-112, 412
Ratledge Chiropractic College, standards-raising
    campaign and, 191-192
Receptor tonus technique, 256
Research, 205-211
Rich, Earl A., 412-413
Ridgway, Eleanor S., 458
Riely, Joe Shelby, 113-114
Rogers, Loran M., 413
  National Chiropractic Association and, 172-175
Ross, N.C., American Chiropractic Association of,
    429-430

Royal Commission review of Canadian chiropractic,
    466-467
Royal Melbourne Institute of Technology - School of
    Chiropractic and Osteopathy, 385-386
Russia, chiropractic in, 487

S

Sacro-occipital technique (SOT), 250-251
Santa Barbara School of Chiropractic, 339
Schillig, Charles, 121
Schillig, Joseph, 120-121
Scholarship, 205-211
Schools/colleges, 338-387; *see also* Education,
    chiropractic
  Angio-European College of Chiropractic, 385
  Canadian Memorial Chiropractic College, 380-382,
    465-466
  Chukyo College of Chiropractic, 386-387
  Cleveland Chiropractic College
    Kansas City, 347-349
    Los Angeles, 350-352
  current, 345-387
  European, establishment of, 473-474
  Institute Francais de Chiropractic, 385
  Life Chiropractic College, 352-353
  Life Chiropractic College West, 353-355
  Logan College of Chiropractic, 355-356
  Los Angeles College of Chiropractic, 357-359
  Macquarie University - Centre for Chiropractic and
    Osteopathy, 385
  medical, 38
  National College of Chiropractic, 359-361
  New York Chiropractic College, 361-363
  Northwestern College of Chiropractic, 363-365
  Palmer College of Chiropractic, 365-368
    West, 369-371
  Parker College of Chiropractic, 371-373
  Pennsylvania College of Straight Chiropractic,
    373-374
  proliferation of, 341-343
  regulation of, 435-440
    Allied Chiropractic Educational Institutions and,
      436
    Chiropractic Research Foundation in, 437-440
    National Chiropractic Association Committee on
      Educational Standards in, 435-436
    North American Association of Chiropractic
      Schools and Colleges in, 440
  Royal Melbourne Institute of Technology - School of
    Chiropractic and Osteopathy, 385-386
  Sherman College of Straight Chiropractic, 373-
    375
  Southern California College of Chiropractic, 376
  Technikon Natal, 386
  Texas Chiropractic College, 376-378

Schools/colleges—cont'd
  Universite du Quebec a Trois-Rivieres, 382-383
  University of Bridgeport - College of Chiropractic, 378, *379*
  Western States Chiropractic College, 379-380
Schulze, William Charles, 106-107, 413-414
Schwartz, Herman S., 414
Science Review of Chiropractic, 207
Scientific conferences and reports, 237-239
Scientific medicine, 52-53
Scoliometer in postural analysis, 265
Searby, Dorothy, 479
Sectarian therapeutics
  after Civil War, 43-46
  bacteriology and, 53
Shamanism, 3-4
Sherman, Lyle W., 414
Sherman College of Straight Chiropractic, 374-376
Sigma Phi Chi, 446
Smallpox vaccination, 34
Smith, Oakley G., 414-415
Social change and policies in New Deal, 171-176
Soft tissue drainage technique, 256
Soft tissue techniques, 255-256
South America, chiropractic in, 485
Southern California College of Chiropractic (SCCC), 188, 376
Spears, Leo L., 415-416
  chiropractic hospital of, 167-168, 182-183, *184*
Spears Painless System, 255
Spine
  first interdisciplinary scientific conference on, 237
  manipulation of
    in Enlightened Age, 17-21
    in Greece, 14-15
    in medieval period, 17
    in sixth century, 15-16
    in western world, 14-21
Spinographer, The, 332
Spinographic Society, 307
Spinography, 295-300
State licensure, 196-202
Steinbach, Leo J., 416
Storey, Thomas H., 104-106
Sturdy, Walter T., 416-417
Subluxation, Meric theory of, 116
Suh, Ching-Ha, research of, 207-209
Summerbell, A.E.P., 478
Surgery, bloodless, Kolar and, 166-167
Surgical procedures in 1800's, 33-34
Sydney College of Chiropractic (SCS), 480
Sydney College of Osteopathy, 480
Synchrotherme (ST), 283, 284

T

Tables, adjusting, 265-274
  Cox-McManus, 274, 275
  Hy-Lo, 267-272
  traction, 272-274
Tasmania, chiropractic in, 478
Technikon Natal, 386
Tetanus antitoxin, 51
Texas Chiropractic College (TCC), 376-378
Thermeter (TM), 283
Thermoelectrical instrumentation, 281-285
Thermoscribe (TS), 283
Theroux, George, 478
Thompson, Ernest A., 417
Thompson, Hazel, 460, 484
Thompson, Robert, 484
Thompson Terminal Point Technique, 257
Thomsonism, 40
Thrust techniques, specific contact, 252-253
Tibet
  medicine in, 9-10
  mythical notions of, 2
Towne, Dorothea, 458, *459*
Traction tables, 272-274
"Tracto-Thrust" system of chiropractic technique, 245
Twentieth century, early, chiropractic i, 90-123

U

United States Commissioner of Education (USCE), Council on Chiropractic Education and, 205
Universal Chiropractic College, 139-143
Universal Chiropractors' Association (UCA), 422-424
  go-to-jail strategies of, 427-428
  model bill legislation of, 428
Universite du Quebec a Trois-Rivieres, 382-383
University of Bridgeport - College of Chiropractic, 378, *379*
Upper cervical adjusting instruments, 276-277
Upper cervical techniques, 253-255

V

Vaccination, smallpox, 34
Vasotonometer (VTM), 283
Vear, Herbert J., 463-464
Vedder, Harry E., 417
Visual nerve tracer (VNT), 280

W

Watking, Claude O., 418
Weiant, Clarence W., 419
Wells, Cecil H., 478
Wells, F. Churchill, 478
Western States chiropractic College (WSCC), 379-380

Wilk's antitrust lawsuit, 219-236
    medical establishment enlightenment and, 227-236
Williams, Harold W., 478
Williams, Nell K., 457
Willis, Reba I., 456
Women, 444-461
    clubs for, 460-461
    compassionate role of, 459-460
    as educators, 456-459
    as groundbreakers, 455-456
    in 1910s, 446
    in 1920s, 446-448
    in 1930s, 448-449
    in 1940s, 449-450
    in 1950s, 450
    in 1960s, 451-452

Women—cont'd
    in 1980s, 452-453
    as pioneers, 453-455
Women's Chiropractic Association, 461
World War II
    chiropractic and, 178-179
    European chiropractic and, 471-472

X

X-ray; *see also* Radiography
    in chiropractic in Australia, 481-482
    discovery of, 290-291
X-ray technology, 115-116

Y

Yerkey, J.G., 478

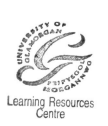

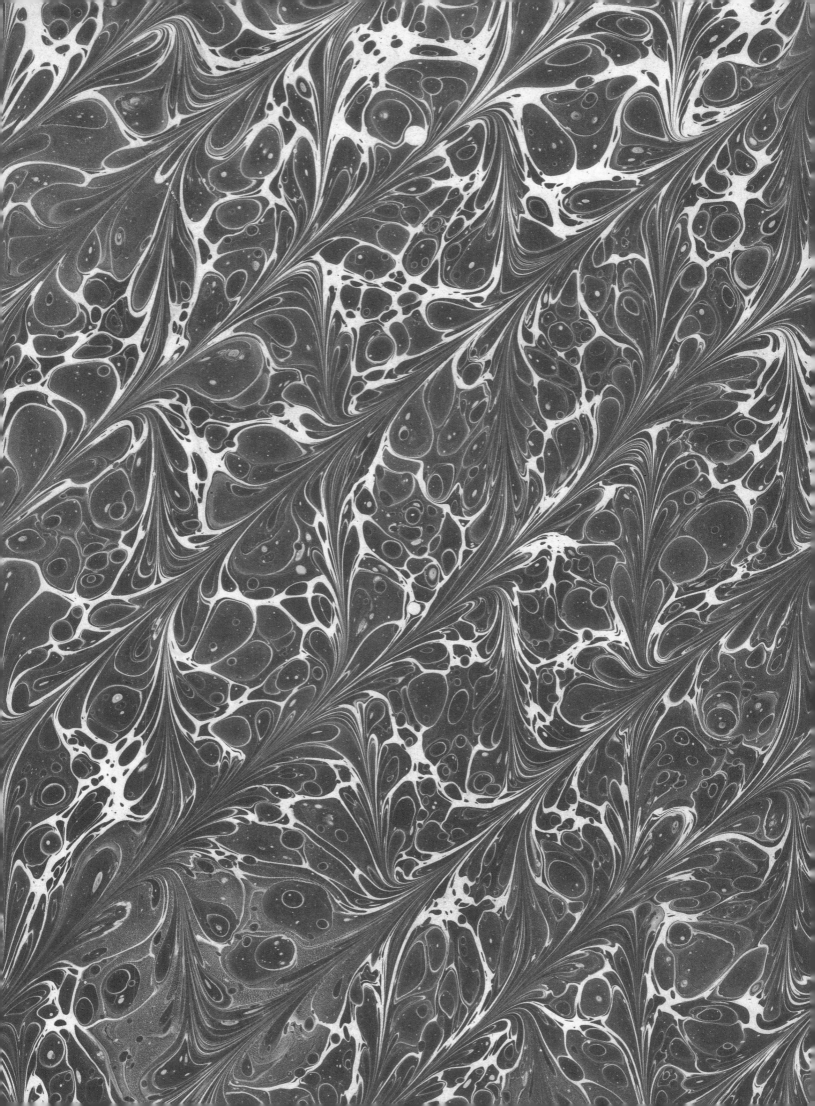